ADJUVANT MEDICAL CARE

Despite tremendous gains in medical knowledge, most conditions are managed, rather than cured, by medications. As a result, countless patients seek supplemental modes of care to better control their symptoms and conditions in order to improve their overall wellbeing. This reality spotlights the need for adjuvant medical procedures.

Adjuvant medical care refers to any supportive therapy that enhances the outcome of medical measures already in place. Adjuvant care does not replace primary or traditional treatments, but instead serves as add-on care to the initial medical treatment plan prescribed by a health care provider.

The addition of one or more non-prescription therapies (e.g., nutritional support, over-the-counter remedies, home care, dietary measures, supplements, etc.) to the primary medical management regimen has become increasingly popular and mainstream thanks to scientific studies that have documented favorable outcomes for many patients.

The verifiable scientific merit of these additional medical treatment options demonstrates their usefulness in the treatment of many medical conditions. The purpose of this handbook is to provide support to doctors and patients who are interested in safe and effective non-prescription and non-pharmacological medical therapies for specific conditions to minimize symptoms and optimize recovery and quality of life.

- The critical information in this book will help doctors and patients discover additional therapies that can reduce pain, advance health outcomes, minimize complications and disability, and extend life.
- Readers will obtain a clearer understanding and deeper knowledge of many safe, reliable, and practical options that are available to reduce symptoms, maximize recovery, and positively augment the management of a variety of conditions.
- Physicians will acquire medical insight into less traditional, yet often effective, supportive options for enhancing and optimizing patient response to care.

This book is a valuable resource for both doctors and patients who are committed to achieving the best possible medical outcomes through a variety of coordinated approaches.

ADJUVANT MEDICAL CARE

Charles Theisler, MD, JD

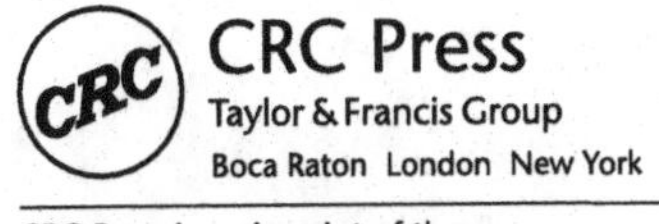

CRC Press is an imprint of the
Taylor & Francis Group, an **informa** business

First Edition published 2023
by CRC Press
6000 Broken Sound Parkway NW, Suite 300, Boca Raton, FL 33487-2742

and by CRC Press
4 Park Square, Milton Park, Abingdon, Oxon, OX14 4RN

CRC Press is an imprint of Taylor & Francis Group, LLC

First edition published by CRC Press 2023

Interior design: Pamela Beaulieu
Cover design: JD&J

This book is not meant to be used to diagnose or treat any medical condition. The content is not intended to be a substitute for professional medical advice, diagnosis, or treatment. This book is sold with the understanding that neither the publisher nor the author is engaged to render any kind of professional advice and are not liable for any damages or negative consequences from any treatment, action, or side effect to any person reading or following the information in this book. Some of the contents may contain information about treatments or uses of supplements or drug products that have not been approved by the U.S. Food and Drug Administration. Neither the publisher nor the author endorses any specific product, service, or treatment. The author and publisher make no representations or warranties of any kind and assume no liabilities with respect to the accuracy, timeliness, or completeness of the contents. Use of this book implies the reader's understanding and acceptance of this disclaimer.

ISBN: 978-1-032-27108-8 (hbk)
ISBN: 978-1-032-27107-1 (pbk)
ISBN: 978-1-003-29138-1 (ebk)

DOI: 10.1201/b22898

Publisher's note: This book has been prepared from camera-ready copy provided by the authors.

Table of Contents

Dedication

It is the bitterness of disease that allows us to fully appreciate the sweetness of health. From a broader perspective, the aim of medical science is to discover and illuminate truth and then to translate those truths into new treatments. Concealing or ignoring the presence of certain studies cannot be a positive influence on medicine, doctors, or patients. Therefore, I thank God for the opportunity to share the knowledge in this book as a blessing to medical practitioners and long-suffering patients who may benefit from the revelations that flow from the work of medical researchers.

Acknowledgment

My sincere gratitude goes to medical researchers whose valuable insights, expertise, patience, and planning yield the revelations that go into unraveling medical mysteries. Their hard work and dedication to detail open new and better avenues of care for those negatively affected by the ravages of disease.

Introduction

DESPITE TREMENDOUS GAINS in medical knowledge, most conditions are managed, rather than cured, by medications. As a result, countless patients seek supplemental modes of care to better control their symptoms and condition in order to enhance their quality of life.

Adjuvant Medical Care describes treatment options that enhance the outcome of medical measures already in place. These methods may help to lessen the severity of symptoms and hasten improvement in recovery from a targeted condition. Essentially, these therapeutic strategies make medical treatments work better. The procedures outlined in this handbook/manual are not designed to compete with existing medical management techniques but rather serve to facilitate the goals of those medical measures. Some of these procedures are stand-alone first-line treatments. Others may have documented clinical and empirical evidence of therapeutic effectiveness that may allow them to function as supplemental measures or reliable second-line treatments.

It has become relatively routine practice for physicians to prescribe clinically meaningful assistive treatment regimens such as dietary modifications or nutritional supplements, particularly the use of daily vitamin, herbal, or mineral products. This book allows doctors to identify and integrate the best documented, most beneficial nonprescription and nonpharmacologic care options to supplement conventional medical treatments and better meet their patients' needs. This work is intended to facilitate and aid in that process.

This book includes straightforward explanations of clinical studies and verifiable scientific research on different modes of adjuvant medical care and the supporting medical rationale for using them in language that patients and doctors both understand.

Unless otherwise stated, therapies and dosing ranges listed are for adults without any contraindications by way of their medical history, medications, or conditions. To avoid possible contraindications or unwanted adverse side effects from any cited therapy, patients should always consult their doctor before employing any nonprescription treatment options in the self-care of their condition. These scientific reviews are intended to be helpful and provide guidance. They are not a substitute, however, for the expertise, skill, knowledge, and judgment of a licensed healthcare practitioner.

MEDICAL CONDITIONS

Acetaminophen (Tylenol) Poisoning

Acetaminophen (Tylenol) overdose, or poisoning, is one of the most common poisonings. Mild poisoning may not cause any symptoms. When present, however, symptoms of acute acetaminophen poisoning are typically minor until about 48 hours or longer after ingestion. Symptoms include anorexia, nausea, vomiting, and right upper quadrant abdominal pain. Acetaminophen toxicity in the U.S. has replaced viral hepatitis as the most common cause of acute hepatic failure and is the second most common cause of liver failure requiring transplantation.[1]

MEDICAL MANAGEMENT TECHNIQUES

Activated Charcoal: Patients who have taken significant overdoses need further measures to prevent absorption or to increase elimination of the drug.

The American Academy of Clinical Toxicology recommends taking oral-activated charcoal 50 gm (orally or by nasogastric tube) if ingestion of a substantial amount of drug has taken place within the past one hour.

Methionine: For acetaminophen (Tylenol) poisoning, 2.5 gm of the amino acid methionine every four hours for four doses is used to prevent liver damage and death. Methionine must be given within 10 hours of taking the acetaminophen. This should be done by a healthcare professional.[2]

In Europe, oral methionine (10 gm over 12 hours) is approved as an agent to restore depleted glutathione stores and to prevent hepatotoxicity after large acetaminophen ingestions.[3]

Oral methionine is as effective as acetylcysteine in preventing severe liver damage and death after acetaminophen overdose. However, as with acetylcysteine, it must be given within 10 hours of ingestion to be effective.[3]

N-acetylcysteine, a derivative of the amino acid L-cysteine, taken within eight hours of a Tylenol overdose mitigates liver toxicity[4] and is effective in reducing the death rate and preventing the permanent harm caused by acetaminophen poisoning. For this use, N-acetylcysteine given by mouth (140 mg/kg, followed by 70 mg/kg every four hours for three days)[5] is as effective as when given intravenously.[1] N-acetylcysteine remains the preferred antidote for acetaminophen overdose in the U.S., Canada, Scotland, and most of England.[6,7] Taking both Tylenol and NAC together can provide a convenient and effective way of preventing toxicity associated with large doses of acetaminophen.[8] As a caution, taking N-acetylcysteine at the same time as activated charcoal may decrease the effectiveness of NAC to prevent poisoning.

Acne Vulgaris

Acne vulgaris is the most prevalent chronic skin disease in the U.S. It is the most common chronic skin disorder among the adolescent age group, affecting 90%–95% of the midteen population. Acne also affects young adults and can persist into the 30s and 40s.[1] It is characterized by areas of pimples (e.g., blackheads, whiteheads, pustules, cysts, etc.), greasy skin, and possible scarring. Acne is primarily thought to be due to overactivity of the sebaceous (oil) glands in the skin where sebum and dead skin block pores and become inflamed. Outbreaks tend to occur where sebaceous glands are most numerous on the face and upper chest, back, or shoulders. Complications include scarring, cutaneous abscesses, and acneiform lesions.

With most prescription acne drugs, results may not be apparent for four to eight weeks, and the skin may get worse during that time. A chronic persistent clinical course along with the emergence of resistance to common antibiotics has led to trials of numerous novel agents in acne management.

MANAGEMENT OPTIONS

Benzoyl Peroxide: Medical treatment should begin with a benzoyl peroxide agent because these are available over the counter and have an extensive history of safety and efficacy. Products are available in a wide range of vehicles (soaps, lotions, gels) and strengths vary from 2.5% to 10%. Higher strengths dry the skin but otherwise are no more effective against acne than the lower strengths.[2] Individuals with acne vulgaris should be aware that benzoyl peroxide reflects the base of treatment upon which other agents are added. For example, benzoyl peroxide plus oral and topical antibiotics and/or retinoids are often combined in more severe cases.[3]

Soap: Mild, non-comedogenic opaque or glycerin facial soap or gentle cleanser (e.g., Cetaphil) is recommended.[4]

Peeling Agents: Products containing salicylic acid (0.5%–10%)[5] or alpha hydroxy acids such as glycolic, malic, lactic, or citric acids have been shown to be effective as peeling agents to remove dead skin cells.[6,7]

Retinoids/Antibiotics: Retinoids are a form of vitamin A. Topical retinoids, either prescription or over-the-counter, along with benzoyl peroxide are typically employed for noninflammatory acne. Oral antibiotics are often used in combination with benzoyl peroxide, retinoids, and topical antibiotics for moderate to severe acne vulgaris.[8]

Zinc: Zinc is a promising alternative to other acne treatments owing to its low cost, efficacy, and lack of systemic side effects. Zinc has been employed extensively both topically and systemically for the management of acne vulgaris.

The efficacy of topical anti-acne medications containing zinc acetate or octoate with or without erythromycin is either equal to or superior to erythromycin, tetracycline, or clindamycin used alone in reducing the severity of acne and the number of lesions.[9]

Oral zinc sulfate is reportedly more effective in the treatment of severe acne than for the treatment of mild to moderate acne, but nausea, vomiting, and diarrhea occur frequently.

Acne treatment with oral zinc salts appears to be equally effective compared with systemic tetracyclines (minocycline, oxytetracycline).[1]

Niacin: Studies have shown that using both niacin (2,000 mg/day) and nicotinamide (600 mg/day) for 12 weeks can improve acne. The authors of one study concluded that niacin (500 mg q.i.d.) is an effective drug in the treatment of moderate and severe acne and that the therapeutic effect of niacin is more effective than nicotinamide.[10]

5% Nicotinamide Gel: 5% nicotinamide gel was as effective as 2% clindamycin gel for the treatment of mild to moderate acne vulgaris. No side effect was observed during the treatment.[11] In another study, 4% nicotinamide gel was of comparable efficacy to 1% clindamycin gel in the treatment of acne vulgaris.[12]

Azelaic Acid: A 20% azelaic acid cream (Azelex) was found to be an effective acne treatment when used twice a day for at least four weeks. It is even more effective when used in combination with erythromycin.[13]

Diet: Studies failed to support a link between the consumption of chocolate or sugar and acne. However, there is strong evidence that low glycemic index diets show favorable improvements. Dairy products should be limited or eliminated because there is evidence that milk and whey proteins increase the number of acne lesions.[14]

Ketogenic Diet: Insulin, due to a number of factors, combined with skin that is colonized with *Cutibacterium acnes* can lead to an inflammatory skin response and acne vulgaris. A ketogenic diet could help ameliorate acne because it results in minimal insulin secretion.[13,15]

Combination Therapy: The combination of 5% benzoyl peroxide and 3% erythromycin (Benzamycin) is a highly effective acne treatment. The combination of 5% benzoyl peroxide and 1% clindamycin in a premixed gel has also been studied and was found to be superior to either agent alone in the treatment of inflammatory and noninflammatory lesions.[16]

Stress, Hygiene, and Diet: Many people think that acne is caused by stress, lack of hygiene, or diet, but no studies support these associations.[16]

Cosmetics: Affected individuals should use oil-free, noncomedogenic cosmetics. Oil from hair products and suntan lotions can also exacerbate acne.[16]

Vitamins A, D, and E play a role in maintaining healthy skin, so these vitamins may help prevent acne.[17]

Aloe Vera Gel: Applying aloe gel in the morning and evening, in addition to a prescription anti-acne medicine, improved acne by about 35% in both children and adults.[18,19]

Omega-3 Fatty Acids: There is clear confirmation for the reduction of acne with regular consumption of omega-3 fatty acids (2,000 mg/day) or γ-linoleic acid (400 mg/day) for ten weeks.[20]

Acrodermatitis Enteropathica

Primary acrodermatitis enteropathica, also called zinc malabsorption syndrome, is a rare genetic disorder that blocks the absorption of zinc through intestinal cells. There are congenital and acquired forms of the disorder.

The onset of symptoms such as diarrhea, an inflammatory rash around the mouth and/or anus, as well as hair loss is usually seen around four to six weeks after weaning or even earlier in infants not on breast milk. The infant initially becomes irritable and withdrawn and develops photophobia. Later, anorexia, pica, growth impairment, hypogonadism, impaired taste and smell, night blindness, and neuropsychiatric symptoms (mood changes, tremors, dysarthria, and jitteriness) can develop in untreated cases.[1]

THERAPY STRATEGY

Zinc: Treatment with oral zinc (2–3 mg/kg/day) will cure all clinical manifestations within one to two weeks and should be continued up to adulthood for continuous supplementation and favorable long-term prognosis.[1]

Doses of zinc sulphate (220 mg) one hour before or two hours after meals have also been used to treat this condition. Zinc may be taken with food if it upsets the stomach although less will be absorbed.[2] Long-term high zinc doses may interfere with copper metabolism and are only indicated for acrodermatitis enteropathica.[3]

Actinic Keratosis

Actinic keratoses (AKs), also known as sunspots, solar keratoses, or age spots, are raised areas of thick, scaly, or crusty skin. AKs usually develop in areas that have been damaged by years of ultraviolet radiation (sun) exposure. Typically, multiple AKs, which are considered to be precancerous, are present and can develop into invasive squamous cell carcinoma.[1] Because it is not possible to tell which AKs will develop into a carcinoma, all AKs are usually removed as a precaution.

TREATMENT OPTIONS

Zinc Sulphate: A study showed that topical zinc sulphate solution (25%) was an effective, safe, and non-costly therapy, especially in patients with multiple actinic keratosis lesions. Eighteen male patients with 100 AK lesions were included. Patients were instructed to apply zinc sulphate solution (25%) twice daily by cotton tip applicator to their AKs for 12 weeks. Seventy-seven percent of patients showed a statistically significant response.[1]

Nicotinamide: Patients who receive oral nicotinamide, 500 mg bid, significantly reduced the rates of actinic keratoses (precancers) by 11% at three months and by approximately 15% after 12 months of treatment compared with a placebo.[2]

Glycolic Acid: Chemical peels containing 20% to 70% glycolic acid have been used by dermatologists to treat ichthyosis, acne, xerosis, warts, psoriasis, actinic keratosis, and seborrheic keratoses.[3] Glycolic acid lotion applications (e.g., 20% twice a day for three months) have been shown to improve sun damaged skin.[4]

Adult-Onset Spinocerebellar Syndrome

Spinocerebellar ataxias are inherited or acquired neurodegenerative disorders associated with progressive difficulties in muscle coordination (ataxia) causing problems with with gait and balance. Adult-onset spinocerebellar syndrome is similar to Friedreich's ataxia with progressive ataxia, loss of proprioception, and deep tendon reflexes with a positive Babinski sign. Spinocerebellar ataxia syndromes presenting in adulthood have a broad range of causes and, despite extensive investigation, remain undiagnosed in up to 50% of cases.[1] Nongenetic causes of adult-onset ataxia include vitamin deficiency states (e.g., vitamin E deficiency or B1 [thiamine] deficiency)[2] and gluten intolerance in celiac disease.[2]

CARE CONSIDERATIONS

Nonspecific pharmacological agents of potential benefit include alpha-lipoic acid, branched-chain amino acids, creatine, and coenzyme Q10.[2]

Tocopherol: Vitamin E deficiency may cause adult-onset spinocerebellar syndrome. Treatment is with alpha-tocopherol acetate (e.g., Aquasol E capsules or drops).[3]

Thiamine: Fatigue in spinocerebellar ataxia type 2 can be treated with large doses of thiamine (100 mg intramuscularly every 7 days).[4] Some observations indicate that high doses of thiamine may also lead to the partial regression of the symptoms.[4]

Choline Chloride: Previous studies demonstrate that taking choline chloride (12 gm/day) by mouth produces a mild but functionally significant improvement in motor coordination in some patients with cerebellar and spinocerebellar ataxia.[5]

Diet: Gluten-free diets are indicated for gluten ataxia (i.e., celiac disease).[2]

Zinc may have a role in neural plasticity and development. Serum and cerebrospinal fluid (CSF) levels of zinc were low in spinocerebellar ataxia 2 (SCA2) patients. Those patients who received zinc (50 mg/day) demonstrated benefit in gait, stance, posture, and the ability to perform rapid, alternating movements. Slow eye movements improved as well, and the researchers suggested this was the result of improvements in attention and processing associated with zinc supplementation.[6]

Alcohol Withdrawal Syndrome

Alcohol withdrawal is commonly encountered in general hospital settings. Alcohol withdrawal syndrome is a set of symptoms that occur in a predictable pattern following the last drink after a period of excessive use. Symptoms typically include anxiety, shakiness, headache, sweating, vomiting, rapid heart rate, confusion, and a mild fever. Tremors (shakes) usually begin within 5–10 hours after the last alcohol drink and typically peak at 24–48 hours. The most dangerous form of alcohol withdrawal is delirium tremens. Treating alcohol withdrawal is a short-term fix that does not help the core problem. Chronic alcoholism is the seventh leading risk factor for death and disability-adjusted life-years.[1]

THERAPY CHOICES

Alcoholic ketoacidosis is treated with IV fluids and carbohydrates until the person can resume drinking fluids and eating.[2]

Thiamine: Thiamine levels are often low in alcohol-dependent people. Deficiency of this important vitamin could lead to Wernicke's encephalopathy.[3] Patients in alcohol withdrawal should receive supplemental B vitamins, especially thiamine (vitamin B1), either by injection (250 mg/day for 3–5 days) or orally.[2]

L-Carnitine: When given intravenously (1–3 grams) for 10 days then taken by mouth (3 grams) for 80 days, acetyl-L-carnitine helps reduce alcohol withdrawal symptoms and increase the amount of time before another alcoholic drink is consumed.[4,5]

Magnesium: Chronic alcohol use is associated with abnormal magnesium metabolism. Those with neuropathy and presenting with severe withdrawal symptoms are more likely to show low serum magnesium levels.[3,6] Oral or parenteral magnesium supplementation may benefit such patients by reducing the severity and duration of alcohol withdrawal.

Nutritional Support: Thiamine and multivitamins are important in the treatment of ethanol withdrawal.[7] Folic acid (folate), cyanocobalamin (vitamin B12), thiamine (vitamin B1), pyridoxine (vitamin B6), and other water-soluble vitamins are often depleted in persons with chronic alcoholism, who are also frequently malnourished. Replenishing these vitamins can prevent or treat Wernicke-Korsakoff syndrome and high-output CHF (with thiamine), correct megaloblastic anemia (with folic acid and B12), and halt peripheral neuropathy (with vitamin B12).[8,9]

Kudzu: In a pilot study at Harvard Medical School, an extract from the Chinese herb kudzu, known as puerarin, in a dose of 1,200 mg/day helped alcoholics curb the craving for alcohol and drink less. For drinkers who want to reduce their alcohol intake, this may be a benefit.[10]

Lithium Orotate: Lithium orotate (150 mg/day) proved useful as the main pharmacologic agent in the treatment of 42 chronic alcoholism patients. Ten of the patients had no relapse for over three and up to 10 years, 13 patients remained without relapse for one to three years.[11]

Alertness

A state of being readily attentive and responsive is called alertness. It is the ability to perceive quickly and act promptly and appropriately on that perception. Persistent lack of alertness is a symptom of a number of conditions such as narcolepsy, attention deficit disorder, chronic fatigue syndrome, depression, Addison's disease, or sleep deprivation.

Alertness is a term with no precise definition. Well-designed, rigorous clinical studies with specific dosing, and the degree and duration of improvement are lacking on this subject.

STRATEGIES TO INCREASE ALERTNESS

Caffeine: Caffeine can seemingly enhance short-term alertness, but its effects are short lasting. Caffeine is the most widely consumed stimulant to counter the effects of sleep loss.

Ascorbic acid increased alertness and increased IQ scores of children from kindergarten through college.[1]

Black tea and caffeine (chocolate, coffee, energy drinks) increase alertness.[2]

Ginkgo biloba improves alertness.[3,4]

Ginkgo and Ginseng: A combination of ginkgo biloba and ginseng (600 mg) improved both memory and concentration. In one study, a single dose of ginkgo biloba at 9 AM improved participant's concentration and speed and the effects were sustained all day. Ginseng was also shown to improve participant's memory.[5]

Taurine: Previous studies indicate that taking an energy drink containing taurine prior to driving may reduce driver fatigue.[6]

Tyrosine: Taking tyrosine (150 mg/kg) helps people who have lost a night's sleep stay alert for about three hours longer than they otherwise would.[7,8] Also, research studies indicate that tyrosine improves memory and reasoning in people who are sleep-deprived.[8]

Dark chocolate has been shown to boost alertness.[9]

Blueberries: Studies have demonstrated that blueberries in particular are able to increase "concentration and memory" for up to five hours.[10]

Allergies

***See also* Hay Fever**

When the immune system overreacts to a foreign substance, an allergy is present. Many different types of allergies exist. Respiratory allergies are an overreaction by the body's immune system to inhalation of pollen, dander, mold, etc. A skin allergy (contact dermatitis) is a heightened response to chemicals, powders, fibers, plants (e.g., poison ivy), or other substances touching the skin. Food allergies or intolerances are also an immune system overreaction that is becoming increasingly common.

PALLIATIVE CARE

L-Tyrosine: In one study, some 492 patients with symptoms of respiratory or skin allergies were treated with tablets containing L-tyrosine (200 mg), vitamin B6 (2.5 mg), and niacinamide (10 mg). In severe cases, as many as six tablets administered four to six times per day were needed to control symptoms. Individuals with hay fever, hives, allergic headaches, and poison oak dermatitis generally obtained relief within two to five days. When itching was present, it was usually relieved within 4 to 16 hours.[1]

Vitamin C taken at a dose of 2,000 mg/day acts as a natural antihistamine to help ease nasal congestion and stuffiness in respiratory allergies.[2]

Butterbur: A Swiss study with over 330 participants concluded that butterbur extract (Ze 339) 8 mg/day was as effective as Allegra for allergy symptoms and could be an effective herbal treatment for hay fever.[3]

Alopecia Areata/Hair Loss

The term *alopecia* means "localized hair loss." Alopecia areata is also known as spot baldness. When a person has alopecia areata, the hair falls out from the scalp or face or other places in round patches ranging from 1–5 cm in diameter. It is a common autoimmune disorder with numerous treatment modalities, but none is universally effective. This type of hair loss can occur at any age but often begins in childhood. Alopecia is not due to stress nor is it contagious. It is thought to result when the immune system attacks the hair follicles. The following is mostly anecdotal evidence for the treatment of hair loss.

MANAGEMENT OPTIONS

Zinc Sulphate: Zinc deficiency usually manifests as hair loss, mouth ulcers, and dry scaly skin.[1] In a randomized, placebo-controlled, double-blinded crossover study, zinc sulphate was utilized in a dose of 5 mg/kg/day in three divided doses for a period of six months and observed a visible clinical response in 62% of patients with alopecia areata.[2] In another study, five patients with zinc-deficiency related alopecia were treated with oral zinc. All patients were improved or cured.[3]

Vitamin D: Research shows that individuals with alopecia areata have much lower levels of vitamin D than those who do not have alopecia and vitamin D stimulates hair follicles to grow. So, when the body does not have enough of this vitamin, the hair may be affected.[4]

Women with other forms of hair loss also often have lower levels of vitamin D.[5]

Biotin: Biotin (vitamin B7) administration was found to reverse alopecia in children who had been treated with the anticonvulsant, valproic acid. Although hair loss is a symptom of severe biotin deficiency, there are no published scientific studies that support the claim that high-dose biotin supplements are effective in preventing or treating hair loss in men or women.[6,7]

Biotin and Zinc: A deficiency in biotin may lead to hair loss, which indicates that the vitamin is important for hair.[8] Taking biotin (30–100 mcg/day) and zinc by mouth, in addition to applying a cream containing the chemical compound clobetasol propionate (Olux, Temovate) to the skin, might help reduce hair loss.[9]

Para-Aminobenzoic Acid (PABA): PABA has been used to prevent hair loss.[10]

Saw Palmetto: Five randomized clinical trials (RCTs) and two prospective cohort studies demonstrated positive effects of topical and oral supplements containing saw palmetto (100–320 mg) among patients with androgenetic alopecia (affecting both men and women) and telogen effluvium. Sixty percent improvement in overall hair quality, 27% improvement in total haircount, increased hair density in 83.3% of patients, and stabilized disease progression among 52%.[11]

Altitude Sickness

Altitude sickness is the negative effect of low blood oxygen at higher altitudes. Mild altitude sickness is called acute mountain sickness (AMS) and is quite similar to a hangover in that it causes headache, nausea, and fatigue. Acute (sudden) altitude sicknesses can occur as low as 8,000 feet (2,500 meters) above sea level.

PREVENTION STRATEGY

Ibuprofen: In one study, 58 men and 21 women took 600 mg of ibuprofen before climbing to over 8,000 feet. Only 43% who took ibuprofen had altitude sickness symptoms. The researchers also noted less severe symptoms overall in those who took the drug.[1]

Alzheimer's Disease (AD)

Alzheimer's is an irreversible and slowly progressive chronic neurodegenerative disorder characterized by memory problems and dementia. Accumulating brain pathology (e.g., amyloid plaques, neurofibrillary tangles, inflammation, and loss of synapses) leads to declines in cognitive and functional abilities. AD is the sixth leading cause of death in the U.S.[1] It usually starts with mild confusion and difficulty remembering and then progresses, slowly worsening over time. There is unsteady loss of thinking, remembering, and reasoning, and loss of proper behavioral abilities. Memory is eventually destroyed to the point that the patient may not recognize close family members or be able to perform the simplest tasks.

Risks for Alzheimer's include age, genetics, lack of exercise, smoking, and cardiovascular factors such as a stroke, heart disease, diabetes, high cholesterol, obesity, and especially high blood pressure (hypertension).[2]

Complications can include restlessness, agitation, and aggressiveness. Incontinence, falls, depression, and personality changes are also common with this disorder. Alzheimer's disease sufferers have been found to have a lack of the enzyme responsible for converting choline into acetylcholine within the brain. To counteract this deficiency, symptomatic medical care typically involves cholinesterase inhibitors (e.g., Aricept, Exelon).

Keys to maximizing outcomes include regular monitoring of patient's health and cognition, education and support to patients and their families, and initiation of pharmacologic and nonpharmacologic treatments as appropriate.

NUTRITIONAL THERAPY AND SUPPORT TO HELP PREVENT OR DELAY DEMENTIA

Choline: Alzheimer's disease sufferers have been found to have a lack of the enzyme responsible for converting choline into acetylcholine within the brain. Countering this acetylcholine deficiency is the mainstay of medical treatment.[3]

Some medications work by boosting levels of choline to increase acetylcholine levels for improved cell-to-cell communication in the brain.[4] This means that products that can increase choline should produce some positive effects. CDP-choline (citicoline) and choline salts, such as choline chloride and choline bitartrate, are available as supplements.[5,6] In patients with Alzheimer's type senile dementia, citicoline (e.g., 1,000–2,000 mg/day in two divided doses) slowed the disease's evolution.[7]

B Vitamins: B vitamins lower homocysteine, which directly leads to a decrease in gray matter atrophy, thereby slowing cognitive decline. In a study in the *International Journal of Geriatric Psychiatry*, researchers established that vitamin B supplementation, in particular vitamins B6, B9, and B12, significantly improved cognition and memory function of older adults with mild cognitive impairment.[8] Taking vitamins B6 (20 mg), B12 (500 mcg), and folic acid (800 mcg) in medicinal quantities reduced the overall shrinkage of a person's brain by 30% over the course of the two-year study.[9,10]

Nicotinamide: In another study published in the *Journal of Neurology, Neurosurgery and Psychiatry*, researchers concluded that vitamin B3, also called niacin, could be used to resist the effects of neurodegeneration. In particular, they found that individuals with the highest levels of niacin were the least likely to develop Alzheimer's disease and had slower rates of cognitive decline.[11]

Tocopherol: Vitamin E has often been recommended for use as an adjunctive treatment primarily because of its antioxidant properties.[12] A study has given some promise that pharmacologic doses of vitamin E slow the progress of Alzheimer's.[13]

The brain has a high oxygen consumption rate and abundant polyunsaturated fatty acids in the neuronal cell membranes. Researchers hypothesize that if cumulative free-radical damage to neurons over time contributes to cognitive decline and neurodegenerative diseases, such as Alzheimer's disease, then ingestion of supplemental antioxidants (such as vitamin E) might provide some protection. This hypothesis was supported by the results of a clinical trial in 341 patients with Alzheimer's disease of moderate severity who were randomly assigned to receive a placebo, vitamin E (2,000 IU/day *dl*-alpha-tocopherol), a monoamine oxidase inhibitor (selegiline), or vitamin E and selegiline.[13] Over two years, treatment with vitamin E (or selegiline with vitamin E) significantly delayed functional decline, the need for institutionalization, and reduced the mortality rate in mild to moderate AD patients.[13,14]

Ascorbic Acid: The brain maintains high levels of ascorbic acid (AA). When AA, better known as vitamin C, is chemically attached to certain drugs, it allows the drugs to better penetrate the blood brain barrier, reaching more of their target cells.[15] There are also reports that advocate the beneficial effect of vitamin C in neurodegenerative disorders including Alzheimer's disease.[16]

Ginkgo Biloba: Research shows that taking ginkgo for up to one year slightly improves some symptoms of Alzheimer's, vascular, or other dementias. Doses of 240 mg/day might work better than doses of 120 mg/day.[17]

Resveratrol: In 2014, a study was carried out with 119 patients with mild to moderate Alzheimer's disease. Participants took capsules containing a placebo or resveratrol, starting with a dose of 500 mg/day and increasing to 1 gm twice a day. Researchers measured participants' blood levels of beta-amyloid-40, a protein that typically decreases in the blood as Alzheimer's disease progresses. Patients treated with resveratrol showed little to no change in beta-amyloid-40 blood levels, while a decrease was observed in the placebo group.[18]

Acetyl-L-Carnitine: In studies, acetyl-L-carnitine slowed the rate of disease progression, improved memory, and improved some measures of mental function and behavior in some patients with Alzheimer's disease. Acetyl-L-carnitine is more likely to help those with early-onset Alzheimer's disease who are less than 66 years of age and have a faster rate of disease progression and mental decline.[19,20,21] A typical dose was 1,500–3,000 mg/day in divided doses for 3 to 12 months.[22]

Huperzine A: Huperzine acts as an anticholinesterase. The results from a meta-analysis of eight randomized controlled trials showed that Huperzine A (doses ranged from 200–500 μg/day for 12 to 24 weeks) could significantly improve the minimental state examination (MMSE) and activities of daily living (ADL) score of AD patients. Moreover, the results showed that there was significant improvement of cognitive function.[23]

Sodium Oligomannate: Chinese regulators approved an extract of brown algae, sodium oligomannate (GV-971 450 mg twice daily), to decrease amyloid beta-related pathologies as a treatment for mild to moderate Alzheimer's. However, questions remain as to the mechanism of action and the quality of research.[24]

L-Arginine/Nitric Oxide: In a Japanese study, patients with impaired cognitive function were placed on oral L-arginine (1.6 gm/day) for three months. Nitric oxide (NO) is synthesized from L-arginine. Nitric oxide causes blood vessels to open wider for improved blood flow. After three months of treatment with L-arginine, cognitive function improved significantly in all subjects from a mean of 16 to 23. Within three months of stopping L-arginine treatment, the cognitive test scores returned to pre-treatment levels. Lipid peroxide levels (an indicator of oxidative stress) also declined significantly during L-arginine treatment. The authors hypothesized that L-arginine treatment significantly improved cognitive function by increasing blood levels of NO, by reducing oxidative stress, or both.[25]

Diets: According to research, moderate adherence to the hybrid MIND diet—which combines elements of the Mediterranean diet and the Dietary Approaches to Stop Hypertension (DASH) diet—may significantly lower the risk (54%) of developing Alzheimer disease.[26]

Flavonol kaempferol is the most effective of three flavonoids with antioxidant and anti-inflammatory properties in reducing the risk of Alzheimer's disease. The rate of developing AD was reduced by 50% among individuals reporting high intake of kaempferol and by 38% for high intake of the flavonols myricetin and isorhamnetin. Kaempferol is readily available in green leafy vegetables (e.g., kale, beans, tea, spinach, and broccoli), fruits (e.g., grapes and strawberries), and also as a supplement.[27]

Physical activity can help individuals with Alzheimer's function better, decline more slowly, and further help with symptoms like agitation, wandering, and sleeplessness.[28]

PHARMACOLOGIC SUPPORT

Sindenafil (Viagra): A new study at the Cleveland Clinic revealed that patients prescribed sindenafil had a 69% reduced risk of Alzheimer's. It was further found that sildenafil promoted the growth of new nerve projections in nerve cells from patients with the disease. Although further studies are needed, this study supports the concept that sildenafil may be a potential breakthrough preventive treatment.[29]

Amblyopia (Nutritional)

Amblyopia, also known as "lazy eye," is dimness of vision occurring in one eye. Central dimness or paracentral scotomata (a small area of blindness) may be present but without apparent physical defect or disease. The condition is often due to poor nutrition (e.g., persons with a history of alcohol abuse, severe nutritional deprivation, or vitamin B12 deficiency). The condition is generally reversible if treated with proper diet and vitamins within two or three months of the onset of visual loss.

NUTRITIONAL THERAPY

B vitamins are needed for treatment.[1,2]

Amyotrophic Lateral Sclerosis

Amyotrophic lateral sclerosis (ALS), also known as Lou Gehrig's disease, affects nerve cells in the brain and spinal cord that are responsible for voluntary movement. ALS is a progressive neurodegenerative disease and is the most common type of motor neuron disease. The term *amyotrophic* comes from the Greek and means "no muscle nourishment."

The disorder results from a loss of motor neurons in the motor cortex (upper motor neurons) and in the brain stem and central spinal cord (lower motor neurons).[1] ALS usually strikes people between the ages of 40 and 70 and occurs more often in male patients than in female patients.

Presenting symptoms may vary but can include muscle weakness or stiffness, in addition to upper motor neuron signs, sensory symptoms, and tongue fasciculations on examination. As the disease progresses, muscles get weaker and it becomes much more difficult to walk, talk, eat, and breathe. Most patients with ALS die from respiratory failure, usually within three to five years from when the symptoms first appeared.[2]

LIMITING RISK, DELAYING ONSET, AND NUTRITIONAL SUPPORT

Tocopherol: Taking vitamin E supplements (at least 400 IU/day) for more than five years or consuming a diet rich in this vitamin is associated with reduced risk for amyotrophic lateral sclerosis (ALS).[3,4,5]

L-Carnitine: In animal studies, oral administration of 3 gm/day of L-carnitine prior to disease delayed the signs of disease, delayed deterioration of motor activity, and extended life span. Injection of carnitine increased life span of the animals tested even when given after the appearance of signs of disease.[6,7,8]

Resveratrol is a polyphenol found in the skin of grapes, blueberries, raspberries, and mulberries. It is reported to have neuroprotective effects. A few pre-clinical studies have been completed studying the effects of resveratrol.[9,10,11] All studies reported a delay in disease onset and statistically significant increases in survival.

Vitamin D: A small clinical study showed that patients with ALS tended to have low vitamin D levels and that oral vitamin D supplementation with 2,000 IU/day was safe and may be of benefit.[12]

Diet: According to one study, "nutritional care of the patient with amyotrophic lateral sclerosis should include promotion of foods high in antioxidants and carotenes, including fruits and vegetables."[13] In an analysis of cohort studies' data from patients with ALS, higher intake of ω-3 polyunsaturated fatty acids was "associated with higher ALS function."[13]

Anal Fissures

An anal fissure is a very painful condition caused by trauma, or tears in the moist mucosal tissue that lines the anus and anal canal. These tears can be caused by straining to have a bowel movement, hard or large stools, and/or chronic episodes of diarrhea. Symptoms include severe sharp pain with defecation, rectal bleeding, and anal itching.[1]

CARE CONSIDERATIONS

General Procedures: Increase dietary fiber (25–30 gm/day) as well as water intake to augment the bulk of stools, along with sitting in warm-water baths 2–3 times a day. By following these measures, anal fissure symptoms will resolve in approximately half of patients.[2]

Stool softeners and protective ointments (e.g., 0.2%–0.4% nitroglycerin ointment applied tid;[3] a number of individuals may develop nitrate-induced headaches) are also used to treat anal fissures.[4]

Calendula: Applying calendula tincture to the affected area may reduce pain in individuals with anal tears or fissures, even those who do not respond to treatment with sitz baths and/or nifedipine.[5] In one case, a 52-year-old woman with chronic anal fissures was treated with nonpharmacological, pharmacological, and surgical options. Following surgery, her fissures returned, and she began using a calendula tincture applied to the area three times daily with a cotton ball for 4.5 months. She reported improvement in pain with no rectal bleeding thereafter.[6]

Anemia

Anemias are a group of diseases characterized by a significant reduction in the amount of healthy red blood cells or hemoglobin, resulting in a corresponding decrease in the blood's oxygen carrying capacity to the cells and tissues. Anemia is the most common blood disorder in the world, affecting more than three million individuals and is often a sign of underlying pathology. If the anemia onset is gradual, a person may not be symptomatic until the hemoglobin level is less than 8 gm/dL.[1] Symptoms often include fatigue, pale skin, rapid heart beat or palpitations, poor appetite, shortness of breath, and dizziness. There are many different types and causes of anemia.

Anemia (Chronic Kidney Disease)

Anemia due to a lack of red blood cells is common with chronic kidney disease primarily because of a lack of the hormone erythropoietin (EPO) that stimulates red blood cell production. Because EPO is produced in the kidneys, most people with total loss of kidney function, or kidney failure, have anemia. Anemia evaluation and treatment should be initiated in patients with stage 3 CKD (GFR less than 60 mg/dL). Injections of EPO and its analogs may be needed to help treat this type of anemia.

NUTRITIONAL CONSIDERATIONS

Tocopherol: Research shows that taking vitamin E improves the response to EPO, which affects red blood cell production, in adults and children on hemodialysis.[1]

Folic Acid: The vast majority of patients with serious kidney disease have high levels of homocysteine. High levels of homocysteine have been linked to heart disease and stroke. Taking folic acid lowers homocysteine levels in people with serious kidney disease.[2]

L-Carnitine: The concentration of plasma and tissue carnitine in chronic hemodialysis patients decreases severely due to impaired synthesis in the kidney and liver, as well as significant losses during hemodialysis.[3] Carnitine administration has been shown to be effective in many patients for the adjunctive treatment of anemia associated with chronic kidney disease.[4]

Vitamin C supplementation significantly improved patient response to EPO.[5] When subclinical vitamin C deficiency is suspected, CKD patients should receive 1–1.5 gm oral vitamin C per week or 300 mg intravenous ascorbic acid three times a week after each hemodialysis session.[6]

Anemia (Copper Deficiency)

Copper helps form red blood cells. Copper deficiency is an under-recognized cause of reversible microcytic anemia and leukopenia (low white blood cell count). Patients presenting with refractory anemia and leukopenia, with or without associated neurologic deficits, should have copper and ceruloplasmin levels measured as part of their diagnostic evaluation.[1] The association of copper deficiency with the development of concomitant neurologic deficits such as peripheral neuropathies and myeloneuropathy are indistinguishable from the findings seen in vitamin B12 deficiency.[1,2]

When copper levels are deficient, iron levels also fall. The mechanism by which copper deficiency induces anemia is based on the requirement of copper for several enzymes (e.g., ceruloplasmin) involved in iron transport and utilization and, therefore, in heme synthesis.[3]

NUTRITIONAL SUPPORT

Zinc: Zinc-induced copper deficiency leading to anemia and several other cytopenias (reduction in blood cells) have been reviewed.[3,4] Excessive zinc intake can block how much copper is normally absorbed. Therefore, excessive zinc intake must be avoided. Excess zinc elimination from the body, however, is a relatively slow process and until that excess zinc is removed, copper absorption remains blocked.[5]

Copper Supplementation: Six out of seven anemia patients with unexplained anemia and lower than normal copper levels were treated with copper supplementation and had improvement in their hematological abnormalities.[6]

Anemia (Hemolytic)

Red blood cells carry oxygen for every cell (except cartilage and the cornea) throughout the entire body. Hemolytic anemia is a condition in which red blood cells are prematurely destroyed and removed from the bloodstream before their normal lifespan is over. When destruction of red blood cells outpaces the bone marrow's production of these cells, hemolytic anemia occurs. Like other anemias, hemolytic anemia can cause pallor, fatigue, dizziness, and low blood pressure. Yellowing of the skin and whites of the eyes (jaundice), dark urine, shortness of breath, and a rapid heart rate or an enlarged spleen may also occur.[1]

CLINICAL CARE

Prophylactic folic acid is indicated because active hemolysis can consume folate and cause megaloblastosis.[2]

Vitamin E: In premature infants this type of anemia is treated with vitamin E.[3] Vitamin E (300 IU/day) helps prevent hemolysis of RBCs.[4]

Vitamin B12: Hemolytic anemia secondary to vitamin B12 deficiency exists, but is a rare presentation.[5]

Anemia (Macrocytic)

Macrocytic anemia is characterized by large red blood cells, but with reduced hemoglobin levels. This cell malformation is due to inhibition of DNA synthesis during red blood cell production. When DNA synthesis is impaired, the cell cycle cannot progress from the growth stage (G2) to the mitosis (M) stage. This leads to continuing cell growth without cell division, which presents as macrocytosis. Because the cells are abnormally large there are too few of them to carry adequate oxygen.

Low blood oxygen levels can lead to fatigue, pallor, shortness of breath, weakness, diarrhea, anorexia, glossitis, instability when walking, tingling in the hands or feet, and confusion. The two most common causes of megaloblastic anemia are deficiencies of vitamin B12 or folate (vitamin B9). Other causes of macrocytosis include liver disease (alcohol-related), drugs (chemotherapy compounds, anticonvulsants, antibiotics, and HIV medications), bone marrow disorders, hypothyroidism, hemolysis, and pregnancy. Treatment is directed to the underlying cause.[1]

TREATMENT

Vitamin B12: If deficient, supplementation with the proper vitamin is required. Vitamin B12 deficiency must be ruled out prior to supplementation with folate. Failure to do so can mask a concomitant B12 deficiency and lead to progression of neurologic complications.[2] B12 1,000–2,000 mcg orally can be given once a day to patients who do not have severe deficiency or neurologic symptoms or signs.[3]

Oral folic acid supplementation 400–600 mcg/day should be instituted in the wake of a deficiency.

Thiamine: Some inborn errors of metabolism can respond to pharmacologic doses of thiamine. This includes megaloblastic anemia, for which the mechanism of action is unknown.[4]

Anemia (Microcytic)

Microcytic anemia is any of several types of anemia characterized by small red blood cells.

Iron deficiency (e.g., due to blood loss, iron deficient diet, or celiac disease) is the most common cause of anemia in the world. Other causes of microcytic anemia include copper and pyridoxine deficiencies, thalassemia, pregnancy, chronic diseases (infections, inflammation, celiac disease, and cancer), and lead poisoning. Symptoms include thin or brittle fingernails, pale skin, fatigue, weakness, shortness of breath after exercise, resting tachycardia (rapid heartbeat) >100 bpm, cold skin, and loss of appetite.[1]

ADDRESSING DEFICIENCIES

Vitamin B6 deficiency induced in infants is associated with a hypochromic microcytic anemia. A malnourished patient with a hypochromic anemia who failed to respond to iron therapy but subsequently responded to the administration of vitamin B6 has also been described. Occasionally, patients receiving therapy with antituberculosis agents, such as isoniazid, which interfere with vitamin B6 metabolism, develop a microcytic anemia that can be corrected with large doses of pyridoxine. Some patients with sideroblastic anemias (*see* Chap. 64) respond to the administration of pyridoxine even though these patients are not deficient in this vitamin.[1]

Copper Deficiency: *See* Anemia (Copper Deficiency).

Iron: In most cases, oral administration of iron therapy with soluble iron salts ($Fe2+$ sulfate, succinate, lactate, fumarate, glycine sulfate, glutamate, and gluconate, since all are about equally absorbed) at a dose of 325 mg two to three times a day is appropriate. It is generally recommended that approximately 200 mg of elemental iron be administered daily.[2]

Ascorbic Acid: Giving vitamin C along with iron increases how much iron the body absorbs in adults and children.[3] A prospective, randomized, crossover study evaluated 27 hemodialysis patients with functional iron deficiency. All patients who were administered 500 mg of intravenous vitamin C three times weekly for three months had significant increases in hemoglobin and transferrin saturation. Both hemoglobin and transferrin saturation declined after cessation of vitamin C therapy. Researchers also reported a significant increase in hemoglobin concentration and a decrease in the needed dose of recombinant human erythropoietin (EPO) in 36 hemodialysis patients whose ferritin level was >500 gm/L after eight weeks of treatment with vitamin C at a dosage of 1 gm/wk.[4]

Taurine: Previous clinical studies demonstrate that taking iron with 1,000 mg of taurine improves red blood cell counts and iron levels in women with anemia due to iron deficiency.[5]

Anemia (Normochromic and Normocytic)

In normocytic and normochromic anemia, blood cells are of normal size and have adequate hemoglobin concentration, but are present in insufficient quantities to transport normal amounts of oxygen to the tissues. Normocytic anemia has many causes, the most common being anemia of chronic diseases (e.g., kidney disease, cancer, RA, and thyroiditis), but also includes blood loss or hemolysis, bone marrow suppression, man-made heart valves, or drug therapy. Normocytic anemia also commonly develops due to aging and is more likely to affect women over the age of 85.[1] Normocytic anemia symptoms are not very prominent as the condition will usually tend to build up gradually over a period of time. However, when it has fully progressed, the condition will present with typical symptoms of pallor, tiredness, and weakness, etc.[1]

MANAGEMENT

The management of normocytic normochromic anemia depends on treating the underlying cause of anemia.[2]

Aneurysms

See also **Aortic Aneurysms**

An aneurysm is an abnormal bulge or ballooning in a weakened area of an arterial wall. Smoking and high blood pressure are the two major risk factors for the development of an aneurysm. A family history of aneurysms and being over 40 years of age are also factors. Aneurysms can occur anywhere in the body but are more frequent in the brain, aorta, legs (behind the knee), and spleen. Most aneurysms remain asymptomatic unless they grow unusually large or rupture.

MANAGEMENT METHODS

Nicotine: Smoking damages the walls of arteries making them weaker and more likely to bulge.

Blood Pressure: Blood pressure must be controlled to reduce the risk of an aneurysm in any location from rupturing.

Potassium: A lower level of serum potassium and higher level of C-reactive protein are independent risk factors for giant aneurysms in Kawasaki disease.[1]

Angina Pectoris

Angina pectoris is chest pain that occurs when the coronary blood supply is temporarily insufficient to meet the oxygen needs of the heart muscle (hypoxia). The pain can be accompanied by a feeling of heaviness or tightening in the chest. Angina is not a condition; it is a symptom of coronary heart disease or blocked arteries. Angina can also be a warning sign that there is an increased risk for a heart attack. Nitroglycerine is the primary medical treatment for angina.

MODIFY RISK FACTORS

Blood pressure and lipids should be well-controlled and smoking should cease.

NUTRITIONAL AND OTC SUPPORT OPTIONS

Aspirin: Enteric-coated aspirin at a dose of 81 mg/day is advised for all patients with stable angina who have no contraindications to its use.[1]

Magnesium Oxide: For chest pain due to coronary artery disease, 800–1,200 mg of magnesium oxide taken daily for three months can be effective.[2]

L-Carnitine: Carnitine supplementation (1 gm twice a day) improved exercise capacity in individuals with angina.[3] 22.7% of the patients were free of angina while taking carnitine, compared with only 9.1% during the placebo treatment.[4]

Half of 160 men and women diagnosed with a recent MI were randomly assigned to receive 4 gm/day of oral L-carnitine in addition to standard pharmacological treatment. After one year of treatment, mortality was significantly lower in the L-carnitine supplemented group compared to the control group (1.2% vs. 12.5%), and angina attacks were less frequent.[5]

One randomized, placebo-controlled study in 200 patients with exercise-induced stable angina found that supplementing conventional medical therapy with 2 gm/day of L-carnitine for six months significantly reduced the incidence of premature ventricular contractions at rest and also improved exercise tolerance.[6]

EPA/DHA: Thirty-nine patients with angina were given either 10 gm/day of fish oil (MaxEPA brand) or a placebo (olive oil). After 12 weeks, the average number of angina attacks fell significantly by 41% in the fish-oil group but did not change in the placebo group. The need for nitroglycerin (a medication used to treat angina) also fell in the fish-oil group, but not in the placebo group.[7,8]

Folic Acid: High-dose folic acid reduced the need for prescription medication in patients with angina.[9]

Vitamin C appears to help sustain the long-term effectiveness of anti-pain therapies that patients may be using (for angina).[10] Taking 500 mg of vitamin C per day significantly improved vasodilation.[11]

NAC: Taking N-acetylcysteine (NAC) by mouth or injecting it intravenously can improve chest pain when used with the drug nitroglycerin. Intravenous N-acetylcysteine is a significant aid in preventing nitroglycerin tolerance.[12]

L-Arginine: Arginine supplementation has been effective in the treatment of angina in some, but not all, clinical trials. In an uncontrolled trial, seven of 10 people with intractable angina improved dramatically after taking 9 gm of arginine per day for three months.[13] Supplementation of L-arginine 700 mg orally four times daily prevented nitrate tolerance when transdermal nitroglycerin was given continuously.[14]

Coenzyme Q10: Five small placebo-controlled studies have examined the effects of oral CoQ10 supplementation (60–600 mg/day) in addition to conventional medical therapy in patients with chronic stable angina. In most of the studies, CoQ10 supplementation improved exercise tolerance and reduced or delayed electrocardiographic changes associated with myocardial ischemia compared to a placebo.[15]

Bromelain: Research indicates that bromelain prevents or minimizes the severity of angina pectoris. After discontinuing bromelain, angina attacks reappeared after a variable period of time.[16,17] It is thought that the best results occur at a dose of 750–1,000 mg/day in divided doses.[18]

Anorexia Nervosa

Anorexia means loss of appetite and is an eating disorder. Anorexia nervosa is a potentially life-threatening disorder that is characterized by being drastically underweight and having an intense fear of becoming fat. The disorder is diagnosed when a person weighs at least 15% less than his or her normal or ideal body weight. Sufferers see themselves as fat even when they are very thin. Thus, there is typically very little eating, often to the point of starvation, excessive exercise, and a distorted body image. Malnutrition is a core feature of anorexia nervosa. Severe malnourishment can lead to multiple organ damage or death.

NUTRITIONAL CONSIDERATION

Zinc: The rate of weight gain measured as the increase in BMI was significantly greater in a zinc supplemented group than in a placebo group.[1,2,3] Taking zinc supplements by mouth can help to increase weight gain and improve depression symptoms in teens and adults with anorexia.[4]

Thiamine: Deficiency of thiamine (vitamin B1) causes a range of neuropsychiatric symptoms that resemble those reported in patients with anorexia nervosa.[5] For chronic anorexia, thiamine (e.g., 100–500 mg/day) has been used, even without definite proof of a deficiency. Symptoms improve dramatically if thiamine deficiency has been causative.[6]

Antacids

Antacids are medications that neutralize acid in the stomach. They are frequently used to treat heartburn or indigestion. Antacids such as Tums, Di-Gel, Dulcolax, Mylanta, etc., are different from acid reducers or blockers. Aluminum hydroxide gel in antacids (e.g., Equate) can combine with phosphorus to form a complex that is excreted in the feces. This is a valuable feature for reducing phosphate levels in hyperphosphatemia. However, aluminum-containing antacids can precipitate, leading to decreased absorption of vitamin A.[1]

SUPPLEMENTATION

Vitamin A supplementation should be considered in patients who frequently use antacids with aluminum hydroxide.

Anticonvulsants

Anticonvulsants are also known as antiseizure or antiepileptic drugs and are used to reduce the frequency and severity of epileptic convulsions. Anticonvulsant drug-induced disorders in mineral and bone metabolism are quite common. Current evidence indicates that these drugs derange bone metabolism, both through induction of increased hepatic catabolism of vitamin D, as well as by direct effects on membrane cation transport systems.[1] All patients receiving chronic anticonvulsant drug therapy should be carefully evaluated for the presence of drug-induced osteomalacia and treated appropriately with vitamin D.[1]

COUNTERING ADVERSE EFFECTS OF ANTICONVULSANTS

Calcium and Vitamin D: Current evidence indicates that appropriate vitamin D (600–800 IU/day) and calcium supplementation (800–1,200 mg/day) can significantly reduce the clinical complications of seizures. Vitamin D 600–1,000 IU/day plus calcium 1,000–2,000 mg/day should be prescribed whenever necessary.[2]

Anxiety

Anxiety disorders are the most common psychiatric disorders in North America. Anxiety is feelings of excessive worry, fear, apprehension, and uncertainty without a known stimulus. Experiencing anxiety from time to time is a normal part of life. Anxiety can be accompanied by physiological changes such as sweating, pallor, rapid heart beat (>100 BPM), or tremor. Anxiety is often present when facing a problem at home or at work, before and after making an important decision, or before taking a test or having a job interview. Individuals should seek medical help when intense anxiety or panic interferes with daily tasks.

MANAGEMENT CHOICES

Niacinamide: Anti-anxiety medications like Valium, Librium, and Xanax are well known and effective. More naturally, the effects of niacinamide closely resemble the actions of these benzodiazepines. Anti-anxiety doses for niacinamide range from 500 mg, twice a day, to 1,000 mg, three times a day.[1]

Magnesium is indicated for anxiety to help alleviate symptoms.[2] Several forms of magnesium supplements are effective, including magnesium oxide and magnesium lactate; the latter has more magnesium per dose.[3]

Inositol[4] and **kava**[5] may also be helpful. An additional benefit of inositol, which is rare for any nootropic or supplement, is a decrease in panic attacks. One month-long study showed that 18 gm of inositol per day (a large dose) was more effective than the currently prescribed drug, fluvoxamine.[6]

Ginkgo Biloba: Research shows that taking a ginkgo extract for four weeks can reduce symptoms of anxiety.[7]

Arginine and Lysine: A week of treatment with 2.64 gm of lysine and 2.64 gm of arginine per day reduced the stress-induced anxiety state and basal cortisol levels in healthy humans with stress and anxiety.[8]

Glycine: Glycine is a nonessential (or neutral) amino acid that has profound anti-anxiety properties. When an individual experiences anxiety or panic, norepinephrine is released, creating feelings of anxiety and panic. Glycine (e.g., 3–4 gm/day) antagonizes the release of NE, thus mitigating anxiety and panic and feelings of over-arousal.[9]

GABA, also known as gamma-aminobutyric acid, was utilized in a clinical trial where researchers used EEG to measure participants' brain waves after taking either GABA or a placebo. Just one hour after taking GABA (100–200 mg) they saw a significant increase in alpha waves, which caused feelings of calm and relaxation.[10]

Kava inhibits the limbic system, suppressing emotional excitability and mood enhancement. Kava has been used to treat anxiety disorders. The recommended dosage is 100 mg three times per day.[11]

Valerian binds to specific neurologic receptors and acts in a competitive action with any benzodiazepine. It is used for anxiety, and stress in recommended dosages of 200–300 mg two times per day.[12]

Aortic Aneurysm

An aortic aneurysm is an abnormal bulging or "ballooning" of a weakened area in the wall of the body's largest artery. Aneurysms in the abdominal portion of the aorta are more common than in the thoracic area. Typically, there are no symptoms unless the aneurysm grows large (i.e., over 5 cm in diameter). Then it can cause pain or rupture resulting in dangerous bleeding and death. Smoking, genetics, injury, and high blood pressure are risk factors for developing an aortic aneurysm.

GENERAL CONSIDERATIONS

Avoidance of Nicotine: Smoking can damage and weaken the walls of the aorta. Smoking should be avoided or cut down to a minimum.

Control of High Blood Pressure: High blood pressure must be well managed as it can further strain the weakened walls of the aortic artery, allowing an aneurysm to grow larger or rupture.

Copper: Copper is a trace element that acts as an essential cofactor in multiple enzymatic reactions critical to the normal functioning of vascular, hematological, skeletal, and neurological systems.[1] In one study, the concentration of copper in the liver of individuals with aortic aneurysms was 74% lower than those without aneurysms. A mutation affecting copper metabolism may be present on the X chromosome. Men with a personal or family history of aortic aneurysm should take a 2–4 mg/day dose of a copper supplement.[2,3]

Diet: A high consumption of fruits may help to prevent many vascular diseases. One study suggests that a lower risk of abdominal aortic aneurysm is among these benefits.[4] Swedish researchers followed 80,000 men and women and found that those who ate the most fruits, which amounted to about two servings a day or more, excluding juice, were 25% less likely to have an abdominal aortic aneurysm and 43% less likely to have one rupture compared to those who ate less than one serving of fruit.[4]

Arsenic Toxicity

Acute arsenic toxicity is most frequently caused by accidental ingestion of pesticides or an attempted suicide. Complications of acute arsenic toxicity may include hemolysis, skin rash, Mees lines in the nails, toxic cardiomyopathy, vomiting, loss of appetite, and abdominal pain, diarrhea, and black water urine (dark urine). In acute poisoning, hemodynamic stabilization is of primary importance. Acute arsenic poisoning can lead to cancer, liver disease, coma, and death. Medical treatment of arsenic poisoning typically involves bowel irrigation, medication, and chelation therapy.

MANAGEMENT OF TOXICITY

Arsenicum Album-30: A homeopathic product, Arsenicum Album-30, was administered to a group of patients adversely affected by groundwater arsenic. The results were highly encouraging and suggest that the drug can alleviate arsenic poisoning in humans.[1]

Mineral Supplements: Mineral supplements can lower the risk of potentially fatal heart rhythm problems as a result of arsenic poisoning.[2]

Selenium: Multiple studies have shown that low-dose selenium (Se) supplementation exerted a protective effect against arsenic, or cadmium, induced toxicity.[3] However, selenium has an exceptionally narrow range between therapeutic and toxic concentrations.

Ascorbic Acid: Arsenic induced hepatotoxicity has been reported by recent experimental studies which have suggested that vitamin C supplementation improves mitochondrial structure and function, along with restriction of apoptosis due to caspase-3 inhibition in arsenic trioxide exposed rat liver. The overall report suggests that vitamin C and vitamin C-rich fruits such as gooseberry provide protection against metal induced hepatotoxicity.[4]

Asthma/Bronchial Asthma

Asthma is a chronic, or long-term, condition that is characterized by intermittent episodes of sudden violent coughing, wheezing, difficulty breathing, chest tightness, and breathlessness. Chronic inflammation narrows the airways (bronchoconstriction) in the lungs and produces thick, excess mucus. The bronchioles (smaller branches of the bronchial airways) narrow even further in response to certain stimuli (e.g., pollen, dust, mold, aspirin, exercise, gastroesophageal reflux, respiratory infections, etc.), resulting in periodic attacks. Attacks are complicated by mucus plugs in some of the bronchioles. Symptoms can range from mild to severe. This condition interferes with daily activities and can lead to an acute life-threatening episode.

Asthma is the leading chronic illness among children (20%–30%).[1] The cause of asthma is unknown. Asthma is not curable and has become a serious challenge to clinical medicine with an increase in incidence, morbidity, and mortality in the past two decades.[2] Goals in treating asthma include preventing asthma symptoms, maintaining nearly normal pulmonary function and activity levels, preventing asthmatic exacerbations, and avoiding adverse effects from asthma medications.

SUPPORTIVE TECHNIQUES

Cessation of Smoking: All nicotine products should be avoided, including second-hand smoke. Obtain smoking cessation counseling when appropriate.

Allergen or Irritant Avoidance: Sufferers should stay away from circumstances or triggers that are known to incite an attack. Common triggers include tobacco smoke, infections, exercise, weather changes, pollen, animal dander, dust mites, outdoor air pollution, wood stoves, and mold. Some patients with asthma experience symptoms with use of aspirin or nonsteroidal anti-inflammatory medications (NSAIDs) or with consumption of beer or red wine; some women report worsening symptoms with menses.[3]

Magnesium sulfate ($MgSO_4$) is a moderately potent bronchodilator, similar to aminophylline,[4,5] relaxing smooth muscle, reducing inflammation, and improving peak expiratory flow rate and forced expiratory volume in one second.[6] Magnesium supplementation also reduces hospital admissions.[6] Therefore, $MgSO_4$ is often used in the emergency department and is considered an adjunct therapy for severe and life-threatening asthma exacerbation.[4] It has been reported that patients having diets low in Mg have more bronchial symptoms and self-reported wheezing.[7] In a recent study patients receiving 340 mg/day had less reactive airways (decreased odds of airway hyperactivity) and improved peak expiratory flow rates (PEFR) and reported improved asthma control and quality of life within six months.[3] In another study, forced expiratory volume increased in relation to magnesium intake up to 400 mg/day.

Vitamin B12 may work against asthma in several different ways. One effect is to detoxify asthma-causing chemicals known as sulfites. Even if sulfites are absent from the daily diet, the body manufactures some every day as a natural byproduct of metabolism. Research has shown that vitamin B12 supplements (e.g., 1,000 mcg or higher/day) protect against sulfite-induced asthma attacks.[8,9]

Of 85 asthmatics given vitamin B12 injections one to three times a week, 48 (56%) improved. Children tended to respond to the vitamin better than adults.[10] In another study, daily injections of large amounts of vitamin B12 for 15 to 20 days relieved asthma in 10 of 12 patients.[11]

Reduced Salt Intake: Asthmatics who restrict their salt intake often experience symptom relief and require fewer asthma medications.[12,13]

Ascorbic Acid: A direct association exists between vitamin C intake and forced expiratory volume (FEV1).[14] Evidence for the beneficial effect of vitamin C on respiratory health comes from a meta-analysis of three randomized controlled trials (RCTs) that evaluated the effect of vitamin C on exercise-induced bronchoconstriction. The trials encompassed 40 asthmatic participants who received either vitamin C (0.5 gm dose on two subsequent days in one trial, a single dose of 2 gm in the second trial, 1.5 gm daily for two weeks in the third trial) or a placebo before exercise. Compared to a placebo, vitamin C administration significantly reduced the exercise-induced decline in FEV_1 by 48% (95% CI: 0.33–0.64).[15]

Exercise Induced Asthma: Evidence is strong that vitamin C supplementation at doses of 1–2 gm/day may be helpful.[16]

Spinal Manipulation: Spinal manipulative therapy (SMT) is an underutilized conservative noninvasive treatment for patients with asthma. The use of osteopathic or chiropractic spinal manipulative techniques including rib elevation and myofascial release may decrease mortality and morbidity rates in this patient group.[17,18] A total of 140 pediatric cases were studied. Notable improvements (25% to 70%) in patients' peak expiratory flow rates (PEFs) have been reported following the use of manipulative therapy.[17] This study demonstrates that spinal manipulation procedures may significantly improve pulmonary function for pediatric patients with asthma.[19]

Choline: Taking choline appears to lessen symptoms and the number of days that asthma is a problem for some asthma sufferers. It also is reported to reduce the need to use bronchodilators. There is some evidence that higher doses of choline (3 gm daily) might be more effective than lower doses (1.5 gm daily).[20]

Beta-carotene by mouth appears to reduce asthma attacks that are triggered by exercise.[21]

Vitamin D: Studies on the role of vitamin D in respiratory diseases have consistently indicated that low vitamin D levels may be associated with higher incidence, greater severity, or poorer treatment responses in various respiratory diseases, including asthma.[22,23] A Cochrane systematic review reported that supplementation with vitamin D (range 400–4,000 IU/day) reduced asthma exacerbations requiring systemic steroids by 30% overall in adults and children with mild to moderate asthma.[24]

Oxygen: Although no evidence exists to support the use of oxygen in acute asthma, nonetheless it should be administered when oxygen saturation levels fall below 94%.[25]

Inhalers: Little evidence supports the use of inhaled bronchodilators, yet they remain one of the first-line treatment choices for acute asthma.[25] Primatene Mist is FDA approved for the treatment of asthma symptoms and is available over the counter.

Ataxia

Ataxia is the term for a group of neurological diseases that negatively affect movement and coordination. Awkwardness of movements creates difficulty in getting dressed, walking, swallowing, eye movements, speech, activities of daily living, etc. Ataxia can arise from disorders that involve cerebellum, spinal cord, brain stem, vestibular nuclei, thalamic nuclei, cerebral white matter, cortex (especially frontal), and peripheral sensory nerves.[1]

Different conditions can cause ataxia including vitamin B1, vitamin E, and possibly zinc deficiency,[2] alcohol abuse, medications, strokes, tumors, cerebral palsy, brain degeneration, and multiple sclerosis.[1] Inherited ataxia from defective genes also causes the condition. There is no cure for ataxia, but there are symptomatic treatments. The goal of treatment is to manage symptoms and to improve comfort and mobility.[3] Medication typically has minimal impact on slowing ataxia's progression unless it is caused by nutritional deficiencies.[4]

TREATMENT OPTIONS

Tocopherol: The inherited genetic movement disorder called ataxia causes severe vitamin E deficiency. Vitamin E supplements are used as part of the treatment for this type of ataxia.[5]

Children with chronic liver disease, celiac disease, cystic fibrosis, and abetalipoproteinemia have difficulty absorbing vitamin E and have low serum vitamin E levels. Ataxia, areflexia, and loss of proprioception can develop. The neurological deterioration can be partially arrested with vitamin E supplementation.[6]

Choline: Some studies suggest that taking choline chloride (12 gm/day) by mouth daily produces a mild but significant functional improvement in motor coordination in some patients with cerebellar and spinocerebellar ataxia.[7] Other research results dispute this finding.[8]

Diet: A gluten-free diet is recommended because oversensitivity to gluten may develop with ataxia.[9]

Vitamin supplements may also help individuals with a deficiency.[9]

Atherosclerosis

Atherosclerosis, arteriosclerosis, or hardening of the arteries are all terms for the same condition that causes thickening of the arterial walls and loss of elasticity. It happens when plaque, made up of cholesterol, fat, and calcium, collects in the innermost (intimal) arterial layer. Over time, the plaque thickens and hardens, causing the arterial lumen to narrow and the walls to stiffen. This limits the flow of oxygen-rich blood to three major organs (brain, kidneys, heart) and other parts of the body (arms, legs, pelvis).

Risk factors associated with developing atherosclerosis are high fats and cholesterol (LDLs) in the blood, smoking, high blood pressure, sedentary lifestyle, obesity, genetics, and diabetes. Patients with atherosclerosis face higher dangers for heart attack, stroke, peripheral artery disease, and death. Heart disease and stroke remain the most common causes of death in the U.S. Nonsurgical goals in treating atherosclerosis include lowering the risk of blood clots forming, preventing atherosclerosis-related diseases, and reducing risk factors in an effort to slow or stop the buildup of plaque as well as to relieve symptoms.[1]

MANAGEMENT TECHNIQUES

Avoid Nicotine: Smoking is to be avoided or significantly reduced because it is a major preventable risk factor for atherosclerosis. Current research suggests that nicotine itself may also accelerate existing atherosclerotic disease.[2]

Weight Loss/Diet: Diet plays a major role in the etiology of cardiovascular disease and as a modifiable risk factor is the focus of many prevention strategies. Weight management with a healthy diet (no trans fats; fewer saturated fats; more fiber, fruits and vegetables; and moderate [if any] alcohol) and increased physical activity are important treatment options.

Cholesterol: Since high cholesterol and triglycerides are important risk factors, blood levels need to be well controlled. For treatment goals see hypercholesterolemia.

Folic Acid: High-dose folic acid appears to prevent the progression of atherosclerosis. Several studies found that large doses of folic acid promoted the healing of chronic leg ulcers caused by atherosclerosis.[3,4]

Vitamin E: One study demonstrated that supplementation of low-dose vitamin E protects LDL against oxidative modification. The authors concluded that supplementation with low-dose vitamin E would be beneficial for ameliorating atherosclerosis.[5]

Policosanol: Policosanol (5–20 mg/day) is believed to decrease total cholesterol (TC), low-density lipoprotein (LDL), and increase high-density lipoprotein (HDL) by inhibiting cholesterol synthesis and increasing LDL processing. Previous clinical studies demonstrate that taking policosanol, alone or with aspirin, for 20 months can reduce heart disease-related events in individuals with atherosclerosis.[6,7] In another study, 5–10 mg of policosanol/day was effective in lowering LDL-C and TC and increasing HDL-C levels in older patients with CHD, and also showed benefits in the occurrence of cardiac events and overall frequency of serious adverse events of vascular etiology.[8]

Ascorbic Acid: The ability of blood vessels to relax or dilate is compromised in individuals with atherosclerosis. Randomized, double-blind, placebo-controlled studies have shown that treatment with vitamin C consistently results in improved vasodilation in individuals with coronary heart disease, as well as those with angina pectoris, congestive heart failure, diabetes, high cholesterol, and high blood pressure. Improved vasodilation has been demonstrated at an oral dose of 500 mg of vitamin C daily.[9,10,11,12]

Niacin: Niacin has been used for more than 50 years in the treatment of cardiovascular disease and was the first drug to show a reduction in cardiovascular events and mortality in patients with prior myocardial infarction.[13,14,15] Half of the eligible patients in a study were randomly assigned 500 mg extended-release niacin daily or a placebo, both to be taken at night. After 30 days, the niacin dose was raised to 1,000 mg/day and maintained at this dose for one year. Results demonstrated that extended-release niacin slowed the development of atherosclerosis in adults with coronary artery disease, independently from statin therapy.[15] Extended-release niacin (500 mg increased to 1,000 mg taken at night for one year) had positive effects on atherosclerosis measured in terms of carotid intima-media thickness (CIMT), which had decreased by the end of the study.[15]

Vitamin E: Cross-cultural studies in Europe reported that a higher level of plasma vitamin E is associated with a lower mortality rate from CVD.[16]

Fish oil can help reduce atherogenicity.[17] Omega-3 polyunsaturated fatty acids from fish oil slowed atherosclerosis progression in coronary arteries in a randomized, double-blind, placebo-controlled clinical trial.[18]

Oral antiplatelet drugs (e.g., aspirin) 81–325 mg/day, are essential because most complications result from plaque fissure or rupture with platelet activation and thrombosis.[19]

Autism

Autism, or autism spectrum disorder (ASD), refers to a broad range of conditions characterized by challenges with social interaction via limited communication (verbal and nonverbal), and by restricted interests and repetitive behaviors. ASD is a developmental disorder with symptoms typically appearing in the first two years of life. The symptoms interfere with the individual's ability to properly function at school, work, and other areas of life.[1] No current specific medication exists to treat autism and there is no cure. Interventional therapies for behavior and communication or education are a mainstay of medical management.

SUPPLEMENTS AS CARE OPTIONS

Pyridoxine and Magnesium: A placebo-controlled, double-blind study[2] found that pyridoxine (vitamin B6) 300–500 mg/day plus magnesium 200–400 mg/day produced significant improvement in behavior: better eye contact, less self-stimulation, fewer tantrums, more interest in the world, and more frequent speech.

Additional studies confirmed the value of combined magnesium and pyridoxine therapy.[3,4,5] LeLord et al. reports that 47% of autistic patients respond positively to magnesium and vitamin B6 therapy.[6]

Quercetin: Some research indicates that taking quercetin and other ingredients can improve behavior and social interactions in some children with autism.[7] Data from a small, prospective, open-label trial in children with autism spectrum disorder showed significant improvement in adaptive functioning and overall behavior after 26-week administration of a supplement containing luteolin from chamomile (100 mg), quercetin (70 mg), and the quercetin glycoside rutin (30 mg); one capsule per 10 kg of weight was given daily with food. Most clinical studies used quercetin 500–1,000 mg/day in divided doses.[8]

Basal Cell Carcinoma (BCC)/Squamous Cell Carcinoma (SCC)

BCC of the skin is the most frequently occurring form of all cancers, with squamous cell carcinoma being the second most common. BCC often appears as a painless raised area of skin, which may be shiny with small blood vessels running over it, or it may present as a raised area with ulceration. The bottom layer of the epidermis is the basal cell layer. With basal cancer, cells in this layer are the ones that become cancerous. Most basal cell cancers occur on skin that is regularly exposed to sunlight or other ultraviolet radiation.

Squamous cell carcinoma develops in the small, flat squamous cells that make up the middle and outer layers of the skin. SCC typically develops into small, red, rounded skin tumors that can be flat or raised. They tend to grow slowly and may ulcerate. Most of these cancers can be cured with fairly minor surgery and other types of local treatments.[1]

THERAPEUTIC CONSIDERATIONS

Zinc Gluconate: Sharquie et al. observed significant improvement in all 100 lesions of basal cell carcinoma with intralesional 2% zinc gluconate solution without any significant adverse effects in an open-label case interventional study.[2]

Ketogenic Diet: A ketogenic diet has been of interest in oncology research as an adjunctive therapy. The hypothesis is that because cancer cells cannot metabolize ketones, although normal cells can, the Warburg effect (i.e., that most cancer cells rely on aerobic glycolysis) can be taken advantage of through a ketogenic diet to aid in the treatment of malignant disease. Further studies are needed.[3]

PREVENTION

Nicotinamide: Oral nicotinamide prevents common skin cancers in high-risk patients, and reduces costs. An Australian study was conducted involving 386 patients at high risk of developing nonmelanoma skin cancers. Patients who receive oral nicotinamide 500 mg bid for 12 months reduced the rates of new basal cell cancer and squamous cell cancer diagnoses by 23% compared with a placebo. Nicotinamide reduced the rates of actinic keratoses (precancers) by 11% at three months and by approximately 15% after 12 months of treatment compared with a placebo.[4]

Aspirin: A recent a meta-analysis indicates that low-dose aspirin may have a preventive effect on basal and squamous cell cancers.[5]

Vitamin A: Oral ingestion of vitamin A can reduce the risk of squamous cell carcinoma in those at high risk for skin cancer.[6] A cohort study in the U.S. assessed the association between intake of vitamin A and carotenoids and risk of cutaneous squamous cell carcinoma. Results support the protective role of supplemental and dietary vitamin A (900–3,000 mcg/day)[7] against squamous cell carcinoma and that vitamin A may be beneficial in preventing SCC.[8]

Becker's Muscular Dystrophy

Becker's muscular dystrophy is an inherited disorder characterized by slowly progressing muscle weakness of the legs and pelvis. The disorder is similar to Duchenne muscular dystrophy. The main differences are that Becker's gets worse at a much slower rate and is less common. There is no known cure for Becker's muscular dystrophy.

ADDITIONAL THERAPIES

L-Carnitine: Nearly 40% of patients responded to L-carnitine supplementation (e.g., 320–640 mg/day) with increased muscle strength and decreased myoglobinuria.[1,2]

Calcium and Vitamin D: Since corticosteroids are used as a standard treatment, vitamin D and calcium supplementation are indicated to help prevent thinning bones and fractures.

Other treatments may include:[2]

- Amino acids
- Coenzyme Q10
- Fish oil
- Green tea extracts
- Vitamin E

Behcet's Disease

Behcet's disease is a multiorgan vasculopathic inflammatory condition characterized by a triad of recurrent episodes of oral aphthous (mouth) ulcers and genital sores, as well as ocular inflammation (anterior and posterior uveitis). Repeated attacks of uveitis can cause blindness.[1] Additional symptoms can include arthritis, colitis, and CNS involvement. The diagnosis is based on mouth and groin sores recurring at least three times in 12 months. Behcet's disease usually develops in young adults aged 20–30 years, but patients of all ages, gender, and races may be affected. Behcet's disease is not contagious. Treatment of Behcet's disease is symptomatic and is aimed at reducing symptoms and preventing complications.[2,3] Corticosteroids and colchicine are frequently used in medical treatment.

PREVENTING BONE LOSS

Calcium and Vitamin D: Because corticosteroid medications cause osteoporosis as a side effect, supplements with calcium (800–1,200 mg/day) and vitamin D (600–800 IU/day) are necessary to minimize bone thinning.

NUTRIPHARMACOLOGY

Zinc Sulphate: Sharquie et al. in a randomized controlled, double-blind crossover trial comprising 30 subjects found 100 mg of oral zinc sulphate given three times daily for three months to be an effective treatment modality for Behcet's disease without any major adverse effects.[2]

Potassium Iodide: 300–900 mg/day can relieve local tenderness, fever, and arthralgias in 24–48 hours. Potassium iodide appears to be particularly effective in conditions where neutrophils predominate in the early stages of the disease.[4]

Belching/Burping

Burping or belching is a normal physiologic mechanism for expelling air through the mouth from an overstretched stomach. It occurs after a large meal or the result of swallowing air along with fluids, especially carbonated drinks, or food. This triggers the lower end of the esophagus to relax, allowing some air to escape up the esophagus and out the mouth. Belching can help relieve bloating and temporarily reduce heartburn. Excessive belching can be a problem especially when paired with additional symptoms such as abdominal pain. *H. pylori* infection, small intestine bacterial overgrowth, food intolerance (e.g., lactose), and hiatal hernia are some medical causes for excessive belching.

SYMPTOMATIC CARE

OTC Products: A variety of over-the-counter products can be effective in relieving excess bloating depending on the cause, such as Lactaid or Dairy Ease to help digest lactose. Products containing simethicone (Gas-X, Mylanta Gas) can help reduce the feeling of bloating. Beano may decrease the amount of gas produced.

Pancreatic Enzymes: Excessive bloating and belching can also be treated with pancreatic enzymes taken before meals:[1]

- Pancreatin 300 mg
- Pepsin 250 mg
- Bile salts 150 mg

Bell's Palsy

Bell's palsy is a lower motor neuron disease of the facial nerve characterized by a transient paralysis. The disorder affects men and women equally and can occur at any age. Bell's palsy is associated with significant edema (swelling) and ischemia (restricted blood supply) of the facial nerve as it passes through its bony canal.[1] The primary cause is often exposure to a viral infection. The main symptom is muscle weakness on one side of the face, causing that side of the face to droop and appear distorted. Additional symptoms which may include pain behind the ear, loss of taste in half the tongue, sensitivity to sound in one ear, or excessive lacrimation in one eye, can be mild to severe.

Most cases recover in two to eight weeks or so, with or without treatment. Healing is occasionally incomplete, resulting in residual nerve dysfunction such as partial palsy or motor synkinesis (involuntary movement accompanying a voluntary one) or autonomic synkinesis (involuntary lacrimation after a voluntary muscle movement). A general rule is that patients with good control of hypertension and no diabetes can usually be expected to have a more complete recovery.[1]

SHORTENING HEALING TIME

Corticosteroids/Antivirals: The use of pharmacologic agents has been controversial in the past owing to inconsistent efficacy and the high rate of spontaneous recovery. Recent studies have shown with increasing confidence that pharmacologic agents, such as corticosteroids and antivirals, can be beneficial and can affect clinical improvements.[2]

Methylcobalamin (Vitamin B12): The results of a nonblinded study indicate that intramuscular methylcobalamin, vitamin B12, 500 (1 gm IM 3x/wk until full recovery or for eight weeks) used alone or in combination with prednisone can shorten the time to recovery.[3]

Beta Thalassemia

Beta thalassemia is an inherited blood disorder that reduces the production of hemoglobin. Low levels of hemoglobin can lead to a lack of oxygen in many parts of the body. Beta thalassemia is classified into two types depending on the severity of symptoms: thalassemia major, also known as Cooley's anemia, and thalassemia intermedia. Of the two types, thalassemia major is more severe.

The signs and symptoms of thalassemia major appear within the first two years of life. Children develop life-threatening hemolytic, microcytic, and hypochromic anemia[1] which can cause pale skin, weakness, fatigue, poor growth, and skeletal abnormalitiess. Individuals with this disorder are at an increased risk of developing abnormal blood clots.[1]

Thalassemia intermedia is milder than thalassemia major. The signs and symptoms of thalassemia intermedia appear in early childhood or later in life. Affected individuals have mild to moderate anemia and may also have slow growth and bone abnormalities.[1]

ALTERNATE MANAGEMENT METHODS

Tocopherol: Taking vitamin E by mouth can benefit children with the beta-thalassemia and vitamin E deficiency.[2]

Folic Acid: Children with thalassemia major become dependent on blood transfusions and, although the transfusions help, they create other problems (e.g., iron overload). So, iron supplements are to be avoided. Folic acid supplementation (1,000 mcg/day for 1-3 months in children) is given daily to help red blood cells develop and to decrease symptoms of bone pain and myalgia.[3,4,5]

For nontransfused thalassemia patients, folate supplementation (1 mg/day) is still recommended.[6]

Black Tea: Drinking black tea with meals is recommended to reduce iron absorption from food.[6]

Vitamin D supplementation (50,000 IU once a week until levels normalize) is recommended for patients with a vitamin D3 level less than 20 ng/dL. Calcium supplementation should also be encouraged if dietary intake is insufficient.[6]

Nutritional deficiencies are common in thalassemia due to hemolytic anemia, increased nutritional requirements, and morbidities such as iron overload, diabetes, and chelator use. Typically, multivitamin supplementation without iron is suggested (e.g., Centrum Silver in tablet or chewable form).[6]

L-Carnitine: Previous clinical studies demonstrate that L-carnitine may reduce symptoms of the blood disorder beta-thalassemia.[7] Both thalassemia and carnitine deficiency represent independent causes of erythropoietin resistance, and thus anemia, in uremic patients. Carnitine administration (2 gm for each hemodialysis session) has been shown to be effective in many patients for the adjunctive treatment of anemia associated with chronic kidney disease.[8] One study suggests that a very long-term carnitine administration (900 mg p.o. daily for 12 months) should be useful also in uremic patients on chronic dialysis affected by beta-thalassemia on target hemoglobin because it reduces the doses of erythropoietin needed to manage the anemia.[9]

Bile Acid Sequestrants

Prescription bile acid sequestrants such as cholestyramine (Cholybar, Questran) and cholestipol (Colestid) are used to reduce low-density lipoprotein (LDL) cholesterol levels. After oral administration, the sequestrants are not absorbed but instead bind to bile acids (which contain cholesterol) in the intestine and prevent their reabsorption into the body.[1] Drugs that sequester bile acids can result in deficiencies of iron, folic acid, and fat-soluble vitamins (A, D, E, and K).[1]

MEDICAL CONCERNS

Vitamin supplements with A, D, E, and K may be needed in the wake of long-term therapy.[2]

Biliary Atresia

Biliary atresia is also known as extrahepatic ductopenia and progressive obliterative cholangiopathy. It is a childhood disease of the liver in which one or more bile ducts are inflamed and blocked or abnormally narrow. This prevents bile from draining out of the liver into the intestines. It is one of the leading causes of cholestasis in a newborn, the foremost reason for cirrhosis and liver-related death in children. Biliary atresia first manifests during the first two to eight weeks of life with jaundice and pale (clay-colored) stools. Additional symptoms such as dark urine along with irritability and weight loss may also be present. Surgical intervention via Kasai portoenterostomy is the medical treatment of choice.[1]

NUTRITIONAL PROTOCOLS

Fat-Soluble Vitamins: Biliary atresia is associated with fat-soluble vitamin deficiencies. Therefore, vitamins A, D, E, and K must be supplemented. 2,000 micrograms of vitamin A per gram = 1 ml = 7,500 IU. Starting dose is 1 ml once daily. Starting dose of vitamin D = 30–50 nanograms/kg once a day rounded to nearest 100 nanograms. Starting dose of vitamin E (d-alpha-tocopheryl acetate) = 50 mg (68 IU) once a day.[2]

Bipolar Disorder

Bipolar disorder, also known by its older name of manic depression, is a mental health condition that causes dramatic mood swings that include emotional highs (mania or hypomania) and lows (depression). This results in extreme shifts in mood with corresponding fluctuations in energy and activity levels. Patients can have manic episodes, depressed episodes, or mixed episodes. These episodes may last several weeks or months, with periods of stability in between. There are four types of bipolar disorder and patients are at higher risk for thyroid disease, migraine headaches, heart disease, diabetes, obesity, and other physical illnesses.[1] The number one long-term treatment goal of bipolar disorder is stability. Despite the number of medications and psychotherapy techniques, the relapse rate is more than 70% over five years.[2]

THERAPY METHODS

Vitamin C: Bipolar patients tend to have excess acetylcholine receptors, which is a major cause of depression and mania.[3,4] Bipolar patients also produce elevated levels of vanadium, which causes mania, depression, and melancholy.[5,6] Vitamin C has been shown to protect the body from the damage caused by excess vanadium. A double-blind, placebo-controlled study showed that a single 3 gm dose of vitamin C/day decreased manic symptoms in comparison to a placebo.[6]

B Vitamin Deficiencies: Eighty percent of bipolar sufferers have some vitamin B deficiencies, often accompanied by anemia.[7] The combination of essential vitamin supplements with the body's natural supply of lithium reduces depressive and manic symptoms of patients suffering from bipolar disorder.[8]

Lithium: Lithium orotate, a low-dose source of lithium, is often prescribed for bipolar disorder. Approximately 3.83 mg of elemental lithium is obtained from 100 mg of organic lithium orotate. Lithium orotate can be used in low doses (e.g., 5 mg) with good results and no side effects.[9,10] Clinical trials involving 150 mg/day doses of lithium orotate administered 4–5 times a week showed a reduction of manic and depressive symptoms in bipolar patients.[10] Lithium orotate is also used as maintenance therapy for patients with a diagnosis of bipolar disorder.[11]

Taurine: Taurine is an amino acid made in the liver from cysteine and is known to play a role in the brain by eliciting a calming effect.[4] Studies have also shown that the amino acid derivative taurine, as an alternative to lithium, blocks the effects of excess acetylcholine that contributes to bipolar disorder.[12]

Black Hairy Tongue

Black hairy tongue is a temporary, harmless oral condition that gives the tongue a dark, furry appearance. Black hairy tongue is a misnomer because no hair growth is involved. What actually happens is that dead skin cells build up on the filiform papillae (tiny bumps on the tongue) and these begin to trap bacteria, yeast, and food, resulting in a black, hair-like appearance. Black hairy tongue is typically caused by bacteria or fungi (yeast) in the mouth, but can also be caused by antibiotics particularly tetracyclines.[1] As a result, the tongue can also turn brown, yellow, green, or other colors. Some patients report a tickling feeling in the back of the roof of the mouth, a metallic taste in their mouth, or nausea.[2]

TREATMENT STRATEGIES

Home Instructions: Brushing the tongue 2–3 x/day with a soft-bristled toothbrush and without any toothpaste helps to remove debris on the tongue and thereby reduces the discoloration.[4] This measure also prevents the growth of fungus and bacteria that may cause infection. Individuals can also use a tongue scraper, but this can irritate the tongue[2,3] and brushing is generally more effective than scraping.[4]

Avoidance of toothpastes and mouthwashes that contain hydrogen peroxide, witch hazel, or menthol and cessation of smoking are recommended.[2,4]

Increased roughage in the diet may be helpful.[2]

Body Odor/Bromhidrosis

Bromhidrosis is a common disorder characterized by foul-smelling sweat. The strong odor is usually associated with a mix of perspiration and increased bacterial flora, typically of *Corynebacterium sp.* Topical antibacterials and antiperspirants are the treatments of choice along with maintaining good hygiene.

MANAGING THE CHIEF SYMPTOM

General Considerations: Washing with antibacterial soap or splashing apple cider vinegar or white vinegar under the arms after showering may be helpful because bacteria cannot thrive in the acidic environment. A strong antiperspirant with aluminum chloride and a deodorant in it may be used once armpits are dry. Applying witch hazel as a natural deodorant and sterilizer is an alternative.[1] Onions, garlic, and spicy foods in the diet should be avoided.

Topical Zinc Sulphate: Owing to its antibacterial action, topical zinc sulphate has been tried and found to be effective in the management of axillary bromhidrosis and foot malodor.[2]

Oral Zinc: Oral doses of zinc 220 mg tid dramatically reduced unwanted axillary perspiration odor in one study. The problem returned within days of discontinuing the zinc dose.[3]

Boils/Styes

Small and painful pus-filled bumps (about the size of a pea) under the skin are known as boils. They are typically red, swollen, and tender and often increase in size over time. Most boils are caused by a staphylococcus infection in a hair follicle or a sweat gland. A boil that occurs on the eyelid is called a stye. Most boils and styes heal on their own within one to three weeks.

CONSERVATIVE APPROACHES

Primary treatments are hot packs and lancing if the boil is soft and often antistaphylococcal antibiotics.[1]

Wheat: There is some anecdotal evidence that eating a small amount of freshly ground wheat each day may successfully treat boils. A woman who had developed 10 boils that failed to respond to medical treatment heard about this approach and decided to try it. Each day she ground up 1–2 teaspoons of wheat and sprinkled it on her breakfast cereal. All of the boils resolved rapidly. The woman's husband, a dentist, recommended the treatment to a number of individuals who had boils and, in each case, it appeared to help.[1,2]

Bronchitis (Acute)

Bronchitis is an infection causing inflammation or swelling of the mucus membranes on the bronchiole tubes (large and medium-sized airways). Cough is the predominant and defining symptom of acute bronchitis.[1] Acute bronchitis also results in excess mucus production. Bronchitis is often caused by bacterial or viral infections and typically is self-limiting with complete healing and return to normal function in two to three weeks. However, because the cough associated with bronchitis is so bothersome and slow to resolve, many patients seek treatment.[1]

Persistent fever may suggest a complication such as pneumonia. Antibiotics are mostly ineffective for treatment of acute bronchitis.[2] In a Cochrane Review, no patients undergoing antibiotic treatment had clinical improvement during follow-up at 2 to 14 days.[3]

ADJUVANT TREATMENT

Over-the-counter medications (e.g., expectorants, suppressants, decongestants, antihistamines, or painkillers) are often recommended as first-line treatment for acute cough.[4]

Bromelain: Combined bromelain and antibiotic therapy was shown to be more effective than antibiotics alone in treating acute bronchitis.[5,6]

Echinacea can be helpful for symptoms of acute bronchitis.[7]

Dark honey for children helps manage symptoms related to bronchitis.[7]

Bronchitis (Chronic)

Chronic bronchitis causes a productive cough on most days over a period of three or more months and recurs at least two years in a row. Chronic bronchitis (CB) is due to inflammation of the bronchial linings in the lungs leading to production of thick excess mucus. CB is a chronic obstructive pulmonary disease (COPD) which is the fourth leading cause of death in the U.S. CB results from repeated irritation and damage to the lung and airway tissues. The end result is hypoxemia (low blood oxygen levels) and CO_2 retention (elevated blood carbon dioxide levels).

Cigarette smoking is the number one cause of chronic bronchitis, although smog, dust, and industrial pollutants also contribute. Chronic bronchitis is a serious, lifelong condition that recurs or never fully resolves. Mortality from COPD has increased steadily over the past three decades. Complications can include breathlessness, pneumonia, pulmonary hypertension, increased ACE levels, respiratory failure, polycythemia, and pneumothorax.

The goals of therapy for chronic bronchitis are to relieve symptoms, improve exercise tolerance, treat exacerbations, prevent complications, slow the progression of the disease, and reduce morbidity and mortality.

TREATMENT OPTIONS

Avoidance of Nicotine: The most critical nonpharmacological intervention is smoking cessation to improve general health and to reduce the risk of future morbidity. Obtain smoking cessation counseling when appropriate. Smoking cessation is the most effective preventative measure for COPD. Nicotine gum or patches may help. Exposure to secondhand smoke and irritants such as occupational dust and chemicals as well as air pollutants should also be avoided or reduced.[1]

Pulmonary Rehabilitation: Personalized treatment programs that teach COPD management strategies and cardiovascular conditioning to improve health-related quality of life, dyspnea, and exercise capacity help to reduce hospitalization rates over a 6–12 month period.

Vitamin D: Serum vitamin D levels are thought to be negatively associated with higher risk and severity of COPD, and poorer treatment response.[2,3,4] Evidence suggests that vitamin D supplementation could help decrease the risk of moderate-to-severe exacerbations in patients with low baseline vitamin D levels.[5,6] For all these reasons, vitamin D supplementation (e.g., 2,000–4,000 IU/day)[7] would seem warranted.

Ascorbic Acid: In a single blind uncontrolled comparative clinical study, 45 patients were divided into two groups. All participants had cough with sputum, dyspnea on exertion, and their FEV1/FVC ratio was less than 70%. Group 1 underwent customary medical treatment while group 2 was given ascorbic acid 500 mg twice a day along with customary therapy. These results demonstrate the positive effects of vitamin C on slowing the decline of lung function in patients with COPD. Ascorbic acid could be considered a component of the recovery program.[1]

Guaifenesin, an expectorant, is used to loosen congestion in the chest and treat cough symptoms by promoting vagally mediated increase in airway secretions.[1] Guaifenesin is available over the counter as Mucinex.

NAC: A derivative of the amino-acid cysteine, N-acetylcysteine (NAC) performs two different functions that may be beneficial for the lungs. First, NAC acts as a mucolytic, a compound which breaks up mucus in the respiratory tract, thereby allowing the mucus to be cleared more easily from the bronchial passages. Second, NAC participates in the synthesis of glutathione, a powerful antioxidant that protects the lungs against toxins and free radicals.[8]

In one study, 1,392 patients with chronic bronchitis received 200 mg of NAC three times per day for two months. Of those patients, 87% showed an improvement in symptoms, including less severe coughing, greater ease of expectorations, and less shortness of breath.[8] NAC 600 mg three times daily is used in those with idiopathic pulmonary fibrosis.[9] Some experts argue that this is a more proper dose for CB. Additional research is needed.

L-Carnitine: L-carnitine 2 gm/day for six weeks improved well-being and function, measured by questionnaires, in patients with chronic obstructive pulmonary disease.[10]

Potassium Iodide: For chronic bronchitis, tenacious secretions can be liquified using potassium iodide as an expectorant.[11]

Black pepper (Piper nigrum) increases absorption and decreases the metabolism of asthmatic preparations.[12]

Bloodroot (Sanguinaria canadensis) and **red puccoon** supplementation act as expectorants.[12]

Gamma-Aminobutyric Acid (GABA): Previous clinical studies demonstrate that taking GABA (1.5–3 gm of a GABA product such as Aminalon for 18 to 20 days) along with medications used for bronchitis increase the amount of time between symptom episodes.[13]

Physical Measures: Therapeutic interventions such as chest PT, high-frequency chest wall oscillation, or the use of a flutter valve are warranted.[1]

Oxygen: Proven benefits of supplemental home oxygen therapy in hypoxemic patients include longer survival, reduced hospitalizations, and better quality of life.[14]

Bronchopulmonary Dysplasia (BPD)

Bronchopulmonary dysplasia is a serious lung condition that affects primarily premature infants born more than 10 weeks before their due dates and weighing less than two pounds at birth who need oxygen therapy. The lungs of premature infants are fragile and often aren't fully developed. They can easily be irritated or injured within hours or days of birth.[1] Most babies diagnosed with BPD get better over time, but they may need treatment for months or even years.[1]

CARE CONSIDERATION

Tocopherol: Bronchopulmonary dysplasia may improve with oral or IM vitamin E therapy[2] or be prevented in some cases with caffeine or vitamin A.[3]

Bulimia Nervosa

Bulimia nervosa is commonly called bulimia. Bulimics have an overwhelming desire to go on excessive eating binges that are often followed by self-induced vomiting or laxative abuse (purging). Patients with bulimia have a fear of gaining weight. More women than men engage in these frequent repeated binge and purge episodes. The cause of this serious eating disorder is unknown. Medical complications from self-induced vomiting include dental erosion or periodontal disease, damage to areas of the pharynx and larynx, GERD, esophagitis, Barrett's esophagus, metabolic acidosis, dehydration, hypotension, hypokalemia leading to arrhythmias, and aspiration pneumonia. Electrolyte imbalances are common, especially from laxative abuse.

TREATMENT PROPOSALS

Tryptophan and B6: Eleven women with bulimia were given tryptophan (3 gm/day) combined with vitamin B6 (45 mg/day). Compared to a placebo, the tryptophan/vitamin B6 group improved mood, eating behavior, and feelings about eating. No side effects were reported.[1]

Burns

When an external heat source (e.g., fire, oven, boiling liquids, chemicals, electricity, etc.) contacts the skin, the skin temperature rises and proteins are at risk of being denatured.[1] This damaging process can cause localized tissue death and swelling. There are three degrees of burns depending on the skin depth and severity of damage. To repair burn damage, collagen, which is the main component of connective tissue and the most abundant protein in the human body, is needed. Burn complications are a major cause of illness and death among burn patients. Complications can include infections, hypovolemia, scarring, hypomagnesemia, hyponatremia, hyperkalemia, and hypernatremia. Treatment needs to be focused on rapid healing and prevention of infection.

NUTRITIONAL SUPPORT

Ascorbic Acid: Vitamin C is necessary to form collagen. Without adequate amounts of vitamin C, the body cannot form collagen to repair the damaged cells. For severe burns, daily oral doses of 1–2 gm of vitamin C are recommended.[1]

DHEA: Progressive ischemia and necrosis of the skin following thermal injury can be reduced by post-burn administration of the steroid hormone dehydroepiandrosterone (DHEA).[2]

Bromelain: The removal of damaged tissue from wounds or second/third degree burns is termed debridement. Bromelain contains escherase and when applied as a cream (35% bromelain in a lipid base) can be beneficial for debridement of necrotic tissue and acceleration of healing.[3] Bromelain agents such as Debriding Gel Dressing (DGD) and Debrase Gel Dressing showed rapid removal of the necrotic layer of the dermis with preservation of the unburned tissues.[4]

Previous clinical studies indicate that applying gel containing bromelain enzymes under a wound dressing helps remove dead tissue from second- and third-degree burns.[5]

Enzymatic debridement using bromelain is better than surgical debridement as surgical incision is painful, nonselective, and exposes the patients to the risk of repeated anesthesia and significant bleeding.[6,7,8]

Calendula: A study found that cleaning burns, venous ulcers, and skin lesions with 10% calendula solution followed by daily application of 2% calendula gel resulted in a greater number of healed wounds, as well as a reduction in the median time to heal when compared to using calendula solution alone.[9]

Glutamine: In patients with major burn injury, plasma glutamine concentration was 58% lower than that in normal controls.[10] Administering glutamine through a feeding tube or intravenously (by IV) can reduce infections, shorten hospital stays, and improve wound healing in burn patients.[11]

Aloe Vera: Applying aloe gel to the skin improves burn healing.[12]

Honey: In clinical practice, honey is used topically for its antibacterial, antiseptic, and anti-inflammatory effects, enhanced wound healing, patient comfort, and pain reduction in the managing burns of various depths. Honey is further known to have a wound debriding action.[13] A 2012 meta-analysis of Cochrane systematic reviews of local and systemic interventions for wounds, found robust evidence for the use of topical honey to reduce healing times in burns.[14]

Vitamin K: Researchers in Sarajevo reported on the effects of vitamin K injection on burn pain. They first determined that (in mice) vitamin K was more effective than morphine in its "thermoanalgesic" properties (relief of pain from burns).[15]

Bursitis

There are more than 150 small synovial fluid filled sacs (bursae) located near the joints where muscles and tendons slide across bone. Bursae help to reduce friction and allow the joints to move more freely. When one or more bursae are inflamed, it is known as bursitis.

This condition causes inflammation, tenderness, and pain in areas around a joint, such as the tendons, ligaments, bursae, and muscles.[1] The condition is painful and may limit or stop the joint from moving and the area may also look swollen or red. Both tendonitis and bursitis are often caused by repetitive activities. Without treatment the tendon can rupture which may need surgery.[1]

THERAPY CHOICES

Relative rest is essential in the treatment of bursitis or tendonitis. Exercises or activities that eliminate painful motions are preferable.

Hot or Cold Therapy: Cold is more effective in the first 48 hours after pain and swelling begin. Thereafter, warm heat (dry or moist) may be more helpful.[2]

Over-the-counter pain reliever (acetaminophen) or anti-inflammatory (NSAID) medications such as ibuprofen, aspirin, or naproxen may help lessen pain and inflammation.[2]

Vitamin B12: Thirty-six patients with bursitis were treated with vitamin B12 injections (1,000 mcg) given intramuscularly each day for 7 to 10 days. This was followed by injections three times a week for two to three weeks, then once or twice a week for two to three weeks. More than 90% of the patients reported pain relief. Complete relief was often noted within several days.[3,4]

Glucosamine Sulfate: Glucosamine sulfate can help reduce inflammation in bursitis. Glucosamine increases the risk of bleeding. Individuals who take blood-thinning medications, such as aspirin, clopidogrel (Plavix), or warfarin (Coumadin), should not take glucosamine.[5]

Ascorbic Acid: Vitamin C with flavonoids helps to repair connective tissue and decreases inflammation.[4]

Bromelain: Bromelain can also reduce inflammation.[4] A typical dose is 750–1,000 mg/day in divided doses.

Cadmium Toxicity

Cadmium is an extremely toxic metal commonly found in industrial workplaces. Similar to lead and arsenic, cadmium causes lipid peroxidative changes in various tissues.

Acute inhalation exposure can result in flu-like symptoms (chills, fever, and muscle pain) and can damage the lungs. Chronic exposure typically results in kidney, bone, and lung damage. Renal injury and mild tubular impairment observed in chronic low-dose exposure situations could be an early warning sign of subclinical or clinical morbidity and mortality.[1]

THERAPEUTIC METHODS

Ascorbic Acid: An experimental study discussed protective the role of vitamin C supplementation in the lung and brain of rats exposed to excessive cadmium. Vitamin C reverted hematological changes in mercury and cadmium-exposed animals. Vitamin C was also observed to be protective against concomitant exposure to heavy metal and radiation in another experimental study.[2]

Lipoic acid (LA) has proven useful in conferring some protection against cadmium poisoning.[3,4]

Vitamins: Vitamins A, C, E, and selenium can prevent or reduce many toxic effects of cadmium on some organs and tissues such as liver, kidney, skeleton, and blood.[5]

Soybeans: In cadmium toxicity, two recent animal studies demonstrated that dietary soybean supplementation helped to prevent arterial and cardiac injury.[6]

Saunas: Cadmium is significantly present in sweat during sauna, which appears to be a moderately successful modality for reducing body burden of cadmium without risk of tubular damage.[7]

Calcinosis Cutis

Calcinosis cutis is a condition where calcium salt crystals accumulate within the dermis (skin). Lesions usually appear as small, firm, white or yellow lumps (papules, plaques, or nodules) on the surface of the skin that may be hard or soft. A solitary lesion may develop, although multiple lesions are more common. Lesions may become tender and ulcerate, discharging a creamy chalk-like material consisting mainly of calcium phosphate with a small amount of calcium carbonate.[1] Calcinosis usually has no symptoms but can be painful in some cases. Calcinosis cutis commonly occurs in patients with systemic sclerosis and dermatomyositis. There are four subtypes of this disorder. Any underlying cause (e.g., hypercalcemia and/or hyperphosphatemia) should be corrected.

MANAGEMENT APPROACHES

Tocopherol: Treatment with oral vitamin E supplementation 300–1,600 IU/day is an effective treatment.[2]

Aluminum Hydroxide: Oral aluminum hydroxide treatment resulted in almost complete clearing of calcinosis after eight months of therapy. There were no adverse effects from therapy.[3] Magnesium or aluminum antacids may be effective phosphate binders in patients with hyperphosphatemia.[4]

Cancer (Bladder)

Bladder cancer is one of the most common cancers in the U.S. each year. Men, Caucasians, and smokers have twice the risk of bladder cancer as the general population. The most common type of bladder cancer is transitional cell carcinoma, also called urothelial carcinoma. If the cancer is confined to the lining of the bladder, it is non-invasive bladder cancer. In most cases, the first sign of bladder cancer is hematuria (blood in the urine).

DESIGNS ON PREVENTION

Nicotine: Those at risk for developing bladder cancer, as well as those patients with bladder cancer, should avoid smoking. Cigarette smokers have a higher risk of bladder cancer than previously thought. A study found that the proportion of bladder cancer due to smoking in women is now the same as for men—about 50%.[1] Former smokers were twice as likely to develop bladder cancer as those who never smoked, and current smokers were four times more likely to do so.[1]

Tocopherol: Taking 200 IU of vitamin E by mouth for more than 10 years appears to help prevent death from bladder cancer.[2,3]

Ascorbic Acid: Taking 1-6 gm of vitamin C per day can help prevent bladder cancer for those who are prone to it.[4,5]

Cancer (Breast)

Most breast cancer forms in the epithelial cells lining the lobules or ducts of the breasts. After skin cancer, breast cancer is the most commonly diagnosed cancer in women in the U.S. Typical symptoms may include a lump in the breast, a change in size or shape of the breast, and/or a discharge from a nipple. Mammograms combined with biopsies can often diagnose the cancer. The strongest risk factor for breast cancer is age because most breast cancers occur in women over 50 years of age.[1] Family, personal history of breast cancer, and gynecologic histories are significant contributors to the risk of developing metastatic breast cancer, as is breast density (the more dense the breast tissue, the higher the risk of breast cancer), alcohol intake, hormone therapy history, and diet, which may contribute to development or growth of breast cancers.[2]

Advanced stages of breast cancer are often indicated by fixation of the mass to the chest wall or overlying skin, satellite nodules or ulcers in the skin, and exaggeration of skin markings (due to skin edema).[3]

PREVENTION

Diet: Eating a plant-based diet as well as higher mushroom consumption were associated with a lower risk of breast cancer.[4,5]

Exercise: At least 150 minutes of moderate intensity exercise per week and maintaining a healthy weight is recommended as a prevention strategy by the American Cancer Society.[6]

Breast Feeding: Multiple studies have found breastfeeding to confer a lower rate of cancer risk, morbidity, and mortality, with a 26% lower lifetime risk for those mothers who breastfeed for 12 months or longer.[7]

Avoid alcohol intake of even one drink per day (10–15 grams), because it represents an elevated risk for breast cancer.[8]

Folic Acid: Breast cancer risk lessens when folate intake increases in heavy drinkers, but not in light drinkers.[8]

Aspirin: Studies have shown that aspirin reduces the risk of breast cancer development.[9] Use of low-dose aspirin (81 mg) at least three times a week was linked to a 20% risk reduction for some types of breast cancer.[10]

Vitamin D: Supplementation with vitamin D3 (2,000 IU/day) reduced the incidence of advanced (metastatic or fatal) cancer in the test group with the strongest risk reduction seen in individuals with normal weight.[11]

Vitamin A: A review of epidemiological studies was conducted to investigate the relationship between β-carotenoids and breast cancer. The evidence from studies confirms that there is an association between β-carotenoids and breast cancer risk; the dietary intake of β-carotenoids or vitamin A may be beneficial in reducing the risk of developing breast cancer.[12]

THERAPEUTIC STRATEGIES

Coenzyme Q10: Two women experienced complete disappearance of breast cancer after taking large doses of CoQ1O. Since that time, two additional patients with metastatic breast cancer were treated with CoQ1O at the same clinic. The results in both of these cases were dramatic.[13]

Comment: A daily dose of 30 mg of CoQ10 can be an effective adjunct to medical treatment. The way in which CoQ10 fights breast cancer is not known.[14]

In a previous report, 32 patients with breast cancer were treated with antioxidants, fatty acids, and 90 mg of CoQ10. Six of the 32 patients reported some signs and symptoms of cancer diminished or showed partial tumor regression. In one of these six cases, the dosage of CoQ10 was increased to 390 mg. In one month, the tumor was no longer palpable, and in another month, mammography confirmed the absence of tumor.[14]

Aspirin: A study in Scotland included 4,627 women who took daily aspirin after breast cancer surgery and found a lower risk of death from breast cancer and all other causes. An observational study of women treated for breast cancer in the U.S. found that those who took a daily aspirin for three to five years following treatment for breast cancer were 60% less likely to experience a recurrence and 71% less likely to die from the disease.[15] Taking aspirin daily always presents a risk for GI bleeding.

Cancer (Esophagus, Oral Cavity, Stomach, Pancreas, Cervix, Colon, Rectum, Breast, Lung, and Prostate)

Cancer refers to any one of a number of diseases of the cells characterized by the development and growth of abnormal cells without regard to normal physiological checkpoints that control and regulate cell growth. Generally, these cells divide uncontrollably and have the ability to invade and destroy normal body tissue.

PREVENTIVE PRINCIPLES

General Measures: Following these general guidelines may lessen the risk of acquiring any type of cancer:[1]

- Avoiding smoking. Smoking is associated with the following cancers: bladder, colorectal, head and neck, kidney and ureter, liver, lung, pancreas, penile, stomach, uterine cervix, and myeloid leukemia.[2,3,4] Complete cessation is recommended to maximize health benefits. Reduce the frequency of alcohol intake.
- Alcohol use is a known risk factor for gastrointestinal (GI) cancers. Higher risk may be associated more with frequent drinking.
- Eating a healthy diet.
- Maintaining a healthy weight.
- Protecting the skin from sun exposure.
- Obtaining hepatitis B and HPV vaccinations.
- Avoiding risky drug and sexual behaviors.
- Getting regular checkups and screening tests.

Ascorbic Acid: The notion that vitamin C may play a preventive role in cancer was first proposed in 1949. It was demonstrated by Cameron et al. that high-dose vitamin C improved the survival rates of patients with terminal cancer.[5,6,7]

In the 1970s, researchers gave 10 gm of vitamin C per day to 100 terminally ill cancer patients and compared their outcome with 1,000 cancer patients who were given conventional therapy. It was observed that 10.3% of cancer patients receiving vitamin C survived. All patients on conventional therapy without vitamin C died.[5] Other studies support these findings. In a Japanese study, patients with uterine cancer were administered 5–30 gm of vitamin C. These patients survived six times longer. When a comparison was made between those supplemented with or without vitamin C, survival rate was 15% higher in those supplemented with vitamin C.[8]

There is considerable evidence that a high intake of vitamin C is linked with a low risk for cancer of esophagus, oral cavity, stomach, pancreas, cervix, rectum, and breast.[9,10,11]

Vitamin D: Recent research suggests that vitamin D supplementation may help reduce the risk of prostate cancer, colon cancer, and other malignancies.[1] Chronic vitamin D deficiency represented a risk factor in the development of more aggressive colon tumors.[12] Evidence suggests vitamin D has antineoplastic effects, and observational studies have shown an inverse association between serum vitamin D levels and colorectal cancer risk. Meta-analysis further demonstrated a clinically meaningful benefit of vitamin D supplementation on colorectal cancer, including metastatic colorectal cancer survival outcomes.[13,14] Researchers have also confirmed the pivotal role of vitamin D, specifically its receptor (VDR), in slowing down the action of a key protein in the carcinogenic transformation process of colon cancer cells. Patients in the initial stages of colon cancer could benefit from being treated with vitamin D3. Typical safe dosing ranges for vitamin D3 are from 5,000–50,000 IU/day.[15]

Selenium: Secondary analysis of a previous study revealed that selenium protected against prostate, lung, bladder, skin, gastric, and colorectal cancers.[16] In a Cochrane review of cancer prevention studies, higher selenium intake (200 mcg/day) had a significantly lower risk of prostate and bladder cancer.[17]

Fiber: Elevated total dietary fiber intake was associated with a significantly reduced risk of incident distal colorectal adenoma. Protective associations were most notable for fiber originating from cereals or fruit. Individuals consuming the highest intakes of dietary fiber have reduced risks of incident colorectal adenoma and distal colon cancer.[18]

Butyrate: At the intestinal level, butyrate, a short-chain fatty acid, suppresses the proliferation of colorectal cancer cells for prevention and inhibition of colonic carcinogenesis.[19] The optimal dosage of butyrate for colon cancer prevention is unknown, but 150–300 mg/day has been used in studies.

Supplements: Research suggests that taking selenium, zinc, vitamin A2, vitamin C, and vitamin E by mouth daily for five years reduces the risk of recurrent large-bowel tumors by about 40%.[20]

Aspirin: Findings from a screening trial found that older adults (>65 years) who regularly took aspirin had a significant reduction in mortality from cancer compared with individuals who did not take aspirin. The greatest reduction in risk was noted for colorectal cancer (CRC) mortality among individuals who used aspirin three or more times per week.[21] Colorectal cancer was the first cancer found to be preventable with aspirin. The use of aspirin for patients with Lynch syndrome to prevent CRC also has strong supporting evidence.[22] A recent observational study indicates that aspirin may have a preventive effect on pancreatic cancers as well.[23]

Avoidance of Hot Beverages: Studies have demonstrated an association between consumption of hot coffee, maté, or tea and esophageal cancer risk.[24] Also, drinker preferences for "very hot" tea, with a temperature of 60°C (140°F) or higher, was associated with a significant increased risk for esophageal basal cell carcinoma.[24]

Methionine: A diet rich in methionine and folate appears to help reduce the chance of colon cancer. This seems to be especially true for people with a family history of colon cancer and people who drink large amounts of alcohol.[25]

Beta-sitosterol (*Asclepias curassavica*) is reported to inhibit the growth of human colon cancer cells.[26]

Coenzyme Q10: Reports of coenzyme Q10 lengthening the survival of patients with pancreatic, lung, rectal, laryngeal, colon, and prostate cancers exist in the peer-reviewed medical literature.[27] These patients also received additional therapies including chemotherapy, radiation therapy, and surgery.

Cancer (Gastric)

Stomach cancer usually begins in the mucus-producing cells that line the stomach. This type of cancer is known as adenocarcinoma. Stomach cancer is difficult to diagnosis because individuals with early gastric cancer often do not have any symptoms. Also, early symptoms that do present, such as fullness, heartburn, or indigestion, are typically nonspecific and mimic other gastrointestinal diseases. The disease is more common among men and those in their 50s. Weight loss and blood in the stool can be key symptoms as the disease further develops. Gastric cancer is the third most common cause of cancer-related deaths in the world.

LOWERING RISK, PREVENTION, AND TREATMENT

Diet: Smoked or pickled foods, as well as salted meats and fish, should be avoided. A diet high in fresh fruits and vegetables can help reduce the risk of stomach cancer.[1]

Aspirin: Using aspirin or other non-steroidal anti-inflammatory drugs (NSAIDs) such as ibuprofen or naproxen appears to lower the risk of stomach cancer.[1] These medicines can also lower the risk of developing colon polyps and colon cancer. The risk of GI bleeding is always a potential risk with aspirin use.

Nicotine: Smoking should be dramatically curtailed or eliminated.

Ascorbic Acid or Beta-Carotene: In a high-risk population with precancerous gastric lesions (i.e., nonmetaplastic atrophy or intestinal metaplasia), combining anti-helicobacter pylori therapy and antioxidant supplementation such as ascorbic acid or beta-carotene appears to be effective in curing these lesions.[2]

Riboflavin and Niacin: Taking riboflavin along with niacin helps prevent gastric cancer.[3]

Selenium: A significant inverse association between low baseline serum selenium levels and deaths from gastric cancer (where the stomach connects to the esophagus) has been reported.[4]

Cancer (Ovarian, Pancreatic, Breast, Mesothelioma, and Incurable Cancer)

ADJUVANT CHEMOTHERAPY METHODS

High-dose ascorbic acid combined with certain categories of chemotherapy can be more effective than chemotherapy alone:

- Ascorbic acid along with arsenic trioxide may be more effective in treating ovarian cancer cells.[1]
- Ascorbic acid plus gemcitabine may be more effective in battling pancreatic cancer cells.[1]
- Ascorbic acid combined with gemcitabine and epigallocatechin-3-gallate (EGCG) may be more effective in malignant mesothelioma cells.[1]

- Intravenous (IV) vitamin C was studied in patients with breast cancer who had been treated with chemotherapy and radiation therapy. The study demonstrated that patients who received IV vitamin C had better quality of life and fewer side effects.[1]
- A study of intravenous vitamin C and high oral doses of vitamin C was done in patients with incurable cancer. Vitamin C was a safe and effective therapy improving the quality of life in these patients, including physical, mental, and emotional functions, symptoms of fatigue, nausea and vomiting, pain, and appetite loss.[1]

Beta-sitosterol in combination with the breast cancer drug tamoxifen appeared to enhance the drug's effectiveness against breast cancer cells.[2] A 2003 study found that beta-sitosterol induced apoptosis, a type of programmed cell death, which is key to halting the spread of cancer cells.[3]

Coenzyme Q10: Anecdotal reports of coenzyme Q10 lengthening the survival of patients with pancreatic, lung, rectal, laryngeal, colon, and prostate cancers exist in the peer-reviewed scientific literature.[4] The patients described in these reports also received therapies other than coenzyme Q10, including chemotherapy, radiation therapy, and surgery.

PREVENTION

Aspirin: A recent limited observational study indicates that daily aspirin may have a preventive effect on ovarian cancer.[5]

Vitamin D: Supplementation with vitamin D3 (2,000 IU/day) reduced the incidence of advanced (metastatic or fatal) cancer in the test group with the strongest risk reduction seen in individuals with normal weight.[6]

Cancer—Prostate (PCa)

The prostate is a small walnut-shaped gland in men located in front of the rectum and behind the bladder. It surrounds the urethra which passes through it and produces seminal fluid to nourish and transport sperm. Prostate cancer is the most common cancer in men over 50 and is the second only to lung cancer as a cause of cancer death among men in the U.S. Prostate cancer usually grows very slowly so there are often no early prostate cancer symptoms. It can often be treated successfully. When symptoms do develop, they are similar to BPH and can include nocturia, hesitancy (i.e., difficulty commencing and maintaining a urine stream), blood in the urine, painful urination, and difficulty achieving or maintaining an erection.

Increasing age, a family history of prostate cancer, and being of African American ancestry increase the risk of developing prostate cancer. According to a cohort study in Sweden, men with infertility also appear to represent a high-risk group for prostate cancer. PCa can often be treated successfully.[1]

TREATMENT STRATEGIES

Vitamin E: The National Cancer Institute reports vitamin E supplementation may be a strong inhibitor of prostatic carcinoma. In a five to eight year study of 29,000 smokers, there was a 33% lower incidence of the disease among those taking supplements (compared to those not increasing their intake). Deaths decreased by 41%. The vitamin E dosage was approximately 50 IU/day.[2]

Saw Palmetto, Lycopene, and Vitamin E: As an adjunct to medical treatment, many patients use vitamin E, saw palmetto, and lycopene to treat prostate cancer.[3] Men participating in several studies had better results when taking saw palmetto as compared to taking a placebo.[4]

Vitamin D: A clinical trial with 143 participants indicated that vitamin D may be effective in treating patients with prostate cancer. Patients were given 4,000–10,000 IU of oral vitamin D3 per day.[5]

PREVENTION

Lycopene: A current review of 26 studies with 563,299 participants found both lycopene supplementation and circulating concentrations exhibited a preventive effect on PCa.[5]

Dose-response meta-analysis further demonstrated that higher lycopene consumption (9–21 mg/day) was linearly associated with a reduced risk of PCa.[6]

Also, the meta-analysis of 21 observational studies from 1950s to 2003 by Etminan et al. demonstrated both the highest category of lycopene intake and circulating concentrations were associated with a significant lower risk of PCa.[7]

Selenium: In a Cochrane review of cancer prevention studies, higher selenium intake (200 mcg/day) had a significantly lower risk of prostate cancer.[2]

Cancer (Skin Cancer)

***See* Melanoma, Basal, and Squamous Cell Carcinomas**

Canker Sores /Recurrent Aphthous Stomatitis (RAS)/ Oral Aphthosis

Canker sores are the most common oral ulcerative condition encountered in clinical practice. The lesions occur on the soft tissues in the mouth or at the base of the gums. They present as recurrent small, round, or ovoid shallow craters or ulcers with yellow or white floors that are surrounded by erythematous (reddened) halos. These painful sores make eating and talking difficult. The treatment of recurrent aphthous stomatitis (RAS) is nonspecific and is based primarily on empirical data. In most cases, treatment is not necessary for minor canker sores, which tend to clear on their own in a week or two.[1]

A diet lacking in vitamin B-12, zinc, folic acid, or iron as well as genetics or sensitivity to chocolate, coffee, strawberries, eggs, nuts, cheese, or spicy or acidic foods can cause canker sores.[2]

MANAGEMENT CONSIDERATIONS

Diet: Acidic (fruit juices, citrus fruits, tomatoes), salty, or spicy foods that can cause further irritation and pain as well as alcohol and carbonated drinks should be avoided.[3]

Mouthwash: A mouthwash containing 0.15% triclosan in ethanol and zinc sulfate reduced the number of new aphthous ulcers in 43% of cases, the pain intensity in 45%, and extended the ulcer-free interval.[4] An antiseptic mouthwash or a homemade rinse made from a small amount of salt and warm water can also help.[5]

Toothpaste: Sodium laurel sulfate-free toothpaste (Rembrandt Canker Sore Toothpaste, Tom's of Maine SLS-free toothpastes, plain baking soda) is recommended.[5]

Topical Treatments: Benzocaine (Anbesol, Kank-A, Orabase, Zilactin-B), fluocinonide (Lidex, Vanos), hydrogen peroxide (Orajel Antiseptic Mouth Sore Rinse, Peroxyl),[1] and 5-amonisalicylic acid reduce the duration from 11 days to 7 days.[1] Rinses with soothing, coating products containing bismuth subsalicylate (Kaopectate) may provide symptomatic relief. Those containing aloe have been reported to promote ulcer healing.[6]

Zinc Sulphate: In canker sore patients with initial serum zinc levels less than or equal to 110 micro ng/dl, all showed improvement with zinc sulfate supplementation up to a total of 660 mg/day.[7] In another study, substantial clinical improvement of oral ulcers occurred in 46.2% of patients who took zinc sulfate.[8]

Sharquie et al. found oral zinc sulphate (100 mg tid) reduced the number and size of recurrent aphthous ulcers in comparison to a placebo.[9] In another double-blind, placebo-controlled study of 15 patients, zinc sulphate had both therapeutic and prophylactic action as it also reduced the relapse rate in recurrent ulcers.[10]

Nutrients: Doctors prescribe important nutrients, such as folate (folic acid), vitamin B6, vitamin B12, or zinc if intake is low.[1,3,11]

Vitamin B12: 1,000 mcg/day has been used successfully as a treatment.[12]

Milk of Magnesia: In the case of minor ulcers, patients can treat these using over-the-counter medications such as "Milk of Magnesia" or "Bonjela."[11]

Dampening the prescription medication sucralfate, also known as Carafate, and dabbing it onto the ulcer several times a day to relieve the pain can make eating far easier. Or use sucralfate 1 gm/10 mL solution two to four times a day. It generally heals the sore within a day or two.[12]

Lysine: Clinical studies indicate that taking 500 mg of lysine daily prevented canker sores and 4,000 mg/day during a breakout decreased the healing time of canker sores.[13]

Vitamin B12: Due to the relationship between RAS and vitamin deficiencies, some authors have reported that treatment with vitamin B12, apart from being simple, inexpensive, and of low risk, proves effective in application to RAS, even independently of the serum vitamin B12 levels of the patient.[14] Other investigators have reported similar results.[15] Vitamin and mineral deficiency replacement is a front-line treatment strategy.[16]

Ascorbic Acid: A recent study explored the effects of daily ascorbic acid 2,000 mg/day over three months for managing minor RAS. A 50% reduction in oral ulcer outbreaks and a significant reduction in pain level was noted in these patients. There is strong evidence to suggest that ascorbate decreases neutrophil-mediated inflammation via modulation of reactive oxygen species (ROS).[17] Ascorbic acid as an adjunctive therapy to topicals should be considered as well because of its relatively benign side-effect profile.[18]

Capillary Fragility

Capillary fragility is characterized by thinning and loss of elasticity in capillary walls. It results in walls being easily injured and more susceptible to rupture and leak. When these small vessels tear and leak, it produces the appearance of petechiae (tiny purple, red, or brown spots) under the skin.[1] A large number of diseases are associated with capillary fragility. There are no serious complications from having capillary fragility, but it may signify a more serious underlying problem. For example, persons with increased capillary fragility (e.g., due to hypertension) are especially predisposed to stroke, retinal hemorrhage, and death.[2]

TREATMENT

NSAIDs should be avoided because of increased bleeding risk.

Vitamin C: Vitamin C is critical in the biosynthesis of collagen, an important component in connective tissues including blood vessels, without which capillary fragility and subcutaneous hemorrhages develop.[3] Supplementation with 1 gm of vitamin C per day for two months improved capillary strength in all diabetic patients tested.[4]

Bioflavonoids/rutin (antioxidants abundant in the pulp and rinds of citrus fruits and other foods containing vitamin C) have been used, particularly in European countries, in the treatment of capillary bleeding.[5] Rutin is a flavonoid reported to reduce capillary bleeding. It has been used in a dose of 60 mg oral (2–3 x/day) along with vitamin C (e.g., Cadisper-C) which is believed to facilitate its action.[6]

Adrenochrome monosemicarbazone, a product of adrenaline (e.g., in the supplement Cadisper-C), is believed to reduce capillary fragility, control oozing from raw surfaces, and prevent microvessel bleeding (e.g., epistaxis [nose bleeds]), hematuria (blood in the urine), and secondary hemorrhage from wounds, etc. Do not take Cadisper-C if pregnant or breastfeeding.[6]

Proanthocyanidins: Taking 150 mg/day of these powerful plant flavonoids can increase capillary strength.[7]

Bromelain: A clinical study demonstrated that bromelain supplementation administered to boxers completely cleared all bruises on the face and hematomas of the orbits, lips, ears, chest, and arms in four days.[8] It is thought that the best results occur at a dose of 750–1,000 mg/day.[9]

Carbon Monoxide Poisoning

The most common symptoms of carbon monoxide poisoning are headache, dizziness, weakness, nausea, vomiting, chest pain, and confusion. High levels of carbon monoxide inhalation can cause loss of consciousness and death. Unless suspected, carbon monoxide poisoning can be difficult to diagnose because its symptoms mimic symptoms of other illnesses. 100% oxygen therapy is the first choice of treatment in medicine.

ADDITIONAL CONSIDERATIONS

NAC: N-acetylcysteine (NAC) is used to help counteract carbon monoxide poisoning.[1]

Ascorbic Acid: F. Klenner, MD, discovered a property of intravenous ascorbate as a "flash oxidizer" of carbon monoxide and a viable treatment option.[2,3] He reportedly counteracted carbon monoxide poisoning with large doses of ascorbic acid (9 gm/day intravenously).

Cardiac Arrythmias

An arrythmia refers to any change from the normal sequence of electrical impulses that affects either the rate or rhythm of the heartbeat. Irregular heartbeats such as atrial fibrillation, bradycardia, tachycardia, conduction disorders, rhythm disorders, ventricular fibrillation, and premature contractions are arrythmias, also known as dysrhythmias. Palpitations are disturbances in the rhythm that can be felt and can make the heart feel like it is beating too hard or too fast, skipping a beat, or fluttering. Symptoms and signs of arrhythmia often include chest pain, dizziness, breathlessness, palpitations, fainting, chest fluttering, tachycardia or bradycardia, and shortness of breath. Arrythmia is the most common cause of sudden cardiac arrest. There are a wide variety of causes for arrythmias, such as myocardial infarction, coronary heart disease (CAD), hypertension (HTN), thyroid problems, drug abuse, diabetes, certain medications, etc. Smoking and excessive alcohol or caffeine use also increase the risk of an arrythmia.

TREATMENT OPTIONS

Avoid Alcohol: Just one alcoholic drink doubles the risk of atrial fibrillation (AF) within the next four hours, and the more alcohol consumed, the higher the risk.[1]

Magnesium is of great importance in cardiac arrhythmias. It increases the ventricular threshold for fibrillation. Sinus node refractoriness and conduction in the AV node are both prolonged.[2]

The potential ability of magnesium supplementation to prevent and/or treat arrhythmias has been recognized in clinical medicine for years. This includes prevention of atrial fibrillation (AF) following cardiac surgery, acute treatment of rapid AF, new-onset and treatment-refractory supraventricular tachycardia (SVT), refractory ventricular fibrillation, and a variety of drug-induced arrhythmias, most notably torsades de pointes (TdP). As a result, the American Association for Thoracic Surgery and European Society of Cardiology have incorporated magnesium into recent guidelines for preventing and managing certain arrhythmias.[3]

Oral magnesium has also been used for many years in patients with symptomatic extrasystoles. Studies show that the incidence of extrasystoles, as well as patients' symptoms, were reduced during oral magnesium therapy.[1] In one study, giving magnesium orally (300 mg/day for at least six weeks) or intravenously was helpful for treating arrythmias.[4,5]

For patients with frequent ventricular arrythmias (PVCs), an increase in the daily oral intake of magnesium and potassium (50% increase in the recommended minimum daily dietary intake of the two minerals for three weeks) in patients with frequent ventricular arrhythmias results in a moderate but significant antiarrhythmic effect.[6]

One study found that administration of prophylactic magnesium reduced the risk of supraventricular arrhythmias after cardiac surgery by 23% (atrial fibrillation by 29%) and ventricular arrhythmias by 48%.[7]

Administering magnesium sulfate (10–15 ml of 20% $MgSO_4$ in one minute and 500 ml of 2% $MgSO_4$ in five hours) was effective in intractable ventricular tachycardia and ventricular fibrillation. It was also effective in ventricular tachycardia characterized by "torsades de pointes" (irregular heartbeat) and in massive digoxin intoxication 1-6 gm of magnesium sulfate given by IV over several minutes, followed by an IV infusion may be beneficial.[8,9]

Taurine dampens activity of the sympathetic nervous system and dampens epinephrine release. 10–20 gm taurine per day reduced premature atrial complexes (extra heartbeats) by 50% and prevented all PVCs, but did not prevent pauses.[10] Adding 4–6 gm of L-arginine immediately terminated essentially all remaining pauses and PACs, maintaining normal cardiac rhythm with continued treatment.

Effects of taurine are useful in preventing arrhythmias and regulating excitability of the myocardium. L-arginine may have anti-arrhythmic properties resulting from its role as a nitric oxide (NO) precursor and from its ability to restore sinus rhythm spontaneously.[10]

Ascorbic Acid: Postoperative patients in whom AF develops have an increased incidence of strokes and perioperative myocardial infarction, are prone to development of congestive heart failure and respiratory failure, and thus are at an increased risk of mortality. The role of vitamin C was studied in 100 randomized patients undergoing coronary bypass surgery.[11] Half received ascorbic acid and a β-blocker preoperatively and postoperatively, and the other half received only a β-blocker. The group that received both vitamin C and a β-blocker had a 4% incidence of AF compared with 25% in the control group. Additional studies have reported similar findings. In a 2005 study on the role of vitamin C in the prevention of early recurrence of AF following cardioversion, AF recurred in 4.5% of patients pretreated with vitamin C, compared with 36.3% in the control group. The control group treated with vitamin C had a significant reduction in serum inflammatory indices, such as white blood cell count, fibrinogen level, and level of C-reactive protein. Taking vitamin C before and for a few days after heart surgery helps prevent irregular heartbeat after heart surgery.[12]

L-Carnitine: A meta-analysis of 13 controlled trials concludes that including L-carnitine among the other therapies given in the acute setting for MI appears to significantly cut all-cause mortality and lead to fewer angina symptoms and ventricular arrhythmias.[13]

Cardiogenic Shock

Cardiogenic shock is a medical emergency resulting from damage to the ventricles from a myocardial infarction (MI). The condition is a medical emergency and is fatal if not treated promptly. Because the damaged ventricles cannot pump an adequate amount of blood, symptoms often include low urine production (<30 mL/hour), rapid heartbeat, weak pulse, pallor, cool arms and legs, rapid breathing, and an altered level of consciousness. Some patients may have a severely low blood pressure and heart rate. Emergency life support treatment is needed.

KEY ADJUVANT MEDICINE CONSIDERATION

L-Carnitine: Cardiogenic shock is fatal nearly three-quarters of the time. In an Italian study, 27 patients with an acute myocardial infarction who had lapsed into cardiogenic shock were given an intravenous injection of 4 gm of carnitine, followed by an additional 6 gm/day intravenously for the duration of the shock condition. After 10 days, 77.8% of the patients were still alive, a dramatic improvement over the expected survival rate of 25%–30%.[1,2]

Cardiomyopathy

Cardiomyopathy is any progressive chronic disease that deforms the heart muscle, making the walls enlarged, inflamed, or brittle, and impairs the heart's ability to efficiently pump blood. The three main types of cardiomyopathy include dilated (with stretched walls and impaired contraction), hypertrophic (usually an enlarged and thick left ventricle), and restrictive (abnormally brittle ventricles that restrict filling). As a result, the heart's function is flawed and it cannot maintain a normal ejection fraction or cardiac output.

Heart conditions such as tachycardia or high blood pressure, viral infections, nutritional (e.g., vitamin B1) deficiencies, and certain diseases are typical causes of cardiomyopathy. Some individuals with cardiomyopathy have no signs or symptoms and need no treatment.[1] For others, symptoms of heart failure develop quickly, are severe, and significant complications can occur. Symptomatic cardiomyopathy is a serious disease associated with high mortality and morbidity. Treatment in asymptomatic individuals with hypertrophic cardiomyopathy is controversial, and no conclusive evidence has been found that medical therapy is beneficial.[2]

MEDICAL MANAGEMENT OPTIONS

Non-Pharmacological Treatment: Salt restriction and alcohol discontinuation.[3]

Selenium deficiency leads to cardiomyopathy that is fully reversible with oral selenium (20–40 mcg/day).[4,5]

Carnitine: In patients with chronic heart disease, administration of L-carnitine (approximately 1 gm L-carnitine per 10 pounds of body weight) over 12 months led to attenuation of left ventricular dilatation and prevented ventricular remodeling while reducing incidence of chronic heart failure and death.[6]

Primary carnitine deficiency (PCD) is an inherited disorder in which patients affected with the disease may present with acute metabolic decompensation during infancy or with severe cardiomyopathy in childhood. Treatment of this disorder with L-carnitine is highly effective in correcting cardiomyopathy and muscle weakness, as well as any impairment in fasting ketogenesis.

The Food and Drug Administration first approved L-carnitine in 1985 for the treatment of PCD. Primary treatment involves supplementation of oral L-carnitine. Typically, a high dose (100–400 mg/kg/day) divided into three doses is required. Treatment with oral L-carnitine at pharmacologic levels is quite effective in treating cardiomyopathy and muscle weakness in children.[7]

Alpha-Lipoic Acid (ALA): Alpha-lipoic acid (ALA) has been described as a therapeutic agent for a number of conditions related to cardiovascular disease. In one study, researchers found that ALA effectively ameliorated cardiac hypertrophy in vivo and in vitro. ALA can reduce the degree of heart hypertrophy.[8]

Taurine: Evidence strongly indicates that taurine (3–6 gm/day for 30 to 45 days) prophylaxis is effective in improving cardiac function[9] and decreasing left ventricular end-diastolic volume.[10] Experimental data indicates that taurine can reverse cardiomyopathic degeneration and death.[11]

Idebenone, 5 mg/kg/day, reduced cardiac hypertrophy in most Friedreich's ataxia patients studied. It is well-tolerated in high doses up to 55 mg/kg/day. The possibility that the current dose or higher doses may improve cardiac hypertrophy in other patients remains to be fully determined.[12]

Magnesium: Patients with hypoparathyroidism can manifest cardiomyopathy, which responds to magnesium supplementation.[13]

CoQ10: Taking statins (Lipitor, Zocor, Crestor, etc.) for high cholesterol has been shown to reduce endogenous coenzyme Q10 levels which may block steps in muscle cell energy generation, possibly leading to statin-related myopathy. For cardiac effects, typical dosages of CoQ10 are 100–600 mg/day given in two or three divided doses.[14]

Carpal Tunnel Syndrome (CTS)

Carpal tunnel syndrome is the most common entrapment neuropathy. Compression of the median nerve in the carpal tunnel of the wrist causes numbness, tingling, and pain on the palm side of the thumb and most fingers, except the small finger. The pain or numbness can be especially bad at night. Women are far more likely than men to develop CTS. Conditions that can lead to developing CTS include trauma, diabetes, hypothyroidism, pregnancy, and rheumatoid arthritis. If left untreated, CTS can cause chronic pain, muscle wasting, and weakness in the affected thumb and fingers leading to impairment and disability.

Conservative treatment should be tried first, with surgical exploration taking place if there is no success or worsening of symptoms occurs. Many physicians utilize orthotic splints, NSAIDs, physical therapy, and steroid injections. While surgical treatment, or carpal tunnel release, is commonplace, the procedure is reported to have up to a 57% failure rate.[1]

NUTRITIONAL SUPPORT

Vitamin B6 is often used as a conservative and adjunct therapy in treatment of carpal tunnel syndrome. Vitamin B6, 200–500 mg/day, can alleviate symptoms of CTS.[2]

Bernstein and Dinesen suggested that vitamin B6 supplementation substantially improved pain scores even though electrophysiologic data showed only mild improvement, supporting the theory that vitamin B6 raises pain thresholds.[3] Ellis et al. found that, in at least seven patients, a primary deficiency (dietary inadequacy) of vitamin B6 was linked to CTS.[4] In a case study, Folkers and colleagues determined that 2 mg/day of vitamin B6 improved patients' clinical condition, but that 100 mg of vitamin B6 daily for a longer period allowed patients to avoid hand surgery.[5]

In a retrospective review of 994 CTS patient charts, Kasdan and Janes found that, in the 494 patients whose treatment included vitamin B6 (100 mg twice daily), the rate of symptom alleviation was much higher (68%) than among patients who did not receive vitamin B6 (14.3%).[6]

Alpha Lipoic Acid/Gamma Linoleic Acid ALA/GLA: While surgery is reserved for the most severe cases, the earlier stages of disease may be controlled by a pharmacological treatment aimed to bring about "neuroprotection" (i.e., limiting and correcting the nerve damage). One study aimed to compare the efficacy of a fixed association of alpha-lipoic acid (ALA) 600 mg/day and gamma-linolenic acid (GLA) 360 mg/day, and a multivitamin B preparation (vitamin B6 150 mg, vitamin B1 100 mg, vitamin B12 500 µg/day) for 90 days in 112 subjects with moderately severe CTS.[7]

A significant reduction in both symptoms scores and functional impairment was observed in ALA/GLA group, while the multivitamin group experienced a slight improvement of symptoms and a deterioration of functional scores. Electromyography showed a statistically significant improvement with ALA/GLA, but not with the multivitamin product.

The fixed association of ALA and GLA proved to be a useful tool and may be proposed for controlling symptoms and improving the evolution of CTS, especially in the earlier stages of disease.[7,8]

Linseed Oil or Flaxseed Oil: Topical linseed oil could be effective in the management of mild and moderate carpal tunnel syndrome, especially in improving the severity of symptoms and functional status.[9] The topical use of flaxseed oil gel was more effective in the improvement of symptoms and function of patients with mild to moderate carpal tunnel syndrome as compared with a hand splint.[10]

Cataracts (Diabetic)

High blood sugar levels raise the risk for senile cataracts by about 40%. Good control of blood pressure and diabetes, including A1c levels, for prevention is the best treatment strategy.[1]

NUTRITIONAL SUPPORT IN LOWERING RISK

Ascorbic Acid: One of the major causes of end-organ damage in diabetes is thought to be intracellular accumulation of sorbitol, a metabolic byproduct of glucose. Because sorbitol is impermeable to cell membranes, it becomes trapped inside the cells of the ocular lens and the peripheral nervous system in general. Sorbitol accumulation leads to osmotic swelling and consequent cell damage. The fluid in the eye that bathes the lens should be high in vitamin C. One study suggests that vitamin C supplementation prevents intracellular accumulation of sorbitol and may reduce the risk of diabetic cataracts.[2]

Women whose diets were highest in vitamin C (about two servings of fruit and two servings of vegetables daily) had a 20% lower risk of developing cataracts than women whose diets were low in vitamin C rich foods. Perhaps higher doses with supplements could lower the risk considerably more.[3]

Vitamin A: Individuals who consume high amounts of vitamin A in their diets appear to have a lower risk of developing cataracts.[4,5]

Cataracts (Prevention)

When a normal clear eye lens gets cloudy and decreases vision, this is referred to as a cataract. The eye's lens is mostly made of water and protein which are arranged in a way that keeps the lens clear and lets light pass through it. As we age, the protein can become less organized, clouding part of the lens. Other causes of cataracts include corticosteroid treatment, trauma, diabetes, and other diseases. Symptoms may include faded colors, blurry vision, seeing halos around lights, and trouble seeing at night. This may result in difficulty driving, reading, or recognizing faces. Cataracts are the most common cause of vision loss in people over age 40 and are the principal cause of blindness in the world.

PREVENTIVE METHODS

Ascorbic Acid: A recent study demonstrated the benefits of taking vitamin C supplements for women 56–71 years old. Those who took vitamin C were less likely to develop "lens opacities" (cataracts).[1]

Riboflavin (vitamin B2) status is poor in cataract patients. Results suggest association between human cataract and nutritional deficiency of riboflavin.[2]

Lutein: Some studies suggest that eating higher amounts of lutein might decrease the risk of developing cataracts. Also, early previous studies indicate that taking lutein three times weekly for up to two years can improve vision in elderly people with cataracts.[3]

Retinoids: Individuals who consume high amounts of vitamin A in their diet seem to have a lower risk of developing cataracts.[4]

Cavities/Dental Caries

A buildup of food and bacteria forms a film called plaque on the teeth. Tooth decay, also known as dental caries or cavities, occurs when bacterial acids in the plaque digest carbohydrates (sugars and starches) left on the teeth. Over time these same acids can dissolve the surface of the tooth causing holes, called cavities, in the enamel and dentin. It is possible to prevent a cavity when decay has made holes in a tooth's enamel but has not yet reached the dentin. Tooth decay is influenced by what we eat and drink and how well we take care of our teeth. If tooth decay is not treated, it can cause pain, infection, and tooth loss.

REDUCING THE RISK OF CAVITIES

Diet: Sugary foods and drinks should be avoided.

Vitamin D: Analysis of clinical research indicates that taking either vitamin D2 or D3 reduces the risk of cavities by 36% to 49% in infants, children, and adolescents.[1,2] Children may need 10 times more than the current recommended dose of 200 IU/day. Children getting 2,000 IU/day showed no signs of toxicity.[3]

Celiac Disease/Nontropical Sprue/Gluten Intolerance

Celiac disease, also known as sprue, is a long-term autoimmune digestive disorder that, over time, damages the small intestine in individuals who cannot tolerate gluten, which is found in wheat, rye, and barley. Celiac disease tends to run in families. It is characterized by imperfect absorption of food elements, especially fat, xylose, and vitamin B12, from the small intestine.

Classic symptoms include gastrointestinal problems such as chronic diarrhea, abdominal distention, malabsorption, and loss of appetite.[1] Neurologic syndromes, including gait and limb ataxia can occur (6%–10% of patients). In children, malabsorption can cause the failure to grow normally. Vitamin and mineral deficiencies such as folate, vitamin K, and vitamin D, as well as iron (leading to iron-deficiency anemia), are common.[2] Treatment goals are to relieve clinical symptoms, replenish vitamin/mineral stores, and prevent complications.

CARE CONSIDERATIONS

Gluten: A strict gluten-free diet is the best management technique.

Vitamins: Many patients may need to supplement their levels of:

- calcium
- folate
- iron
- vitamin B12
- vitamin D
- vitamin K
- zinc[3]

B Vitamins: Malabsorption can be corrected with supplemental vitamin B12.[4] In addition, high doses of vitamin B complex (including 0.8 mg folic acid, 0.5 mg of B12, and 3 mg pyridoxine per day) are also indicated because the disease does not respond to vitamin B12 alone.[5] In one study, patients who initially reported poor well-being showed notable improvements in anxiety and depressed mood with supplementation.[6]

L-Carnitine: Some research shows that taking L-carnitine reduced fatigue associated with celiac disease.[7]

Iron and Vitamin C: Celiac disease causes low iron levels. Adding vitamin C to iron supplementation helps the body absorb iron more efficiently.[8]

Cerebellar Ataxia (Intermittent)

Ataxia is a clinical neurological sign indicating a problem in the central nervous system especially the cerebellum and/or the spinal cord. Intermittent ataxia is a loss of muscle coordination that comes and goes during walking and produces an irregular gait. During an episode, affected individuals may experience dizziness, nausea, vomiting, migraine headaches, impaired vision, slurred speech, and/or ringing in the ears.[1] Deficiencies in cobalamin (vitamin B12), vitamin B1, vitamin E, and possibly zinc can produce cerebellar signs and symptoms.[2] Inborn errors of metabolism (enzyme defects) can also be manifested by intermittent cerebellar ataxia. Therefore, the presence of intermittent ataxia suggests a potentially treatable metabolic disease.[3] A considerable number of other medical conditions can also cause intermittent ataxia.

NUTRIPHARMACOLOGY

Thiamine: Intermittent cerebellar ataxia is an inborn error of metabolism known to respond to pharmacological doses of thiamine.[4,5]

Biotin: Some cases of intermittent cerebellar ataxia are known to respond to pharmacologic doses of biotin.[3]

Magnesium: Cases of intermittent cerebellar ataxia, restless legs, and generalized convulsions associated with hypomagnesemia have been reported. Magnesium supplementation corrected the underlying problems.[6]

Cerebellar Degeneration—Alcoholic

Cerebellar degeneration is a process in which neurons in the cerebellum, which controls coordination and balance, deteriorate and die. Ataxia or loss of coordination in standing and gait typically develop over weeks and months but there can be an acute onset as well. The cause is often alcohol abuse and nutritional deficiencies.

LESSENING AND IMPROVING SYMPTOMS

Thiamine and B Vitamins: For alcoholic cerebellar degeneration, symptoms are often relieved with discontinuation of alcohol abuse, plus a normal diet and dietary supplementation with thiamine given concurrently with other B vitamins.[1,2]

Cerebral Palsy

Cerebral palsy refers to a group of neurological disorders that appear in infancy or early childhood. It is a disorder of posture and movement due to damage, a defect, or lesion in the immature brain before or during birth. Cerebral palsy affects the motor area of the brain's cerebral cortex. The damage may be from lack of oxygen, infection, genetic abnormalities, trauma, or hemorrhage. As a result, there are permanent postural deformities and movement disorders. Symptoms vary among individuals, but some patients can also have seizures, intellectual disability, and impaired vision or hearing, as well as language and speech problems.

CARE CONSIDERATIONS

Physical activity is recommended for people with cerebral palsy, particularly in terms of cardiorespiratory endurance and muscle strengthening.

Magnesium: Premature infants with very low birth weight (less than 1,500 g) are at high risk for developing cerebral palsy. Magnesium helped prevent brain hemorrhage in VLBW infants and may also reduce the extent of brain injury associated with birth asphyxia.[1,2]

GABA: Previous clinical studies demonstrate that taking one to four tablets of a product containing GABA (Gammalon) daily for two months might improve mental development, learning, vocabulary, and physical function in children with cerebral palsy.[3]

Occupational and physical therapy may help manage spasticity. This includes cold, heat, positioning, stretching exercises, and use of orthotic devices.[4]

Cervical Dysplasia

The presence of abnormal or precancerous cells on the surface of the uterine cervix is cervical dysplasia and yields a risk of cervical cancer. Cervical dysplasia can range from mild to severe, depending on the histological appearance of the abnormal cells. Cervical dysplasia is most often asymptomatic. Most women with low grade (mild) dysplasia (LGSIL or CIN1) will undergo spontaneous regression without treatment, so monitoring is indicated.[1] Surgical treatment is appropriate for women with high-grade cervical dysplasia.[1]

REDUCING RISK

Vitamin A: Low dietary intake of vitamin A is associated with a nearly three-fold increase in the risk of cervical dysplasia. Vitamin A supplementation is recommended to lower the risk.[2]

Ascorbic Acid: Relatively low vitamin C levels may predispose women to cervical dysplasia as reported by a study at Albert Einstein College of Medicine. Vitamin C intake less than 50% of the recommended daily allowance yielded a 10-fold increase in risk of cervical dysplasia.[3,4] This study indicated a protective role of supplementary vitamin C for women at high risk of cervical cancer.

Folic Acid: It is known that low red blood cell folate levels enhance the effect of other risk factors for cervical dysplasia.[5] In controlled clinical studies, folic acid supplementation (10 mg/day) has resulted in the improvement or normalization of cytology smears in patients with cervical dysplasia. When patients were treated with folic acid, the regression-to-normal rate, as determined by colposcopy/biopsy examination, was observed to be 20% in one study,[6] 63.7% in another,[5] and 100% in yet another.[7]

Chediak-Higashi Syndrome

Chediak-Higashi syndrome is an autosomal recessive disease characterized by fair skin and white or light-colored hair and light-colored irises (oculocutaneous albinism), immune deficiency, coagulation deficiency (tendency to bruise and bleed easily), and neuropathy. Immune deficiency results in recurrent infections and is caused by a mutation of a lysosomal trafficking regulator protein, which leads to a decrease in phagocytosis.

NUTRITIONAL SUPPORT

Ascorbic Acid: Primary abnormalities on neutrophil locomotion are completely or partially corrected following ascorbate therapy.[1] Supplementation at 1–2 gm/day to enhance compromised wound healing is recommended.

Cheilitis/Angular Cheilitis

Erythema (redness), painful cracking, scaling, bleeding, and ulceration at the corners of the mouth (labial commissures) is known as angular cheilitis. Cheilitis can be a presenting sign of nutritional deficiency of iron, riboflavin (B2), folate (B9), cobalamin (B12), or zinc. Treatment is toward the underlying cause.[1]

CARE CONSIDERATIONS

Zinc oxide as a barrier paste can be applied frequently over the affected areas.[1]

Emollients: Petrolatum or lip balm can be applied frequently for barrier protection.[1]

Nutritional Deficiencies: Correcting nutritional deficiencies such as riboflavin, iron, zinc, folate, or cobalamin or folic acid deficiency should reverse the inflammatory process.[2]

Iron: In one study, it was shown that iron-replacement therapy for patients suffering from iron-deficiency anemia caused significant regression of angular cheilitis.[3]

Chicken Pox/Varicella

Chicken pox is a highly contagious viral infection. The herpes zoster virus initially causes a skin rash of small itchy pink or red bumps. Later, fluid-filled blisters develop. The rash first appears on the stomach, back, and face, then spreads over the whole body. Finally, the blisters scab over with a crust. Because new bumps tend to appear for several days, all three stages (rash, blisters, and scabs) can be present at the same time.

HASTENING HEALING TIME

General Advice: Calamine lotion and a cool bath with added baking soda, aluminum acetate (e.g., Domeboro), oatmeal, or colloidal oatmeal may help relieve some of the itching. Antihistamines such as diphenhydramine (Benadryl, etc.) can also be used. Avoid aspirin and ibuprofen, if possible, in managing chickenpox symptoms. Tylenol can be used for mild fever.[1,2]

Vitamin A: Ninety-three children with chicken pox who had no clinical evidence of vitamin A deficiency were given vitamin A (a single 200,000 unit dose) and eight exposed siblings who had not yet shown signs of illness were given the same dose of vitamin A during the incubation period. Crusting of the lesions (a sign of recovery) occurred significantly more rapidly in the vitamin A group. Average time to healing was only 5.1 days instead of the usual 5–10 days.[3]

Chilblains/Pernio

Small painful or itchy red or purple bumps that form on the fingers or toes as a reaction to cold temperatures are known as chilblains. Swelling and/or blisters are often present. It is a form of localized vasculitis frequently associated with Raynaud's disease. The disorder affects primarily women, but also children or the elderly, in damp temperate climates.[1] As a rule, chilblains tends to respond poorly to treatment. Existing lesions often clear up in a few weeks with or without active treatment.

MANAGEMENT TECHNIQUES

Prevention by wearing proper clothing and avoiding prolonged exposure to cold is the prime treatment method.

Friar's Balsalm/Iodine: According to the British National Health Service, patients had good results by applying a mixture of friar's balsam and a weak iodine solution. Any physician or pharmacist can assist in procuring this formula.[2]

Lanolin: Chilblains.org recommends the application of a lanolin cream to the hands or feet because it helps retain body heat.[3] This is useful in both treating and preventing chilblains.

Nicotinic Acid: In a limited older study, nicotinic acid proved to be a valuable adjunct in the treatment of chilblains.[4]

Cholera

Cholera is an acute illness due to infection of the small intestine by some strains of the bacterium *Vibrio cholerae*. The bacterial disease is usually spread through contaminated water. Cholera causes profuse amounts of watery diarrhea (rice-water stool) and vomiting, leading to leg cramps, dehydration, and death.[1]

LOWERING FLUID LOSS

Niacin: Taking niacin (2,000 mg/day) by mouth helped to control the loss of fluid (diarrhea) due to cholera.[2]

Bromelain: Bromelain supplementation helped protect animal subjects against diarrhea and fluid loss from *Vibrio cholerae*.[3] Human studies are lacking.

NUTRITIONAL SUPPORT

Rehydration: With timely replacement of water and electrolytes, more than 99% of cholera patients will survive. That's why rehydration is the most important treatment for cholera.

Zinc supplementation (20 mg/day in children six months or older) should be started immediately.[4]

Cholesterol/Hypercholesterolemia/Hyperlipidemia

Abnormally high amounts of any or all fats in the blood, whether cholesterol (hypercholesterolemia), triglycerides (hypertriglyceridemia), or related compounds, is hyperlipidemia. Cholesterol is a waxy, fat-like substance produced by the liver and found in cell walls and nerves. Both cholesterol and its derivatives are important parts of healthy cell membranes, bile acids, and hormones and allow the body to produce vitamin D. High cholesterol has no signs or symptoms, but excess cholesterol forms fatty deposits in the walls of the arteries. Over time, as the cholesterol accumulates, it causes atherosclerotic plaques to form, which thicken and harden the artery walls. This is referred to as atherosclerosis. High serum cholesterol and its subtypes, especially low-density lipoproteins (LDLs), which transport cholesterol to the tissues increase the risk for developing atherosclerosis, coronary artery disease, heart attack, and ischemic stroke.

Both genetics and an unhealthy lifestyle (e.g., poor diet or obesity) play significant roles in developing hypercholesterolemia. Secondary causes of elevated cholesterol include hypothyroidism, type 2 diabetes, alcohol excess, obstructive liver disease, nephrotic syndrome, renal failure, and certain medications. General goals of treatment are to lower total and LDL cholesterol to reduce the risk of first or recurrent events such as MI, angina, heart failure, ischemic stroke, or peripheral arterial disease.[1]

CLINICAL TREATMENT GOALS

Total cholesterol:	< 200 mg/dL
LDL (bad cholesterol):	< 100 mg/dL
HDL (good cholersterol):	> 45 mg/dL
Triglycerides:	< 150 mg/dL

ADDITIONAL OPTIONS FOR MEDICAL MANAGEMENT

Nonpharmacologic therapies such as weight loss, smoking cessation, and exercise are the mainstays of treatment.[2]

Aspirin: For decades, low-dose aspirin (75–100 mg/day) has been widely administered for prevention of atherosclerotic coronary vascular disease (ASCVD). By irreversibly inhibiting platelet function, aspirin reduces risk of atherothrombosis but at the risk of bleeding, particularly in the gastrointestinal (GI) tract. Aspirin is well established for secondary prevention of ASCVD and is widely recommended for adults aged 40–70 years who are not at increased bleeding risk.[3]

Diet: In a meta-analysis of RCTs comparing low-fat and low-carbohydrate diets, it was reported that low-fat diets had the most favorable effects on total cholesterol and LDL cholesterol levels, whereas low-carbohydrate diets had the most favorable effects on triglyceride and HDL cholesterol levels.[4]

Exercise (e.g., aerobics 120 minutes per week) can help manage hyperlipidemia.[5]

Statins (e.g., Lipitor or Crestor) **and niacin** (the nicotinic acid form of vitamin B3) are medications used to treat high cholesterol. Both medications lower LDL (bad) cholesterol and raise HDL (good) cholesterol.[6,7]

Nicotinic acid (vitamin B3) is the most powerful agent currently available for raising low levels of good cholesterol (HDL-C).[7] Niacin and statins also lower triglycerides (fats) in the blood.[6,7] There is some indication that patients on statins benefit further from niacin supplementation to slow the progression of heart disease.[8]

Nicotinic acid or niacin (other forms of niacin, such as niacinamide or nicotinamide, do not lower cholesterol) 1.5–3 gm/day in sustained or extended-release capsules is indicated as an adjunct for reduction of:[9]

- Elevated VLDL.
- Total cholesterol, LDL cholesterol, Apo B and triglyceride levels in adults with hypercholesterolemia and dyslipidemia (Types IIA and IIB).
- Total and LDL cholesterol levels in adults with hypercholesterolemia.
- Very high triglyceride levels (Types IV and V hyperlipidemia) that do not respond to determined dietary effort to control them.

Therapeutic levels of niacin may require up to 2 gm tid with a daily maximum of 9 gm.[10] After cholesterol levels decrease to an acceptable level, a maintenance dose of 1,000–2,000 mg at bedtime is recommended. Niacin should be avoided in patients with gout, liver disease, active peptic ulcers, and uncontrolled DM.[11]

Plant Sterols: Ingestion of 2–3 gm daily of plant sterols (i.e., phytosterol) reduces LDL by 6%–15%. They are usually available in commercial margarines.[12]

Soy Protein: Increasing soybean protein (25–47 gm/day) or taking a phytoestrogen pill (40 gm/day) demonstrated significant lowering of cholesterol levels including lowering HDLs and raising LDLs.[13,14,15,16]

Ascorbic Acid: A meta-analysis of 13 randomized controlled trials (RCTs) assessed the effect of vitamin C supplementation on serum cholesterol and triglycerides—established risk factors for cardiovascular disease (CVD).[17] The analysis included 549 hypercholesterolemic subjects, with an age range of 48–82 years, who received vitamin C supplements or a placebo at doses ranging from 500–2,000 mg/day for 4–24 weeks. Overall, vitamin C supplementation significantly reduced serum levels of low-density lipoprotein cholesterol (LDL-C) and serum triglycerides.[17]

Magnesium: One gm of magnesium oxide daily for six weeks has been employed successfully as a treatment.[18]

Copper: Data (animal studies) supports the hypothesis that elevated levels of hepatic HN'1G-CoA reductase seen with copper deficiency are associated with an increased rate of whole body and hepatic cholesterol synthesis.[19]

Policosanol: Cuban researchers found 5-20 mg/day of policosanol to be effective at improving serum lipid profiles. A starting dose is 2–10 mg/day, taken with the evening meal. Policosanol is believed to decrease total cholesterol (TC) and low-density lipoprotein (LDL) and to increase high-density lipoprotein (HDL) by inhibiting cholesterol synthesis and increasing LDL processing.[20]

Lipid profile improvements were also seen in healthy volunteers, patients with type II hypercholesterolemia, type 2 diabetics with hypercholesterolemia, postmenopausal women with hypercholesterolemia, and patients with combined hypercholesterolemia and abnormal liver function tests. Additionally, policosanol has performed as well as or better than simvastatin, pravastatin, lovastatin, probucol, or acipimox with fewer side effects in patients with type II hypercholesterolemia.[20]

Pantethene: Evidence indicates that taking pantethine, a product of panthothenic acid (vitamin B5), by mouth can modestly lower triglycerides, total cholesterol, and low-density lipoprotein (LDL) cholesterol as well as triglycerides and can raise high-density lipoprotein (HDL) cholesterol levels.[21]

Clinical studies have used pantothenic acid 600–1,200 mg/day for dyslipidemia.[22]

Berberine: Taking berberine 500 mg/day tid for 12 weeks was significantly more effective than ezetimibe (Zetia) in lowering LDL cholesterol and was better tolerated.

Patients taking berberine were able to reduce their LDL cholesterol by 31.7% and LDL levels fell below 130 mg/dl in more than twice as many subjects as those taking Zetia.[22]

Vitamin D3 levels less than 30 ng/mL were associated with highly significant increases in the prevalence of diabetes, hypertension, hyperlipidemia, and peripheral vascular disease.[23]

Garlic has lipid-lowering and antithrombotic properties and when used to treat hyperlipidemia some modest short-term improvements in lipid measures were found, but its effects on cardiovascular outcomes is unknown. The product must contain allicin, the active ingredient in garlic. Fresh garlic is the most effective (one clove a day). The recommended supplemental dose is 600–800 mg/day.[24]

Chronic Obstructive Pulmonary Disease (COPD)

***See* Chronic Bronchitis**

Cluster Headaches

In cluster headaches, excruciating pain is typically experienced in or around one eye while the eye tears and the same eyelid droops. Nasal congestion accompanies the watery eye. Headaches occur in cycles, often waking afflicted individuals in the middle of the night and reoccurring at fairly regular intervals every day thereafter. Patients are typically forced to pace the floor pressing on the painful area. The pain usually resolves in an average of 45 minutes, but the discomfort can last up to three hours. Bouts of frequent headache attacks last roughly 6–12 weeks and then go into remission. Risk factors include genetics, gender (male), smoking, and head trauma. Oral prescriptions and over-the-counter pain medications are not effective for treating a cluster headache because the drugs cannot be absorbed fast enough.

MANAGEMENT

Verapamil: The prescription medication verapamil is considered to be a first-line treatment for preventing cluster headaches (minimum dosage of 240 mg/day and a typical dose is between 360 and 560 mg/day.)[1,2]

Lithium: A literature review by Peatfield determined that lithium carbonate (900 mg–2.2 gm/day) was effective in both chronic and episodic forms of cluster headache.[3]

Oxygen Therapy: Individuals with acute cluster headache respond very well to oxygen inhalation to abort an attack. This is usually prescribed as 100% oxygen at 10–12 L/min for 15–20 min.[4]

Melatonin: Blood levels of melatonin have been found to be low in patients with cluster headaches, particularly during attacks.[5]

Twenty patients who were experiencing cluster headaches received 10 mg of melatonin or a placebo once a day (in the evening) for 14 days. Headache frequency was significantly reduced in the melatonin group, whereas no significant improvement was seen in the placebo group. Of the 10 patients who received melatonin, headaches disappeared after three to five days of treatment, and no further attacks occurred until melatonin was discontinued.[5]

Magnesium: Giving magnesium sulfate intravenously lessens the pain of acute headaches, including cluster headaches.[6,7]

Lifestyle: When suffering a bout of cluster headaches, attacks can be triggered by alcohol, food containing nitrates (e.g., bacon, hot dogs, and cured meats), nitroglycerin (a vasodilator), and strong odors such as petroleum, paint, and nail varnish.[8] Therefore, it is best to try to avoid these triggers during those times.

Spinal Manipulation: Spinal manipulative therapy directed to the upper cervical nerves may enhance proper function of the cervical sympathetic nerves and help correct cervicogenic pathologies (e.g., via the greater and lesser occipital nerves) contributing to cluster headaches.[9,10]

Occipital Nerve Block: A greater occipital nerve block (with a local anesthetic and a corticosteroid) can provide prompt temporary prevention.[11]

Cognitive Impairment (Mild)

Mild cognitive impairment (MCI), also known as incipient dementia and isolated memory impairment, is a neurological disorder that causes the loss of intellectual functions pertaining to the mental processes of perception, language, memory, judgment, and reasoning. These alterations are serious enough to be noticed by the individuals experiencing them or to others, but the changes are not severe enough to interfere with daily life or independent function.

MCI can be thought of as the stage between the average mental decline of normal aging and dementia. All patients who will acquire dementia go through a period of MCI. Patients with MCI are at higher risk to develop Alzheimer's disease, although in some individuals, the MCI can return to normal cognition or remain stable.

THERAPY CHOICES TO HELP PREVENT PROGRESSION

Diet: Increased intake of polyunsaturated fatty acids (PUFAs), particularly omega 6, is associated with improved cognitive function in older adults.[1]

Choline: A meta-analysis of small randomized, placebo-controlled trials reported a positive impact of citicoline (1,000 mg/day, administered for 28 days to 12 months) on memory and behavior in subjects with cognitive deficits associated with cerebrovascular disorders.[2]

In another study, the authors recommend citicoline (1,000 mg bid) for long-term preventive treatment in high-risk age-related MCI populations for Alzheimer's disease.[3]

A six-month, multicenter observational study enrolled 197 stroke subjects (mean age, 81.5 years) with a progressive decline of their mental health and general confusion and/or stupor who were initially administered citicoline for 5 or 10 days (2,000 mg/day, by intravenous infusion) within a four-month period, and then for 21 days (1,000 mg/day by intramuscular injection), repeated once after a seven-day washout period.[4] Citicoline treatment was found to be associated with higher scores on cognitive and functional evaluation scales when compared to baseline measurements.

Vitamin E: In the most recent multicenter, randomized, double-blind, placebo-controlled study, supplemental vitamin E (2,000 IU/day) for over two years significantly delayed functional decline, as determined by the (in)ability to perform basic activities of daily living, and reduced the annual mortality rate in mild and moderate Alzheimer's disease.[5]

B Vitamins: B vitamins lower homocysteine, which directly leads to a decrease in gray matter atrophy, thereby slowing cognitive decline. In one study, researchers established that vitamin B supplementation, in particular vitamins B6, B9, and B12, significantly improved cognition and memory function of older adults that exhibited mild cognitive impairment.[6]

Folic Acid: Sixteen patients whose impaired intellectual function, confirmed on neuropsychological testing, were strikingly improved after 6–12 months of folic acid therapy. On the basis of clinical, neuropsychological, computed tomography, and radionuclide cisternographic findings, researchers concluded that chronic folate deficiency could induce cerebral atrophy.[7]

Alcohol: In a cohort study, low to moderate alcohol consumption (10–14 drinks per week) was associated with protecting cognitive function and better individual cognition domain results for word recall, mental status, and vocabulary among middle-aged or older adults.[8]

Flavonoids: There is mounting evidence suggesting flavonoids (600 mg/day of flavones, flavanones, or anthocyanins) are powerhouses when it comes to preventing thinking skills from declining as a result of aging.[9]

Sindenafil (Viagra): To help prevent deterioration to dementia/Alzheimers consider asking your physician for a sildenafil (Viagra) prescription. A new study at the Cleveland Clinic revealed that patients prescribed sindenafil had a 69% reduced risk of Alzheimer's. It was further found that sildenafil promoted the growth of new nerve projections in nerve cells from patients with the disease. Although further studies are needed, this study supports the concept that sildenafil may be a potential breakthrough preventative treatment.[10]

Colds/Coryza

Many types of viruses cause the common cold, with rhinoviruses being the most common. The virus typically causes a sore throat, sneezing, a stuffy runny nose, sinus congestion, and coughing. It is probably the most common human illness. The average cold lasts 7-10 days. Complications of the common cold can be bacterial sinusitis, middle ear infection, asthma attacks (especially in children), or a worsening of chronic bronchitis.

MANAGEMENT TECHNIQUES

Zinc acetate or gluconate lozenges (13.3 mg zinc) taken every 2–3 waking hours significantly reduced the duration of the common cold by about 50%. Zinc gluconate is effective, whereas zinc picolinate, zinc citrate, and zinc aspartate are not. It is important to begin treatment at the first sign of a scratchy throat.[1,2,3,4,5]

A Cochrane review also concluded that zinc (lozenges or syrup) may reduce the duration and severity of the common cold if it is taken within 24 hours of the first symptoms.[6]

Vitamin C: Overall, there is evidence that regular use of vitamin C supplements shortens the duration of the common cold.[5] Taking 1–3 gm of vitamin C appears to shorten the course of the cold by one to one and a half days. Taking vitamin C does not appear to prevent colds.[2,7]

Cold Sores/Herpes Simplex/Herpes Labialis

Herpes labialis, also known as cold sores or fever blisters, is a common viral infection. The blisters are caused by the herpes simplex virus (HSV). Symptoms usually begin with a tingling or burning sensation on or near the lips. This is followed by the appearance of small, painful, fluid-filled blisters that are single or can be grouped together form on and around the lips. A breakout is often seen after a fever or exposure to wind or sun. The majority of individuals with HSV will not show any symptoms at all between flare-ups. Herpes labialis is contagious for individuals who have not been previously infected by the virus and for those with weakened immune systems. Fewer breakouts and shorter duration for outbreaks are the treatment goals.

MANAGEMENT CONSIDERATIONS

Excessive wind and sun exposure should be avoided.

Cold Sore Ointments: Docosanol (Abreva) is an over-the-counter cream for cold sores that has been approved by the FDA to shorten the outbreak. Zilactin and Campho-Phenique are topical over-the-counter treatments that lessen discomfort during the outbreak.

Ascorbic acid with bioflavonoids (600 mg) t.i.d for a minimum of three days if started in the prodromal phase shortens the duration of pain and reduces vesiculation and disruption.[1]

A published literature review further supports these findings along with the use of lysine and zinc.[2]

L-lysine at least 1,000–1,248 mg (four 312 mg tablets) per day for six months, was found to reduce the frequency of outbreaks.[3] In a separate study, lysine appeared to reduce the frequency, duration, and severity of outbreaks.[4] Overall, lysine's efficacy for herpes labialis may lie more in prevention than treatment.[5]

Zinc, in the form of topical zinc gluconate, citrate, sulfate, picolinate, or chelated zinc, has been used to treat herpes outbreaks and to speed the healing process.[2,6]

Zinc oxide and glycine cream (applied every two hours during the day, starting as soon as possible after the first symptoms appear and continuing until the complaints disappear) shortens the duration of the outbreak.[7] Zinc sulfate (1%) gel applied in a similar fashion was studied in 79 patients. After five days, 50% of the patients in the treatment group were symptom-free, compared with 35% in the placebo group.[8]

The application of aqueous zinc gluconate solution relieved pain, itching, tingling, burning, and shortened healing time, while also reducing recurrence rates.[9] The zinc gluconate solution must be kept in contact with the infected tissues for about 30 minutes to an hour and is repeated frequently (4–9 times a day) until the sores are gone.[10]

Complex Regional Pain Syndrome/ Reflex Sympathetic Dystrophy

Complex regional pain syndrome (CRPS), also called reflex sympathetic dystrophy, is a chronic pain condition in which near maximum levels of intense pain impulses are sent to an affected site. The condition is characterized by excruciating pain, hypersensitivity, vasomotor changes, and functional loss of the affected limb. There is extreme tenderness and swelling of the affected extremity with varying degrees of sweating, warmth and/or coolness, flushing, discoloration, and shiny skin. The goals of treatment are to decrease pain and other symptoms, restore function to the affected limb, and maintain a reasonable quality of life.

PREVENTION AND TREATMENT STRATEGY

Ascorbic Acid: Taking vitamin C after orthopedic surgery or injury to the arm or leg is reported to help prevent complex regional pain syndrome from developing.[1] Studies have shown that individuals who took a daily minimum dose of 500 milligrams of vitamin C after a wrist fracture had a lower risk of complex regional pain syndrome compared with those who did not take vitamin C.[2,3] Additionally, a number of recent clinical studies have shown that vitamin C administration to patients with chronic regional pain syndrome decreases their symptoms.[4]

Conjunctivitis/Pinkeye

Pinkeye is an inflammation of the conjunctiva, the thin, clear tissue that lines the inside of the eyelid and the white part of the eyeball. This inflammation makes blood vessels more visible and gives the eye a pink or reddish color. Causes include viral infection (especially adenoviruses), bacterium, allergy, irritants (e.g., smog, chlorine in swimming pool water), and riboflavin (vitamin B2) deficiency. Pinkeye, whether due to a viral or bacterial infection, is very contagious.

Conjunctivitis from a viral infection usually clears up in about two weeks with or without treatment. Mild bacterial conjunctivitis may get better without antibiotic treatment and without causing any complications. It often improves in 2–5 days without treatment but can take two weeks to go away completely.[1] Antibiotics may help accelerate healing from bacterial conjunctivitis, especially if there is a discharge of pus from the eye. An eye doctor needs to be consulted if the eye is red, there is moderate to severe pain, or there is sensitivity to light or blurred vision.[2]

NUTRITIONAL CONSIDERATION

Riboflavin: Riboflavin deficiency usually occurs with other B vitamin deficiencies. Symptoms and signs include conjunctivitis, sore throat, lesions of the lips and mucosa of the mouth, glossitis, seborrheic dermatitis, and normochromic-normocytic anemia.

Treatment for riboflavin deficiency is with B complex and riboflavin, 5–10 mg once/day, given until recovery is achieved.[3] Ariboflavinosis has also been implicated in a type of allergic conjunctivitis known as vernal conjunctivitis.[4] Allergic conjunctivitis has been reported to successfully respond to 1–5 mg folic acid daily.[5] In a report by Castellanos, 92% of 105 patients improved within a short time (35.7% in three to four days and 65% in 10 to 15 days) when one to three mg of riboflavin were given daily by mouth.[6]

Constipation

Constipation is when bowel movements become infrequent or difficult to pass, typically due to hardened feces. A person can be considered to be constipated when bowel movements are less than three times per week and result in passage of small amounts of hard, dry stool. The stools are hardened because food is traveling too slowly, and/or the colon is absorbing too much water from the fecal material in the colon. Constipation can cause a feeling of lower abdominal discomfort or bloating in addition to hard or lumpy stools. Constipation can also alternate with diarrhea.

There are many causes of constipation, such as irritable bowel syndrome, a primary or secondary motor disorder of the colon, a defecation disorder, a large number of diseases that affect the colon (e.g., bowel obstruction or stricture, colon or rectal cancer, anal fissures, etc.), adverse events of medications (e.g., opiates, iron, calcium channel blockers, etc.), or low fiber diets. In most cases, a specific disorder is not diagnosed.

MANAGEMENT METHODS

Dietary Modifications: Fiber is the laxative most doctors recommend for normal and slow-transit constipation. The most important aspect of the therapy for constipation is dietary modification to increase the amount of fiber consumed. Gradually increase daily fiber intake to 20–25 gm, either through dietary changes or through fiber supplements. Fruits, vegetables, and cereals have the highest fiber content. When added to the diet, wheat bran, whole grain bread (e.g., whole-wheat bread), cereals, and pastas, also draw water into the intestinal tract and speeds transit to help treat constipation.[1]

Bulk Forming Agents: The basis for treatment and prevention of constipation should consist of bulk-forming agents in addition to dietary modifications that increase dietary fiber and soften feces in 1–3 days. Soluble fiber supplements add water and bulk to the stool. Supplements include psyllium (Metamucil, Konsyl), calcium polycarbophil (FiberCon), and methylcellulose fiber (Citrucel).[2] In a meta-analysis, dietary fiber alone increased stool frequency in patients with constipation, but did not improve stool consistency, laxative use, or painful defecation.[3] This further underscores the need for adding bulk-forming agents.

Stimulants: Stimulants including rhubarb, aloe, castor oil, bisacodyl (Ducodyl, Dulcolax, Correctol), and senna (Senokot, Fletcher's Castoria, Ex-Lax regular strength pills) cause the intestines to contract.[2] There is strong evidence that aloe juice (100–200 mg/day), which contains latex is a powerful laxative.[4] Bisacodyl taken by mouth should produce a bowel movement within 6–12 hours. Senna is an FDA-approved over-the-counter (OTC) laxative. The herbal liquid laxative senna (5–15 mL once or twice a day) is commonly used to relieve constipation.[5] Senna can be used with psyllium or the stool softener docusate (Colace, DulcoEase) in adults, including the elderly, and is considered safe and effective in children.[6] It is also effective for treating constipation in people who have undergone anorectal surgery.[7]

Osmotic Agents: Osmotic laxatives help fluids move through the colon. Examples include prescription strength polyethylene glycol (Golytely, Nulytely)[8] or over-the-counter products such as lactulose (Kristalose, 10–20 gm/day) and polyethylene glycol (Miralax). Magnesium oxide is a useful supplement in treating constipation.[9] Typically, to relieve constipation, doses range from 1,000–2,000 mg/day. Magnesium citrate (citrate of magnesia, Citroma, 240 ml orally one time) is effective and has a number of health benefits, including improved calcium absorption, increased gastrointestinal motility, stool softening, and others.[9] Magnesium hydroxide (2.4–4.8 gm) in the form of milk of magnesia can also be effective.[10] Magnesium sulfate (10–30 gm) in the form of salts should only be used for occasional treatment of constipation, and doses should be taken with a full 8 oz. glass of water.[10,11]

Lubricants: Lubricants such as mineral oil enable stool to move more swiftly and easily through the colon.

Stool Softeners: Stool softeners such as docusate sodium (Colace), and docusate calcium (Surfak) moisten the stool by drawing water into the intestines, making it easier to pass.[2] Docusates are not effective in treating constipation but are used mainly to ease the discomfort in passing stool and to prevent constipation. Polyethylene glycol (PEG) and sorbitol, as well as glycerin or bisacodyl suppositories, can also soften stool.[1,12]

ADDITIONAL MANAGEMENT OPTIONS

Enemas and Suppositories: Acute constipation may be relieved by the use of a tap water enema or a glycerin (e.g., 2–3 gm) suppository. If neither is effective, the use of oral sorbitol, low doses of bisacodyl or senna, or saline laxatives (e.g., milk of magnesia) may provide relief.[13] Sodium phosphate (Fleet) or soapsuds enemas can be useful to soften hard stools and help produce a more comfortable bowel movement.[2]

Water: Dehydration is a common cause of chronic constipation. Increased intake of water helps with hydration.

Caffeinated Coffee: One study found that caffeinated coffee can stimulate the intestines the same way as a meal can. This effect is 60% stronger than drinking water and 23% stronger than drinking decaffeinated coffee.[8]

Exercise: Regular physical exercise, such as a walk for 30 minutes to one hour daily, and abdominal exercises are helpful.

Dexpanthenol: Previous clinical studies demonstrate that taking dexpanthenol, a chemical similar to pantothenic acid, by mouth daily or receiving dexpanthenol injections can help treat constipation.[14]

Lactobacillus: As a longer range strategy, probiotics containing lactobacillus taken for four to eight weeks can reduce symptoms of constipation including stomach pain and discomfort, bloating, and incomplete bowel movements.[15]

Squatting: Studies have shown that squatting during defecation straightens the anorectal angle to reduce straining.[16] At present, there is only anecdotal evidence to support the use of squatting devices, but they can be tried with little or no risk to individuals with constipation.[17]

Thiamine: For obstinate constipation, thiamine has been used, even without definite proof of a deficiency. Symptoms improve dramatically if thiamine deficiency has been causative. Thiamine is nontoxic and doses of 100–500 mg/day produced no adverse side effects.[18,19]

Corneal Ulcer/Keratitis

A corneal ulcer is an open sore on the cornea of the eye. Although there are many different causes, keratitis is frequently caused by a virus or bacterial infection. The cornea covers the iris and the round pupil. Symptoms can include red, watery, or itchy eye with a burning or stinging sensation, sensitivity to light, and a pus-like discharge. The infection can lead to loss of vision or blindness, and so requires immediate medical care.[1]

TREATMENT OPTIONS

Ascorbic Acid: In one study, 51 cases of small acute corneal ulcers were examined. Half the patients received an oral ascorbic acid dose of 1,500 mg/day until healing was complete. The administration of ascorbic acid was found to significantly accelerate the healing of deep ulcers.[2]

A double-masked study was conducted to evaluate the effects of topical ascorbate on alkali burns utilizing rabbit eyes. The study showed that topical 10% ascorbate administered 14 times per day to alkali-burned eyes significantly reduced the incidence of corneal ulceration and confirmed prior studies demonstrating that subcutaneous administration of ascorbate decreases corneal ulcerations after alkali burns.[3]

Vitamin A Deficiency: Vitamin A deficiency is the leading cause of preventable childhood blindness in the developing world. In the U.S., vitamin deficiency is a rare condition, but is more common in anorexia nervosa, chronic alcoholism, and cystic fibrosis. The results can be devastating. A case of bilateral corneal ulceration was reported with successful treatment with vitamin A. The oral dosage regimen to achieve that goal was 200,000 IU vitamin A in oil, followed the next day with an additional dose of 200,000 IU. If patients have severe corneal disease or malabsorption, the preferred dose is 100,000 IU water-miscible vitamin A administered intramuscularly.[4]

Coronary Heart Disease/Coronary Artery Disease (CAD)/ Ischemic Heart Disease/Coronary Atherosclerosis

Coronary arteries are the blood vessels that deliver oxygenated blood to the heart. Coronary atherosclerosis, also commonly known as coronary artery disease and coronary heart disease, is a >50% narrowing of any coronary artery. When cholesterol, fat, and calcium plaque builds up and hardens within the innermost layer (intima) of the coronary arteries, the wall becomes thicker and more stiff. This reduces or blocks the flow of rich oxygenated blood that can reach the heart. The resulting myocardial ischemia can lead to shortness of breath, palpitations, chest pain (angina), heart attack, arrhythmias, and heart failure.

Coronary atherosclerosis is the leading cause of cardiovascular disability and death in the world. Modifiable risk factors for developing CAD include smoking, high blood pressure, high cholesterol (LDL), diabetes, sedentary lifestyle, and obesity.

Complications include acute coronary syndrome (angina, heart attack), arrhythmia, heart failure, cardiogenic shock, and sudden cardiac arrest.[1]

Treatment goals include lowering LDL to 70–100 mg/dL, triglycerides less than 150 mg/dl, and total cholesterol below 200 mg/dL typically using statins as a first-line treatment, while also lowering blood pressure below 140/90 mm Hg. A variety of medications are available to treat CAD. A primary goal in treatment is to reduce modifiable risk factors.

MANAGE SYMPTOMS AND REDUCE THE RISK OF FURTHER PROBLEMS

Weight Loss/Diet: *See* Atherosclerosis.

Cessation of smoking reduces the risk of heart disease and its complications. Even after a heart attack, stopping smoking lowers the risk of another heart attack in the future.

Aspirin (75–162 mg/day) reduces cardiovascular events including repeat revascularization, MI, and cardiac death by approximately 33%.[2] According to *The Washington Manual*, low-dose aspirin (75–325 mg/day) for CAD is one of the most cost-effective treatments in medicine.[3] Currently, low-dose aspirin is recommended for individuals with a higher risk of CVD, ages 40–70 who are not at increased risk of bleeding.[4]

Tocopherol: Several epidemiologic studies have indicated that high dietary intake of vitamin E is associated with high serum concentrations of alpha tocopherol, as well as with lower rates of ischemic heart disease.[5] The Cambridge Heart Antioxidant Study supported these findings.[6]

In one study, 2,002 patients with coronary atherosclerosis were randomly assigned to receive vitamin E (400 or 800 IU/day) or a placebo. Vitamin E supplementation substantially reduced the rate of nonfatal myocardial infarction in patients with proven symptomatic coronary atherosclerosis. For the vitamin E group, risk of "cardiovascular end points" (i.e., cardiac-related deaths) were reduced by 47%.[6]

In a study from the United Kingdom, high doses of vitamin E, much higher than the current RDA, drastically lowered nonfatal and fatal myocardial infarction in persons with angiographically documented coronary heart disease.[6]

EPA/DHA: Epidemiological studies and dietary trials in humans suggest that alpha-linolenic acid (EPA/DHA) is a major cardio-protective nutrient.[7] High dietary intake of alpha-linolenic acid reduced the amount of "plaque" in arteries serving the heart.[8] Increased intake of N-3 fatty acids in fish oils or alpha-linolenic acid (e.g., 1.5 gm/day) was associated with anti-arrhythmic activity, decreased platelet aggregation, slowed atherosclerotic progression, and decreased rates of sudden death in patients with known coronary artery disease.[9,10]

The DART study demonstrated the efficacy of fish oil on CAD. The fish oil group consumed 200–400 gm/week of fatty fish (2 portions of fish per week) or 0.5 gm/day of Maxepa fish oil supplement. At two years, the end point of all-cause mortality was reduced by 29% in the fish oil group.[11] Fish oil 4 gm/day has since been shown to reduce triglyceride levels by at least 30% in patients with triglycerides of 500 mg/dL or greater.[12] Prescription omega-3 fatty acids are also available.

Folic Acid: In another study, a total of 165 deaths were observed due to coronary heart disease (CHD). A statistically significant association between the risk of fatal CHD and low serum folate levels was found.[13] The data indicates that low serum folate levels are associated with an increased risk of fatal CHD. Folate consumption has been found to be a determinant of homocysteine-related carotid artery thickening.

Folic acid 30 mg bid in patients with coronary heart disease acutely lowered blood pressure and enhanced coronary dilation in patients with coronary artery disease.[14]

Nicotinic Acid: Niacin has been used for more than 50 years in the treatment of cardiovascular disease, including preventing coronary heart disease,[15] and was the first drug/supplement to show a reduction in cardiovascular events and mortality in patients with prior myocardial infarction.[16,17,18] Even with optimal LDL cholesterol lowering, patients with coronary artery disease retain significant cardiovascular risk. Based on epidemiological and animal studies, increasing HDL cholesterol has become a target goal. Nicotinic acid is the most powerful agent currently available for raising low levels of HDL-C.[19]

In the Coronary Drug Project, niacin treatment was associated with significant reductions in CV events and long-term mortality, similar to the reductions seen in the statin monotherapy trials. In combination trials, niacin plus a statin or bile acid sequestrant produces additive reductions in CHD morbidity and mortality and promotes regression of coronary atherosclerosis.[19]

Ascorbic Acid: Randomized, double-blind, placebo-controlled studies have shown that treatment with vitamin C consistently results in improved vasodilation in individuals with coronary heart disease, as well as those with angina pectoris, congestive heart failure, diabetes, high cholesterol, and high blood pressure.[20] Improved vasodilation has been demonstrated at an oral dose of 500 mg of vitamin C daily.[21]

Furthermore, researchers have observed that vitamin C administration causes a significant reduction in LDL and an increase in HDL and thereby provides protection against CAD.[22]

Vitamin D: Low serum vitamin D3 levels were highly associated with coronary artery disease, myocardial infarction, heart failure, stroke, and incident death.[23]

Berberine (e.g., 500 mg tid) is effective in the prevention of coronary artery diseases and helps decrease total cholesterol and triglyceride levels.[24]

Cracked Skin/Tennis Shoe Dermatitis

For many people, cracked skin appears or gets worse during the winter, when air is drier. This primarily affects the hands, feet, and lips.[1] Most deep fissures are found on the feet or hands. The soles of the feet and especially the heels and big toes are most commonly involved. Deep cracks are very painful and can bleed. The main cause is wearing wet or sweaty socks or swimming a lot. Excessive bathing with soap (soap dermatitis—soap removes the natural protective oils from the skin), winter weather, and eczema all can cause cracked skin.[2]

MANAGEMENT TECHNIQUES FOR SHALLOW CRACKS ON THE FEET AND HANDS

Change socks in the middle of the day or whenever they are wet. Wear socks without shoes, if possible.[2]

Vaseline: Cracks heal faster if protected from air exposure and drying. Therefore, keep the cracks constantly covered with petroleum jelly (such as Vaseline). Put it on the cracks three times a day.[2] Do not use lotions as they usually contain too much water.

Polysporin: If the crack seems mildly infected, an antibiotic ointment such as Polysporin can be applied three times a day.[2] Do not use ointment or creams and liquid bandage together.

Band-Aid or Sock: Covering the Polysporin ointment with a bandage (e.g., a Band-Aid or sock if on the feet) further speeds recovery.[2]

Liquid plastic skin bandage works better than a Band-Aid or a sock.

MANAGEMENT TECHNIQUES FOR DEEPER CRACKS ON THE FEET AND HANDS

Liquid Plastic Skin Bandage: Apply two layers of liquid plastic skin bandage to seal the crack. Thereafter an extra layer can be added if needed.[2]

Crohn's Disease

Crohn's disease, also known as regional enteritis or ileitis, belongs to a group of conditions known as inflammatory bowel diseases, or IBD. Crohn's causes chronic inflammation and irritation through all the wall layers of the intestinal tract, leading to ulcerations of the small and large intestines. The disease can affect any area from the mouth to the anus, but typically affects the ileum (end of the small bowel) and beginning of the colon (large bowel) while sparing the rectum.

Transmural (across the entire intestinal wall) inflammation usually occurs with signs of mucosal cobblestoning on endoscopy due to nodules from submucosal edema along with ulcerations. Patches of "skip areas," or healthy tissue, are scattered in between areas of inflammation. This can lead to primary symptoms of cramping and abdominal pain with perianal disease. Additional symptoms can include diarrhea (sometimes with blood) and urgency along with nausea and lack of appetite leading to weight loss and/or malnutrition. Anemia, fatigue, and fever or night sweats are also common. Intestinal complications of Crohn's include subacute or acute bowel obstruction, ulcers, malnutrition, fistulae, abscesses, and bowel perforation. Extraintestinal complications can involve inflammation of the eyes, joint arthritis, osteoporosis, skin rashes, kidney stones, and liver disease. Crohn's disease can be both painful and debilitating. Patients with this disorder can have severe symptoms followed by periods of minimal to no symptoms that can last for weeks or months. Men and women are affected equally.

The diagnosis is often clinical as there is no single test to diagnose Crohn's disease. Currently, fecal calprotectin is one of the more useful tests to help diagnose or rule out Crohn's disease in adults.

Patients at higher risk for progression of the disease include those who smoke, have inflammatory arthritis or other associated immune-mediated disease, ileocolonic or perianal disease, and individuals who require corticosteroids in order to maintain remission.[1] Treatment goals are to decrease inflammation, prevent or reduce the number of flare-ups, and to prolong remissions.

THERAPY STRATEGIES

Smoking cessation should be a top priority.[1]

Diet: Protein-energy malnutrition and suboptimal weight is reported in up to 85% of patients with Crohn's disease.[2] A low-roughage diet that is high protein, low fat, and milk free often provides symptomatic relief in patients with mild to moderate disease or in patients with strictures.[3]

Nutritional Support: Adequate nutrition is critical to promote healing. Sufficient protein and calories limit the stress on an inflamed and often strictured bowel. Those with steatorrhea benefit from decrease in fat intake to less than 80 gm/day. Elemental diet preparations, such as Ensure, Sustacal, or Isocal, have been found to induce remission, improve symptoms, and decrease disease activity in patients with acute disease.[4] Administration of vitamin B12, folic acid, fat-soluble vitamins, and iron may be needed to prevent or treat deficiencies.[5]

EPA/DHA: Crohn's disease is a common and sometimes serious disorder in which the intestinal lining becomes inflamed, resulting in abdominal pain, diarrhea, and bleeding.

Previous studies have proposed a protective role from supplementary dietary intake of PUFAs (EPA and DHA) in inflammatory bowel disease (IBD). The results are potentially comparable to the effects of mesalazine, which has clear efficacy in the treatment of acute ulcerative colitis and in the maintenance of its remission.[6]

In one study, 78 patients with Crohn's disease that was currently in remission were randomly assigned to receive 4.5 gm/day of a fish-oil concentrate or a placebo for one year, in a double-blind study. Of the patients in the fish-oil group, 28% had relapses during the study compared to 69% in the placebo group (a statistically significant difference). This study demonstrated that fish oil can prevent relapses in patients with Crohn's disease.[7]

In another study, 18 patients with ulcerative colitis were given 3.2 gm of EPA and 2.16 gm of DHA daily for four months. The treatment group showed a 61% reduction in leukotriene B4 compared to a 2% reduction in the placebo group. Seven patients who received concurrent treatment with prednisone were able to reduce their medication by 50%.[8]

Similarly, 11 patients with ulcerative colitis received 2.7 gm of EPA or 1.8 gm EPA or a placebo for eight months. Mean disease activity decreased 56% in the treatment group and only 4% in the control group.[9]

B12: Crohn's disease can cause vitamin B12 deficiency due to a lack of absorption. Vitamin B12 1,000–2,000 mcg/day helps prevent pernicious anemia, promotes normal growth and development, and is essential for proper nerve function.[10] Vitamin B12 and folate should be administered as indicated.[11]

Calcium and Vitamin D: Crohn's disease and steroids used to treat it can increase the risk of osteoporosis, so patients may need to take a calcium supplement with added vitamin D.[10] Calcium carbonate and calcium acetate (e.g., 365–500 mg with each meal) are used to restrict oxalate absorption to minimize the risk of kidney stones.[12]

Iron and Vitamin C: Chronic intestinal bleeding may allow iron deficiency anemia to develop and the need to take iron (ferrous sulphate) supplements.[10] Vitamin C supplementation helps with iron absorption.[13]

Probiotics: *Boswellia serrata* has been featured in several studies on Crohn's disease.

A randomized, double-blind controlled study comparing *Boswellia serrata* extract H15 with mesalamine in patients with Crohn's disease demonstrated no statistical difference in the Crohn's Disease Activity Index, indicating *Boswellia serrata* is as effective as mesalamine.[14] Other studies have shown possible effectiveness of *Boswellia serrata* gum resin in patients with ulcerative colitis. Proposed mechanisms of effect of *Boswellia serrata* include inhibition of 5-lipoxygenase.[15]

Iron and Vitamin E: A significant proportion of patients with Crohn's develop iron-deficiency anemia secondary to blood loss. Iron supplementation, however, may worsen inflammation. A study done by Carrier and colleagues demonstrated that supplementation with vitamin E plus iron reduced the adverse effect that iron had on colitis disease activity.[16]

Vitamin D: In a pilot study, incremental daily doses of vitamin D3, from 1,000 IU up to 5,000 IU, were administrated over a 24-week period to 18 patients. The overall improvement in vitamin D status was associated with a significant decrease in disease severity as assessed by Crohn's Disease Activity (CDAI) scores. Patients who achieved vitamin D3 levels greater than 40 ng/mL were most likely to benefit.[17] Vitamin D3 has been shown to reduce symptoms. This compound also has been shown to be an immunosuppressant, and has demonstrated positive effects in a variety of diseases believed to be mediated by autoimmune processes.[17]

Low levels of vitamin D below 15 ng/mL are associated with increased risk of Crohn's disease relapse, more hospitalizations, more active disease activity, and heavier use of corticosteroids than in patients with moderate deficiency in the 15-30 ng/mL range.[1,18]

Wormwood: In this double-blind study in Germany, 40 patients suffering from Crohn's disease receiving a stable daily dose of steroids at an equivalent of 40 mg or less of prednisone for at least three weeks were administered a herbal blend containing wormwood herb (500 mg tid) or a placebo for 10 weeks. At the end of week 10, all patients were steroid free, but there was a steady improvement in CD symptoms in 90% of patients who continued to receive wormwood. The results indicate that wormwood reduced the amount of steroids needed to treat Crohn's.[19]

Strawberries: Recent research suggests that eating about 3.5 ounces of strawberries per day can reduce inflammation and improve IBD symptoms.[20]

Thiamine: Fatigue in inflammatory bowel diseases can be treated with large doses of thiamine.[21]

Sitz baths, analgesics, hydrocortisone creams, and local heat may provide symptomatic benefit in perianal CD, in conjunction with conventional systemic therapy.[22]

Cryptosporidiosis

Cryptosporidium is a microscopic parasite that affects the distal small intestine and causes the diarrheal disease cryptosporidiosis. It is acquired by drinking contaminated water, swimming or wading in contaminated recreational water sources (i.e., pools, waterparks, lakes), eating contaminated food, or contact with infected animals. *Cryptosporidium* is a leading cause of waterborne disease among humans in the U.S.

THERAPY PROPOSAL

DHEA: Up-regulation of the immune system by exogenous DHEA may be useful in the treatment and palliation of cryptosporidiosis.[1]

Cushing's Syndrome/Hypercortisolism

Cushing's syndrome most often affects adults aged 30–50, but can also occur in children. Too much cortisol, whether originating from long-term, high-dose corticosteroid use, adrenal gland tumors, certain types of cancer, or the result of a pituitary adenoma secreting ACTH (adrenocorticotropin), typically causes weight gain and fatty deposits. The hallmark signs of Cushing's syndrome are a fatty hump between the shoulders and obesity of the face, neck, and abdomen while the limbs remain comparatively thin. Purple stretch marks are common, especially on the abdomen. Symptoms include extreme fatigue, muscle weakness, anxiety, irritability, and loss of emotional control. Three times more women are affected than men.

Cushing's disease must be differentiated from polycystic ovary syndrome and metabolic syndrome. The syndrome is associated with increased mortality and impaired quality of life because of the occurrence of comorbidities. Cushing's disease can result in cardiovascular disease, high blood lipid levels, central obesity, high blood pressure, bone loss, and less often type 2 diabetes.[1]

GENERAL ADVICE

The individual's general condition should be supported by high protein intake and appropriate administration of potassium.[2] Low blood potassium is a common feature in patients with Cushing's syndrome. Mild to moderate hypokalemia is treated with potassium tablets (72–96 mmol/day).[3]

REDUCING CORTISOL

Gamma-Aminobutyric Acid (GABA): Previous clinical studies demonstrate that taking 1–3 gm of GABA (Aminalon) daily for one month reduces the excessive release of the hormone cortisol that causes Cushing's disease.[4]

Cutaneous Amyloidosis

Primary cutaneous amyloidosis is a form of amyloidosis, where clumps of the abnormal amyloid proteins are deposited in the skin (between the epidermis and dermis), but without associated deposits in internal organs as in other forms of amyloidosis. This gives the skin an abnormal texture or color. There are three types of cutaneous amyloidosis: (1) amyloid type produces symptoms similar to eczema with reddish or brown scaly spots and can be very itchy; (2) macular is less common and less itchy than amyloid but looks very similar; (3) nodular causes red, pink, or brown lumps to form but may not cause any symptoms. Diagnosis is via skin biopsy. Itching is the primary symptom.

THERAPY APPROACHES

Tocoretinate is a hybrid compound of retinoic acid and tocopherol. In a study designed to evaluate the effects of topical tocoretinate on lichen amyloidosis and macular amyloidosis, it was concluded that topical tocoretinate reduces the clinical symptoms of lichen and macular amyloidosis.[1]

DMSO: Several case reports suggest that DMSO, applied in creams or taken by mouth, may help treat cutaneous amyloidosis.[2]

Menthol Cream: Cooling topical applications such as menthol cream may help distract from the itching sensation.[3]

Capsaicin Cream: For macular amyloid, capsaicin cream can be effective if applied regularly for several weeks.[3]

Strong Topical Corticosteroid Creams with or without wrapping or wet wrap treatment can be helpful.[3]

Cutaneous Leishmaniasis

Sandfly bites, typically in the tropics and subtropics, can transmit a parasite (*Leishmania*) that produces skin ulcers. Initially, papules evolve into nodules, then break down to form ulcers on exposed parts of the body such as the face, arms, and legs. The lesions heal with scarring. Leishmaniasis is a major health problem that causes significant morbidity due to a long clinical course and residual scarring. It occurs worldwide, especially in countries having tropical climatic conditions, and is a significant problem among returning travelers.[1]

CLINICAL CARE

Zinc Sulphate: In one study, oral zinc sulphate in doses of 2.5, 5, and 10 mg/kg/day for 45 days was an effective and safe treatment option. Cure rates in these groups ranged from 83.9%, 93.1%, and 96.9% respectively. Clinical cure with 2% intralesional zinc sulphate was comparable to meglumine antimoniate.[1,2]

Cyanide Poisoning

Cyanide poisoning is a condition that develops when a person inhales, touches, or swallows cyanide, which prevents the body from using oxygen. Smoke from fires or cigarettes can also cause cyanide poisoning.

EMERGENCY CARE

Vitamin B12A (hydroxocobalamin) is a specific antidote for cyanide poisoning, along with oxygen, that has been successfully used in Europe (Cyanokit®) and is now approved for that use in the U.S.[1,2]

Cystic Fibrosis

Cystic fibrosis (CF) is an inherited disorder that causes severe damage to the lungs and also to the pancreas, liver, and intestine. Unusually thick secretions of mucus, sweat, and digestive fluids plug up tubes, ducts, and passageways, especially in the pancreas and lungs. Individuals with CF are at greater risk of getting lung infections because thick, sticky mucus builds up in the lungs, trapping and allowing germs to thrive and multiply.

Lung infections, caused mostly by bacteria, are a serious and chronic problem for many patients living with this disease. Inflammation, damaged airways, hemoptysis, pneumothorax, and respiratory failure are additional possible complications. Most individuals with CF also have digestive problems leading to diarrhea, malnutrition, poor growth, and weight loss. Some patients have significant problems from birth while others have a milder version of the disease that may not show up until they are teens or young adults. Available treatments for CF display incomplete efficacy. Treatment goals are to maintain lung function as near to normal as possible, administer nutritional therapy (*see below*), and manage complications.[1]

SUPPORTIVE CARE

Medical Nutrition: Optimal nutritional support has been integral in the management of cystic fibrosis since the disease was initially described. Maximizing nutritional status through pancreatic enzyme replacement and vitamin and nutritional supplements is necessary for normal growth and development and for maintaining long-term lung function.[2]

Diet: A high-calorie, high-fat diet, with 40% of total calories from fat is generally recommended.[3]

Fat-Soluble Vitamins: Cystic fibrosis frequently results in a deficiency of essential fatty acids and fat-soluble vitamins (A, D, E, and K) as well as fats, proteins, and calcium. The body cannot absorb them without digestive enzymes from the pancreas. For that reason, fat-soluble vitamins, calcium, and exocrine digestive enzymes are required as supplements.[4]

Taurine: Taurine supplementation might be useful along with usual treatment to reduce fatty stools (steatorrhea) in children with cystic fibrosis.[5] In one study, eight patients with CF and fat malabsorption received taurine (30 mg per kg of body weight per day) or a placebo, each for one week. Taurine supplementation significantly improved the absorption of fats.[4,6]

Magnesium: Serum magnesium levels decrease with age in patients with cystic fibrosis (CF) and hypomagnesemia occurs in more than half of patients with advanced CF.[7] Oral magnesium supplementation (300 mg/day for eight weeks) in children with cystic fibrosis improved clinical and functional variables (e.g., respiratory muscle strength).[8]

Vitamin D deficiency is common among individuals with CF, especially at northern latitudes. Low vitamin D status is associated with reduced lung function in people with CF and supplementation may help.[9]

Darier's Disease/Keratosis Follicularis

Darier's disease, also known as keratosis follicularis, is an inherited skin condition characterized by small, thin, greasy bumps that are yellow to brown in color and can emit a strong unpleasant odor. The skin lesions generally develop a brown, greasy crust and become thickened, warty (hyperkeratotic), scaly, and darkened. The lesions slowly grow bigger, eventually coming together (coalescing) to form discolored, warty plaques that may cover extensive areas of the body particularly on the trunk.[1] The most common sites for blemishes are the scalp, forehead, upper arms, chest, back, knees, elbows, and behind the ear. The nails and mucous membranes are also affected in most cases.[1]

CARE CONSIDERATIONS

General Measures: Sunscreen use, cool cotton clothing, and avoidance of hot environments can help prevent flares, especially during the summer.[2]

Moisturizers: Moisturizers with urea or lactic acid can reduce scaling and hyperkeratosis.[2]

Vitamin A: In Darier's disease, vitamin A topically or systemically (e.g., 25,000 IU given twice daily) leads to distinct improvement of the skin lesions.[3]

Three patients with Darier's disease were treated with 1,000,000 IU of orally administered vitamin A daily for 14 days. In all patients, a 50% to 80% improvement in the skin lesions was noted.[4]

Twin sisters were treated with oral vitamin A 100,000 IU and vitamin E 1,600 IU/day and within two months of uninterrupted therapy responded well.[5] Vitamin E promotes storage and utilization of retinol (vitamin A1) and decreases its toxicity.[6]

Deep Vein Thrombosis (DVT)

A DVT is a serious condition that is caused by deposits of fibrin, RBCs, platelets, and WBC components in a vein, causing vessel wall inflammation and/or obstructing venous outflow in one or more of the larger deep calf, thigh, or pelvic veins. The clot, or thrombus, prevents the normal flow of blood through the vein, increasing venous pressure. Symptoms are not always present but, typically, the reduced blood flow or blood backing up in the vein can cause swelling, hypoxia, pain, redness, and warmth.

Complications from a DVT include a pulmonary embolism, which can be fatal if a clot fractures and migrates into the inferior vena cava and ultimately the lungs. In the lungs, the unattached mass, or embolus, can become wedged in a vessel too small to allow further passage, blocking blood flow. Another possible complication of DVT is post-thrombotic syndrome, or symptomatic chronic venous insufficiency, after a DVT which can lead to pain, swelling, skin sores and ulcers, darkened skin, and varicose veins. DVTs can cause serious illness, disability, and death.

DVT is often associated with long distance air travel, women who smoke and take birth control pills, the elderly, hospitalized as well as post-surgical patients, and other situations that involve being immobile for long periods of time (e.g., those with obesity, congestive heart failure, severe respiratory disease, or recovering from an illness). Venous ultrasonography is the test of choice to detect proximal DVT.

The goals of treatment for DVT are to:

- Stop the blood clot from getting bigger.
- Prevent the clot from breaking off and traveling to the lungs where it could lead to pulmonary embolism.
- Reduce the chance of developing another clot.
- Minimize the risk of developing other complications.[1]

PREVENTIVE APPROACHES

Anticoagulants are the cornerstone therapy for thrombosis prevention and treatment. This includes aspirin (81 mg/day up to 325 mg bid) which has been found to be safe and effective in DVT prophylaxis.[2]

Minimize Risk Factors: Many risk factors increase the likelihood of developing DVT, but can be minimized. These include avoiding prolonged bed rest, injury or surgery, and sitting for prolonged periods of time. Obesity, pregnancy, oral contraceptives, smoking, being older than 60, having Crohn's disease or heart failure, and a history of some forms of cancer are additional risk factors.[3]

Vitamin E: Obviously, no one taking prescription blood thinners to prevent deep vein blood clots should stop taking them. One study found that taking vitamin E appeared to cut the clot risk in half among women with genetic mutations that increased their risk.[4] Another study demonstrated that vitamin E (600 IU/day) may prevent deep vein clots for women in general. Female patients who took vitamin E were 21% less likely to develop venous thromboembolism than women who did not, but the reduction was more than double this (44%) among the women who had a history of clots.[5]

Iron: Low levels of iron in the blood are associated with an increased risk of dangerous blood clots that form in veins.[4] One study of 609 patients with hereditary hemorrhagic telangiectasia (HHT) who have an increased risk for blood clots found that those who took iron supplements did not have a higher risk for blood clots. In patients with HHT, a low level of iron in the blood is a potentially treatable risk factor for blood clots. This suggests that treating iron deficiency may help prevent DVT in the general population.[6]

Rutin is a bioflavonoid that inhibits platelet aggregation and clotting.[7,8] Rutin successfully treated and prevented blood clots in both arteries and veins.[7] In another study, rutin was found to effectively inhibit fibrin clotting and thrombin activity as well as thrombosis and acute thromboembolism. Clinical studies are still needed to confirm these promising results.

Dementia/Cognitive Decline

***See also* Alzheimer's Disease**

Dementia is an umbrella term for a broad range of brain disorders that cause a chronic, usually irreversible, deterioration in the ability to efficiently remember, think, reason, and socialize. Other symptoms may include emotional problems, personality changes, difficulties with language, and a decrease in motivation. Dementia, including Alzheimer's, accounts for more than one half of nursing home admissions.[1]

Everyone loses some neurons as they age, but individuals with dementia experience far greater losses. There are many medical causes of dementia, which can cause serious impairment and loss in quality of life. Alzheimer's disease is the most common cause of progressive dementia followed by vascular dementia, dementia with Lewy bodies, Parkinson's, and frontotemporal dementia.[2] Age is the strongest risk factor for developing dementia, but risks also include genetics, smoking, obesity, diabetes, and cardiovascular factors. Vitamin D deficiency and chronic sleep deprivation may also increase the risk of dementia.[3] Certain medicines, other vitamin deficiencies, excess alcohol, hypothyroidism, hypoglycemia, and kidney problems can also cause dementia. Delusions and hallucinations are not uncommon in dementia-related psychosis. Dementia shortens life expectancy.

Goals of treatment are to maintain function, manage behaviors, and to reduce comorbid emotional disorders. It is in the sufferer's best interests to minimize or eliminate sedating drugs and anticholinergics.[4]

PROTECTIVE LIFESTYLES

Physical activity seems to be protective against developing dementia. Education, ongoing intellectual stimulation, and social engagement may also be protective.[3]

Saunas: In a Finnish study, frequent use of saunas (9–12 times per month) was associated with a reduced risk of dementia over a 39 year follow-up period.[5]

NUTRITIONAL SUPPORT

Nutritional Deficiencies: A recent study showed a strong link between dementia and a vitamin D deficiency.[6] Adults should increase their daily dose to 600–800 IU/day.[7] Deficiencies in vitamin B1, vitamin B12, vitamin B3 (pellagra), or protein-calorie malnutrition are also known causes of dementia.[8]

Coffee Restriction: Drinking six or more cups of coffee per day is associated with smaller brain volume and a 53% increased risk for dementia compared with light coffee consumption (1–2 cups per day).[9]

Cyanocobolamin: Metabolic disorders such a vitamin B12 deficiency cause dementia and must be corrected if present.[8] Older adults on a vegetarian or vegan diet have an increased risk of vitamin B12 deficiency. Certain drugs (metformin, proton pump inhibitors, and histamine [H-2] receptor antagonists) can also lead to a B12 deficiency. A typical dose for vitamin B12/cyanocobolamin is 1,000–2,000 mcg/day.

Tocopherol: A deficiency of vitamin E accelerates cerebral aging.[10] The precise implications for dementia sufferers are not known. It is known that patients with severe, prolonged deficiency may develop dementia, blindness, and cardiac arrhythmias. Treatment must be tailored to the underlying cause of vitamin E deficiency and may include oral or parenteral vitamin supplementation.[11]

Endocrine Causes: Eliminating or controlling potential endocrine causes, such as Addison's and Cushing's disease as well as hypothyroidism and repeated episodes of hypoglycemia, can be beneficial.

Ginkgo Biloba: Some research shows that taking ginkgo for up to one year slightly improves some symptoms of Alzheimer's, vascular, or other dementias. Doses of 240 mg/day may work better than doses of 120 mg/day.[12]

Folic Acid: Folate deficiency is associated with depression and dementia.[13] Sixteen patients, whose impaired intellectual function was confirmed on neuropsychological testing, had striking improvement after 6–12 months of folic acid therapy. On the basis of clinical, neuropsychological, computed tomography, and radionuclide cisternographic findings, researchers concluded that chronic folate deficiency could induce cerebral atrophy.[14] Runcie described 10 cases and reviewed the medical literature, emphasizing that the syndrome of folate responsive dementia and depression was much more common in geriatric and psychogeriatric units than is recognized.[15]

Flavonoids (e.g., 600 mg/day) have shown positive effects against dementia and Alzheimer's disease, reversing age-related declines in neurocognitive performances.[16]

Depression

Clinical depression is a common but serious mood disorder with persistent feelings of sadness and loss of interest. If those feelings persist for at least two weeks, they qualify as a major depressive disorder. Major depression is characterized by a sense of inadequacy, despondency, decreased activity, pessimism, anhedonia, and sadness where these symptoms severely disrupt and adversely affect the person's life, sometimes to such an extent that suicide is attempted or occurs.[1] Neurotransmitters, especially serotonin, norepinephrine, and dopamine are associated with depression. Depression can exist independently or can co-occur with other serious medical illnesses such as diabetes, cancer, heart disease, and Parkinson's disease.

ADJUVANT THERAPY OPTIONS

Magnesium: Researchers studied the effects of 150–300 mg of magnesium (as glycinate or taurinate) given with each meal and at bedtime to patients with major depression. The results showed rapid recovery from major depression in less than seven days. Magnesium was typically found to be effective for treatment of depression in general use. Related and accompanying mental illnesses in case histories including traumatic brain injury, headache, suicidal ideation, anxiety, irritability, insomnia, postpartum depression, cocaine, alcohol and tobacco abuse, short-term memory loss, and IQ also improved.[1]

St. John's Wort: St. John's wort is a monoamine oxidase (MAO) inhibitor. It inhibits reuptake of serotonin, noradrenaline, adrenaline, and dopamine. Numerous studies of St. John's wort (e.g., 900 mg/day for 4–12 weeks) in patients with depressive disorders have shown that it is more effective than a placebo and as effective as antidepressants (e.g., Prozac or Zoloft).[2,3] Unlike prescription MAO inhibitors, individuals taking St. John's wort do not have to avoid tyramine-rich foods.[4]

DHEA (dehydroepiandrosterone) is a hormone produced by the adrenal glands and is available as a supplement. DHEA helps produce other hormones, including testosterone and estrogen. DHEA is a glucocorticoid antagonist and is effective in treating mild to moderate depression.[5,6]

DHEA also appears to be effective in the treatment of major depression.[7] Treatment with DHEA significantly improved mood scores compared with baseline and placebo conditions. In one study, patients were given 90 mg/day (low dosage) and 450 mg/day (high dosage), for three weeks each. DHEA is an effective monotherapy for the treatment of both major and minor depression of moderate severity occurring at midlife in men and women.[8] The product is available as a supplement.

EFA/DHA: Omega-3 fatty acids play a critical role in the development and function of the central nervous system. There is enough epidemiological and laboratory evidence to show that depressed patients appear to have lowered omega-3 status and enough clinical evidence to suggest that omega-3 fatty acids may play a role in certain cases of major depression. Epidemiological and laboratory studies demonstrate that fish oil supplements are well-tolerated and without significant side effects. Generally, according to the medical literature, omega-3 supplements are inexpensive and therapeutic at doses of 4-9.6 gm/day, which makes them an attractive option as an adjuvant to standard care.[9]

Vigorous exercise at least three times a week and **light therapy** are standard non-drug treatments for mild to moderate depression.

Curcumin: Most available research shows that taking curcumin, a chemical found in turmeric, reduces depression symptoms in those already using an antidepressant.[10]

Folic Acid and B12: Low folate status has been linked to depression and poor response to antidepressants in some, but not all, studies.[11] Randomized controlled trials that involve folate and B12 suggest that patients treated with 800 mcg of folic acid/day or 400 mcg of vitamin B12/day will exhibit decreased depression symptoms.[12] Additionally, Botez et al. reported improvement in both mood and neuropsychological function in a controlled trial of folic acid (15 mg/day) for four months without other drugs for depression.[13]

L-Methylfolate: Having either a folate deficiency or a problem with malabsorption is associated with poor response to antidepressant medications. L-methylfolate is the only form of folic acid that crosses the blood-brain barrier and plays a role in neurotransmitter synthesis. It indirectly facilitates the synthesis of serotonin, dopamine, and norepinephrine, three neurotransmitters involved in mood regulation. Several studies have shown that L-methylfolate (15 mg/day) enhanced the efficacy of selective serotonin reuptake inhibitors (SSRIs) and serotonin-norepinephrine reuptake inhibitors (SNRIs).[14]

Zinc: The highest amount of zinc in the body is found in the brain, particularly in the hippocampus. Research suggests that zinc levels are lower in patients with depression. The lower the zinc levels, the worse the depression.[15] Ingesting zinc (25 mg/day) for 12 weeks along with antidepressants improved patients with major depression.[15] Zinc can also improve depression in patients who do not respond to treatment with antidepressants alone.[16]

Vitamin B1: One symptom of thiamine deficiency is depression.[17] Thiamine (e.g., 50–100 mg/day) is a natural alternative to antidepressants.[18]

Vitamin D: A randomized study of individuals with major depression treated with oral vitamin D was conducted. Vitamin D supplementation (50,000 IU/day over three months) improved symptoms of major depressive disorder, especially in female patients, through a serotonin-dependent mechanism.[19]

L-tryptophan, the amino acid precursor of serotonin, is not widely used as an adjunctive treatment despite its recommendation in treatment-resistant depression. Results support the use of L-tryptophan (e.g., 8–12 gm/day in divided doses) as an augmentation strategy in treatment-resistant depression. Tryptophan compares favorably to the published 50%–60% response rate with lithium augmentation.[20]

Diabetes Mellitus Type 1 (DM1) /Juvenile Diabetes/ Insulin Dependent Diabetes Mellitus (IDDM)

In type 1 diabetes, the pancreas produces little or no insulin. Juvenile-onset diabetes is usually caused by an autoimmune process wherein the immune system begins destroying healthy insulin-producing pancreatic beta cells within the islets of Langerhans. This destructive process can go on for months or years before symptoms appear, often relatively suddenly. Eventually, without adequate amounts of insulin, glucose cannot enter into the body's cells. Thereafter, blood sugar levels build up and remain high, causing symptoms such as increased thirst, fatigue, unintended weight loss, mood changes, excessive urination, and increased hunger.

In treating DM1, especially in patients taking insulin, episodes of hypoglycemia can lead to seizures, loss of consciousness, or death since low blood glucose can precipitate major cardiovascular and cerebrovascular events. Diabetic ketoacidosis, which can cause brain swelling, is another serious complication associated with DM1. Long-term complications from diabetes are the chief threats from this disorder. These include heart and blood vessel damage (heart attack, heart failure, and stroke), nerve damage (neuropathy), kidney damage (nephropathy), and eye damage (retinopathy).

Lowering hyperglycemia and avoiding hypoglycemia are key goals in long-term diabetes management.

CLINICAL THERAPEUTICS

Medical nutrition therapy is recommended for all patients to achieve and maintain healthy body weight. A well-balanced, nutritious diet remains a fundamental element of therapy. The meal plan should be moderate in carbohydrates and low in saturated fat, with a focus on balanced meals.[1]

Niacinamide: Sixteen type 1 diabetics were given either a compound related to niacin known as niacinamide at 3 gm/day or a placebo, beginning one week after the start of insulin therapy. The diabetes improved enough to warrant stopping the insulin in 86% of the niacinamide-treated patients. Three of the seven patients who received niacinamide remained in remission for more than two years (remissions from DM1 are rare.[2] Other studies have shown that niacinamide can preserve pancreatic beta-cell function in cases of early type 1 diabetes.[3,4]

Biotin plays a role in the metabolism of glucose within the cell.[5,6,7,8] In human studies, seven insulin-dependent diabetics were removed from insulin therapy and treated with biotin (16 mg/day) or a placebo for one week. Fasting blood-glucose levels rose significantly in patients given the placebo but decreased significantly in those treated with biotin.[5] In another study, 18 diabetics were given 9 mg/day of biotin for one month, along with an antibiotic that prevents biotin from being degraded by intestinal bacteria.[6] After one month, the average blood glucose level had fallen by 45% in the group receiving biotin.

Taurine: Platelet aggregation is excessive in patients with diabetes. Hyper-reactivity of platelets may contribute to some of the complications of diabetes, particularly atherosclerosis and kidney damage. When these individuals were given 500 mg of taurine three times a day for 90 days, taurine levels and platelet aggregation both became normal.[9]

These findings suggest that insulin-dependent diabetics are deficient in taurine and that the deficiency causes excessive activity of platelets.

Magnesium: Correction of hypomagnesemia in type 1 diabetic children with oral magnesium (300 mg/day) is associated with optimization of glycemic control and reduction of atherogenic lipid fraction as well as an increase in protective lipid fraction.[10]

Vanadium Compounds: Vanady sulfate can be used to mitigate insufficient insulin response in diabetes mellitus type 1 and can reduce reliance on exogenous insulin.[11] A normal dose is up to 1,800 mcg/day, but doses to treat diabetes can be considerably higher (e.g., up to 10 mg/day which is equal to 2 mg of vanadium).[12]

Diabetes Mellitus Type 2 (DM2)/Adult Onset Diabetes

DM2 is the most common form of diabetes. In type 2 diabetes, also known as adult onset diabetes, the pancreas makes adequate amounts of insulin, but the cells resist the effect of insulin to allow glucose into the cells. Too much glucose stays in the blood and not enough enters the cells. The end result is high blood sugar levels. Symptoms include increased thirst, excessive urination, increased hunger, poor healing, and frequent infections. Obesity (especially abdominal) and smoking increase the risk for developing both DM2 and hypertension. Hypertension is present in about 75% of patients with DM2 and further increases the risks of cardiovascular disease, which is a leading cause of death for individuals with DM2.[1] Typically, DM2 develops after the age of 45. However, more children are being diagnosed with this disorder due to childhood obesity.

Because diabetes accelerates atherosclerosis, long-term complications include heart and blood vessel damage (heart attack, heart failure, and stroke), nerve damage (neuropathy), kidney damage (nephropathy), eye damage (retinopathy), and peripheral vascular disease with reduced blood flow to the legs and feet possibly leading to amputations. There is also an increased risk for vascular dementia.[2] Poor glycemic control leads to an increase in the severity of the aforementioned complications.[3]

Hypoglycemia is another important and serious complication of glucose-lowering medications since low blood glucose levels can precipitate major cardiovascular and cerebrovascular events. A recent study suggests avoiding drugs associated with increased risk of hypoglycemia (i.e., insulin, sulfonylureas, or others) to avoid and minimize the risk of cardiovascular events.[4] Ketoacidosis is reported to occur with greater frequency in DM2 patients than previously thought.

MANAGEMENT GOALS[4]

- Healthy eating/weight loss: Avoid sugary foods and soft drinks. Eat less fat. For obese patients, the goal of calorie restriction is to achieve a 5%–10% weight loss.[5]
- Regular exercise: DM2 patients can lower their risk for death from any cause by up to a third by exercising at a moderate to high level or by cycling.[6]
- Smoking cessation (smoking makes glycemic control in diabetics more difficult and increases diabetes-related complications)
- Possibly, diabetes medication or insulin therapy
- Blood sugar monitoring
- Avoiding hypoglycemia
- Normalizing blood pressure
- Elevating low-density lipoprotein cholesterol

MEDICAL MANAGEMENT OPTIONS

Deficiencies of certain minerals, such as potassium, magnesium, and possibly zinc and chromium, may aggravate carbohydrate intolerance.[7]

Chromium: Beneficial effects on glycemia from chromium supplementation have been reported.[7]

Calcium: A daily intake of 1,000–1,500 mg of calcium, especially in older subjects with diabetes, is recommended.[7]

Ascorbic Acid: Supplementation of Vitamin C reduces blood glucose and improves HbA1c levels in DM2.[7]

Vitamin C is known for its beneficial effects on serum lipids and HbA1c. A strong association between vitamin C levels and glycemic control was found in a study involving 84 patients with DM2. Patients who were given 1,000 mg of vitamin C daily demonstrated a significant decrease in fasting blood sugar, HbA1c, and serum insulin.[8] The relationship between vitamin C and glucose levels was also demonstrated in a large sample of U.S. adults without a history of diabetes in which serum vitamin C concentrations were inversely associated with HbA1c levels.[9] An observational study on the use of vitamin C supplements demonstrated that a significantly lower risk of diabetes was associated with the use of daily vitamin C supplements when compared to nonusage.[10] An improvement was seen in fasting glucose and HbA1c levels with a higher dose supplementation of 2,000 mg of vitamin C per day for 90 days.[11]

Clinical trials have suggested that vitamin C (1,000–2,500 mg/day) reduced the microvascular complications of DM2 such as retinopathy, nephropathy, and diabetic neuropathy. Apart from this, there is another biological significance of vitamin C. Vitamin C in higher doses reduces HbA1c concentration levels and low-density lipoproteins. As such, vitamin C plays a positive role as an adjunct in the treatment of DM2 and atherosclerosis.[12]

Vitamin D: Currently there is widespread occurrence of vitamin D deficiency. It is very difficult to get enough vitamin D from food sources alone. Vitamin D is associated more closely with glucose metabolism than obesity.[13] One study suggests that vitamin D deficiency and obesity interact synergistically to heighten the risk of diabetes and other metabolic disorders.[14] Serum vitamin D3 levels less than 30 ng/mL were associated with highly significant increases in the prevalence of diabetes.[15] There is a strong inverse association between low levels of D3 and diabetes prevalence, meaning that as the deficiency worsened, so did diabetes control.[16,17] A minimum of 800 IU of vitamin D per day is recommended.

Ginseng: Thirty-six diabetics who were not dependent on insulin were randomly assigned to receive ginseng (100 or 200 mg/day). Treatment with ginseng lowered blood sugar levels and improved mood and psychological performance. The 200 mg dose of ginseng was more effective than the lower dose, improving HbA1c levels (a measure of long-term blood sugar control) and increasing physical activity.[18]

Magnesium (Mg): Diabetes is frequently associated with Mg deficit both extracellular and intracellular, especially in those with poorly controlled glycemic profiles. It's important to note that Mg deficiency can be present without low blood levels of magnesium.[19] However, hypomagnesemia, when present, is usually indicative of an important systemic magnesium deficit.[18] The clinical consequence of a chronic Mg deficit is post-receptorial insulin resistance and consequent reduced glucose utilization in the cells, worsening the reduced insulin sensitivity present in DM2.[18] Benefits have been found in most,[20,21,22,23] but not in all clinical studies.[24] In summary, oral Mg supplements (ranging from 400–2,500 mg/day) appear to be useful in persons with DM2 to restore Mg deficiencies, to improve insulin resistance, and to lower oxidative stress and systemic inflammation.[25]

Higher amounts of magnesium are associated with a significantly lower risk of diabetes, possibly because of the important role of magnesium in glucose metabolism. Magnesium deficits and increased urinary magnesium excretion can occur in individuals with insulin resistance and/or DM2. The magnesium loss in DM2 patients appears to be secondary to higher concentrations of glucose in the kidney that increase urine output.[22]

In a small trial in Mexico, participants with DM2 and hypomagnesemia who received a liquid supplement of magnesium chloride (providing 300 mg/day elemental magnesium) for 16 weeks showed significant reductions in fasting glucose and glycosylated hemoglobin concentrations, compared with participants receiving a placebo, and their serum magnesium levels became normal.[24]

The detection and correction of altered Mg status in diabetic patients is clinically appropriate, although many physicians tend to ignore Mg status.[26]

Tocopherol: Plasma levels of vitamin E were found to be significantly lower in a group of type 2 diabetics. In a double-blind study, administration of 900 mg/day of vitamin E for four months to non-insulin dependent diabetics significantly improved both glucose and insulin action.[27] High-dose vitamin E reduced levels of C-reactive protein (CRP), a marker of inflammation and a predictor of cardiovascular disease. The subjects received 1,220 IU of vitamin E supplementation a day for three months.[28,29]

Zinc and Vanadium: Hypersecretion of insulin increases the chance of the incidence of DM2, while inhibiting insulin secretion helps prevent diabetes. Trace elements like zinc and vanadium prevent hyperinsulinemia, partly because of their own insulin activity. In vitro, vanadium salts mimic most effects of insulin and induce a sustained fall in blood glucose levels.[30]

Vanadium compounds (vanadyl sulfate) can be used to mitigate insufficient insulin response in diabetes mellitus.[29] Vanadium can perhaps substitute for oral hypoglycemic agents in DM2. Two small studies have confirmed the effectiveness of vanadyl sulphate at a dose of 100 mg/day in improving insulin sensitivity.[31] Clinical trials with vanadium salts seem promising in type 2 (non-insulin dependent) diabetic patients, indicating the therapeutic potential of vanadium salts. Avoiding deficiencies of trace elements will enable the reduction of the incidence and severity of diabetes.[30]

Chromium and niacin in combination play an important role in carbohydrate metabolisms. In one study, 16 elderly individuals received either 100 mg of niacin, 200 mcg of chromium, or both, daily for 28 days. Fasting blood glucose levels and glucose tolerance were unaffected by either chromium or niacin alone. However, when both nutrients were supplemented, significant improvements were seen in both fasting blood sugar and glucose tolerance.[32]

ALA: There is strong evidence that alpha-lipoic acid (600–1,200 mg/day) for three to six weeks helps with DM2.[32] Several studies have found that ALA lowers insulin resistance.[33]

Chromium Picolinate: Evidence shows that taking chromium picolinate (200–1,000 mcg/day) by mouth, either alone or with biotin, can lower fasting blood sugar, lower insulin levels, and help insulin work in those with DM2. Also, chromium picolinate might decrease weight gain and fat accumulation in patients with DM2 who are taking sulfonylureas.[34]

Thiamine: Previous clinical studies demonstrate that taking high-dose thiamine (100 mg three times daily) for three months decreases the amount of albumin in the urine in individuals with DM2. Albumin in the urine is an indication of kidney damage.[35]

Biotin: In a small randomized, placebo-controlled intervention study in 28 patients with DM2, daily supplementation with 9 mg of biotin for one month resulted in a mean 45% decrease in fasting blood glucose concentrations.[36]

Aloe Vera: Nine studies were included in a meta-analysis involving the fasting blood glucose (FBG) and HbA1c parameters. The results support the use of oral aloe vera (2 tablespoons of 80% aloe vera juice/day) for 2–3 months to significantly reduce FBG (46.6 mg/dL) and HbA1c (1.05%). The analysis shows that patients whose fasting blood glucose (FBG) is above 200 mg/dl may benefit the most from treatment with oral aloe vera.[36,37] The types of aloe vera utilized ranged from aloe vera extract, raw crushed aloe leaves, aloe vera gel powder, and freshly extracted aloe vera juice.[38]

Ketogenic Diet: Low-carbohydrate nutritional programs including ketosis reduce insulin resistance. A ketogenic diet was used to treat individuals with diabetes before the advent of insulin. The American Diabetes Association has updated its guidelines to include low-carbohydrate eating patterns for type 2 diabetes treatment. Results from several studies have shown positive outcomes.[39] Additionally, preliminary results from the Indiana Type 2 Diabetes Reversal Trial involving 465 patients demonstrated reduced A1c levels, lower insulin resistance, lower insulin use or elimination, reduced need for medication across the board. Reversal of diabetes was achieved for 55% of patients who completed the low-carbohydrate diet patterns.[39] Lowering a patient's insulin resistance through a ketogenic diet may also help prevent or treat diabetic skin disease.[40]

Berberine: Studies have found that berberine, a chemical found in certain plants, can have positive effects on blood sugar, triglycerides, and insulin.[41] Research indicates that taking berberine 500 mg tid for two to three months can control blood sugar as effectively as sulfonylureas, metformin, and rosiglitazone.[42]

Cinnamon: A study of 60 people with type 2 diabetes, 30 men and 30 women, was undertaken. Those subjects who consumed cinnamon (1–6 gm/day) for 40 days had reduced mean fasting serum glucose (18%–29%), triglycerides (23%–30%), LDL cholesterol (7%–27%), and total cholesterol (12%–26%) levels. No significant changes were noted in the placebo groups.[43]

Low-dose aspirin therapy (75–162 mg) is appropriate for primary prevention in patients with diabetes and older than 40 years or who have other risk factors.[44]

Diabetic Neuropathy

See also Peripheral Neuropathy

In diabetes, high blood sugar and decreased blood flow can damage and injure nerves throughout the body. That damage is known as neuropathy. Of the four types of neuropathy, peripheral neuropathy is the most common type and occurs primarily in the lower extremities (legs and feet). Typical symptoms include symmetrical numbness and tingling in the toes, foot pain, foot ulceration, and other problems. These symptoms are induced by the abnormal function of small peripheral sensory fibers. Factors other than diabetes such as high blood pressure, high cholesterol, and smoking may further contribute to nerve damage.

Preventing neuropathy by properly managing and controlling blood sugar levels is the primary goal. Once established, sensory diabetic neuropathy is persistent even if hyperglycemia is controlled after the diagnosis is established. Therefore, other methods in addition to lowering and stabilizing blood glucose levels must be employed.

ADJUNCTIVE APPROACHES

Pyridoxine: Serum pyridoxal (a form of vitamin B6) levels were measured in 50 patients with significant diabetic neuropathy. The level of B6 was significantly lower in these patients when compared with randomly selected diabetic patients matched for age and sex without clinical evidence of neuropathy. The results indicate an association between pyridoxal deficiency and neuropathy in diabetic patients.[1]

Nine patients with diabetic neuropathy were treated with pyridoxine 50 mg tid. Six of those nine noted significant improvement in their neuropathy symptoms.[2]

Evening Primrose Oil (EPO): In a recent study, 111 patients with mild diabetic neuropathy were randomly assigned to receive six capsules of evening primrose oil twice a day providing 480 mg/day of gamma-linolenic acid, a component of evening primrose oil, or a placebo for one year, in a double-blind trial. A total of 16 parameters were measured and all 16 improved during treatment with EPO. EPO was significantly more effective than a placebo for 13 of the 16 parameters measured.[3]

In a double-blind, placebo-controlled study, 22 patients with diabetic polyneuropathy received 360 mg of gamma-linoleic acid for six months. Compared with the placebo group, patients on linoleic acid demonstrated significant improvement in neuropathy symptoms and nerve conduction tests.[4]

In an interventional study, 80 patients with DM2 neuropathy were given vitamin E 400 mg and evening primrose 500–1,000 mg/day for 14 weeks. Eighty-eight percent of the patients reported relief from "burning pain."[5]

Thiamine: Low plasma thiamine concentrations have been found in patients with type 1 and type 2 diabetes mellitus. In a small placebo-controlled study, benfotiamine, a related vitamin B1 substance, 100 mg given four times daily by mouth significantly improved neuropathic pain in patients with diabetic polyneuropathy.[6]

For repeated episodes of severe neuropathy, administering thiamine 500 mg/day was observed to resolve neuropathy symptoms within two weeks (as opposed to two months without thiamine). In addition, the frequency of illness was two to four episodes per year without thiamine, compared to no more than one seasonal illness per year with thiamine. Thiamine was also effective in preventing further episodic neurologic attacks.[7]

Acetyl-l-carnitine at a dose of 1–2 gm/day may be effective in treating peripheral neuropathies, especially diabetic neuropathies.[5] In a study involving 294 patients with peripheral neuropathy, acetyl-l-carnitine 1,000 mg/day was injected intramuscularly followed by an oral dose of 2,000 mg/day for 355 days. The authors concluded that carnitine was effective and well-tolerated in improving neurophysiological parameters and in reducing pain over a one-year period.[8]

Two large studies have demonstrated that a dosage of 500–1,000 mg tid resulted in significant pain reduction, improved vibratory perception, improved nerve conduction velocity, improved nerve amplitude and nerve regeneration in the neuropathic patient.[9,10]

Biotin: In one study, three patients with severe diabetic peripheral neuropathy were given high doses of biotin (10 mg IM daily for six weeks; then 10 mg IM three times per week for six weeks, and then 5 mg/day orally). These biotin dosages were 50–100 times higher than the recommended daily allowances.[11] Within four to eight weeks after the biotin administration, there was objective improvement in the symptoms of peripheral neuropathy, specifically painful muscle cramps, paresthesias, ability to stand, walk, and climb stairs, and disappearance of restless leg syndrome in all patients.[11]

Ascorbic Acid: Clinical trials have suggested that mega doses of vitamin C (1,000–2,500 mg/day) reduce the microvascular complications of DM2 such as retinopathy, nephropathy, and diabetic foot. Apart from this, there is another biological significance of vitamin C. Vitamin C in higher doses reduces HbA1c levels and low-density lipoproteins, or bad cholesterol.[12]

Palmitoylethanolamide (PEA): A number of patients not responding well to conventional therapy were started on PEA 600 mg sublingually twice daily for quick absorption and to avoid first-pass effects. After 10 days, they were switched to tablets of 600 mg PEA twice daily, and if pain was sufficiently reduced, the dose was thereafter reduced to 300 mg twice daily. In case studies of patients suffering with metastatic prostate cancer pain, failed low-back surgery, diabetic neuropathy, polyneuropathy, and a female with partial vulvectomy from vulvar intraepithelial neoplasia II, all responded to the previous regimen. Most results were seen between weeks one and three of treatment, but some cases improved only after five weeks of treatment.[13]

Alpha lipoic acid (ALA), also known as thioctic acid, is a vitamin-like chemical that plays an essential role in mitochondrial bioenergetic reactions. It has gained considerable attention for use in managing diabetic complications. It appears that the clearest benefit of lipoic acid supplementation (600–1,800 mg/day) is in patients with diabetic neuropathy.[14]

Studies found that alpha-lipoic acid (600–1,200 mg/day for three to six weeks) can help with neuropathy caused by diabetes or cancer treatment. Alpha lipoic acid reduces symptoms such as pain, tingling, and prickling in the feet and legs.[15]

A short-term study of 24 patients with DM2 found that the symptoms of peripheral neuropathy were improved in patients who took 1,800 mg/day of oral lipoic acid (LA) for three weeks compared to those who took a placebo.[16] More recently, a randomized, double-blind, placebo-controlled trial in 181 patients with diabetic neuropathy found that oral supplementation with 600 mg/day, 1,200 mg/day, or 1,800 mg/day of LA for five weeks significantly improved neuropathic symptoms. The authors concluded that an oral dose of 600 mg once daily appears to provide the optimum risk-to-benefit ratio.[17]

CoQ10: Research shows that taking CoQ10 improves nerve damage and nerve pain in individuals with nerve damage caused by diabetes.[18]

Methylcobalamin: Methylcobalamin (MeCbl) is the activated form of vitamin B12. Clinical evidence proved that MeCbl has the capacity to inhibit the neuropathic pain associated with diabetic neuropathy.[19,20,21]

Vitamin D: Recent research showed that a single, high dose of intramuscular vitamin D was safe and effective for patients with painful diabetic neuropathy. In that study, 143 patients with predominantly DM2 neuropathy pain received a single intramuscular injection of 600,000 IU vitamin D. Significant effects were seen on the McGill pain score and the McGill Pain Questionnaire Score after 10 weeks.[22,23]

Magnesium: Hypomagnesemia is currently considered an accurate predictor of progression of diabetic nephropathy. Mg deficits have also been associated with cognitive decline, multimorbidity, and aging.[24]

Diaper Rash/Diaper Dermatitis/Contact Dermatitis

Diaper rash is marked by red, irritated, or tender-looking skin in the diaper region (i.e., buttocks, thighs, and genitals). It results from contact with urine and feces that inflames the skin and breaks down outer skin layers. Another contributing factor to diaper dermatitis is *Candida albicans*. Diaper dermatitis can cause diffuse reddening of the skin with papules, vesicles, edema, and scaling of the involved areas as well as psoriasiform lesions, secondary erosions, and ulcerations.[1]

MANAGEMENT TECHNIQUES

Clean: Use water and a soft washcloth or cotton balls to clean the affected area, then pat dry. Disposable diaper wipes without alcohol and that are fragrance-free may be used. The area should be allowed to fully dry by air.

Air Exposure: Air exposure to the diaper region can be increased by:

- Letting the baby go without a diaper and ointment for short periods of time, perhaps three times a day for 10 minutes each time, such as during naps.
- Avoiding airtight plastic pants and diaper covers.
- Using diapers that are larger than usual until the rash goes away.[2]

Zinc oxide cream or paste (Desitin, Balmex, Triple Paste) is a first line therapy and has been used for the treatment of diaper dermatitis for decades. It is a useful, soothing, and antipruritic agent that has been time-tested.[3]

Vitamin E: Application of acetate tocopherol ointment has been evaluated in the neonatal intensive care unit (NICU) setting and proved to be safe and more effective than the commonly used skin ointments in the topical treatment of exulcerative skin lesions in neonates.[4]

Ointments, Creams, or Lotions: Over-the-counter products include vitamin A and D ointment, and Lotrimin for yeast infections. Pharmacists can often advise caregivers on the best option.[5]

Witch Hazel: A study indicated that applying an ointment made with witch hazel to diaper rash helped. The study included 309 children.[5] Witch hazel is available in ointment, cream, gel, or salve for topical use.

Calendula: Some clinical studies suggest that applying a calendula ointment (1.5%) to the skin for 10 days improves diaper rash comparable to or better than aloe gel.[6,8]

Bentonite: A study that included 60 infants showed that shampoo clay (bentonite) was effective in healing diaper rash and that it worked faster than calendula.[7]

Aloe Vera: A study comparing aloe vera and calendula in the treatment of diaper rash in children found each to be an effective treatment for diaper rash.[8]

Zinc Gluconate: Giving zinc gluconate orally to infants appears to accelerate the healing of diaper rash.[9]

Colloidal Oatmeal Bath: Colloidal oatmeal can reduce the inflammation and irritation that atopic dermatitis can cause.[10]

Diarrhea (Acute)

Diarrhea is an increased frequency and decreased consistency of fecal discharge. Generally, it can be defined as three or more loose or runny (more liquid than solid) stools per day. Diarrhea is typically associated with urgency as well. Everyone gets occasional diarrhea, but most diarrheal illnesses are self-limited or viral-induced and nearly 50% last less than one day.[1] There are many causes of diarrhea including viruses, bacteria (e.g., *Clostridium difficile*), parasites, food poisoning, irritable bowel syndrome, malabsorption syndromes, colon cancer, hyperthyroidism, Addison's disease, and drugs (e.g., magnesium supplements, antibiotics, quinidine, metoclopramide, Cytotek, NSAIDs), etc.[2]

Dehydration is the leading complication of acute diarrhea because copious amounts of fluid and electrolytes (e.g., sodium, potassium, magnesium, chloride) can be lost. Vascular or circulatory collapse with the sudden loss of blood flow to the brain and other organs, causing altered mental status and hypotension, is a serious complication of dehydration.[3] Other possible complications can include hypokalemia, hyponatremia, hypomagnesemia, and metabolic acidosis.[2,3] Hypomagnesemia after prolonged diarrhea can further cause tetany. Unfortunately, patients with magnesium deficiency are particularly susceptible to digoxin-related arrhythmia. Acute diarrhea is most often self-limiting, subsiding within 72 hours, but if it lasts more than two weeks further medical investigation is needed.[4]

Most healthy adults with diarrhea do not develop dehydration or other complications and can be treated symptomatically by self medication. Children are more susceptible to dehydration (particularly when vomiting occurs) and may require medical attention.[5]

THERAPEUTIC CHOICES

Symptom control is via hydration and antidiarrheal agents (e.g., bismuth subsalicylate [Pepto-Bismol] 2 tablets by mouth every hour as needed or loperamide [Imodium] 4 mg initially, then 2 mg by mouth as needed, maximum 16 mg/day). Do not use antidiarrrheal agents in the presence of bloody diarrhea (e.g., due to Crohn's, ulcerative colitis, salmonella, shigella, *Campylobacter*, or other bacterial infection).[6]

Diet: Management of the diet is a first priority for treatment of diarrhea. Most physicians recommend stopping solid foods for 24 hours and avoiding dairy products.[7] Bland foods are advised. These include bananas, white rice, hot cereals (oatmeal, cream of wheat, rice porridge), bread or toast, applesauce, boiled potatoes, or unseasoned crackers.[8]

Liquids: If no nausea is present, the first priority in treatment is to replace fluids and salt. It is beneficial to drink small amounts of clear liquids only, such as herbal tea, ginger ale, broth, juice, or gelatin until diarrhea stops.[9] Apple juice may make diarrhea worse and should be avoided.

Caffeine and alcohol should be avoided.[9]

Oral rehydration solutions (Pedialyte) can be used for moderately severe diarrhea that is accompanied by dehydration in children older than 10 years of age and in adults. These solutions are given at 50 ml/kg over 4–6 hours for mild dehydration or 100 ml/kg over 6 hours for moderate dehydration.[10]

Zinc: Diarrhea is typically more persistent and severe in infants and young children with malnutrition than in children who are not malnourished. Children with severe zinc deficiency commonly have chronic diarrhea, immune deficiency, and growth retardation.[11]

Zinc supplementation in a largely malnourished group of children was associated with a statistically significant reduction in the severity and duration of diarrhea.[8] Zinc supplementation lowers the incidence of diarrhea by 25% according to an analysis of studies on children in developing countries.[12] The World Health Organization recommends a daily dose of 10–20 mg of zinc (based on age) for 10 to 14 days for management of acute diarrhea.[13]

Probiotic products for bacterial replacement are helpful because lactobacillus strains (*Lactobacillus acidophilus, Lactobacillus bulgaricus*) help prevent diarrhea caused by antibiotics in adults and children. Lactobacillus reduced the chance of diarrhea by about 60% to 70% when started within two days of beginning antibiotic treatment and continued for at least three days after finishing the antibiotics.[14] Also for *Clostridium difficile*-associated diarrhea, probiotics containing *Sac. boulardii* are an effective adjunctive treatment.[15]

Bulk forming agents (soluble fiber) such as methylcellulose (Citrucel), psyllium fiber (Metamucil), or polycarbophil (Fibercon) help to absorb excess fluid in the large bowel and slow transit in the intestinal tract, thus helping to solidify loose stools. To help regulate the bowels, women should take 7 gm/day and build to 25 gm/day. Men can build up to 38 gm/day.[16]

Adsorbents such as kaolin-pectin (30–120 mL after each loose stool), bismuth subsalicylate (*see* Pepto-Bismol *above*), and attapulgite (1,200–1,500 mg after each loose bowel movement or every 2 hours, up to 9,000 mg/day) absorb fluid to help manage diarrhea.

Diarrhea (Chronic)

Chronic diarrhea is defined as frequent attacks of loose or runny stools that persist for more than four weeks. There are many possible causes of chronic diarrhea including diabetes, medications, IBD, malabsorption, infections, and excessive alcohol or caffeine intake. Treatment is aimed at correcting the cause of diarrhea whenever possible, firming up loose stools, and dealing with any complications. The most serious complication of chronic diarrhea is dehydration, which can be life-threatening.

MANAGEMENT STRATEGIES

Hydration and nutritional support (e.g., Pedialyte).[1]

Diet: Avoidance of excess intake of alcohol or caffeinated beverages. Sugars such as sorbitol (candies, chewing gum, and other sugar-free items), mannitol, fructose (fruit and honey) should be reduced or eliminated. Avoiding fatty foods and dairy products can also help relieve diarrhea.[2,3]

Medications: Common medications can cause diarrhea. Taking a new medication just prior to the onset of diarrhea may be the culprit.[2]

Psyllium: Some fiber supplements, such as psyllium, can relieve chronic diarrhea. They may be especially helpful for those with IBS or other digestive conditions that cause loose stools.[2]

Imodium A-D: Chronic diarrhea sufferers should take 4 mg orally after the first loose stool, then 2 mg orally after each unformed stool until diarrhea is controlled. Maximum dose: 16 mg/day.[4]

Folic Acid: In an older study, six patients with chronic diarrhea due to various causes were treated with 40–60 mg/day of folic acid. In each case, bowel movements became normal within two to five days.[5]

Diarrhea (Traveler's)

Traveler's diarrhea, also known as Montezuma's Revenge or Delhi belly, is defined as three or more episodes of watery diarrhea in 24 hours with at least one other accompanying symptom such as abdominal cramping, nausea, vomiting, or fecal urgency. Infectious agents such as *E. coli*, shigellae, and salmonellae account for 80% of cases.[1] Those who take H-2 blocker medications or antacids are at increased risk because a decrease in stomach acidity allows higher survival rates for many infectious agents.[2]

PREVENTION AND TREATMENT OPTIONS

Fluid replacement is the primary treatment.

Imodium A-D: Mild traveler's diarrhea can usually be managed with the judicious use of antimotility agents such as loperamide (Imodium A-D) in a dosage of two 2 mg tablets initially, then one tablet after each loose stool (maximum 24-hour dosage: 8 mg).[3]

Bismuth subsalicylate (BSS), as in Pepto-Bismol, may be considered for any traveler to prevent traveler's diarrhea. BSS has been studied using four divided doses of either 2.1 gm/day or 4.2 gm/day (with meals and at bedtime). A lower divided dose of 1.05 gm/day has also been shown to be preventive, although it is unclear whether it is as effective as the higher doses.[4] Research shows that taking bismuth subsalicylate the day before traveling and continuing until two days after returning home reduces the risk of traveler's diarrhea by up to 41%.[5]

Digitalis Toxicity

Digitalis toxicity can arise from long-term drug therapy (Lanoxin, Digoxin) as well as taking an excessive amount of the drug at one time. Digitalis toxicity is serious and can be life-threatening. Symptoms can include headache, confusion, anxiety, or hallucinations; loss of appetite, nausea, vomiting, or diarrhea; fast or slow palpitations or irregular heartbeat; blurred vision and seeing halos around bright lights. Severe toxicity requires hospital admission.

MEDICAL CONSIDERATIONS

Magnesium: Digitalis toxicity is more likely to develop in people who take digoxin and have a low level of magnesium in their body.[1] Magnesium supplementation would seem warranted.

Potassium supplementation is often required to prevent hypokalemia and digitalis toxicity in patients taking digoxin and diuretics. A potassium-sparing diuretic and a potassium supplement may also be prescribed.[1]

Disc Desiccation/Disk Degeneration

Healthy intervertebral disks act as spinal spacers, stabilizers, and shock absorbers. The intervertebral disc is the largest structure in the body with no blood supply.

Normal aging damages intervertebral disks to the extent that they dehydrate and degenerate. Disk degeneration is common and results from replacement of the hydrophilic glycosaminoglycans within the nucleus pulposus with fibrocartilage. Disk dehydration does not result in the loss of disk height, which is a result of annular bulging and vertebral endplate bowing.[1] The key is to stabilize and slow the desiccation process down if possible.

TREATMENT AND DELAYING STRATEGIES

General Advice: Lose weight, stay active, do stretching and exercises, use heat or ice, improve posture, and obtain joint manipulation or distraction.[2]

Medications: Treating symptoms of degenerative disc disease often includes over-the-counter pain medications and anti-inflammatories.

Vitamin C: Supplementation with vitamin C may help ameliorate disc disease by increasing the strength and resilience of disc cartilage. A number of years ago, a Texas orthopedist observed that patients with early disc disease could frequently avoid surgery by taking 750–1,000 mg/day of vitamin C. He later discovered that doses of 1,500–2,500 mg/day or more were even more effective.[3]

Avoidance of Nicotine: Smoking should be eliminated or significantly reduced because it leads to advanced degenerative disk disease throughout the spine by speeding up the processes which make discs lose height, diameter, and mass, and prematurely dehydrate.

Diuretics (Loop and Thiazide Diuretics)

Prescription loop diuretics (Lasix, Bumex) and thiazide diuretics (Microzide, Thalitone) increase the urinary excretion of sodium, potassium, and magnesium. Loop diuretics increase excretion of calcium as well, while thiazide diuretics decrease calcium excretion.

NUTRITIONAL SUPPORT

Potassium and Magnesium: Because of increased excretion with diuretics, patients should be advised to take in foods rich in potassium and magnesium or take supplements of the same.[1]

Potassium supplements may be prescribed if a patient must take diuretics and digitalis together.[2]

Calcium: Patients on loop diuretics may also need calcium supplementation.

Diverticulitis

To understand diverticulitis, it is necessary to first understand diverticulosis. Diverticulosis is the development of small pouches in the wall at the last part of the large intestine (sigmoid colon). If a local pouch, or diverticulum, gets inflamed or infected, this is known as diverticulitis. Approximately 1%–10% of patients with diverticulosis may develop diverticulitis. Some literature states the number could be as high as 25%, but studies have not confirmed this.[1] Typical symptoms include lower left-sided, crampy abdominal pain, bloating, tenderness, possible low grade fever, nausea with vomiting, and constipation or sometimes diarrhea.

Approximately 15% of diverticulitis patients will experience complications, which can include an abscess (collection of pus) in the pelvis if and where the diverticulum has ruptured, colonic obstruction due to extensive inflammation, fistula, generalized infection of the abdominal cavity (bacterial peritonitis), or bleeding into the colon.[2] Complicated diverticulitis needs immediate medical care. The goal of treating diverticulosis is to prevent the pouches from causing symptoms or problems.

PREVENTION

Fiber: Increasing fiber to at least 30 gm/day, supplemented by psyllium seed preparations or bran, helps treat diverticular bleeding[3] and prevents bouts of diverticulitis.[4]

Probiotics: Some studies show that probiotics (containing *Lactobacillus*, *Bifidobacterium*, or *Saccharomyces boulardii*) may help with diverticulosis symptoms and may help prevent diverticulitis due to their anti-inflammatory effects and ability to maintain an adequate bacterial colonization in the colon.[5] In one study, both *Lactobacillus casei* (subsp. *DG*) administered as a single sachet containing 24 billion CFUs/day for 10 days/month and mesalazine administered at a dose of 1,600 mg/day for 10 days/

month, prevented the recurrence of symptoms. After one year, approximately 14% in each of the probiotic and mesalamine groups experienced a recurrence of symptoms, compared to 46% of those in the placebo, and 0% in the combination group.[4]

In another study, a probiotic containing *Lactobacillus paracasei* B21060 (5 billion CFUs/day) combined with a high fiber diet (at least 30 gm of fiber daily) decreased abdominal pain and bloating.[4]

Vitamin D: Vitamin D has a role in maintaining colonic homeostasis and mucosal integrity and in modulating inflammation in the gut.[1] People with low vitamin D levels have been found to be more likely to develop diverticulitis and complications of diverticulitis. Perhaps that is why diverticulitis is more likely to occur in darker winter months. A typical adult dose of vitamin D is 5,000 IU of vitamin D3 daily which should be taken with a meal for better absorption.[4]

TREATMENT OF ACUTE ATTACK

Many cases of diverticulitis are uncomplicated and require only at-home treatment.

Bed rest is indicated for 2–3 days.

Liquid Diet: The bowel will also need some time to rest. A clear liquid diet should be instituted for the first 2–3 days.[6]

Stool Softeners: For mild diverticulitis, stool softeners are recommended.[7]

Low-Residue Diet: During flare-ups, a low-residue diet is often required. This may include grain products, fruit, vegetables, meats or other protein, and dairy. If the low-residue diet is needed for an extended period of time, vitamin and mineral supplementation may be needed.[8]

Antibiotics may also be needed.

Fiber: There should be a slow reintroduction of fiber into the diet.[6] After a few days, the patient can start a soft, low-fiber diet and use a psyllium seed preparation (e.g., Metamucil or Citrucel) daily to keep the stool soft; after one month, patients can begin a high-fiber diet.[8]

Dizziness/Vertigo/ Benign Paroxysmal Positional Vertigo (BPPV)

Dizziness describes the sensation of lightheadedness, disequilibrium, feeling wobbly, or being unsteady. Causes of dizziness include medications such as drugs to treat seizures (carbamazepine, phenytoin), certain antibiotics (gentamicin, streptomycin), antidepressants, sedating drugs, and alcohol.

Vertigo is typically a disorder of the inner ear, resulting in repeated episodes of a false sensation of movement (i.e., spinning, swaying, or tilting or falling to one side), often precipitated by head movements. This includes the individual feeling like he or she is spinning (subjective vertigo) or the room is spinning (objective vertigo). Symptoms can range in severity from mild dizziness to debilitating episodes that may induce nausea or vomiting and significantly hinder daily functioning.[1] A virus affecting the inner ear (labyrinthitis) is a common cause. Other causes include diabetes, Meniere's disease, tumors (acoustic neuroma), decreased blood flow to the base of the brain, multiple sclerosis, head trauma, multiple sclerosis, and migraine headaches.

Benign positional paroxysmal vertigo (BPPV) is the most common type of vertigo and is seven times more likely in individuals over the age of 60.[2] Benign paroxysmal positional vertigo (BPPV) is characterized by recurrent episodes of vertigo lasting for seconds. The episodes are precipitated by changes in head position, especially neck extension, bending down, lying supine with the affected ear down, rising from bed, and rolling over in bed to the affected side. Symptoms can be reproduced by performing the Dix-Hallpike test. BPPV has a favorable prognosis, with nearly 25% of patients experiencing spontaneous resolution by one month and up to 50% at three months.[1]

MANAGEMENT OPTIONS

Home Instructions: Bed rest and avoiding alcohol, bright lights, and reading are important tools in mitigating symptoms. It is prudent to be and stay well-hydrated to minimize dizziness and balance problems.[3]

Diet: Caffeine, salt, alcohol, and tobacco should be avoided.

Meclizine: Meclizine (Bonine) 25–100 mg/day by mouth in a single daily dose or divided q 6–12 hours is a first-line treatment for vertigo.[4]

Dimenhydrinate (Dramamine) 25–100 mg orally every four to eight hours. Dramamine may cause drowsiness.[5]

Ginkgo biloba is known for resolving the symptoms of vertigo. It works by improving blood flow to relieve dizziness and balance issues. Ginkgo biloba (120 mg bid) is just as effective as the medication betahistine in managing vertigo.[6]

Almonds: Eating a daily handful of almonds can help with vertigo symptoms. How almonds help is unknown.[7]

Apple Cider Vinegar and Honey: Both apple cider vinegar and honey are believed to have beneficial effects for vertigo. Two parts honey and one part apple cider vinegar can prevent and treat vertigo symptoms.[7]

Bioflavonoids: In addition to standard medicines for nausea and dizziness, bioflavonoids have been recommended.[8]

Vestibular rehabilitation exercises are commonly included in the treatment of vertigo.[9]

BPPV MANAGEMENT OPTIONS

Epley Maneuver: One of the first treatments is the Epley maneuver which involves a series of positions that are performed before bedtime each night until the symptoms of vertigo resolve for at least 24 hours.[4]

Ginger root tea can reduce the effects of vertigo better than manual repositioning, such as the Epley maneuver, alone.[4] Ginger root can be steeped in a cup of boiling water for five minutes. Honey can help with the bitter taste. Drinking ginger tea twice a day may help dizziness, nausea, and other vertigo symptoms.[4]

Dry Eye Syndrome/Keratoconjunctivitis Sicca/Xerophthalmia

Dry eyes are a common symptom and occur in up to 30% of those older than 50 years.[1] Unfortunately, the medical literature is confusing regarding terminology with the term *dry eye syndrome* often used interchangeably with dry eye symptoms. Dry eyes from most causes is keratoconjunctivitis sicca. Sjögren's syndrome, systemic lupus erythematosus, and rheumatoid arthritis can cause dry eyes.[2]

The term *xerophthalmia* means "dry eye" and is a late manifestation of severe vitamin A deficiency that causes abnormal dryness of the conjunctiva and cornea of the eye, associated with inflammation and ridge formation. Xerophthalmia is a major problem in developing countries as a leading cause of preventable blindness.[3]

TREATMENT METHODS

The first line of treatment in all cases of dry eyes is the use of artificial tears.

Fish oil may also be beneficial. Several studies have established an association between decreased dietary intake of omega-3 fatty acids and dry eye syndrome. A small randomized, double-blind trial of patients with mild to moderate dry eye syndrome used a daily dose of fish oil that contained 450 mg of eicosapentaenoic acid, 300 mg of docosahexaenoic acid, and 1,000 mg of flaxseed oil. After 90 days, those in the treatment group had a notable increase in tear volume compared with the placebo group. Furthermore, 70% of the treated group had become asymptomatic compared with only 37% of those who took a placebo.[4,5]

Vitamin A: Treatment is both practical and inexpensive as a treatment for xeropthalmia. Oral administration of 200,000 IU vitamin A on two successive days to be followed by a similar dose several weeks later has been beneficial.[2,6]

In a controlled trial, 60 children with corneal xerophthalmia were given 200,000 IU oil-miscible vitamin A by mouth and a matched group of 45 children were given 100,000 IU water-miscible vitamin A intramuscularly. Oral administration of vitamin A was not only more practical but appeared to be just as effective as parenteral administration in the treatment of severe xerophthalmia.[7,8]

Duchenne Muscular Dystrophy

Duchenne muscular dystrophy is a rare progressive genetic disorder that occurs primarily in males and which eventually causes muscle degeneration and weakness. It is caused by a lack of the protein dystrophin. Symptoms first occur in childhood between the ages of three and five and involve the muscles of the shoulders, hips, and thighs. The child may typically have difficulty jumping, running, and walking along with enlarged calves due to fat deposits or fibrotic tissue. All voluntary muscles are eventually affected. In later stages, muscle degeneration involves the heart and breathing muscles.[1]

TREATMENT OPTIONS

L-Carnitine: In patients with Duchenne's, 40% responded to L-carnitine (1,200–1,800 mg/day) with increased strength and decreased myoglobinuria.[2,3]

Idebenone: There is some evidence that taking idebenone (an analogue of CoQ10) improves airway function and prevents airway infections in children and teens with Duchenne muscular dystrophy who are not already being treated with steroids.[4]

Dumping Syndrome

Dumping syndrome is a group of symptoms such as bloating, nausea, diarrhea, dizziness, weakness, sweating, and rapid heartbeat after eating. Dumping syndrome most frequently occurs in patients who have undergone major gastric or esophageal surgery. Symptoms are due to rapid emptying of the stomach contents into the duodenum that can result in stomach cramps, nausea, and diarrhea. This may occur as quickly as 30 to 60 minutes after eating a meal, but can also occur as late as two to three hours after eating.

MANAGEMENT METHODS

Diet: Six small meals should be eaten daily to avoid overloading the stomach. More protein, fiber, and fat, and fewer carbohydrates is recommended as is avoiding sweets and sugars because they aggravate the dumping syndrome.[1] Fluids should be limited to 4 oz. (1/2 cup) during mealtimes. This prevents the rapid movement of food through the upper gastrointestinal tract and allows adequate absorption of nutrients. Liquids should be consumed 30 to 45 minutes before eating and one hour after eating, rather than with meals. Individuals can rest or lie down for 15 minutes after a meal to decrease movement of food from the stomach to the small intestine. This decreases the severity of symptoms. Very hot or cold foods or liquids may increase symptoms in some patients.

Supplements such as pectin, guar gum, black psyllium, and blond psyllium can be taken to thicken the digestive contents and to slow its progress through the intestines.[2]

Dupuytren's Contracture/Palmar Fibromatosis

Dupuytren's contracture causes bundles of connective tissue fibers (palmer and digital fascia) on the palm side of the hand to thicken and harden. As the cords tighten over time, they become shorter, typically resulting in one or two fingers (most often the fourth and fifth digits of both hands) being pulled into a permanently bent position at the metacarpal-phalangeal junction, resulting in hand deformity. The disorder is essentially painless but results in abnormal appearance and loss of function.

NONSURGICAL CARE CONSIDERATIONS

Vitamin E is perhaps the most universally prescribed and used substance for early treatment of Dupuytren's contracture and the lump it causes on palm of hand. Vitamin E is perhaps the most important of all scar reduction therapies. Reported to reduce plaque and fibrous tissue infiltration in damaged arterial walls, studies suggest vitamin E can reduce scar and fibrous tissue buildup in other parts of the body. Vitamin E is also a first-line early treatment option for Dupuytren's contracture and Peyronie's disease.[1] The British Journal of Medicine[2,3] and others[4,5,6,7,8,9] recommended up to 2,000 IU of vitamin E bid along with topical vitamin E in the early stages of the disease process.

Stretching, steroid injections, or enzyme injections (i.e., collagenase clostridium histolyticum [CCH] which is approved by the Food and Drug Administration) can be effective.[10]

Dysgeusia/Abnormal Taste

Dysgeusia, also known as parageusia, is a distortion or perversion of the sense of taste. It often causes a lingering foul, rancid, metallic, or salty taste perception.[1] Dysgeusia is the most frequent form of taste disturbance and is often idiopathic. The condition has been attributed to certain diseases, vitamin deficiencies, prescription medications, and cancer treatment.[1] Treatment must address the underlying problem whenever possible. In two-thirds of cases, dysgeusia resolves spontaneously after about 10 months.[2]

TREATMENT OPTIONS

Topical Anesthetics: In cases of severe dysgeusia, topical anesthetics either as solution, spray, or gel (lidocaine 2%, lidocaine spray 10%, or lidocaine gel) may be helpful.[2]

Zinc Gluconate: 140 mg/day has been tested and recommended. This intervention has been moderately effective, with improved taste, mood, and dysgeusia in 50% of patients. Heckman randomized 50 patients with idiopathic dysgeusia to 140 mg zinc gluconate/day or a placebo. Zinc appeared to improve general gustatory (taste) function with subjects rating the dysgeusia as less severe with treatment.[3,4]

Alpha Lipoic Acid: In an open observational study in 44 patients with burning mouth syndrome, treatment with alpha-lipoic acid (200 mg tid) for two months significantly improved taste function as measured by symptoms scores.[5]

Dysmenorrhea

Painful menstruation that typically involves painful abdominal cramps that occur prior to or during the menses is referred to as dysmenorrhea. Many women routinely suffer from cramps which affect the lower abdomen or back just before or during the menses. Cramps are caused by uterine contractions and can range from mild to severe in intensity.

Primary dysmenorrhea (from the menstrual cycle) usually begins during adolescence. Associated symptoms may include headache, nausea, vomiting, flushing, or diarrhea. Physical findings of a pelvic mass, abnormal vaginal discharge, or pelvic tenderness that is not limited to the time of the menstrual period suggest a diagnosis of secondary dysmenorrhea where symptoms arise from pelvic pathology.

MANAGEMENT CONSIDERATIONS

EPA/DHA: Dysmenorrhea is a common gynecologic complaint in adolescents. After ovulation, fatty acids build up in the phospholipid layer of the cell membrane. In one study, the authors concluded that dietary supplementation with omega-3 fatty acids (2 gm/day for more than two months) was effective in relieving dysmenorrhea in adolescents.[1]

Vitamin D3: A study found that high doses of vitamin D3 led to a significant decrease in menstrual cramps. In one Italian study, 40 women were split into two groups. One group received a single oral dose of 300,000 IUs of vitamin D3 and the other received a placebo five days before the expected start of their menstrual periods. The pain score in the first group dropped by 41%, while those in the placebo group reported no change in their pain scale.[2] Typical safe dosing ranges for vitamin D3 are from 5,000–50,000 IU/day.[3]

Vitamin B12 and EPA/DHA: In a study involving dysmenorrheic Danish women, 78 were given five capsules a day of either fish oil, fish oil with vitamin B12, seal oil, or a placebo during a three to four month intervention period covering at least three menstrual periods. Results from fish oil alone and seal oil were only borderline significant. Highly significant reductions in reported pain grade were reported in the fish oil with B12 group. Based on these results, dietary supplements with fish oil enriched with or in combination with vitamin B12 can substantially reduce menstrual discomfort.[4]

Vitamin supplements have been used medically to treat dysmenorrhea.[5,6] Pyridoxine (vitamin B6), magnesium, and vitamins D and E are key considerations.[7,8,9]

Black cohosh has vascular and estrogenic activity. Some studies have shown that black cohosh binds to estrogen receptors.[10] Therefore, black cohosh is used for dysmenorrhea and is recommended for this indication by the German Commission which establishes guidelines for the proper use of herbs.[11] The recommended dosage is 20–160 mg/day.[10]

Magnesium is a natural calcium antagonist that can influence the intracellular calcium concentration in the myometrium.[12] Magnesium decreases the frequency and intensity of uterine contractions and abolishes myometrial hyperexcitability, anoxia, and pain.[13] The University of Maryland Medical Center recommends supplementation for menstrual cramps in the form of magnesium 360 mg, once daily for three days. If possible, patients should begin one or two days before bleeding starts.[14]

Ginger: Another study suggests that ginger powder may help if taken during the first three to four days of the menstrual cycle.[15]

Vitamin E (400–800 IU) for two days before and for three days after bleeding begins can decrease pain severity and duration and reduces menstrual blood loss.[16]

Thiamine: Taking thiamine (100 mg/day) alone or with 500 mg of fish oil/day for 90 days was found to be effective in treating dysmenorrhea in a double-blind random controlled trial in girls and young women 12–21 years old.[17,18]

Boron: Some research shows that taking boron 10 mg by mouth daily around the time of menstrual bleeding reduces pain in young women with painful periods.[19]

Pain Relievers: Over-the-counter pain relievers such as ibuprofen (prescription dose: 800 mg tid) and naproxen (prescription dose: 500–550 mg bid) are specifically approved by the FDA for treatment of dysmenorrhea.[20] Aspirin and acetaminophen (Tylenol) are also used to treat the discomfort of dysmenorrhea.[20]

Diet: A crossover study with a low-fat vegetarian diet showed decreased duration and intensity of dysmenorrhea.[21]

Dyspraxia

Dyspraxia is a form of developmental coordination disorder (DCD) affecting fine and/or gross motor coordination in children and adults. Children with dyspraxia are typically late in reaching milestones (e.g., rolling over, sitting, standing, walking, writing, riding a bike, speaking, and self-care). Dyspraxia primarily impacts an individual's ability to plan and process motor tasks. It results in lifelong impaired motor, memory, judgment, processing, and other cognitive skills. Dyspraxia also impacts the immune and central nervous systems.[1]

NUTRITIONAL SUPPORT

Tocopherol: Taking vitamin E by mouth together with evening primrose oil, thyme oil, and fish oils ostensibly improved movement disorders in children with dyspraxia.[2]

Eczema/Atopic Dermatitis

Eczema is a condition that causes skin to become dry, itchy, red, swollen, cracked, and rough. "Eczema" is derived from a Greek word meaning "to boil over," which is an apt description for the inflamed, red, itchy patches that occur during flare-ups. Red rashes on the scalp, forehead, face, inside the elbows, behind the knees, and on the hands and feet are common. For babies, the condition appears most often on the face and scalp. A history of eczema increases the risk of fungal, viral, and bacterial infections due to an impaired protective skin barrier. Eczema is common in childhood but can occur at any age. Atopic dermatitis is long-lasting, tends to flare periodically, and can persist into adulthood. The goals of treatment are to clear the skin, reduce itching, prevent flares-ups, and repair and maintain the skin barrier.

THERAPEUTIC OPTIONS

Topical agents are the mainstay of treatment for mild-moderate AD and include application of topical corticosteroids once or twice a day to actively inflamed areas.[1]

Emollients: Moisturize the skin and better maintain the skin barrier with liberal use of emollients. Occlusive emollient ointments are generally preferable. Seek your pharmacist's advice.[1]

Harsh soaps should be avoided.[2] Contact with solvents, detergents, perfumes, and wool should be eliminated, if possible.

Zinc Sulphate: A statistically significant improvement was observed with a combination cream containing zinc sulphate (2.5%) and clobetasol (0.05%) over plain clobetasol (0.05%) cream in 47 patients with chronic hand eczema in a double-blind, right to left, prospective clinical trial.[3]

EPA/DHA: Omega-6 (n-6) and omega-3 (n-3) polyunsaturated fatty acids (PUFAs) play a critical role in normal skin function and appearance. Consuming oils rich in n-6 and n-3 fatty acids can alter the fatty acid composition and eicosanoid content of the epidermis. A deficiency of essential fatty acids is characterized by dermatitis. Supplementation with n-6 fatty acids (linoleic acid) alleviates symptoms associated with skin sensitivity and inflammatory skin disorders.[4,5,6] In most but not all studies, administration of γ-linoleic acid (GLA) has been found to improve the clinically assessed skin condition, the objectively assessed skin roughness, and the elevated blood catecholamine concentrations of patients with atopic eczema.[4]

Vitamin D: In a small randomized, double-blind, placebo-controlled study in 45 patients with atopic dermatitis and low vitamin D status (70% of subjects had serum vitamin D3 concentrations <20 ng/mL), daily administration of 1,600 IU of oral vitamin D3, alone or together with 600 IU/day of vitamin E, for a period of 60 days significantly reduced the extent and intensity of eczema, as assessed by the SCORAD

(SCORing Atopic Dermatitis) score.[7,9] Vitamin D3 (1,600 IU/day for 60 days) also improved vitamin D status and reduced disease severity in 53 patients with atopic dermatitis in another small randomized trial.[8,9]

Avoidance of Triggers: Certain food such as nuts and dairy products, as well as smoke or pollen, can worsen eczema symptoms and should be avoided.[10]

Vitamin B12: In one study, vitamin B12 cream was applied to the scalp twice daily for eight weeks. The authors concluded that topical vitamin B12 demonstrated a significant superiority in comparison with a placebo with regard to the reduction of the extent and severity of atopic dermatitis.[11]

Ehlers-Danlos Syndrome

Ehlers-Danlos syndrome causes overly flexible joints and stretchy, fragile skin. This group of disorders affects connective tissues supporting the skin, bones, blood vessels, and many other organs and tissues. Defects in connective tissues cause the signs and symptoms of these conditions which range from mildly loose joints to life-threatening complications. Complications include pneumothorax, blue sclera, aneurysms, optic atrophy, lens dislocation, GI bleeding, ligamentous laxity, and bladder diverticulum.[1]

No medical treatment is currently available for this disorder. Aspects of nutritional management are based on: (1) increasing scientific evidence that nutrition may be a major factor in the pathogenesis of many disorders once thought to result from defective genes alone; (2) the recognition that many of the symptoms associated with Ehlers-Danlos syndrome are also characteristic of nutritional deficiencies; (3) the synergistic action within the body of appropriate combinations of nutritional supplements in promoting normal tissue function.[2]

MANAGEMENT CONSIDERATIONS

The main goal of treatment for Ehlers-Danlos syndrome (EDS) is to prevent injury and complications.[2]

Nutrition: The following combination of nutritional therapeutic interventions in daily doses has been proposed.[2] Symptoms associated with Ehlers-Danlos syndrome may be successfully alleviated using a specific (and potentially synergistic) combination of nutritional supplements, comprising calcium, carnitine, CoQ10, glucosamine, magnesium, methyl sulphonyl methane, pycnogenol, silica, vitamin C, and vitamin K, at dosages that have previously been demonstrated to be effective against the above symptoms in other disorders.[3]

- Vitamin C 1,500 mg/day
- γ-linolenic acid 240 mg/day
- CoQ10 100 mg/day
- Calcium 500 mg/day

- Magnesium 200 mg/day
- Carnitine 250 mg/day
- Glucosamine 1,500 mg/day
- Vitamin K 35 mcg/day
- Methyl sulphonyl methane (MSM) 1,500 mg/day
- Silica 3 mg/day
- Pycnogenol 80 mg/day

These supplements are generally well-tolerated, have a good safety record in terms of low toxicity, and in general do not interact adversely with prescription drugs.[3]

Zinc therapy has also shown promise.[4]

Calcium and **vitamin D** supplements should be taken to help strengthen the bones.

Ehlers-Danlos Syndrome (Type VI)

Ehlers-Danlos syndrome type VI is a rare genetic connective tissue disorder characterized by lax joints, scoliosis, fragile sclera of the eye, and progressive kyphoscoliosis.

NUTRITIONAL STRATEGY

Ascorbic Acid: Genetic impairment of collagen synthesis has been observed to be responsive to ascorbic acid supplementation in an 8-year-old boy with Ehlers-Danlos syndrome type VI. Four grams of ascorbic acid daily produced a significant improvement in the quality of newly synthesized collagen but did not alter collagen formed prior to the supplementation of C.[1,2]

Eosinophilic Pneumonia/ Acute Eosinophilic Pneumonia or AEP

AEP is a severe and rapidly progressive lung disease of unknown etiology that can cause fatal respiratory failure. Most patients are non-smoking, middle-aged females. All patients exhibit typical clinical features including acute-onset respiratory distress with fever, diffuse pulmonary infiltration, and elevated proportions of eosinophils in bronchoalveolar lavage fluid. There are acute and chronic types of AEP and many patients have recurrent eosinophilic pneumonia. Patients with AEP typically have a rapid and good clinical response to intravenous corticosteroids.

ADJUVANT CARE

Vitamin D: Research studies point to a relationship between low vitamin D levels and the development or outcomes of respiratory diseases.[1] Studies on the role of vitamin D in respiratory diseases have consistently indicated that low vitamin D levels may be associated with a higher incidence, greater severity, or poorer treatment responses in various respiratory diseases, including pulmonary tuberculosis (PTB), respiratory tract infections, chronic obstructive lung disease, and asthma.[1] Studies are needed on the relationship between vitamin D supplementation and respiratory diseases, including AEP, but supplementation would appear to be warranted to help facilitate recovery and prevent more frequent relapses in chronic AEP.[1]

Epidermolysis Bullosa

Epidermolysis bullosa (EB) is a genetic condition that causes fragile, blistering skin, especially on the hands and feet. Blisters may not appear until a toddler begins to walk or engages in new physical activities that increase friction on the feet.[1] There are different forms of this genetic disease, depending upon where the blistering occurs within the different skin layers. Infection is the chief complication associated with EB. In recessive dystrophic epidermolysis bullosa, a good nutritional balance is necessary to obtain adequate healing of chronic skin wounds.[2]

CONSERVATIVE CARE

Nutritional Deficiencies: Involvement of the oral mucosa and esophageal stenosis may be responsible for severe nutritional deficiencies. Most patients have significant growth retardation. Iron, vitamin D, C, B3, B6, zinc, and selenium deficiencies exist in 36%–70% of EB patients.[2]

Niacinamide/nicotinamide is recommended in bullous diseases. The mechanism of action is unknown.[3]

Tocopherol: Eleven patients with epidermolysis bullosa simplex and two patients with EB dystrophica were treated with vitamin E (α tocopherol). The preliminary results showed that blisters were less numerous, they were smaller and healed quicker, and the patients better resisted mechanical trauma (activity, occupation, games, manual labor).[2]

In various case studies, EB was well controlled in patients using 400 IU d-alpha tocopherol acetate q.i.d. for four months.[4,5,6]

Epilepsy/Seizures

Epilepsy, or seizure disorder, is characterized by recurring seizures and is the fourth most common neurological disorder. Common causes of epilepsy are idiopathic (65% of cases), vascular abnormalities (11%), congenital malformations (8%), and trauma (5%).[1] A person is diagnosed with epilepsy if they have two unprovoked seizures not caused by some known and reversible medical condition like alcohol withdrawal or extremely low blood sugar. There are two main types of seizures: (1) generalized seizures affect the whole brain and (2) partial or focal seizures that affect just one part of the brain. A generalized seizure that causes loss of awareness or control can be dangerous, leading to vehicular accidents, falls, drownings, etc.

According to the Epilepsy Foundation, the goal of treatment is to enable patients with epilepsy to lead lifestyles consistent with their capabilities. Antiseizure medications are the mainstay of medical treatment. Men who take antiseizure medications for epilepsy have higher rates of psychiatric comorbidities and erectile dysfunction.[2] Patients who are seizure-free for a certain period of time can be reevaluated to determine whether the drug can be discontinued or the dose reduced. Despite the development of new anticonvulsant agents in recent years, many epileptic patients continue to have seizures.[3]

ADJUNCTIVE MANAGEMENT CONSIDERATIONS

Tocopherol: Twenty-four children (aged 6–17 years) with epilepsy who had failed to respond to antiepileptic drugs received 400 IU/day of vitamin E or a placebo for three months in a double-blind trial. Ten of the 12 patients given vitamin E had a greater than 60% reduction in seizure frequency, compared to none of 12 patients in the placebo group.[4]

A double-blind, placebo-controlled trial was carried out on 65 epileptic patients with chronic antiepileptic intake. The subjects received 400 IU/day of vitamin E or a placebo for six months. Vitamin E administration also caused a significant decrease in the frequency of seizures and improved EEG findings. The authors concluded that the results of this study indicate that coadministration of antioxidant vitamin E with antiepileptic drugs improves seizure control and reduces oxidative stress.[5]

Manganese: In human studies, blood levels of manganese were lower in epileptic children than in healthy children.[6,7,8,9,10] Other nutrients may be lacking as well.

Magnesium: For almost a century, magnesium (Mg) has been used as prophylaxis and treatment of seizures associated with eclampsia. Mg is a CNS depressant.[11] In one study, 22 cases of drug-resistant epilepsy received daily oral magnesium oxide supplementation of 420 mg bid which was associated with a significant decrease in the number of seizure days per month. Thirty-six percent of patients had a response rate of 75% or greater at the second follow-up. Two patients reported freedom from seizures.[11]

Clinical and experimental investigations have shown that magnesium depletion causes a marked irritability of the nervous system, eventually resulting in epileptic seizures. Epileptic patients have lower magnesium levels than in controls.[12,13] The lower the magnesium blood levels, the more severe the epilepsy. Researchers surmise that epilepsy itself does not cause Mg depletion, but that anticonvulsant drug therapy may.[14,15]

Taurine: Research has shown that taurine (375–8,000 mg/day) can help prevent seizures.[16]

Dimethylglycine (DMG), sometimes called vitamin B15, is a normal body constituent formed in the metabolism of homocysteine to methionine. It is commercially available without a prescription and may be helpful in selected patients with seizures.[17] One patient had a dramatic reduction in his seizure frequency after starting DMG 90 mg bid. Doses as high as 600–1,000 mg/day have been reported.[18]

Thiamine: Seventy patients in a study were divided into four groups. In one group, administration of thiamine (50 mg/day for six months) improved neuropsychological functions in both verbal and nonverbal IQ testing.[19,20]

Additional nutrients that may reduce the frequency of seizures include vitamin B6, taurine, and omega-3 fatty acids.[19]

Supplementation with folic acid, vitamin B6, biotin (B7), vitamin D, and L-carnitine may be needed to prevent or treat deficiencies resulting from the use of anticonvulsant drugs.[19]

Ketogenic Diet: The ketogenic diet (KD) can be an efficacious treatment for intractable epilepsy, especially in children, and is associated with infrequent side effects.[21] KD, a restrictive, high-fat, low-carbohydrate, and protein diet, has been a successful treatment for intractable epilepsy in children and adults with drug refractory epilepsy.[22,23] Ketogenic dietary therapies should be strongly considered in a child who has failed two antiseizure drugs.[24] A standard approach to treatment includes a two-year diet period if the diet is successful, or the diet can be stopped after three months if unsuccessful.[24] The International Ketogenic Diet Study Group recommends that children with epilepsy "should take daily multivitamins and calcium with adequate vitamin D" in addition to ketogenic dietary therapy.[24]

Gluten-Free Diet: Among children with intractable seizures and chronic gastrointestinal symptoms, adherence to a gluten-free diet may reduce seizure burden. Early screening for celiac disease in pediatric patients with epilepsy, specifically with temporal EEG findings and intractable epilepsy, is warranted.[25]

Choline: There are reports that taking high doses of choline might be helpful for some people with a type of seizure called complex partial seizures.[26,27]

Gamma-Aminobutyric Acid (GABA): Previous clinical studies show that taking GABA (2.5–3 gm) along with medication (phosphatidylserine) for three to eight months reduces the frequency of absence seizures in some individuals, but does not benefit those who have seizures triggered by lights or other visual causes.[28]

Pyridoxine: There appears to be a link between seizures associated both with pyridoxine deficiency and pyridoxine dependency.[26] Seizures from pyridoxine deficiency respond well to anticonvulsants or pyridoxine. For pyridoxine dependency, the response to anticonvulsants is poor but large doses of pyridoxine (14 mg/kg of body weight per day) produce a cessation of seizures.[29]

Cilantro: Cilantro is an herb often used in making salsa and in pickling. It also has a folk medicine history as an anticonvulsant. Researchers at the University of California,

Irvine (UCI), reported that the cilantro leaf, or *Coriandrum sativum*, harbors a potent potassium channel-activating anticonvulsant. A metabolite, (E)-2-dodecenal, activated several potassium channels that regulate electrical activity in the brain. Dodecenal bound to a specific part of the potassium channels, opening them, and reducing cellular excitability and seizure activity.[30] The results provide a molecular basis for the therapeutic actions of cilantro.

Folic Acid: Folate deficiency resulting from long-term phenytoin therapy is a common occurrence. Treatment of 26 folate deficient epileptic patients with 5 mg of folic acid daily for one to three years resulted in improved drive, initiative, alertness, concentration, mood, and sociability in most.[31]

Reduce alcohol intake as heavy consumption (three or more drinks per day) is associated with increased risk of seizures.[32]

Epilepsy—Status Epilepticus (Children)

Status epilepticus (SE) is a single prolonged epileptic seizure, or crisis, lasting more than five minutes or two or more seizures within a five-minute period without the person returning to normal between them. Convulsive status epilepticus requires emergency medical treatment. Status epilepticus may be regarded as the most extreme form of epilepsy. It can cause permanent brain damage or death.

TREATMENT

Pyridoxine, or vitamin B6, (100 mg IV) is a first-line agent to treat status epilepticus in children.[1]

Erectile Dysfunction

Erectile dysfunction (ED), also known as male impotence, is the persistent inability to achieve and maintain an erection firm enough to complete the sex act. Causes include medical problems (e.g., peripheral nerve damage, diabetes, hormone dysfunction, heart disease, hypertension, atherosclerosis, obesity, MS, etc.), alcohol, smoking, and certain drugs (e.g., sleeping pills, amphetamines, SSRIs, tricyclic antidepressants, anti-anxiety medications, opioids, etc.).

METHODS OF MANAGEMENT

Avoidance of Alcohol and Nicotine: Avoiding tobacco products and alcohol is the first step in treating ED.

L-Arginine: Arginine is a precursor of nitric oxide, which helps to dilate blood vessels. It is a commonly used adjuvant to regular medicines for the treatment of erectile dysfunction. In small studies, men were given 2.8–6 gm of arginine per day for several weeks.[1,2,3] Forty percent of the men in one treatment group experienced improvement, compared to none in the placebo group.[2] In a double-blind trial, men with erectile concerns took 5 gm of arginine per day or a placebo for six weeks.[4] Nine of 29 patients (31%) taking L-arginine reported a significant subjective improvement in sexual function.[3]

Pycnogenol/L-Arginine: L-arginine (3 gm/day) has also been studied in combination with pycnogenol (40–120 mg/day) and showed a significant improvement in erectile function.[4,5] Pycnogenol enhances endothelial nitric oxide synthase to produce more nitric oxide from L-arginine.[6]

L-Citrulline: Oral citrulline supplementation raises blood arginine levels more effectively than arginine supplementation itself.[7] In a single blind, short-term study of men with ED (erection hardness score of 3 out of 4), L-citrulline was given at dose of 1.5 gm/day for a month. It was concluded that citrulline was safe and psychologically well-accepted, and reported as very satisfying to the patients.[8]

L-Arginine, Nicotinic Acid and Propionyl-L-Carnitine: The efficacy of a combination of L-arginine, nicotinic acid, and propionyl-L-carnitine (PLC) with and without the PDE-5 inhibitor vardenafil was assessed in men with diabetes and erectile dysfunction. Erectile function, measured by the International Index of Erectile Function (IIEF), improved by two points in those receiving the combination of L-arginine, nicotinic acid, and PLC. A group receiving vardenafil alone demonstrated an improvement in IIEF score by 4 points, and the group receiving L-arginine, nicotinic acid, and PLC plus vardenafil improved by 5 points. Those receiving a placebo did not show an incremental improvement.[9]

L-Carnitine: Studies have shown that L-carnitine (2 gm/day) combined with sildenafil (Viagra) improved erectile function better than sildenafil alone.[9]

Ginseng: One study of Panax ginseng showed it improved sexual function in men with erectile dysfunction. A cream preparation is used to prevent premature ejaculation.[10]

Dehydroepiandrosterone (DHEA): DHEA is converted by the body into testosterone. A group of 20 patients was treated with an oral dose of 50 mg DHEA once a day for six months. Positive results were obtained, but the small size of the study group limits its application to the general population.[11]

Erythema Nodosum (EN)

Erythema nodosum is a skin condition that causes painful swollen red or purple bumps most commonly on the shins. Young women ages 15–30 are five times more likely than men to develop erythema nodosum. Inflammation of the subcutaneous fat causes tender red lumps or nodules of erythema nodosum that range in size from a dime to a quarter. They may be inflamed off and on for a period of weeks, then shrink and become flat, leaving a bruised appearance. This condition is the most common form of panniculitis, or inflammation of the fat layer underneath the skin. EN can develop on its own or in association with certain medical conditions (e.g., sarcoidosis, TB, IBD, etc.) and medications (e.g., penicillin, oral contraceptives with estrogen, salicylates, etc.). Erythema nodosum can go away on its own in three to six weeks. Chronic erythema nodosum is a condition in which additional lesions pop up in different locations for a period of weeks to months or may last for years.[1]

STANDARD MEDICAL CARE

Pain Medications and Anti-Inflammatories: Over-the-counter pain and anti-inflammatory medications are recommended.[2]

Potassium iodide (KI) is a standard treatment (e.g., 400–900 mcg/day for one month) when symptoms begin.[2,3] Oral KI was administered to 15 patients with erythema nodosum. Eleven of those patients demonstrated improvement.[4] Relief of subjective symptoms, including tenderness, joint pain, and fever, occurred within 24 hours. Substantial improvement in the eruption occurred within a few days and the lesions disappeared completely 10 to 14 days after therapy was initiated.

Potassium iodide is used for many inflammatory dermatoses including erythema multiforme, Wegener's granulomatosis, granuloma annulare, Behcet's syndrome, neutrophilic dermatoses (pyoderma gangrenosum, Sweet's syndrome), and panniculitides (erythema nodosum, subacute nodular migratory panniculitis, nodular vasculitis).[5,6]

Erythropoietic Protoporphyria (EPP)

In erythropoietic protoporphyria (EPP), cells are unable to change the chemical porphyrin into heme which is essential for transporting oxygen and for breaking down certain compounds in the liver. This is due to an inherited deficiency of the enzyme ferrochelatase which causes a buildup of the chemical protoporphyrin in the skin, bone marrow, red blood cells, blood plasma, skin, and eventually the liver. This results in photosensitivity (i.e., the skin is damaged by sunlight). The first symptoms usually appear in infancy or early childhood and present as an uncomfortable or painful burning sensation of the skin after sun exposure that may be accompanied by swelling and redness.[1] The major complaint from this disorder is severe pain on exposure to sunlight and some types of artificial light, such as fluorescent lights (phototoxicity).[2] The hands, arms, and face are the most commonly affected areas. Microcytic hypochromic anemia, gallstones, liver damage, and enlargement of the spleen are common in patients with EPP.[1] Life expectancy is shortened.[1]

SYMPTOM MANAGEMENT

Avoidance of sunlight will benefit affected individuals and can include the use of clothing styles with long sleeves and pant legs, made with double layers of fabric or of light-exclusive fabrics, wide-brimmed hats, gloves, and sunglasses.[3] Tinting or placing a film over car and/or house windows can also be of benefit.

Skin protection with opaque sunscreens is vitally important.

Diet: Fluids and glucose along with a high-carbohydrate diet are needed to boost carbohydrate levels, which helps limit the production of porphyrins.[4]

Activated Charcoal: Oral activated charcoal may be taken to reduce protoporphyrin accumulation in the liver in patients with liver disease.[5]

Beta-Carotene: Beta-carotene exhibits provitamin A (retinol) activity. It can delay the onset of erythema in solar urticaria and is effective in light-sensitive skin diseases such as polymorphic light eruption.[6] It also reduces the risk of sunburn.[2] When administered in sufficiently high doses, beta-carotene be an effective therapy for ameliorating the photosensitivity associated with EPP.[7]

Oral beta-carotene (Solatene) (60–180 mg/day) was given to 133 patients suffering from erythropoietic protoporphyria (EPP), 27 patients with polymorphous light eruption, six patients with solar urticaria, three patients with hydroa aestivale, one patient with porphyria cutanea tarda, and two patients with actinic reticuloid to relieve the photosensitivity associated with these diseases. Eighty-four percent of the patients with erythropoietic protoporphyria increased by a factor of three or more their ability to tolerate sunlight.[8]

Cysteine: Oral cysteine has also been used and is thought to have a similar mechanism of action as beta-carotene without the yellow-orange discoloration of the skin.[1]

Intravenous vitamin E was reported in a case as being effective for reversing liver disease from increased protoporphyrin.[1]

Vitamin D and Calcium: Because EPP patients avoid sunlight, deficiency of vitamin D is likely, A supplement with vitamin D and calcium is recommended for bone health.[9]

Iron: EPP patients often have iron deficiency. An iron supplement may be advisable if the serum ferritin is below about 20 ng/mL.[9]

Facial Neuralgia (Atypical)

Facial neuralgia is a severe stabbing, burning, or shocking pain due to an irritated or damaged nerve. Persistent burning or lancinating paroxysmal pain in the facial region typically follows along the anatomical course of a damaged nerve. When patients present with symptoms and no clear etiology, one should consider neuropathic pain such as sphenopalatine or glossopharyngeal neuralgia in the diagnosis.[1]

CARE FOR THIS DISORDER

Vitamin B12 deficiency may cause isolated facial neuralgia, independent of trigeminal neuralgia.

A group of 17 patients all of whom had low levels of serum B12 (on average, 186.7 pg/mL; reference range, 300–900 pg/mL), received intramuscular or subcutaneous injections of 1,000 mcg vitamin B12, once a week for four weeks. The dose was subsequently tapered down to two-week intervals for eight weeks, and then once a month for a year, at which point treatment with B12 injections was found to alleviate the condition.[2]

Familial Mediterranean Fever (FMF)

Familial Mediterranean fever, also known as periodic peritonitis, is characterized by recurrent episodes of pain in the abdomen, chest, joints, pelvis, and/or muscles, accompanied by fever. It is an inherited disease prevalent among Eastern Mediterranean populations, mainly non-Ashkenazi Jews, Armenians, Turks, and Arabs. The goals of treatment are to control symptoms and to reduce the number of attacks because there is no cure for this condition.

NUTRITIONAL MANAGEMENT APPROACHES

Diet: A low-fat diet may reduce the number and severity of attacks.[1]

Vitamin D: Vitamin D levels are lower in children with FMF than in healthy controls. Researchers conclude that scientific research has not clarified whether vitamin D deficiency is a consequence or a cause of inflammatory disease and surmise that vitamin D levels should be carefully examined. Nutritional supplementation may be required in patients with FMF.[2]

Colchicine is the front-line medical treatment for FMF. Resistance to colchicine is observed in up to 30% of patients and is an ongoing problem. Vitamin D deficiency appears to be a factor in colchicine resistance.[3] This is another reason to recommend vitamin D supplementation in patients with FMF. Colchicine is highly effective in preventing acute attacks, but it may also disrupt the intestinal absorption of vitamin B12. Patients treated with colchicine for a prolonged period of time could develop deficiency of vitamin B12 and need supplementation.[4]

Fanconi Syndrome

Fanconi syndrome (FS), also called Fanconi's renotubular syndrome, is a kidney disorder in which excess amounts of glucose, cysteine, galactose, fructose, bicarbonate, phosphates (phosphorus salts), uric acid, potassium, and certain amino acids are lost in the urine to be excreted. Normally, these substances are reabsorbed back into the bloodstream by the proximal tubules in the kidneys. A child with FS may experience slow growth, failure to thrive, and chronic kidney disease along with increased urine production, weakness, and bone abnormalities.[1] There are hereditary and acquired forms of this disorder. In general, treatment involves maintaining fluid balance through replacement of the nutrients lost in the urine. In severe cases, some people may develop kidney failure and need a kidney transplant.[1]

CLINICAL CARE

Sodium Bicarbonate: FS causes metabolic acidosis due to loss of bicarbonate. Acidosis may be lessened by giving tablets or solutions of sodium bicarbonate (e.g., 3–10 mg/kg/d in divided doses), potassium bicarbonate, sodium citrate, or potassium citrate (e.g., Shohl's solution with sodium citrate and citric acid).[2] To help prevent diarrhea and stomach upset, take each dose after a meal, mixing the prescribed dose of medication in a full glass (4–8 ounces or 120–240 milliliters) of cold water or juice just before taking. Drink the entire mixture slowly. Ask your doctor or pharmacist for further instructions.[3]

Phosphate and Vitamin D: Correction of metabolic acidosis is beneficial but is not sufficient for the treatment of bone disease. Phosphate and vitamin D3 supplementation are necessary for improved bone strength.

Normalization of serum phosphate levels may be achieved by administering 1–3 gm/day of supplemental phosphate. Administration should start at the lower level and be slowly increased over several weeks to minimize GI symptoms.[4]

Vitamin D deficiency is one of several causes of Fanconi syndrome.[2] Vitamin D should be administered as 1,25-dihydroxyvitamin D3 or 1α-hydroxyvitamin D3. The latter is preferred because liver and/or renal hydroxylation may be impaired in patients with Fanconi syndrome.[4]

Fatigue/Chronic Fatigue Syndrome

Fatigue is described as an extreme physical and mental tiredness that does not go away with rest or sleep. A person with fatigue feels weak, tired, and lacks energy and motivation on a regular basis. The syndrome implies incredible fatigue and inability to do even the simplest of tasks without becoming exhausted, inability to cope with any stress, and insomnia. Society often looks upon fatigue as weakness and a lack of motivation. Individuals with this disorder often lose jobs, feel socially isolated, and have less quality to their lives. Fatigue is a symptom, not a diagnosis, but chronic fatigue syndrome is recognized as an illness by the Centers for Disease Control.

Medical causes of fatigue include depression, sleep apnea, anemia (e.g., iron deficiency anemia), cardiac failure, chronic diseases (e.g., COPD or hypothyroidism), and drug therapy, (e.g., antidepressants, antihypertensives, cytokines/interferon, and anticancer medications). If fatigue is the result of an underlying condition, then treatment depends upon that condition. Any comorbidity identified should be treated.

Chronic fatigue syndrome, in many cases, is caused by inefficient energy production at the cellular level. Intracellular magnesium deficiency is now believed to be the most critical single factor in this disorder.[1]

The following interventions relate to chronic fatigue from unknown causes.

RESEARCH ANALYSIS

Magnesium is required for the synthesis of ATP, the biochemical "storage battery." Fifteen patients, randomly chosen, received magnesium sulfate intramuscularly once a week for six weeks while the remaining 17 received injected water. Energy levels, pain levels, and emotional reactions were significantly better in the treated patients.[1]

For chronic fatigue syndrome (CFS), a solution containing 1 gm of magnesium sulfate has been given as a shot once weekly for six weeks.[2]

Aspartate is converted within the cell to a compound called oxaloacetate. Oxaloacetate stimulates the Krebs cycle, the main biochemical pathway whereby fuel is converted to energy.[3,4]

Potassium-Magnesium Aspartate: In a study, 80 patients who experienced persistent fatigue and weakness were treated with potassium-magnesium aspartate at a dose of 1 gm twice a day. Complete relief of fatigue occurred in 94% of the patients within 3 to 14 days.[3]

In another study of 200 individuals with chronic fatigue, most improved after receiving potassium-magnesium aspartate.[4] These preliminary results were confirmed by three double-blind, placebo-controlled studies.[5,6,7,8]

Pyridoxine: Data provides preliminary evidence of reduced functional B vitamin status, particularly of pyridoxine, in CFS patients.[9]

Pyridoxine, Riboflavin, Thiamine: A placebo-controlled, double-blind study of a supplement including pyridoxine, riboflavin, and thiamine has shown significant improvements, particularly fatigue scores, after six weeks of treatment.[10]

Thiamine: Fatigue in spinocerebellar ataxia type 2 and in inflammatory bowel diseases can be treated with large doses of thiamine.[11,12]

L-Carnitine: Previous clinical studies demonstrate that taking L-carnitine (2–3 gm/day) for two months can improve symptoms of fatigue.[13]

Glycine: In a blinded and controlled study, using 3 gm of glycine an hour before bed for four days appeared to promote sleep quality associated with reduced sleep latency and reduced time to reach slow wave sleep, which resulted in improved daytime fatigue scores and cognition scores.[14]

Fibrocystic Breasts/Cystic Mastitis/Mammary Dysplasia

Fibrocystic breasts typically cause swelling, pain, and tenderness that gets worse premenstrually, but can remain throughout the month. The breasts are composed of tissue that feels lumpy, granular, or hard, or has a rope-like texture. The exact cause of this disorder is unknown. Fibrocystic breasts are the most common cause of noncancerous breast lumps in women between 30 and 50 years of age. It is thought that more than half of women will develop fibrocystic breast disease at some point in their lives, but that many will not have any associated symptoms.

STRATEGIES BASED ON RESEARCH

Evening Primrose Oil (EPO): Evening primrose oil benefits clinical mastalgia.[1] It can change the balance of fatty acids in the cells and may reduce breast pain.[2] EPO 3,000 mg/day (in divided doses) decreased breast pain and patients continued to improve after three months of treatment.[3]

Vitamin E: Doses of vitamin E (400–600 mg/day) have been reported to afford symptomatic improvement in fibrocystic breast disease.[4] Studies have also shown a beneficial effect of vitamin E on breast pain in premenstrual women who experience breast pain that fluctuates during the menstrual cycle.

In one study, 200 international units (IU) of vitamin E taken twice daily for two months improved symptoms in women with cyclic breast pain.[1]

In another study, women with mammary dysplasia were followed and 85% of the patients receiving tocopherol therapy showed objective and subjective remission from the disease.[5]

Abrahms also reported an excellent clinical response rate in a series of patients treated with vitamin E (600 IU/day), which alleviated fibrocystic breast pain and tenderness in approximately 70% of those patients.[6]

For adults older than 18 years, pregnant women, and breastfeeding women, the maximum dose of vitamin E is 1,000 milligrams daily (or 1,500 IU).[2]

Iodine: Breast tissue has a high concentration of iodine, especially during pregnancy and lactation. In a double-blind study, researchers randomly assigned 56 women with fibrocystic breast disease to receive daily supplements of iodine (70–90 mcg I_2/kg body weight). At treatment completion, 65% of the women receiving iodine reported decreased pain compared with 33% of women in the placebo group.[7]

In another study, after five months of treatment, women receiving doses of 3,000 or 6,000 mcg iodine had a significant decrease in breast pain, tenderness, and nodularity compared with those receiving a placebo or 1,500 mcg iodine. The researchers also reported a dose-dependent reduction in self-assessed pain. None of the doses was associated with major adverse events or changes in thyroid function test results.[8]

Avoidance of Nicotine: Patients with mastalgia should stop smoking, or at least reduce the number of cigarettes taken daily, based on a study that identified smoking as a factor associated with mastalgia.[9]

Ginkgo Biloba: Taking ginkgo leaf extract by mouth reduces breast tenderness and other symptoms associated with PMS when started during the 16th day of the menstrual cycle and continued until the fifth day of the following cycle.[10]

Exclusion of caffeine is beneficial for some patients.[11]

Fibromyalgia

Widespread chronic muscle pain, fatigue, sleep problems and a heightened pain response to pressure tenderness in local areas are signs of a long-lasting condition known as fibromyalgia. Emotional and mental distress can also be associated with fibromyalgia. Fibromyalgia can cause pain, disability, major depression, and lower quality of life. The cause of fibromyalgia is unknown and there are no definitive diagnostic tests. Fibromyalgia affects about four million adults in the U.S. Women are more likely to develop this disorder than men. Individuals with lupus or rheumatoid arthritis are also more likely to develop fibromyalgia.[1] Because no known cure exists, the goal of treatment is to mitigate symptoms.

CONSERVATIVE THERAPY

Magnesium abnormalities are associated with previously reported impairment of thiamine metabolism in patients with fibromyalgia.[2]

Taking magnesium hydroxide with malic acid (Super Malic tablets) by mouth can reduce pain related to fibromyalgia.[3] Taking magnesium citrate 300 mg/day for eight weeks is also reported to improve some symptoms of fibromyalgia.[4]

Creatine: Patients with fibromyalgia often suffer from chronic pain, fatigue, difficulty sleeping and depression. A strong overlap has been reported between fibromyalgia and post-traumatic stress disorder (PTSD). In an 8-week open label study of creatine, significant improvements were observed in quality of life, sleep patterns, and pain in patients with fibromyalgia. These improvements deteriorated four weeks after stopping creatine therapy.[5,6]

In a small study, researchers found that creatine 20 gm for five days then 5 gm/day thereafter increased muscle strength in patients with fibromyalgia.[7]

5-HTP: 5-hydroxytryptophan may help to increase deep sleep and reduce pain. In one study, researchers reported that supplementation with 5-HTP may improve symptoms of depression, anxiety, insomnia, and fibromyalgia pain. However, other studies disagree.[8]

Chiropractic and osteopathic treatment have been used frequently to manage the symptoms of fibromyalgia.[9,10]

Coenzyme Q10: Research shows that taking CoQ10 improves nerve damage and nerve pain in individuals with nerve damage caused by diabetes.[11]

Thiamine: Oral therapy with 600–1,800 mg/day of thiamine led to an appreciable attenuation of chronic widespread pain, fatigue, and all other symptoms in all patients within a few days.[12]

Fire Ant Bites

Red fire ants inject toxic proteins into their victims. The stings are immediately and intensely painful. Wounds quickly develop into red pus-filled blisters. Thereafter, pain tends to subside into an itching or burning sensation which can last for days.

REMEDIAL MEASURES

General measures include cold compresses, a hydrocortisone cream or antihistamine (e.g., Benadryl) to decrease itching, an oatmeal bath, or applying a triple antibiotic ointment to help prevent infection.

Ammonia: One remedy for fire ant bites is the application of straight ammonia solution to all bite sites. *Caution:* Ammonia can be irritating to skin and mucous membranes and should be used with caution, especially in children. Fumes should not be inhaled.[1]

Fish Odor Syndrome/Trimethylaminuria

This syndrome results in body odor analogous to rotting fish. This is due to a genetic inability to convert trimethylamine into the compound choline and carnitine to trimethylamine N-oxide. This results in an excessive excretion of trimethylamine (TMA) in the urine, sweat, and breath of affected individuals. The odor interferes with relationships, social life, and career. Some individuals with trimethylaminuria experience marked depression and social isolation as a result of this condition.

MANAGEMENT CHOICES

Diet: Affected individuals must lower intake of chemical precursors to trimethylamine such as choline, lecithin, and carnitine (e.g., saltwater fish, liver, kidneys, eggs, peas, and soybeans) consumption.[1]

Activated charcoal (750 mg bid for 10 days) is reported to reduce the offensive odor.[2] Charcoal can bind trimethylamine in the gut to reduce the amount available for absorption.

Chlorophyllin Copper: A recent study in a small number of Japanese patients with trimethylaminuria found that oral chlorophyllin (60 mg three times daily) for three weeks significantly decreased urinary trimethylamine concentrations.[2]

Riboflavin (vitamin B2) supplements (30–40 mg taken 3–5 times per day with food) enhances existing amounts of FMO3 enzyme so that larger amounts of trimethylamine are converted to its odorless form of oxide.[3]

Slightly acidic soaps and body lotions can convert trimethylamine on the skin into a less volatile form that can be removed by washing. Slightly acidic detergents may also help reduce the intensity of the odor.[4]

Antibiotics: Taking low doses of antibiotics can reduce the amount of bacteria in the gut and suppress the production of trimethylamine.[5]

Folic Acid Deficiency

Folate deficiency means there is a lower than normal amount of folic acid (vitamin B9) in the blood. Isolated folate deficiency is uncommon. Folate deficiency usually coexists with other nutrient deficiencies because of its association with a poor diet and/or alcoholism. Long-term anticonvulsant therapy, oral contraceptives,[1] and losses of folic acid due to disorders such as Crohn's disease or untreated celiac disease or using diuretics also cause deficiencies. Megaloblastic anemia is a late finding in folate deficiency. Vitamin B12 deficiency must be ruled out before any folic acid treatment can begin.

TREATMENT

Folic Acid: For folic acid deficiency, at least 400 mcg/day is recommended. If megaloblastic anemia is present, then 1 mg/day is the usual dose.[2]

Methotrexate Side Effects: Methotrexate is an effective rheumatoid arthritis medication, but can remove folate from the body, causing gastrointestinal symptoms. Studies indicate that folic acid supplementation can reduce side effects from this medication by around 79%.[3]

Foot Odor/Bromodosis

Unpleasant foot odor is caused by moisture (sweat) mixed with bacteria on the skin. Foot odor is a common condition especially in teens and adults whose feet sweat into their socks and shoes on a daily basis.

CLINICAL APPROACHES

Home Instructions: Offensive foot odor can be managed by dusting the feet in the morning with a moisture-absorbing powder (e.g., cornstarch, which is highly absorbent and can be used daily). Changing socks and re-powdering the feet midway through the day helps eliminate the moisture that bacteria need to cause foot odor.[1]

Zinc Sulphate: Sharquie et al. in a single-blinded placebo-controlled therapeutic trial studied the efficacy of 15% zinc sulphate solution for foot malodor. Zinc sulfate solution 15% was applied to the soles and toe-webs once daily for two weeks and three times per week for next two weeks, followed by a single weekly application as maintenance after the clearance of odor for a period of two months. Fifty-eight patients received zinc sulphate solution while the other 50 patients received a placebo solution. Thirty-five of the 50 patients (70%) who completed the study showed complete clearance of foot odor as compared to only one subject (2%) in the placebo group, making the difference statistically significant.[2,3]

Exfoliation: Using a scrub or pumice stone helps to remove dead skin cells that bacteria like to feed on. An individual with smelly feet should use a pumice stone 2–3 times each week to avoid buildup.[4]

Salt Soaks: Soaks are potentially useful, especially as part of an exfoliating routine. One-half cup of Epsom salts can be dissolved in a bowl or tub of warm water. After soaking for 10–20 minutes, the feet should be thoroughly dried.[4]

Antiperspirants: Using an over-the-counter antiperspirant (e.g., with aluminum chloride) on the feet 2–3 times per week can help reduce the amount of sweating.[4]

Friedreich's Ataxia

In Friedreich's ataxia (FA), nerve fibers in the spinal cord and peripheral nerves degenerate, becoming thinner.[1] The cerebellum also degenerates, but to a lesser extent. Nonetheless, cerebellar damage results in awkward, unsteady movements and impaired sensory functions. FA is an autosomal recessive inherited disease and is caused by a defect in a gene labeled *FXN*, which carries the genetic code for a protein called frataxin. Although rare, the disorder is the most common form of hereditary ataxia in the U.S., affecting about one in every 50,000 people.

Onset is typically between the ages of 2 and 25 years. Kyphoscoliosis is an early sign. Hypertrophic cardiomyopathy is a prominent feature with diabetes mellitus occurring in later stages in approximately 25% of patients.[2] Generally, within 10 to 20 years after the appearance of the first symptoms the patient is confined to a wheelchair. FA can shorten life expectancy, with heart disease as the most common cause of death.[1] Monitoring for cardiomyopathy and diabetes should be undertaken at least yearly.[2]

CARE CONSIDERATIONS

Coenzyme Q10: A randomized double-blind controlled trial, involving high doses of CoQ10/vitamin E or low doses of coenzyme CoQ10/vitamin E determined that high doses of CoQ10 and vitamin E given daily over two years modified the disease progression in patients with genetically proven Friedreich's ataxia.[3]

Tocopherol: Ataxia typically causes low levels of vitamin E. Vitamin E supplements, a special diet, or both may help. Sensitivity to gluten can occur with ataxia, so a gluten-free diet may also help.[4]

Choline (6–12 gm/day) was given to eight patients with Friedreich's ataxia. A noticeable improvement in upper limb coordination was noted in approximately 50% of patients receiving 6 or 12 gm of choline a day. Choline chloride produced a mild but functionally significant improvement in motor coordination in some patients with cerebellar and spinocerebellar ataxia.[5,6]

Lecithin: In one study, two patients in stage I and, to a lesser degree, one patient in stage IV showed better scores for muscle strength and some motor accuracy and coordination tests with lecithin.[7] Lecithin contains choline chloride which is a precursor for the neurotransmitter acetylcholine.

Copper levels were significantly lower in the heart cells of patients with FA and cardiomyopathy. In conclusion, the decrease of copper may be important in consideration of the potential benefit of copper supplements in FA cardiomyopathy.[8]

Idebenone, 5 mg/kg/day, reduced cardiac hypertrophy in most patients studied but does not halt progression of ataxia. However, it is well-tolerated in high doses up to 55 mg/kg/day. The possibility that these higher doses may improve neurologic function remains to be fully determined.[2]

Gallbladder–Biliary Dyskinesia/ Functional Gallbladder Disorder/Cystic Duct Syndrome

The gallbladder is a four-inch long, pear-shaped organ under the liver on the right side of the upper abdomen that stores bile from the liver, which digests fats. Biliary dyskinesia, where bile does not drain out of the gallbladder properly, is an increasingly common functional disease of the gallbladder. Patients with this condition present with gallbladder (biliary-type) pain, but show no evidence of gallstones in the gallbladder. In classic biliary colic, or a gallbladder attack, the pain is identical to a symptomatic gallstone. (*See* Gallstone Disease *below.*) Attacks are often brought on by a heavy or fatty meal.

MANAGEMENT TECHNIQUES

Diet: Regular ingestion of food in the digestive tract counteracts the stagnation of bile. Food should be consumed in small portions (e.g., every four hours) since overeating can provoke pain. Patients should also avoid excessively cold drinks and dishes (otherwise, spasm in the sphincter of Oddi may result or intensify), refractory fats (lamb, beef, duck, pig, goose, sturgeon, etc.), and fried foods. Products with a high content of essential oils (garlic, radish, etc.), smoked products, spicy seasonings (mustard, horseradish, etc.), pickles, marinades, and alcohol-containing beverages should also be avoided.[1]

Spinal Manipulation: Surgery to remove the gallbladder is not effective for all patients and conservative measures should be undertaken initially. As such, manipulative treatment especially of the T6-T9 segments can and should be considered in the management of biliary dyskinesia. This treatment can remove the feedback related to the somatic component of the viscerosomatic reflex, thereby reducing nociceptive facilitation at the spinal level and allowing the body to restore autonomic balance.[1]

Vitamins E and D: The fat-soluble vitamin E along with vitamin D when supplemented orally or parenterally is effective in improving the status of deficiency in chronic conditions of cholestasis.[2]

Curcumin from turmeric has been shown to increase gallbladder contractions, gallbladder emptying, and gallbladder refilling. A 20 mg amount of curcumin was capable of contracting the gall bladder by up to 29% within an observation time of two hours.[3] A dosage of curcumin capable of producing a 50% contraction of the bladder was 40 mg.[3]

Coffee: Coffee (1–2 cups per day) induces cholecystokinin release and gallbladder contraction and colonic motor activity.[4]

Gallstone Disease/Cholelithiasis/Cholecystitis

***See also* Biliary Dyskinesia**

Gallstones are composed of cholesterol, bile pigments and calcium salts. Gallstones form because of abnormally slow gallbladder emptying and bile that is saturated with cholesterol which leads to crystal formation.[1] These crystals then form into larger aggregates and finally into gallstones. Stones can be the size of a small grape pit or as large as a cherry tomato. However, when multiple small stones or a larger one block bile ducts (especially the cystic duct), bile or digestive enzymes can become trapped within the duct. This causes inflammation of the gallbladder (cholecystitis) and severe pain in the upper right abdomen (biliary colic). The pain progressively worsens and can radiate around the abdomen to the back causing nausea, vomiting, and fever.

Biliary pain is often instigated by a fatty or heavy meal, is usually severe, and lasts from 30 minutes to several hours. Stones that block the common bile duct can cause jaundice, infection, and pancreatitis. In addition to pain, there may be fever, chills, nausea or vomiting, and dark urine. If a patient has an acute attack of severe gallbladder pain, hospitalization is necessary. Being overweight or obese increases the chances of developing gallstones as does losing weight rapidly.

MANAGEMENT METHODS

Food Allergies: James Breneman, MD, studied the relationship between food allergy and gall bladder disease in 69 patients.[2] The most common symptom-provoking foods were eggs, pork, and onions. Patients followed an allergy elimination diet consisting of beef, rye, soy, cherries, peaches, apricots, beets, and spinach for one week. All 69 patients were relieved of their symptoms after one week on the diet.

Dietary Factors: There is evidence that a diet low in refined sugar and high in fiber may help prevent gallstones by enhancing the flow of bile. Gallstones are extremely rare in Africa and other parts of the world where the diet is high in fiber and low in refined sugar.[3]

Stomach Acid: In a study of 50 patients with gallstones, more than half had co-existing hypochlorhydria (low stomach acid).[4] When hypochlorhydria was identified and treated with hydrochloric acid supplements, so-called gallbladder symptoms often improved.

Nutritional Supplements: Lecithin is found naturally in bile, where it helps to keep cholesterol in solution. In theory, supplementing with lecithin might help prevent cholesterol from crystallizing in the gall bladder. In one study of eight patients with gallstones who took lecithin for 18–34 months, the stones decreased in size in one case and remained the same in others.[5,6]

Taurine is a normal component of bile. Taurine binds to certain bile salts and therefore enhances their ability to digest fat.[7] Animal studies have shown that taurine supplementation can inhibit gallstone formation. This effect may be due to an improvement in the flow of bile[8] or to a change in the chemical composition of bile.[9]

Vitamins E and D: Fat-soluble vitamins E and D, when supplemented orally or parenterally, were effective in improving the deficiency status in children with chronic cholestasis.[10]

Ascorbic Acid: Vitamin C deficiency in animals leads to cholesterol supersaturation of bile and formation of cholesterol gallstones. Ascorbic acid (vitamin C) appears to help break cholesterol down in bile. Vitamin C deficiencies have been associated with a higher risk for gallstones. Sixteen patients with gallstones who were scheduled for surgery received 500 mg of vitamin C four times a day for two weeks prior to surgery. The treatment resulted in a significant decrease in phospholipid concentration in bile.[11]

A study with over 13,000 subjects that was published in the Archives of Internal Medicine (2000) found that vitamin C offered greater protection for women than men against both known gallbladder disease and undetected gallstones (patients had gallstones but had reported no abdominal pain).[12] Women with higher blood levels of vitamin C were half as likely to develop gallstones.

Regular vitamin C supplementation and, to a lesser extent, increased physical activity and higher total cholesterol levels were associated with a reduced prevalence of gallstones.[13]

Dissolving Stones: Irish researchers developed a mixture of six naturally occurring plant-derived compounds: menthol, menthone, pinene, borneol, camphene, and cineol (Rowachol®). This formula is reported to shrink or dissolve gallstones in some patients and appears to be free of adverse effects.[14]

Gastritis

Gastritis is a general term for a group of conditions that cause inflammation, irritation, or erosion of the mucosal barrier lining the stomach. Pain or discomfort in the upper abdomen is the most common symptom. However, symptoms do not necessarily correspond to the extent of physical changes in the stomach lining. Severe gastritis may be present on endoscopy without the patient having any symptoms. Conversely, severe symptoms may be present with minimal or no changes visible in the lining. Gastritis, whether associated with an autoimmune process, chemical injury, or *H. pylori* infection, underlies the development of peptic ulcer disease and gastric cancer. The goals of treatment are to reduce gastric inflammation, relieve symptoms, and eliminate the underlying cause, if possible.

THERAPEUTICS

Antacids neutralize existing stomach acid and can provide rapid pain relief.[1] Over-the-counter products that neutralize stomach acid include aluminum hydroxide (Amphojel, AlternaGEL), magnesium hydroxide (Phillips' Milk of Magnesia), aluminum hydroxide and magnesium hydroxide (Maalox, Mylanta), calcium carbonate (Rolaids, Titralac, Tums), and sodium bicarbonate (Alka-Seltzer).[1]

Acid blockers, also called histamine (H-2) blockers, reduce the amount of acid released into the digestive tract, which relieves gastritis pain and encourages healing. Available by prescription or over-the-counter, acid blockers include ranitidine (Zantac), famotidine (Pepcid), cimetidine (Tagamet HB), and nizatidine (Axid AR).[1] Recently the FDA alerted the public that the drug ranitidine (Zantac) can contain a cancer-causing impurity called N-nitrosodimethylamine (NDMA). No recall of the drug has been issued.

Proton pump inhibitors reduce acid by blocking the action of the parts of cells that produce acid. These drugs include the prescription and over-the-counter medications omeprazole (Prilosec), lansoprazole (Prevacid), and esomeprazole (Nexium).[1]

Diet: Affected individuals should avoid spicy foods, alcohol, coffee and caffeinated drinks, fatty, and fried foods.[1]

Drugs: NSAIDs should be taken with food and/or antacids. Another option is to cut down or switch from aspirin or NSAIDs to acetaminophen. Patients should NOT stop any prescribed medication without first talking to their doctor.[1]

Ascorbic acid plays a key role in healing and protection of the gastric mucosa from injurious insults. Vitamin C deficiency has repeatedly been linked with peptic ulcer disease and its complications.[2] Increased consumption of ascorbic acid seems warranted with gastritis.

Gastroenteritis (Viral)

Gastroenteritis, also called stomach flu, is inflammation of the stomach and intestines, typically resulting from a viral infection. Acute diarrhea and vomiting are most frequently infectious in origin with viral gastroenteritis being the second most common illness in the U.S. It is common in children and presents most often as diarrhea. Symptoms of acute gastroenteritis in adults are pathogen dependent and frequently include vomiting, diarrhea, abdominal and headache pain, and fever.[1] Gastroenteritis can lead to dehydration, morbidity, and in some countries substantial mortality.

CARE CONSIDERATIONS

Antidiarrheal agents (e.g., bismuth subsalicylate or loperamide) should be considered if there is no suspicion of *C. difficile* or *E. coli* O157:H7 infection.[2]

Zinc sulphate has been used successfully to treat this condition. The World Health Organization and UNICEF recommend daily 20 mg zinc supplements for 10 to 14 days for children with acute diarrhea, and 10 mg/day for infants under six months old, to curtail the severity of the episode and prevent further occurrences in the ensuing two to three months, thereby decreasing the morbidity considerably.[3] This medication should be taken one hour before or two hours after meals. Zinc may be taken with a small amount of food to help avoid or diminish stomach upset.[4]

A pooled analysis of all published and unpublished randomized controlled trials of zinc supplementation in children up to five years old with acute or persistent diarrhea found that zinc-supplemented children had a 15% lower probability of continuing diarrhea on a given day in the acute-diarrhea trials.[1] Similarly, there was a 24% lower probability of continuing diarrhea and a 42% lower rate of treatment failure or death in the persistent-diarrhea trials.[3] A more recent meta-analysis reported zinc supplementation reduced the incidence of diarrhea by approximately 20%, especially in children older than one year.[5]

Genital Herpes/Herpes Genitalis

Genital herpes is one of the most common sexually transmitted diseases in the U.S. Herpes genitalis can be caused by herpes simplex virus (HSV-1), but is mostly caused by HSV-2, and is characterized by a high rate of recurrences. Most people with the virus don't have symptoms. When symptoms do occur, they typically include small blisters in the genital region that break open to form painful ulcers. Even without signs of the disease, herpes can still be spread to sex partners.[1]

MANAGEMENT APPROACHES

Zinc Sulphate ($ZnSO_4$): In vivo use of zinc acetate gel has been found to be effective in preventing sexual transmission of HSV-2 and HIV infections.[2]

Topical 1%, 2%, and 4% zinc sulphate for three months was effective in treating and preventing herpes genitalis.

Topical $ZnSO_4$ has been found to be an effective therapeutic modality not only for treatment but also for prolonging remissions. It has been found to be the most efficacious of the three concentrations and without any side effects.[3]

Aloe Vera: Evidence shows that applying an aloe extract 0.5% cream three times daily increases healing rates in men with genital herpes.[4]

Geographic Tongue

Geographic tongue is characterized by irregular patches on the surface of the tongue. This gives the tongue a map-like appearance. It is caused by a loss of the tiny, finger-like projections, called papillae, on the tongue. Geographic tongue usually has no symptoms. Occasionally geographic tongue may cause a burning or smarting sensation of the tongue causing patients to seek treatment. In most cases, there is no need for treatment.

TREATMENT OPTIONS

Diet: Avoidance of alcohol, hot, spicy, and sour foods, and acidic fruits and beverages is recommended to help prevent worsening of symptoms.[1]

B Vitamins: Geographic tongue may be caused by a lack of vitamin B6 or B12.[2,3,5]

Zinc supplements have been used to treat geographic tongue.[4,5]

Vitamin E: Oral doses of vitamin E have also been used to treat this condition.[6]

Folic acid deficiency has been associated with geographic tongue.[7,8]

For symptomatic lesions, topical corticosteroids, antihistamines, vitamin A, zinc, and acetaminophen have been shown to be effective.[1]

Gingivitis

Gingivitis is the most common form of mild periodontal disease. It causes inflammation, redness, and swelling of the gingiva, or part of the gum, around the base of the teeth. Bleeding gums are a sign of gingivitis, or inflammation of the gums. It is a common and mild form of gum disease caused by a buildup of plaque at the gumline. The goal of treatment is to reverse the damage from gingivitis and to prevent progression to periodontitis because gum disease is the leading cause of tooth loss in adults.

RESEARCH STUDIES

Ascorbic acid and its relationship with periodontal disease is well-documented. In periodontal disease, vitamin C concentration is low in the blood plasma.[1] Ascorbic acid deficiency has been shown to be a conditioning factor in the development of gingivitis.[2] When humans are placed on ascorbic acid-deficient diets there is increased edema, redness, and swelling of the gingiva,[3] which demonstrates that too little vitamin C can cause ascorbic acid-deficiency gingivitis.[4] An older study demonstrated that 14 of 14 patients with gingivitis treated with large doses of ascorbic acid had favorable results.[5]

Guava and Vitamin C: In a population of young non-smoking adults, consumption of either 200 gm guava/day or 200 mg synthetic vitamin C/day, prior to and during the oral hygiene abstention period, was shown to have a preventive effect on the development of experimental gingivitis as compared to the control group that developed the usual amount of experimental gingivitis.[6]

Calendula, Rosemary, and Ginger: A combination mouthwash containing calendula, rosemary, and ginger for two weeks decreased plaque, gum inflammation, and bleeding compared to a placebo mouthwash. The combination mouthwash worked as effectively as chlorhexidine mouthwash.[7]

Zinc: Using toothpastes containing zinc, with or without an antibacterial agent, can help prevent plaque and gingivitis.[8]

Aloe Vera Juice: In a mouth rinse study of 300 healthy people, researchers compared 100% pure aloe vera juice with the standard mouthwash ingredient chlorhexidine. After four days of use, the aloe vera mouth rinse appeared to be just as effective as chlorhexidine in reducing dental plaque.[9]

Glaucoma

Glaucoma is a group of eye conditions that damage the optic nerve, leading to loss of vision or blindness. Glaucoma develops often as a result of abnormally high pressure in the anterior chamber of the eye. However, not every person with increased eye pressure will develop optic nerve damage.[1]

There are two major types of glaucoma: open angle and closed angle. Open angle is the most common form, accounting for 90% of all cases. At first, open-angle glaucoma has no symptoms. It causes no pain and vision stays normal. Nonetheless, over time and without treatment, increased intraocular pressure damages the optic nerve. In closed-angle glaucoma, drainage canals are blocked so pressure in the eye increases. Individuals with glaucoma gradually lose their peripheral (side) vision. If glaucoma remains untreated, objects to the side and out of the corner of the eye can be missed. In more advanced cases, patients often report that their vision is like looking through a tunnel. Over time, central vision may also decrease until no vision remains.[1]

Glaucoma is a leading cause of blindness in patients over 60. In glaucoma, the progressive deterioration of the optic nerve is caused by loss of a specific neuronal population known as retinal ganglion cells (RGC). People with the highest risk of developing glaucoma are African Americans over 40, everyone over the age of 60 (especially Mexican Americans), and patients with a positive family history of glaucoma.[1] Eye drops, medications, and surgery are standard treatments.

PREVENTIVE PROPOSALS

Diet: Large amounts of caffeine may increase eye pressure and should be avoided.[2]

Exercise: Regular exercise may reduce eye pressure in open-angle glaucoma.[2]

Ascorbic Acid: Although effective prescription medications are available for this problem, vitamin C may provide additional benefit. In one study, patients with elevated intraocular pressure who took at least 10 gm/day of vitamin C had a significant reduction in eye pressure. The average decline was 5.6 mm Hg, which is a medically significant improvement.[3]

Choline: A study treating open angle glaucoma used citicoline (1,000 mg/day by intramuscular injection) or a placebo. Citicoline was found to enhance retinal function and neural conduction along post-retinal visual pathways, such that responses of the visual cortex to stimuli were significantly improved compared to a placebo.[4]

Citicoline: Oral citicoline (four cycles of 500 mg/day for four months followed by a two-month washout period) was also found to significantly reduce the rate of visual field loss and the level of intraocular pressure in 41 patients with progressive glaucoma.[5]

CDP-choline (citicoline) and choline salts, such as choline chloride and choline bitartrate, are available as supplements.[5,6]

Bilberry: Research indicates that taking 60 mg anthocyanin, a type of flavonoid from bilberry, bid for 12 months or more, can improve vision in individuals with glaucoma.[7]

Glomerulosclerosis

Glomeruli are the functional units of the kidneys that enable nephrons to filter waste products such as urea out of the blood. Glomerulosclerosis is scarring or hardening of the glomeruli. This damage can result in proteinuria (loss of large amounts of protein [i.e., albumen] from the blood into the urine), microscopic hematuria (blood and casts in the urine), hypertension, and the nephrotic syndrome (proteinuria plus low albumen and high fat in the blood along with edema in the legs feet or ankles). Glomerulosclerosis may develop in children or adults. African Americans are at higher risk.

Glomerulosclerosis frequently complicates diabetes and severe hypertension. Other causes of this disorder include lupus, sickle cell anemia, drugs (heroin, bisphosphonates, anabolic steroids), infections, segmental glomerulosclerosis (FSGS), and obesity. Glomerulosclerosis can lead to kidney failure, requiring dialysis or a kidney transplant. The best treatment for glomerulosclerosis depends on what caused the scarring. The FDA has not approved any drug specifically for treatment of glomerulosclerosis.

CONTROLLING AND PREVENTING GLOMERULOSCLEROSIS

Nonpharmacologic Measures: To help prevent and control glomerulosclerosis, consider vitamin E because it blunts the rise in mesangial diacylglycerol levels induced by high blood sugar; lipoic acid's potent antioxidant activity antagonizes the impact of oxidant stress on TGF-beta expression; pyridoxamine inhibits production of advanced glycation endproducts; arginine, high-dose folate, vitamin C, and salt restriction may support glomerular production of nitric oxide; and soy isoflavones may induce nitric oxide synthase.[1]

Tocopherol: There is some evidence that taking vitamin E by mouth may improve kidney function in children with glomerulosclerosis.[2]

Glossalgia

Pain in the tongue is known as glossalgia, or burning mouth syndrome. It is described as a burning sensation, discomfort, pain, irritation, or rawness of the tongue, lips, or oral cavity, often without organic cause.

PALLIATIVE PROCEDURES

Riboflavin and folic acid have been recommended as treatments for this disorder.[1]

Oils: Lubricating the tongue with a liquid version of vitamin A, peach oil, or with a solution of citral, trimecaine, or rosehip oil can help relieve pain, soothe mucous membranes, heal wounds, and help with overall dryness by increasing salivation.[2]

Glucose-6-Phosphate Dehydrogenase (G6PD) Deficiency

Glucose-6-phosphate dehydrogenase deficiency is a genetic disorder that occurs almost exclusively in males. This condition mainly affects red blood cells. G6PD deficiency along with other provoking factors can cause the sudden premature destruction of red blood cells, leading to hemolytic anemia with jaundice. Recurring brief episodes of hemolytic anemia are the hallmark of the disease.

Symptoms during a hemolytic episode may include dark urine, fatigue, paleness, rapid heart rate, shortness of breath, and yellowing of the skin (jaundice).[1] In patients with glucose-6-phosphate dehydrogenase deficiency, hemolytic anemia is most often triggered by bacterial or viral infections or by certain drugs (antibiotics and medications used to treat malaria). A hemolytic episode can also occur after eating fava beans or inhaling pollen from fava plants (a reaction called favism).[1] In the U.S., G6PD deficiency is more common among males (particularly African Americans).

MANAGEMENT TECHNIQUES

Diet: Fava beans and all other legumes (e.g., beans, peas, and lentils) should be avoided as they tend to cause a hemolytic crisis.

Medicines that provoke red blood cell destruction, especially oxidative drugs, should be stopped.[2] A list of medications to be avoided can be found on the website listed in the References section.[2]

Folic acid and iron are potentially useful in minimizing hemolysis.[2]

Tocopherol: Research shows that taking vitamin E by mouth, alone or together with selenium, may benefit those diagnosed with G6PD deficiency.[3,4,5] Prolonged treatment with at least 100 mg/day increases the survival time of erythrocytes.[6]

Glutaric Acidemia/Glutathione Synthetase Deficiency

Glutaric acidemia types I (80%–90%) and II (10%–20%), also known as glutaric aciduria, are inherited disorders in which the body is unable to process certain fats and proteins properly. Because the enzyme glutathione synthetase is deficient, infants with glutaric acidemia type I (GAI) cannot break down the amino acids lysine, hydroxylysine, and tryptophan, which are building blocks of protein.[1] Normally these amino acids are broken down into a substance called glutaric acid which is then converted into energy. The breakdown products resulting from incomplete processing of these amino acids can damage the brain.

For most children with GAI, if untreated, an infection or fever will trigger an episode that causes serious damage to the basal ganglia.[2] Hemolytic anemia and metabolic acidosis often occur in the mild form of GAI.[1] Signs and symptoms first occur in infancy or early childhood but in a small number of affected individuals, the disorder first becomes apparent in adolescence or adulthood. The disease is characterized by an enlarged head (macrocephaly), drowsiness, decreased muscle tone (hypotonia), developmental delay, vomiting, and excess acid in the blood.[1]

THERAPY CHOICES

Diet: High-protein foods such as meat, fish, cheese, eggs, and nuts need to be eliminated.[3] Strict dietary control may help limit progression of the neurological damage. Restriction of lysine, hydroxylysine, and tryptophan is essential. Supplementation with amino acid based formulas provide energy, nitrogen, vitamins, and minerals which can promote anabolism and growth.[4]

L-Carnitine/Riboflavin: In addition to restricting amino acids, supplementation with L-carnitine (100 mg kg-1 day-1) and riboflavin (100–300 mg/day) has been successful in treating GA types I and II.[4] L-carnitine and riboflavin may arrest the neurologic deterioration in type I.[5] For type II early adult onset, in one case study riboflavin therapy and a fat-restricted, carbohydrate-enriched diet resulted in dramatic improvement.[6]

Sodium bicarbonate is used to correct metabolic acidosis.[7,8]

Vitamins E and C: Supplemental therapy with vitamins E and C, which have antioxidant properties, should also be given.[7,8]

Tocopherol: Several studies report that vitamin E can be of benefit in the treatment of glutathione synthetase deficiency.[9,10,11]

Gluten Enteropathy

See **Celiac Disease**

Goiter (Endemic Goiter)

A goiter is an abnormal enlargement of the thyroid gland. Endemic goiter is an iodine-deficiency disease (IDD). Endemic goiters occur in those areas where the iodine content of the soil is so low that insufficient iodine is obtained through food and water and when no provision is made for supplying iodized salt. In the U.S., where the use of iodized salt is common, a goiter is most often due to Grave's disease, Hashimoto's disease, multinodular goiter, solitary thyroid nodules, or thyroid cancer.[1]

MEDICAL MANAGEMENT

Iodine: Treatment depends upon the cause of the enlargement.[2] Effective prevention of endemic goiter is the regular consumption of iodized table salt. A dose of iodine, 150 mcg/day[3] up to 400 μg/day,[4] is sufficient for normal thyroid function.

Gout

Gout, or acute gouty arthritis, typically presents as an excruciating attack of pain, usually in a single joint of the foot or ankle. Gout is the most common inflammatory arthritis of men and is increasing in prevalence.[1] Gout is associated with an overproduction (10% of patients) or decreased renal excretion (90% of patients) of purines. Because the end product of purine metabolism is uric acid, gout is characterized by elevated blood uric acid levels.[2] Needle-like uric acid crystals form in joint spaces resulting in episodes of sudden excruciating pain, swelling, redness, warmth, and tenderness. Chronic inflammation and clumps of crystals (tophi) can lead to permanent joint damage, deformity, and stiffness. Tophi can also form in white chalky nodules on the helix of the ear. These tophi typically become painful before or during gout attacks.

Gout most frequently affects the metatarsal-phalangeal joint at the base of the big toe and accounts for half of all cases. Other common sites include midtarsal joints, ankles, knees, and fingers. Gout is a relatively common disease that occurs in about 4% of American adults, and is more frequent in men than women. However, women are more susceptible to gout after menopause. Gout occurs more commonly in those who regularly eat meat or seafood, drink beer, or are overweight.[3]

Gout is associated with a higher incidence of diabetes, hypertension, atherosclerosis, hyperlipidemia, kidney stones, and kidney damage.[4] Goals of treatment are to terminate the acute attack, reduce pain, prevent or reduce the number of recurrent attacks, and prevent complications associated with chronic deposition of urate crystals in tissues.

MINIMIZING PAIN

Local ice application, or an ice water soak, is an effective adjunctive treatment during an attack.[5]

NSAIDs have largely supplanted colchicine as the treatment of choice and have excellent efficacy and minimal toxicity with short-term use.[6] Naproxen (Aleve) (e.g., 500 mg twice daily) has Food and Drug Administration (FDA) approval for treating gout.[5]

OPTIONAL PREVENTIVE TREATMENTS

Recurrent gout attacks can be prevented by maintaining low uric acid levels.[5]

Alcohol restriction is important because consumption correlates with gout attacks.[5]

Folic Acid: Dr. Krut Oster treated more than 180 patients with large doses of folic acid (up to 80 mg/day) and found that it reduced serum uric acid levels in most cases.[7] Earlier studies had suggested that folic acid inhibited zanthine oxidase, the enzyme in the body that manufactures uric acid. Later studies showed that it was not folic acid itself, but a breakdown product of folic acid (pterin aldehyde) that inhibits xanthine oxidase.[8]

Vitamin C: In a study that included healthy individuals and patients with gout, a single 4 gm dose of vitamin C resulted in a three-fold increase in the urinary excretion of uric acid. In addition, daily ingestion of 8 gm of vitamin C for three to seven days produced sustained increases in uric acid excretion and significantly lowered serum uric acid levels.[9]

More recently, a prospective study that followed a cohort of 46,994 men for 20 years found that total daily vitamin C intake was inversely associated with incidence of gout, with higher intakes being associated with greater risk reductions. The results of this study also indicated that supplemental vitamin C may be helpful in the prevention of gout.[10]

Vitamin C may reduce the risk of developing gout in men. One strategy to prevent gout attacks is to reduce the amount of uric acid in the body by promoting its excretion in the urine. One study found that men who had the highest vitamin C intake were up to 45% less likely to develop the painful condition than those who had the lowest.[11]

Cherry Juice: In a 1950 study, 12 patients with gout ingested one-half pound of cherries per day. In all 12 cases, serum uric acid levels fell to normal and no further attacks of gout occurred. Cherry juice appeared to be as effective as whole cherries.[12] It is not known how cherry juice works or what the active ingredient is. Cherries or cherry extract reduced the risk of gout attacks by 35%–40% and when combined with allopurinol, risks were reduced by 75%.[13]

Diet: Losing weight reduces the number of gout attacks. A gout diet may help decrease uric acid levels in the blood to help lower the risk of recurring gout attacks and slow the progression of joint damage.[12] Patients with gout should limit their intake of purine rich animal protein (e.g., organ meats, anchovies, sardines, tuna, beef, lamb, pork, shellfish).[14,15] Saturated fats from red meat, fatty poultry, and high-fat dairy products should be avoided and replaced by lean meats and poultry, low-fat and non-fat dairy products, vegetables, and lentils as sources of protein. Reducing or avoiding beer and distilled liquors decreases the risk of gout and recurring attacks, as does limiting or avoiding sugar-sweetened foods such as sweetened cereals, baked goods, and candies.[15,16] Consumption of vegetables and low-fat dairy products is encouraged.[5]

Corn Syrup Restriction: All patients with gout should be advised to make dietary changes to limit or eliminate high fructose corn syrup. Dietary intake of high fructose corn syrup has been shown to increase uric acid production as a byproduct of adenosine triphosphate catabolism.[14]

Citric acid is used to make the urine less acidic. Less acidic urine helps the kidneys get rid of uric acid and thus helps to prevent gout and certain types of kidney stones (urate). Potassium citrate is a citric acid supplement commonly used to prevent and treat gout flare-ups by lowering blood uric acid levels. At a dose of 3 gm/day for 12 weeks, uric acid levels were significantly reduced.[17]

Granuloma Annulare (Localized)

Localized granuloma annulare is characterized by the presence of small, raised, red bumps (nodules or papules) that generally appear arranged in a ring on the skin, although the ring may not always be closed. This chronic degenerative skin disorder affects twice as many women as men. In most cases, granuloma annulare is asymptomatic and no treatment is required because the patches disappear by themselves in a few months, leaving no trace. Nonetheless, treatment is often sought for cosmetic reasons. In some cases, the lesions can last for years. While granuloma annulare resembles a tinea infection, also known as "ringworm," there is no itching or scaling.

THERAPEUTIC NUTRITION

Vitamin E has been used to treat granuloma annulare.[1]

In one study, 30 patients applied vitamin E topically, two to three times a day for three months. Complete resolution of lesions was observed in 57% of those patients.[2] The authors of the study concluded that vitamin E for granuloma annulare allows fast and uncomplicated administration of the vitamin to the lesion, has a good therapeutic ratio without any adverse effects, can be used in children without precautions, and is also cost-efficient.[2]

Topical or oral vitamin E are possible alternatives to consider in the treatment of recalcitrant generalized granuloma annulare.[3]

Vitamin D: In one instance, a case of granuloma annulare resolved with oral-activated vitamin D. The patient was a 40-year-old woman who had a 12-year history of the disease on her legs.[4] She was effectively treated with .25 micrograms of vitamin D3 per day.

Gray Hair

At some stage in their lives, both men and women will experience the onset of gray hair. Premature graying of hair is a cosmetic concern for a number of individuals. Gray hair can be harder to color as it is more resistant to hair dye due to a decreased amount of melanin. Gray hair can also be the result of a medical condition. Deficiencies of vitamin B6, B12, biotin, vitamin D, or vitamin E can contribute to premature graying as can thyroid disease or vitiligo.[1,2] Low levels of serum ferritin (iron) and low levels of the good cholesterol (HDL-C) were found to be common in affected individuals with premature hair graying.[1] Finally, smokers are 2½ times more likely to start graying before age 30 as non-smokers.[1]

COSMETIC CONSIDERATIONS

Avoidance of Nicotine: Smokers are four times more likely to have gray hair than non-smokers and smoking has been conclusively linked to accelerated hair loss.[1]

Para-Aminobenzoic Acid (PABA): PABA 6–24 gm/day taken orally for six weeks restored hair color for about 25% of subjects.[2,3] In a previous study, 200 mg of PABA per day administered to 30 patients for two months darkened hair color for all participants.[4,5]

A typical therapeutic dosage is 300–400 mg/day. Side effects have been noted in doses above 8,000 mg/day.[6]

Vitamin Deficiencies: When vitamin deficiencies (e.g., vitamin B6, B12, vitamin D, biotin, or vitamin E) contribute to prematurely white or gray hair, then correcting these deficiencies may reverse the problem or prevent it from worsening.[1,7]

Gynecomastia

Gynecomastia is a benign proliferation of glandular breast tissue in boys or men. Gynecomastia can affect one or both breasts. Shifting hormone levels in puberty or middle age (physiologic gynecomastia), too much alcohol, street drugs (amphetamines, heroin, marijuana, and methadone), and many different classes of prescription medications can cause this condition. A number of medical conditions can also cause this disorder. As a rule, no treatment is required for physiologic gynecomastia[1] and many cases of asymptomatic gynecomastia in adults resolve without any treatment in six months to two years.[2] Even for symptomatic male breast tissue enlargement, in most cases over time fibrotic tissue replaces the symptomatic proliferation of glandular tissue, meaning that the pain and tenderness will resolve.[3]

CARE FOR THIS DISORDER

Any known causative medications should be withdrawn and illegal drug use must be stopped. Most other cases remit spontaneously or disappear after any causative drug (except perhaps anabolic steroids) is stopped or the underlying condition is treated.[4]

Diet: It is best to avoid food and drink items that are high in phytoestrogens (e.g., flax-seeds, soybeans, wheat, beans, carrots, nuts, potatoes, coffee, alcohol, and marijuana) so that the condition will not worsen.[5]

Underlying causative medical conditions (e.g., hyperthyroidism, hyperprolactinemia) should be addressed.[5] Hormonal dysfunction is common in men with renal failure because of the overall suppression of testosterone and testicular damage due to uremia. Treatment should be directed to improving any underlying illness.[6] One study reported that hyperprolactinemia in uremic men was reduced with zinc supplementation.[7]

McGregor et al. showed that administration of 5 mg/day folic acid to uremic patients could decrease their blood homocysteine level.

Thiamine: Patients with gynecomastia are often responsive to thiamine (vitamin B1) therapy.[8] Adult doses range from 30–100 mg/day.

Diuretics, Salt Restriction, and Tocopherol: Traditionally, diuretics and salt restriction have been recommended. Data concerning the nutritional impact of vitamin E has also been reported.[9]

Surgery is a gold standard therapy for symptomatic gynecomastia that persists for more than one year.[10]

Gyrate Atrophy of the Choroid and Retina

Gyrate atrophy is an inherited disorder of protein metabolism characterized by progressive vision loss. Individuals with this disorder have an ongoing loss of cells (atrophy) in the retina of the eye and in a nearby tissue layer called the choroid.[1] Symptoms such as myopia, night blindness, and loss of peripheral vision develop during childhood. Over time, the field of vision progressively narrows, resulting in tunnel vision. These vision changes may lead to blindness by about the age of 50. Most patients with gyrate atrophy have no symptoms other than vision loss.[2]

Gyrate atrophy is caused by an ornithine aminotransferase (OAT) gene mutation (located on chromosome 10), which is responsible for making the enzyme ornithine aminotransferase. The OAT enzyme helps in energy production in the cells. Because of this deficiency, there is a 10- to 20-fold increase of ornithine concentrations in body fluids that can cause a variety of signs and symptoms such as numbness, tingling, or pain in the hands or feet.[2]

TREATMENT MEASURES

Dietary Restriction: Limiting arginine, which is a precursor to ornithine, intake through proteins in the diet benefits some gyrate atrophy patients. However, this diet is difficult to maintain and must be monitored by pediatricians with experience in this metabolic disease.[3,4]

Vitamin B6 therapy in individuals who respond can help decrease ornithine levels in the blood. In one case study, a patient was treated with a high-dose pyridoxine supplement (300 mg/day for six months) and the ornithine level of his serum was successfully reduced.[5]

H. Pylori Infection

H. pylori is thought to be responsible for at least half of all peptic ulcer disease and most ulcers not due to NSAIDs.[1] *H. pylori*, previously known as *Campylobacter pylori*, is a common type of gram negative bacteria that grows in the digestive tract and has a tendency to attack the stomach lining. It infects the stomachs of roughly 60% of the world's adult population. Most people never suspect they have an *H. pylori* infection, because they do not have signs or symptoms. When symptoms do occur, they mimic gastritis with stomach discomfort, bloating, frequent burping, or nausea. In addition to peptic ulcers, *H. pylori* can also cause gastritis and stomach cancer. The goals of therapy are to maintain the microorganism at a low level or eliminate it, prevent complications, and to reduce morbidity.

MEDICAL MANAGEMENT TECHNIQUES

Avoidance of Alcohol and Nicotine: Alcohol intake and smoking should be reduced or eliminated.

Eradication of *H. pylori* is typically attempted with clarithromycin triple therapy (consisting of a PPI, clarithromycin, and amoxicillin or metronidazole for 14 days). The treatment success of standard triple therapy has, however, recently declined to unacceptable levels (i.e., 80% or less).[2]

Reduce NSAID (e.g., aspirin, ibuprofen, naproxen sodium) intake, if possible, in favor of Tylenol (acetaminophen).

Vitamin C: Omeprazole (Prilosec) used to treat *H. pylori* infection can worsen stomach inflammation. Taking vitamin C may decrease this side effect.[3] The role of vitamin C as an anti-*H. pylori* agent in peptic ulcer diseases appears to be more preventive rather than curative. It is preferable to complete the conventional therapy followed by vitamin C supplementation for an extended period to prevent reinfection in susceptible individuals.[4] A preliminary study showed that vitamin C supplementation at a dose of 500 mg bid following triple therapy can be quite effective.[5]

Bismuth compounds (e.g., Pepto-Bismol) have been shown to be effective the treatment of *H. pylori* infection of the stomach.[6]

Taurine: Previous clinical studies have demonstrated that taking 500 mg of taurine twice daily together with conventional treatments for six weeks reduces *H. pylori* infection and improves ulcer healing.[7]

Probiotics: A meta-analysis showed that supplementation with *S. boulardii* significantly increased the *H. pylori* eradication rate and reduced the risk of overall *H. pylori* therapy-related adverse effects.[8]

N-Acetylcysteine (NAC) pretreatment before a culture-guided antibiotic regimen is effective in overcoming *H. pylori* antibiotic resistance.[9] NAC is a natural antioxidant and mucous-dissolving nutrient that destroys the biofilm of *H. pylori*. *H. pylori*'s biofilm helps it to survive in the stomach and resist antibiotic treatment. Like probiotics, NAC supplementation has been shown to help treat *H. pylori* infection and overcome antibiotic resistance.[10] A typical recommended dose is 600 mg three times daily between meals.[10]

Beer or Wine: In one study, individuals with a moderate consumption of beer or wine had no stomach complaints. It was found that drinking six or more glasses of beer or wine per week decreased *H. pylori* infection rates by 17%. Drinking wine and beer may even help some patients eliminate the *H. pylori* infection entirely.[11] Consuming hard liquor, however, showed no benefit.[11]

Avoidance of Caffeine: Caffeine can irritate the lining of the stomach whether *H. pylori* is present or not, so patients should avoid it.[12]

Korean Red Ginseng: In a previous clinical study, a supplementary administration of Korean red ginseng increased the eradication rates of *H. pylori*, reduced gastric inflammation, and decreased oxidative DNA damage and apoptosis.[13,14]

Cistus Laurifolius: The chloroform extract of *Cistus laurifolius* holds a significant anti-*H. pylori* effect. Accordingly, isolated flavonoids can be used as an alternative or supplement compound to the current treatment of *H. pylori* infection.[15]

Honey: One study showed that Manuka honey suppressed the growth of *H. pylori* in gastric epithelial cells.[16]

Aloe Vera: In another study, aloe vera gel was effective in both inhibiting growth of and killing of *H. pylori* strains, even those that were drug-resistant in a laboratory environment. This suggests that aloe vera could be effective against *H. pylori* infection especially when used in combination with antibiotics.[16]

Hailey-Hailey Disease

Hailey-Hailey disease, also known as familial benign pemphigus, is an inherited skin disorder. Signs and symptoms include a painful rash, blistering, and erosions in skin folds such as the armpits, groin, neck, under the breasts, and between the buttocks.[1] Symptoms are typically relapsing and remitting and are often worse in summer months due to increased heat, sweating, sunburn, infections, and friction.[1,2] The lesions may develop a yellow, crusty, overlying layer. Bacterial overgrowth can cause a bad odor and social isolation in severe cases. Treatment focuses on reducing symptoms and preventing flare-ups.

TREATMENT MEASURES

Triggers: Triggers as summarized above should be avoided. Affected areas should be kept dry. Addressing sweating with topical aluminum chloride (Drysol, Xerac AC) can be helpful. Using sunscreen and moisturizing creams, wearing loose clothing, and avoiding excessive heat may help prevent outbreaks.[1]

Cool compresses and dressings may be effective in treating mild cases.[2]

Tocopherol: Ayres and Mihan reported the successful control of the conditions of three patients with Hailey-Hailey disease by the oral administration of vitamin E in the form of d-α-tocopheryl acetate in doses of 800–1,200 IU/day. Exacerbation occurred on several occasions when the dose was notably reduced, or when the treatment stopped.[3]

Hartnup Disease

Hartnup disease, or pellagra-like dermatosis, is an inherited disorder. The majority of affected individuals have no apparent symptoms. Typical symptoms of a red, scaly, light-sensitive rash can develop on the face, arms, legs, or other exposed areas of skin. Most individuals experience their first symptoms between the ages of 3–9.[1] Cerebellar ataxia (uncoordination), spasticity, photophobia, personality changes, and gross aminoaciduria are possible. It is due to an inborn metabolic disorder caused by the body's inability to reabsorb certain amino acids, especially tryptophan, in the kidney tubule. As a result, the concentration of tryptophan increases in the urine and decreases in the blood, so there is less tryptophan available for the synthesis of niacin.[2]

Affected individuals are not able to use these amino acids to produce other substances, such as vitamins and proteins.[3]

THERAPY CHOICES

Nicotinic acid or nicotinamide (50–300 mg/day) provides relief from both the skin and neurological manifestations.[4] In one study, a 10-year-old girl who suddenly developed diarrhea and psychiatric symptoms, confusion, agitation, abnormal tone of speech, and abnormal flinging of the limbs over 15 days was suspected of having Hartnup disease. She responded dramatically to the administration of niacin 50 mg twice a day and was discharged from the hospital after seven days.[3]

Niacin (40–200 mg/day) may be required with Hartnup disease and in the carcinoid syndrome.[5]

Diet: Hartnup disease can be reduced or avoided by maintaining good nutrition, including a high protein diet, to help overcome the deficient transport of neutral amino acids in most patients.[6,7]

Avoidance of certain drugs such as sulphonamides helps to reduce outbreaks.[7]

L-Tryptophan: According to the medical literature, at least one individual showed an improvement of symptoms after treatment with the compound L-tryptophan ethyl ester. An oral challenge with 200 mg/kg of tryptophan resulted in a prompt increase of tryptophan levels in both serum and cerebrospinal fluid. Sustained treatment with 20 mg/kg q 6h resulted in normalization of serum and cerebrospinal fluid tryptophan concentrations.[1,7]

Hay Fever/Allergic Rhinitis

Hay fever, or allergic rhinitis, is inflammation of nasal mucous membranes in sensitized individuals when inhaled allergenic particles contact those membranes. Basically, the immune system overreacts to the allergens. It is the fifth most common disease in the U.S. Seasonal allergic rhinitis is more common in the spring, summer, and early fall.[1] In the spring, for example, weeds, trees, and grasses release pollen that gets into the nose and throat and can trigger an allergy. Signs and symptoms are similar to the common cold and include a runny or stuffy nose, sneezing, sinus pressure, and red, itchy, and watery eyes. Hay fever can also cause itching of the nose, throat, or the roof of the mouth.

SYMPTOMATIC CARE

Antihistamine Tablets: Second-generation, non-sedating antihistamines are the mainstay of medical treatment and many former prescription drugs (e.g., cetirizine, fexofenadine, and loratadine) are now available over the counter.

Decongestants: Many different brands of oral decongestants or nasal sprays can help relieve the stuffiness and pressure caused by swollen nasal tissue. Cromolyn is a non-sedating OTC nasal spray that is effective in both early and late phases of allergic rhinitis, reducing symptoms of nasal congestion, runny nose, and sneezing.[2]

Methylsulfonylmethane (MSM): One preliminary study found that taking 2,600 mg of MSM per day for 30 days reduced symptoms of seasonal allergies. Additional research is needed.[3]

Curcumin, a chemical found in turmeric, reduces hay fever symptoms such as sneezing, itching, runny nose, and congestion.[4]

Calcium: A placebo-controlled, double-blind, crossover study showed that 1,000 mg calcium administered orally significantly inhibited the allergen-induced swelling of the nasal mucosa in the allergen provocation test.[5]

L-Tyrosine: In a different study, some 492 patients with symptoms of respiratory or skin allergies were treated with tablets containing L-tyrosine (200 mg), vitamin B6 (2.5 mg), and niacinamide (10 mg). In severe cases, as many as six tablets four to six times per day were needed to control symptoms. Individuals with hay fever obtained relief within two to five days.[6] Higher doses of these vitamins and L-tyrosine would negate the need to take so many tablets to achieve the desired effect.

Lactobacillus: Taking two billion colony-forming units of lactobacillus daily for five weeks can improve quality of life by almost 18% in individuals with grass pollen allergy that doesn't respond to the anti-allergy drug loratadine.[7]

Vitamin C taken at a dose of 2,000 mg/day acts as a natural antihistamine to help ease nasal congestion and stuffiness.[8]

Butterbur: A Swiss study with over 330 participants concluded that butterbur extract (Ze 339) 8 mg/day was as effective as Allegra and is an effective herbal treatment for hay fever.[9]

Honey: Consuming local raw honey is believed to help with seasonal allergies. Honey also has antiseptic and antibacterial properties.[10] Children under the age of one should not be given honey.

Complementary medicine therapies, such as acupuncture, biofeedback, chiropractic manipulation, bromelain, gingko, ginseng, licorice, pycnogenol, and quercetin, are also used by individuals with allergic rhinitis.[11]

Hearing Loss/Presbycusis

Hearing loss is when an individual is unable to partially or completely hear sound in one or both ears. Hearing loss can be acute, gradual, permanent, or temporary. It is the third most common health problem in the U.S.

Presbycusis is the bilateral and symmetrical cumulative gradual hearing loss from inner ear damage occurring as a result of age or regular exposure to loud sounds, illness, and genetics. It usually occurs after the age of 50. Initially, changes in the inner ear, such as degeneration of hair cells and changes in the basilar membrane, lead to decreased hearing at higher tones and a decline in pitch discrimination. Sounds gradually become muffled, distorted, or obscured by background noises. As hearing continues to be lost, lower pitch tones also become harder to hear.[1]

Conductive hearing loss is a mechanical problem and occurs when structures cannot properly transmit sounds from the ear canal to the inner ear (cochlea) (e.g., due to wax buildup in the ears, fluid from infections or allergies, otosclerosis, cholesteatoma, and scarring).

More sudden sensorineural (inner ear) ear damage is due to the inability to transmit neural impulses from the inner ear to the brain (auditory cortex). Medical reasons underlying sudden hearing loss (e.g., head trauma, Meniere's disease, acoustic neuroma, ototoxic medications, or very loud noises) may be a medical emergency. Hearing typically returns to normal in about 50% of patients and is partially recovered in others. Sudden sensorineural deafness typically affects only one ear.[2]

CARE CONSIDERATIONS

Noise-induced hearing loss from regular activities such as target shooting, snowmobile riding, listening to music at high volume, or attending loud concerts can cause ear damage and hearing loss. The best preventatives are to wear protective earmuffs/earplugs, avoid loud noises, or to turn down the volume, if possible.[3]

Removal of ear canal obstructions, when possible, is the treatment for conductive hearing loss.

Vitamin B12: One study followed a group of 113 army personnel who had been exposed to military noise and developed noise-induced hearing loss and tinnitus. These patients had a significant decrease in blood vitamin B12 levels compared to individuals without hearing loss. These observations suggest a relationship between vitamin B12 deficiency and dysfunction of the auditory pathway.[4]

In another study, 55 women aged 60–71 years of age with presbycusis had significantly lower serum B12 levels and red blood cell folate levels. Poor vitamin B12 and folate status is thought to be associated with age-related auditory dysfunction.[5]

Magnesium: A study group included 133 patients. Of those, 73 were treated with carbogen inhalation and intravenous $MgSO_4$. The authors found that magnesium improved hearing recovery in cases of idiopathic sudden hearing loss.[6]

Taking magnesium by mouth helps prevent hearing loss in individuals who are exposed to loud noise. Also, intravenous injection of magnesium improves hearing loss that is not related to loud noise.[7] Magnesium aspartate (167 mg) mixed in 200 mL lemonade, taken daily for eight weeks, has been used to treat hearing loss.[7]

Vitamin D deficiency was diagnosed in 27 patients with bilateral deafness in a period of just over three years. Therefore, deficiency of vitamin D should be considered in the differential diagnosis of unexplained bilateral cochlear deafness. Treatment with vitamin D may prevent progressive hearing loss. It may also treat hearing loss that may, on occasion, be partially reversible.[8]

EPA/DHA: Regular fish consumption and higher intake of long chain omega-3 polyunsaturated fatty acids (PUFAs) have been associated with lower risk of hearing loss in women.[9]

Antioxidants: Research studies administered antioxidants, beta-carotene and vitamins C and E, in addition to magnesium. When administered prior to exposure to loud noise, the supplements prevented both temporary and permanent hearing loss in test animals.[10]

Folic Acid: According to the British Dietetic Association (BDA), folic acid is vital for preventing and treating age-related hearing loss.[11]

No Available Treatment: Many causes of hearing loss have no cure. Treatment involves compensating for the hearing loss with hearing aids.[12]

Heart Disease

Heart disease, also known as cardiovascular disease, comprises a range of conditions such as heart attack, heart failure, coronary or valvular heart disease, arrythmias, cardiomyopathies, and congenital heart defects. Heart disease is the leading cause of death for both men and women in the U.S. The most common cause of heart disease is coronary artery disease, which is narrowing or blockage of the coronary arteries. Coronary atherosclerotic heart disease also comprises the most common cause of cardiovascular disability. Specific treatment is contingent on the type of heart disease diagnosed.

TREATMENT GOALS

Goals of treatment are to treat symptoms as well as the underlying cause, lessen risks, and prevent progression.

Minimize Risk Factors: Being overweight is a significant risk factor for developing or worsening of heart disease. Normalizing body weight is a goal for both preventing and treating heart disease as it reduces the workload on the heart. Salt should be restricted to about 2 gm/day. Smoking is another primary risk factor for heart disease. Therefore, quitting is a major step in reducing the risk of cardiovascular disease, as is normalizing blood pressure and cholesterol.[1]

NUTRITIONAL SUPPORT TO LOWER RISKS

Magnesium: *See also* Cardiac Arrythmias.

Magnesium can perform many of the actions attributed to a diverse array of cardiac medications.[2] Magnesium (like aspirin) inhibits platelet aggregation, enhances fibrinolysis (like the "clot-busting" drugs), blocks calcium channels (like drugs such as Procardia), and dilates blood vessels (like ACE inhibitors such as Vasotec). Magnesium also improves the efficiency of heart muscle function, thereby allowing an oxygen-deprived heart to get by with less oxygen.

B Vitamins: Most researchers agree that there is enough evidence to suggest a causal relationship between hyperhomocysteinemia and coronary artery disease.[3] For decades, physicians have known that a rare, inherited form of severe hyperhomocysteinemia causes premature heart attacks and strokes. The *Journal of the American Medical Association* was the first to share that the majority of patients with hyperhomocysteinemia also had B vitamin deficiencies.[4] This study looked at 1,160 adults aged 67–96 years and found that 29.3% had homocysteine levels greater than 14 umol/L. Low levels of B vitamins played a role in 67% of these cases. Individuals can safely reduce their homocysteine level with B vitamin supplements.

Folic acid (vitamin B9) (500 mcg folic acid per day) now appears to lower the risk of heart disease by decreasing homocysteine levels.[5] Researchers believe that a daily dose of folic acid could reduce a person's risk of heart disease and stroke by about 20%.[6]

Riboflavin (Vitamin B2): High levels of homocysteine are linked to early development of heart disease. Taking riboflavin by mouth for 12 weeks decreases levels of homocysteine by up to 40% in some individuals. In addition, taking riboflavin along with folic acid and pyridoxine lowers homocysteine levels by 26% in patients with high homocysteine levels caused by medication that is used to prevent seizures.[7]

Ingestion of 75 mg of riboflavin, 400 mcg of folic acid, and 120 mg of pyridoxine acid a day for 30 days has been used to decrease homocysteine levels.[8]

L-Carnitine: A meta-analysis of 13 controlled trials concluded that including L-carnitine, in addition to other therapies in the acute setting for a heart attack (myocardial infarction), appeared to significantly cut all-cause mortality and lead to fewer angina symptoms and ventricular arrhythmias.[9]

Heart Failure/Congestive Heart Failure

Heart failure (HF) results in difficulty breathing, fatigue, and fluid retention (e.g., swollen ankles). It is one of the most serious consequences of cardiovascular disease. HF is primarily a chronic progressive condition that begins when the heart cannot pump enough blood to supply the body's needs and slowly worsens over the course of years. The heart's inability to efficiently deliver blood can be due to any structural or functional abnormality in the heart's mechanical performance (e.g., a stiff ventricle unable to allow a normal amount of blood into the chamber, or a contraction too weak to expel the needed blood volume).

Heart failure has a number of common medical causes including coronary artery disease (nearly 70% of all cases), high blood pressure, heart attack, type 2 diabetes, valvular disease, infections (cardiomyopathies), and cardiac arrhythmias.[1] Risk factors for developing heart failure are hypertension, smoking, coronary artery disease, diabetes, valvular diseases, and obesity.

Two major types of heart failure are left- and/or right-sided ventricular heart failure. Left-sided heart failure can further be divided into systolic and diastolic failure. High-output and low-output failure, as well as acute and chronic, are other useful clinical descriptions. Symptoms of heart failure (shortness of breath, fatigue, ankle swelling, etc.) can range from mild to severe, and may come and go initially.[2]

In left-sided heart failure, the left ventricle is too weak or stiff to properly circulate blood. As a result, fluid backs up in the pulmonary veins carrying blood away from the lungs back to the heart. The increased pressure forces fluid out of the veins and into the lungs' air sacs. This causes difficulty breathing (dyspnea) and shortness of breath, especially when lying flat. Shortness of breath is the main symptom of left-sided heart failure.

Right-sided heart failure usually occurs as a result of left-sided failure. Congestive heart failure and right-sided heart failure are different terms describing the same circumstance where the comparatively thinner right ventricle is too weak to efficiently pump blood returning to the heart through the lungs. This causes a back-flow of blood overfilling and distending veins (systemic venous congestion) which is one of the hallmarks of right-sided heart failure.[3] Increased venous pressure forces fluid to leak out into the tissues. The consequences are increased lung congestion; an enlarged, swollen liver; and edema (fluid) in both feet, ankles, and legs, as well as the abdomen.[4]

Because of decreased circulation and fluid buildup, symptoms such as shortness of breath (principally when lying down), fatigue, and breathlessness on exertion (e.g., climbing stairs or exercise) can develop. A dry cough may be present, especially at night. CHF is a serious chronic progressive condition that has four stages based on the severity of symptoms (e.g., shortness of breath on exertion, lying down, or just sitting). In the late stages, elevated venous pressure in the superior vena cava can cause engorged neck (internal jugular) veins.

Congestive heart failure is the most common cause of hospitalizations in elderly Americans and is associated with a poor quality of life and shortened survival. Complications include lung congestion, arrhythmias, pulmonary hypertension, angina, heart attacks, impaired liver or kidney function due to decreased blood flow leading to edema and weight gain, etc. Heart failure is associated with a pneumonia rate almost three times greater than expected and a mortality rate four times higher for a first episode of pneumonia.[5]

Reversible underlying causes of HF such as thyroid disease, tachycardia, anemia, HTN, kidney disease, CAD, valvular disease, alcohol or cocaine abuse, malnutrition, SLE, hemochromatosis, and sarcoidosis should be attended first.[6] Thereafter, the goals of treatment are to reduce symptoms, stop heart failure from getting worse, increase lifespan, and improve the quality of life.

ADDITIONAL MEDICAL MANAGEMENT CHOICES

Dietary Sodium Restriction: Sodium and water retention contribute to volume overload in HF. Therefore, salt and fluid restriction is often necessary to help avoid or minimize congestion. A low sodium diet (4 gm/day) means a no-added salt at the table diet and eliminating highly salted food such as deli meats, potato chips, pretzels, canned soups, bacon, flavor packets, etc.[7]

Regular exercise and quitting smoking are mainstays of treatment for all stages of heart failure.

Treatment of high blood pressure and high cholesterol is essential in all stages of heart failure. Lowering blood pressure in hypertensive patients and lipids in hyperlipidemic patients is important not only to help prevent heart failure but to further reduce the incidence of myocardial infarction and death.[8] For hypertension this includes dietary salt (sodium) restriction to 2–3 gm/day.

Low-Dose Aspirin: 81 mg of aspirin per day is part of guideline-directed medical therapy for heart failure and is associated with a significant reduction in mortality and morbidity risk.[9]

Coenzyme Q10 increases cardiac cell adenosine triphosphate (energy) levels by preventing the loss of the adenine nucleotide pool.[10] This enzyme also indirectly stabilizes calcium channels to decrease calcium overload.[10] Lower levels of myocardial CoQ10 are associated with increased worsening or severity of HF.[11,12] Long-term CoQ10 treatment of patients with chronic HF is safe, improves symptoms, and reduces major adverse cardiovascular events.[11]

In patients with congestive heart failure, myocardial CoQ10 content tends to decline as the degree of heart failure worsens. A number of controlled pilot trials with supplemental CoQ10 in heart failure found improvements in functional parameters such as ejection fraction, stroke volume, and cardiac output, without side effects.

An initial meta-analysis by Soja and Mortensen reported that, compared to HF patients in the placebo group, patients treated with CoQ10 achieved a better ejection fraction, stroke volume, cardiac output, cardiac index, and end diastolic volume index.[13]

By using a CoQ10 dosage of 100–200 mg/day to obtain a positive clinical effect (a dose of 100 mg twice daily provided a better absorption and a higher serum level compared with 200 mg once daily) patients achieved significant reductions in hospital stays for worsening of CHF and reduced incidence of serious complications.[14] Cardiovascular deaths were reduced by 43% and all-cause mortality by 42% in a study. Furthermore, CoQ10 supplementation improved the patients' symptoms according to the NYHA functional classification after two years.[11]

Many patients with mild CHF are given 300 mg/day of CoQ10 in divided doses.[13] More recently, larger doses were found to be effective for patients with more severe CHF.[12,15] The recommended dose is 100–1,200 mg/day.[16]

Results demonstrate that treatment with CoQ10, in addition to standard therapy for patients with moderate to severe HF, is safe, well-tolerated, and associated with a reduction in symptoms and major cardiac events.[11,17] A meta-analysis supported the use of combined CoQ10 with standard therapy in HF to reduce mortality.[12,15,18] In addition, three meta-analyses showed a significant improvement in ejection fraction, cardiac output, and stroke volume.[12,15,19]

Thiamine: Thiamine deficiency does not appear to be uncommon in patients with HF, and timely thiamine replacement promptly reverses cardiac failure resulting from severe thiamine deficiency.[20] Supplementation with thiamine (e.g., 100 mg 2–3 x/day) has been shown to improve cardiac function, urine output, weight loss, and signs and symptoms of HF.[19] Clinical trials in patients with congestive heart failure have shown that thiamine supplementation increases the systolic, diastolic, and central venous pressures, with a decline in heart rate and an increase in left ventricular ejection fraction (LVEF). Thiamine acts as a vasodilator and reduces the afterload on the heart, thus improving cardiac function.[21] Thiamine has also been reported to increase diuresis and natriuresis in patients with heart failure receiving diuretics.[21,22]

Taurine is an amino acid. Taurine is not typically considered an "essential" amino acid, since it can be manufactured in the body from the amino acid cysteine. It comprises more than 50% of the free amino acids in the heart.[23] In animal studies, taurine has been demonstrated to slow the rapid progression of heart failure and consequently prolonged life expectancy.[23] Human studies demonstrated taurine to be safe and effective in the treatment of congestive heart failure.[24,25,26]

A randomized, single-blind, placebo-controlled clinical trial was conducted on 29 patients with HF with left ventricular ejection fraction (LVEF) less than 50%. A total of 15 patients received taurine supplementation 500 mg three times a day. Taurine supplementation significantly increased exercise capacity.[27]

In a double-blind study, 58 patients with congestive heart failure received taurine (2 gm, three times a day), or a placebo, each for three weeks.[28] After treatment with taurine, there were significant improvements in shortness of breath, swelling, palpitations, and general functioning. Taurine was effective regardless of whether patients were taking digitalis, or whether the heart failure was due to impaired blood flow or to heart-valve disease.[28,29]

The results indicate that addition of taurine to conventional therapy is safe and effective for the treatment of patients with congestive heart failure.

Taking 2–3 gm of taurine by mouth one to two times daily for six to eight weeks improves heart function and symptoms in patients with moderate heart failure

(New York Heart Association [NYHA] functional class II) to severe heart failure (New York Heart Association [NYHA] functional class IV).[30]

Magnesium: The heart needs magnesium to pump efficiently. Magnesium is an arterial dilator and as such decreases the load on the heart. Patients with CHF have demonstrated plasma depletion of magnesium.[31] Magnesium sulfate and captopril reduced cardiac preload and afterload, which improved heart function.[32]

Magnesium therapy has also been effective in the prevention of arrhythmias. In patients with heart failure, low blood magnesium levels predispose to low potassium, therefore increasing the chance of developing ventricular arrhythmias and hemodynamic derangements.[33] Magnesium has also has been shown to be therapeutically helpful in patients treated with diuretics associated with the Mg^{2+}/K^{+}balance.[34]

In severe CHF, magnesium orotate (6,000 mg/day for one month, 3,000 mg/day for about 11 months) resulted in improvement in nearly 40% of patients. In patients who did not receive magnesium, 56% deteriorated. Overall, magnesium orotate increased the survival rate and improved clinical symptoms and patient's quality of life.[35]

L-carnitine deficiency has been associated with heart failure.[36] Addition of L-carnitine to standard medical therapy for heart failure has been evaluated in several clinical trials. A randomized, placebo-controlled study in 70 heart failure patients found that three-year survival was significantly higher in the group receiving oral L-carnitine (2 gm/day) compared to the group receiving a placebo.[37] Also, 5 gm of L-carnitine has been given by IV daily for seven days in addition to conventional treatment with good results.[38]

L-arginine has demonstrated improvement in cardiac performance in patients with severe congestive heart failure (CHF).[39,40,41] Infusion with L-arginine (20 gm of L-arginine by intravenous infusion over 1h at a constant rate) reduced arterial pressure, reduced heart rate (from an average of 88 beats per minute to 80 beats per minute), increased right arterial pressure, increased cardiac output, and increased stroke volume.[42] Treatment with L-arginine improved overall cardiac performance.[43]

Fifteen patients with moderate-to-severe heart failure were given the amino acid L arginine hydrochloride or a placebo, each for six weeks in a double-blind study. The initial dosage was 5.6 gm/day but was later increased arbitrarily to 12.6 gm/day. L-arginine significantly reduced the number of heart-disease-related limitations. L-arginine treatment also significantly increased the distance patients could walk in six minutes and increased the rate of blood flow during exercise.[44]

Vitamin D: Low serum vitamin D3 levels were highly associated with heart failure and with incident death, coronary artery disease/myocardial infarction, and stroke.[45] Previous clinical studies demonstrate that taking vitamin D3 supplements may decrease the risk of death in people with heart failure.[46]

Heartburn/Acid Reflux/Indigestion/Dyspepsia/Pyrosis/GERD

There are many different functional disorders in gastroenterology, including heartburn and indigestion. Indigestion or dyspepsia is recurrent discomfort or pain in the upper abdomen, often described as fullness, bloating, nausea, or heartburn. When acidic gastric contents flow backwards into the esophagus, it produces the symptom of burning pain in the upper abdomen or behind the lower sternum and is known as heartburn. The discomfort may rise into the chest or throat and may be accompanied by belching, a bitter taste in the mouth, regurgitation, or water brash.

Heartburn and indigestion are quite common and are seen in people of all ages. Causes include overeating, NSAIDs, obesity, diet (*see below*), drinking alcohol, smoking, excess stomach acid secretion, ulcer, loss of lower esophageal sphincter pressure, and low levels of exercise. Symptoms are usually aggravated by overeating, bending over, or lying down, which leads to worsening of symptoms at night.

Occasional heartburn is normal and no cause to seek medical attention. Frequent heartburn (more than twice a week) that interferes with normal daily routines is considered to be chronic acid reflux or gastroesophageal reflux disease (GERD) due to lower esophageal sphincter malfunction. More than half of all patients report treatment resistant GERD.[1] Follow-up studies indicate that 70% to 90% of patients will relapse within one year of discontinuation of therapy, regardless of what therapeutic regimen had been used to induce remission.[2]

Complications from long-term acid exposure include esophagitis, esophageal strictures, Barrett esophagus, and esophageal adenocarcinoma. The goals of treatment are to reduce or eliminate symptoms, decrease frequency and duration of gastroesophageal reflux, promote healing of injured mucosa, and prevent development of complications.[3]

SYMPTOM MANAGEMENT

Nicotine and alcohol should be avoided or reduced because both interfere with the proper functioning of the lower esophageal sphincter.[4]

Diet: Losing weight helps lessen heartburn symptoms. It's best to refrain from eating within three to four hours of going to bed. Eating large meals as well as foods that result in heartburn (e.g., spicy foods, tomatoes, coffee, caffeine, and citrus) or foods that decrease lower esophageal sphincter pressure (e.g., fatty or fried meals, garlic, onions, chili peppers, chocolate, peppermint, spearmint, coffee, cola, and tea) should be avoided.[5] Include protein-rich meals to increase lower esophageal sphincter pressure.[6]

NSAIDs (e.g., aspirin, ibuprofen, or naproxen) are a significant risk factor for GERD symptoms and should be minimized or eliminated if possible. When ingested, they should be taken with food and/or with an antacid to help protect the gastrointestinal lining.

Antacids: Antacids provide immediate symptomatic relief for mild GERD and are often used concurrently with acid blockers.[6] For acid reflux, antacids are usually taken orally one and three hours after meals and at bedtime. In general, antacids should be ingested in liquid form because this probably has a greater acid neutralizing capacity than powder or tablet dosage forms.[7] Over-the-counter products that neutralize stomach acid include aluminum hydroxide (Amphojel, AlternaGEL, Gaviscon), magnesium hydroxide (Phillips' Milk of Magnesia), aluminum hydroxide and magnesium hydroxide (Maalox, Mylanta), calcium carbonate (Rolaids, Titralac, Tums), and sodium bicarbonate (Alka-Seltzer).[4,8]

Acid Blockers: Acid-suppressing therapies are the mainstay for treatment of GERD. H2-receptor antagonists in divided doses are effective in treating patients with mild to moderate GERD.[9] H-2 acid blocking products including Zantac (ranitidine 150 mg), Axid (nizatidine 150 mg), Tagamet (cimetidine 400 mg), and Pepcid (famotidine 20 mg) to reduce acid production may be taken up to twice daily for 6–12 weeks.[4,10] Recently, the FDA alerted the public that the drug ranitidine (Zantac) can contain a cancer-causing impurity called N-nitrosodimethylamine (NDMA). No recall of the drug has been issued.

Proton Pump Inhibitors (PPIs): For GERD, proton pump inhibitors provide the greatest relief of symptoms and the highest rates of healing, especially in patients with erosive disease or moderate to severe symptoms.[11] Drugs that block acid production such as Prilosec (omeprazole), Prevacid (lansoprazole), or Nexium (esomeprazole) may be taken once daily for 4–8 weeks for symptomatic GERD.[4,8,10] Symptom response to a therapeutic trial of PPIs can be diagnostic, but a negative response does not exclude GERD.[12]

Magnesium: Magnesium is a widely accepted and effective approach to treat dyspepsia or indigestion and taking it by mouth as an antacid reduces the burning symptoms.[13] Various magnesium compounds can be used, but magnesium hydroxide (e.g., Milk of Magnesia 311 mg taking 2–4 chewable tablets every four hours up to four times per day)[14] appears to work the fastest. A liquid form is also available. Taking 800 mg of magnesium oxide daily may also be beneficial.[15]

Licorice: Taking Iberogast made in Germany and containing licorice root with glycyrrhizic acid improved symptoms of heartburn. Licorice improved heartburn by 40% over placebo treatment.[16]

Heat Intolerance/Heat Stroke

Heat intolerance includes symptoms of exhaustion, fatigue, nausea, vomiting, or dizziness in response to moderately warm temperatures. Certain disease symptoms (e.g., multiple sclerosis) typically worsen with increased body temperature. Other conditions such as diabetes, Parkinson's, Grave's disease, and Guillain-Barré syndrome as well as certain medications can cause heat intolerance.

Heat exhaustion is caused by a failure of the body's cooling mechanism to maintain a normal core temperature. Symptoms of heat exhaustion include weakness, nausea, cramps, anxiety, excess sweating, syncope (fainting), rapid breathing, and a fast, weak pulse. These result in extreme exhaustion and an inability to exert oneself further. Heat exhaustion also results in water depletion or salt depletion and can lead to heatstroke, which is more serious and can be life threatening.[1]

Heat stroke, or sunstroke, is a life-threatening condition in which the body temperature rises to 104°F or higher and causes additional signs of rapid pulse, difficulty breathing, confusion, and possible coma. Complications may include seizures, rhabdomyolysis, or kidney failure. Heat stroke is relatively common in sports and is the cause of about 2% of deaths.

MEDICAL MANAGEMENT OF HEAT EXHAUSTION

First Aid: The first-line of treatment includes relocating an individual to a cool shaded atmosphere, giving water to sip, and loosening clothes. A bath of cold or ice water has been proven to be the most effective way of quickly lowering core body temperature.[2] Additional recommendations include administering 40 gm of ascorbic acid intravenously.[2]

PREVENTION OF HEAT EXHAUSTION

Ascorbic Acid: Since the symptoms and findings of heat exhaustion resemble those of circulatory collapse, it has been reasoned that ascorbic acid might be used as a preventive against heat illness in industrial workers exposed to high temperatures and high humidity in whom heat exhaustion occurred in a known incidence. Even though workers were exposed to temperatures of 100°F–120°F for 29 consecutive days, none of those who took 100 mg of vitamin C/day plus seven grains of sodium chloride with three grains of dextrose hourly in the form of tablets showed any signs of heat illness.[2]

Fluids: Additional measures for prevention include drinking plenty of fluids and drinks that contain electrolytes to help prevent dehydration.[3]

Alcohol: Alcohol should be avoided in hot weather.[4]

Clothing: Light-colored, loose fitting clothing should be worn in hot weather.[4]

Sunlight: Direct sunlight should be avoided.[4]

Heavy Metal Poisoning

See also Arsenic Toxicity, Cadmium Toxicity, and Lead Poisoning

The heavy metals most commonly associated with poisoning of humans are lead, mercury, arsenic, and cadmium. Heavy metal poisoning may occur as a result of industrial exposure, air or water pollution, foods, medicines, improperly coated food containers, or the ingestion of lead-based paints.

TREATMENT PROTOCOLS

Chelation therapy is the standard medical treatment.

Ascorbic Acid: Vitamin C supplements and vitamin C rich fruits such as gooseberries provide protection against metal induced hepatotoxicity.[1] Apart from its well-established antioxidant properties, vitamin C has been reported to act as a chelating agent of lead (Pb), with a similar potency to that of EDTA. Probably due to this chelating capacity, a significant decrease in blood Pb was observed in a study of 75 adult smokers receiving 1 gm vitamin C daily for one week.[2]

Vitamin C also reverted hematological changes in mercury and cadmium-exposed animals.[3]

Alpha Lipoic Acid (ALA): Studies show that ALA binds with toxic metals such as mercury, arsenic, iron, and other metals that act as free radicals.[4]

Hemorrhoids

Hemorrhoids are dilated veins (submucosal vascular tissue) in the rectum and distal anal canal. Hemorrhoids develop when the venous drainage of the anus is altered, causing the venous plexus and connecting tissue to dilate. This connective tissue, when weakened, leads to descent or prolapse of the hemorrhoids.[1] Affected veins become more swollen due to increased pressure from pregnancy, being overweight, or from chronic constipation, or straining at the stool.

Internal hemorrhoids are typically painless. In contrast, external hemorrhoids cause pain, itching, bleeding, and possible swelling in the anal region. Hemorrhoids are one of the most common causes of rectal bleeding. Rarely dangerous, hemorrhoids usually clear up in a few weeks. For pregnant individuals, most hemorrhoids regress after childbirth. The most common and serious complications of hemorrhoids include perianal thrombosis and incarcerated prolapsed internal hemorrhoids with subsequent thrombosis. They are characterized by severe pain in the perianal region possibly with bleeding.[1]

CLINICAL TREATMENT OPTIONS

General Instructions: Symptomatic, painful hemorrhoids may be managed with stool softeners (e.g., docusate, psyllium) and warm sitz baths (i.e., sitting in a tub of tolerably hot water for 10 min) after each bowel movement and as needed thereafter. Anesthetic ointments containing lidocaine or witch hazel compresses may be utilized, as well as soothing wipes (Tucks), creams, or salves.[2]

Diet: The American Gastroenterological Association recommends increased fluid intake, adding fiber (25–25 gm/day) to the diet to minimize constipation with its associated prolonged straining, and moderate exercise to stimulate bowel function as the mainstays of medical management.[3,4,5] Soluble fiber supplementation decreases bleeding of hemorrhoids by 50% and improves overall symptoms.[6]

Cold Compress: A cold compress to the affected area can reduce swelling and moist towelettes can be substituted for dry toilet paper.[4]

Nitroglycerine Ointment: Dr. Stephen Gorfine at Mount Sinai School of Medicine reduced hemorrhoid pain by about 60% using topical nitroglycerine ointment.[7,8]

The nitroglycerin ointment application works by relaxing the internal sphincter muscle, which becomes abnormally tight when a thrombosed external hemorrhoid occurs. When the sphincter muscle tightens, it cuts off the amount of blood to the anal lining, resulting in acute pain.[7,8,9,10]

Methylsulfonylmethane (MSM): Research shows that applying a specific gel containing MSM together with hyaluronic acid and tea tree oil (Proctoial) for 14 days can reduce pain, bleeding, and irritation in patients with hemorrhoids.[11]

Hepatic Encephalopathy

Hepatic encephalopathy (HE) is a neuropsychiatric condition characterized by transient, gradual, or complete loss of consciousness (hepatic coma) and decline in brain function as a result of liver failure. HE describes a range of reversible neuropsychiatric abnormalities. Hepatic encephalopathy as a result of cerebral edema and intracranial hypertension is a significant cause of morbidity and mortality in advanced cirrhotic patients. Acute HE usually develops in a clinically stable cirrhotic patient as the result of an acute precipitating event such as hypovolemia, metabolic disturbances, gastrointestinal bleeding, infection, and constipation. These precipitating factors should be managed and controlled. Chronic HE, by definition, occurs and persists in the absence of precipitating factors.[1]

CARE CONSIDERATIONS

Nutrition: Protein intake up to 1 gm/kg/day. Lactulose 30 g by mouth q.i.d. as needed and titrate to 2–4 bowel movements/day.[2]

Medications that depress central nervous system function, especially narcotics and benzodiazepines, should be avoided.[1]

Carnitine: Although the mechanisms by which carnitine provides neurological protection are unknown, a systematic review of the literature confirmed that L-acetylcarnitine is promising as a safe and effective treatment for HE.[3,4] L-carnitine or a placebo was administered to 120 patients with hepatic encephalopathy for 60 days. Fasting serum ammonia levels were significantly lower at 30 and 60 days compared to baseline and placebo. Mental function was also significantly improved by L-carnitine in cirrhotic patients.[5]

Ornithine: Ornithine is used for reducing glutamine poisoning in the treatment of hepatic encephalopathy.[6]

Zinc deficiency is a near-constant finding in advanced stages of liver disease.[7]

Herpes Zoster

See **Postherpetic Neuralgia**

Hexane Inhalation

Hexane is used as a cleaning agent or to extract edible oils from seeds and vegetables as a special-use solvent. Acute (short-term) inhalation exposure of humans to high levels of hexane causes mild central nervous system (CNS) effects, including dizziness, giddiness, slight nausea, and headache. Longer exposure may result in nerve damage and paralysis of the arms and legs.[1]

CONSERVATIVE CARE

Lipoic acid (LA) has demonstrated usefulness in conferring some protection against hexane inhalation.[2,3]

Hiccups (Persistent)

Hiccups, also known as hiccoughs or singultus, are repetitive involuntary spastic contractions of the diaphragm. As the diaphragm contracts, the glottis (opening between the vocal cords) snaps shut to check the inflow of air and makes the distinctive hiccup sound. Distention of the esophagus or stomach with air or food, drinking hot fluids, alcoholic or carbonated beverages, gastroesophageal reflux, and angina pectoris can all cause hiccups.[1] Irritation of the phrenic nerves from the neck to the diaphragm, damage to the vagus nerve, and some medications can also cause hiccups.[1] Fortunately, hiccups are usually temporary, but some cases can last inordinately long.

TECHNIQUES TO ALLEVIATE LONG-TERM HICCUPS

Simple Remedies: A number of choices may be helpful for individuals with benign acute hiccups. (1) Irritation of the nasopharynx by tongue traction. (2) Lifting the uvula with a spoon. (3) Eating 1 teaspoon (7 gm) of dry granulated sugar.[2] In Sweden, people put a teaspoon of sugar into vinegar and swallow it to alleviate hiccups.[3]

Breathing into a Paper Bag: Hiccups commence most often during inspiration and are typically inhibited by elevations in the partial pressure of carbon dioxide in arterial blood (PaCO2); this serves as the basis for breath holding or breathing into a paper bag as a common therapeutic intervention.[4]

Valsalva's Maneuver: The patient can employ the Valsalva maneuver where the nose is pinched and the lips are sealed tightly. Then the patient bears down as if straining to induce a bowel movement for 10–15 seconds.

A nasogastric tube can be inserted as far as the stomach and immediately removed. The hiccups should stop at once. If not, the procedure may be repeated.[5]

Physical Maneuvers and Folk Remedies for Hiccups[1,6]

Maneuver	Effect
Scaring the patient	Vagal stimulation
Rapid uninterrupted drinking	Stimulating nasopharynx and esophagus
Eyeball compression	Vagal stimulation
Breath holding	Interruption of respiratory cycle
Supramaximal inspiration	Inducing hypercapnia
Intranasal vinegar instillation	Stimulating nasopharynx
Swallowing sugar	Stimulating nasopharynx and esophagus
Biting a lemon	Stimulating nasopharynx and esophagus
Carotid massage	Vagal stimulation[6]

Homocystinuria

Homocystinuria is an inherited disorder that prevents the full breakdown of methionine and the proper use of its breakdown product, homocysteine. This leads to an abnormal and harmful buildup of homocysteine in the blood and urine and may also cause low levels of cysteine. The disorder is characterized by myopia, dislocation of the lens in the eye, an increased risk of abnormal blood clots, brittle bones, Marfan-like features, and sometimes problems with development and learning. One type of homocystinuria results in poor metabolism of folate (vitamin B9) which also leads to excess homocysteine levels. Nutritional causes of hyperhomocysteinemia are vitamin B6 or B12 deficiency and, less often, folate deficiency.[1] These disorders can cause intellectual disability, seizures, problems with movement, and megaloblastic anemia. Homocystinuria usually does not show symptoms in a newborn baby. A goal of treatment is to decrease elevated homocysteine blood levels. In general, there are three possible therapeutic approaches to homocystinuria: (1) restriction of substrate (low methionine diet), (2) replacement of missing products (e.g., cystine), and (3) supplementation with coenzymes (pyridoxine, betaine anhydrous).[1] Nutritional causes should be handled appropriately or ruled out.

NUTRITIONAL SUPPORT

Pyridoxine is the drug of choice. Eleven patients were treated with pyridoxine (300–450 mg/day) with six of those patients achieving normal or near-normal homocysteine levels.[2] Folic acid should be given in all cases where pyridoxine is used because it causes further biochemical improvement in pyridoxine responsive patients and subjective clinical improvement in all.[3] Pyridoxine at 10 mg/kg/day up to a maximum of 500 mg/day for six weeks is recommended for infants with homocystinuria.[1] About 50% of patients have a form of cystathionine beta-synthase deficiency that improves biochemically and clinically through pharmacologic doses of pyridoxine (50–500 mg/day) and folate (5–10 mg/day).[4,5,6]

Cysteine: Vitamin B6 nonresponders may benefit from supplementation with cysteine.[7] Treatment for B6 nonresponders is multifaceted, also including supplementation with pyridoxine (vitamin B6), vitamin B12, folate, and betaine.[5,6]

Betaine: The vitamin betaine is also useful in reducing plasma methionine levels by facilitating a metabolic pathway that bypasses the defective enzyme.[6]

Diet: Dietary restriction of methionine, which is converted to homocysteine, is necessary for B6 nonresponders. This includes milk and dairy products, eggs, chicken, beef, pork, fish (halibut, salmon, sardines, mackerel), nuts, cereals, etc. Good compliance with methionine restrictions prevented ectopia lentis, osteoporosis, and thromboembolic events, and patients exhibited normal levels of intelligence.[4]

Hot Flashes/Hot Flushes/Menopausal Symptoms

Hot flashes are intense waves of heat felt over the face, neck, and chest. Hot flashes and sweating, especially night sweats, are the most common symptoms of menopause and perimenopause. Mood and sleep disturbances are also frequent complaints. Menopause marks the end of the menstrual cycles and is diagnosed after a woman has gone 12 months without a menstrual period. Some hot flashes pass in a few seconds, while others may last for more than 10 minutes. Overall, episodes of hot flashes can last several months or years. African American and Hispanic women tend to experience hot flashes for more years than white and Asian women. Researchers do not know the exact causes of hot flashes.

TREATMENT PROTOCOLS

Avoidance of Common Triggers: Alcohol, smoking cigarettes or breathing secondhand smoke, eating spicy foods, wearing tight clothing, or bending over should be avoided.[1]

Estrogen replacement is the standard medical treatment. Isoflavones (soy foods) and black cohosh (*see below*) are natural alternatives to estrogen replacement.[2] Some antidepressants may help as well.

Panax ginseng is widely used by perimenopausal women for improving energy and relieving hot flashes. It contains an active ingredient that is chemically similar to estrogen.[3]

B complex vitamins, vitamin E, and ibuprofen may be helpful.[4]

Black Cohosh: The American College of Obstetrics and Gynecology guidelines on the use of black cohosh for menopausal symptoms support its use for up to six months, especially in treating the symptoms of sleep and mood disturbance and hot flushes.

Therefore, black cohosh (20–160 mg/day) is used for the management of vasomotor menopausal symptoms. Maximum effect usually occurs in four to eight weeks.[5] Clinical studies have demonstrated that black cohosh (40–200 mg/day) is effective for hot flashes and other menopausal symptoms and is a "safe and effective alternative to estrogen replacement therapy."[6]

Soy isoflavones may have benefits for hot flashes.[7] Asian women who consume a plant estrogen known as soy isoflavones regularly are less likely to report hot flashes and other menopausal symptoms than women in other parts of the world. It is possible that this is related to the estrogen-like compounds in soy.[8]

Vitamin E: A double-blind, placebo-controlled trial was conducted. Women who took 400 IU vitamin E daily for four weeks reported statistically significant reductions in their hot flashes severity score and their daily frequency. Based on these results, the authors recommended vitamin E for the treatment of hot flashes.[9]

Another study evaluated 800 IU of vitamin E per day for survivors of breast cancer who also had hot flashes. The results showed a statistically significant reduction in hot flashes compared to a placebo.[10]

St. John's wort (e.g., 900 mg/day in divided doses) significantly reduced hot flashes (severity, duration, and frequency) compared to a placebo when used for up to 16 weeks.[11]

Nonprescription agents for hot flushes include dong quai, evening primrose oil, melatonin, red clover isoflavones, and wild yam.[12]

Huntington's Chorea

Huntington's chorea, or Huntington's disease (HD), is a devastating hereditary and progressive disorder that causes the death of neurons in parts of the brain (striatum and cortex) and results in uncontrolled jerking or writhing movements (chorea). Most patients develop signs and symptoms in their thirties or forties. The ability to function gradually worsens. Impairments in voluntary movements tend to have a great impact on an individual's ability to work, communicate, and perform daily activities. There is no treatment that can stop or reverse the course of HD. Death may ensue from pneumonia, injuries, or complications from the inability to properly swallow.

CARE CHOICES

Vitamin E: Natural vitamin E (RRR-alpha-tocopherol) can improve symptoms in people with early Huntington's disease. However, it does not seem to help people with more advanced stages of the disease.[1,2] Using a controlled double-blind crossover technique, researchers in one study demonstrated that large doses of vitamin E acetate (1,200–3,200 IU/day) had a positive effect on the symptoms of the disease.[3]

Exercise: It is extremely important for patients to maintain physical fitness as much as possible. Individuals who exercise and keep active tend to do better than those who do not.

Coenzyme Q10: Numerous studies conducted in the past decade show that CoQ10 may prove to be effective in treating HD because it can enhance ATP production. Animal studies have shown CoQ10 to significantly delay HD symptoms and increase survival.[4]

Creatine: The first clinical trial of a drug intended to delay the onset of symptoms of HD revealed that high-dose treatment with the nutritional supplement creatine was safe and well-tolerated by most participants. In addition, neuroimaging showed a treatment-associated slowing of regional brain atrophy, evidence that creatine might slow the progression of pre-symptomatic disease.[5]

Hypertension/High Blood Pressure

Hypertension, or elevated blood pressure, is the most common cardiovascular disease. It is a serious medical condition that significantly increases the risks of irreversible heart, brain, eye, and kidney damage, as well as other diseases. Hypertension may result from a specific cause (secondary hypertension <10% of cases) such as obstructive sleep apnea, renal artery stenosis, medications, or endocrine disorders, or from an unknown etiology (primary or essential hypertension >90% of cases). Blood pressure is the force of blood against the interior arterial walls. Blood pressure is determined both by the amount of blood the heart pumps and the amount of resistance to blood flow in the arteries.

Hypertension is when the force against the arterial walls is consistently too high. Normal adult blood pressure is 120/80 mm of mercury (mm Hg). Blood pressure is not a steady number; instead, it rises and falls throughout the day with changes in activity or emotion. In general terms, three blood pressure readings of systolic pressure 140 mm Hg or higher is considered to be hypertension, as is diastolic pressure of 90 mm Hg or higher. High blood pressure is known as the "silent killer" since it has no initial symptoms, but can lead to long-term disease and complications such as heart disease, heart attack, stroke, and kidney damage. High blood pressure usually develops over the course of many years and affects nearly everyone.

Men have a greater chance of experiencing high blood pressure before the age of 55. Women are more likely to have high blood pressure after menopause.[1] Smoking is a strong cardiovascular risk factor and increases the risk for developing hypertension. Smoking further exerts a hypertensive effect via the sympathetic nervous system. Hypertensive smokers are more likely to develop severe forms of hypertension, including malignant and renovascular hypertension.[2] Other contributing factors include being overweight/obese, high cholesterol, increased dietary sodium intake, decreased physical activity, increased alcohol consumption (especially binge drinking), drugs (prescription and/or street drugs), and lower dietary intake of fruits, vegetables, and potassium.

The hypertensive process is associated with serious risk of cardiovascular comorbidities such as coronary heart disease, stroke, congestive heart failure, chronic kidney disease, retinopathy, peripheral vascular disease, diabetes mellitus, metabolic syndrome, and dyslipidemia. Reducing those risks is the primary purpose of hypertension therapy.[3] Despite the availability of a wide range of antihypertensive drugs, hypertension remains poorly controlled in a majority of health care settings.[4]

SCIENTIFIC RESEARCH

Nonpharmacological approaches to the treatment of hypertension (*see below*) may suffice in patients with modestly elevated blood pressure. Such approaches also can augment the effects of antihypertensive drugs in patients with more marked initial elevations in blood pressure.[5]

Smoking cessation is the single most effective lifestyle measure for the prevention of a large number of cardiovascular diseases, including hypertension.[2]

Low-dose aspirin (81 mg once/day) appears to reduce the incidence of cardiac events in hypertensive patients.[6] Low-dose aspirin is recommended for individuals with a higher risk of CVD, ages 40–70, who are not at increased risk of bleeding.[7]

Diets: For hypertension, a diet that limits salt (sodium) to 2–3 gm/day and is high in fruit, vegetables, and fiber definitely lowers blood pressure and reduces the incidence of myocardial infarction and strokes.[8,9,10] Dietary or supplemental potassium, calcium, and magnesium consumption also helps to lower BP.[11]

Alcohol: Limit alcohol to no more than two drinks (1 oz or 30 ml ethanol; e.g., 24 oz beer, 10 oz wine, or 3 oz 80-proof whiskey) per day in most men and to no more than one drink per day in women and lighter-weight persons.[12]

Weight Loss/Exercise: Weight reduction even without sodium restriction has been shown to normalize blood pressure in up to 75% of overweight patients with mild to moderate hypertension.[13] Weight loss and sodium reduction together may allow withdrawal of drug therapy.[14] Cardiovascular, or aerobic, exercise (at least 30 minutes a day on most days) can help lower blood pressure, and assist with weight control. Exercise includes raking leaves, mowing the lawn, gardening, washing the floor, climbing stairs, walking, bicycling swimming, tennis, etc.

NSAIDs produce increases in blood pressure averaging 5 mm Hg and are best avoided in patients with borderline or elevated blood pressures.[15]

Magnesium: Magnesium intake of 500 mg/day to 1,000 mg/day may reduce blood pressure (BP) as much as 5.6/2.8 mm Hg. The combination of increased intake of magnesium and potassium, coupled with reduced sodium intake, is more effective in reducing BP than single mineral intake and is often as effective as an antihypertensive drug.[16]

Coenzyme Q10: A systematic review of eight trials using CoQ10 at various doses for essential hypertension, typically as adjuvant therapy, found a mean decrease in systolic and diastolic blood pressure of 16 and 10 mm Hg, respectively.[17] CoQ1O at a dosage of 50 mg bid for 10 weeks resulted in the systolic blood pressure decreasing nearly 20 mm Hg. The reduction in blood pressure was associated with a significant decrease in arterial resistance (i.e., less stiffness of the arteries).[18] The recommended dose is 100–1,200 mg/day.[19]

Ascorbic Acid: A recent meta-analysis of 29 short-term trials indicated that vitamin C supplementation at a median dose of 500 mg/day for eight weeks reduced blood pressure in both healthy, normotensive, and hypertensive adults.[20] Another study also noted that 500 mg/day of vitamin C added to blood pressure medication lowered systolic blood pressure.[21]

Potassium: Low potassium intake is associated with higher blood pressure in some patients; an intake of 90 mmol/day (3,750 mg/day) is recommended.[15] Increased potassium intake further results in the increased excretion of sodium in the urine. This loss of sodium helps reduce water retention, blood volume, and blood pressure.[20] Researchers found an average potassium dose of 60–120 mmol/day (2,500–5,000 mg/day) reduced systolic blood pressure and diastolic blood pressure by 4.4 and 2.5 mm Hg, respectively, in hypertensive patients.[22] Multivitamin-mineral supplements in the U.S. do not contain more than 99 mg of potassium per serving. Potassium supplements are also available as a number of different salts, including potassium chloride, citrate, gluconate, bicarbonate, aspartate, and orotate.[21]

Calcium: Research indicates that a calcium intake at the recommended level of 1,000–1,200 milligrams/day may be helpful in preventing and treating moderate hypertension.[23]

Folic Acid: Research shows that taking folic acid daily for at least six weeks reduced blood pressure in individuals with high blood pressure.[24] In addition, folic acid supplementation reduced the risk of cardiovascular and cerebrovascular events (CVCE) by 12.9% compared with control groups.[25]

Taurine: Previous clinical studies demonstrate that taking 6 gm of taurine daily for seven days or 1.6 gm of taurine daily for 12 weeks reduces blood pressure in individuals with hypertension.[26]

Vitamin D3 inhibits renin synthesis to help decrease blood pressure. Thus, vitamin D deficiency and subsequent upregulation of the renin-angiotensin system may contribute to high blood pressure. The dose-response analysis of a study with 48,633 participants estimated that every 10 ng/mL increase in serum 25-hydroxyvitamin D concentration was associated with a 12% lower risk of hypertension.[27] A meta-analysis of four prospective and 14 cross-sectional studies reported an inverse relationship between circulating vitamin D3 levels and hypertension.[28]

Berberine: Berberine was found to competitively inhibit VSMCα1 receptors, thereby blocking the release of the enzyme adenylyl cyclase.[29] A meta-analysis found that berberine (e.g., 1,000–1,500 mg/day) combined with a blood pressure lowering drug was more effective than the drug alone.[30]

Other Supplements: Olive leaf extract, garlic, potassium chloride, and flax seed have all been reported to be effective in significantly lowering BP.[31]

Hyperthyroidism

Hyperthyroidism is a condition in which the thyroid gland produces more thyroxine, or tetraiodothyronine (T4) and triiodothyronine (T3), than the body needs. Hyperthyroidism can accelerate the body's metabolism significantly causing nervousness, anxiety, rapid heartbeat, hand tremor, excessive sweating, weight loss, heat intolerance, and sleep problems. The most common cause is Graves's disease, followed by toxic nodular goiter, and toxic adenoma. Hyperthyroidism can happen at any age, but in the absence of Grave's disease, is more common in people aged 60 and older. Hyperthyroidism is also more common in women, those with Japanese ancestry, and in patients with a history of taking excess thyroid medication.[1]

MANAGEMENT TECHNIQUES

Calcium: Too much thyroid hormone can prevent the body from absorbing calcium into the bones.[2] The Institute of Medicine recommends 1,000 milligrams of calcium a day for adults ages 19–50 and men ages 51–70. That calcium recommendation increases to 1,200 mg/day for women 51 or older and men who are 71 or older.

Vitamin D: The main role of vitamin D is to maintain calcium and phosphorus homeostasis. Observational studies support a beneficial role of vitamin D in the management of thyroid disease.[3] The Institute of Medicine also recommends 600 international units (IUs) of vitamin D/day for adults ages 19–70 and 800 IUs/day for adults age 71 and older.[4]

Thiamine: Conditions that lead to increased cellular metabolism and therefore to increased demand for essential factors produce a relative deficiency of thiamine. Secondary thiamine deficiency has been reported in hyperthyroidism[5,6] for which the usual supplemental dose is 50–100 mg orally once a day.

L-Carnitine: Nutritional supplementation with L-carnitine (2–4 gm/day in two doses for two to four months) has been shown to have a beneficial effect on the symptoms of hyperthyroiditis including rapid or pounding heartbeat, nervousness, and weakness in individuals with high thyroid hormone levels. L-carnitine may also help prevent bone demineralization caused by the disease.[7,8]

Selenium is required for the metabolism of thyroid hormones. Selenium concentration is higher in the thyroid gland than in any other organ in the body. Among patients on anti-thyroid medications, those taking selenium supplements may achieve normal thyroid levels more quickly than those who do not.[9] A randomized, double-blind, placebo-controlled trial compared the effects of 200 mcg/day selenium (as sodium selenite), 1,200 mg/day pentoxifylline (an anti-inflammatory agent), or a placebo for six months in 159 patients with mild Graves' orbitopathy.[8] Compared with patients treated with a placebo, those treated with selenium reported a higher quality of life. Furthermore, ophthalmic (thyroid eye disease) outcomes improved in 61% of patients in the selenium group compared with 36% of those in the placebo group, and only 7% of the selenium group had mild progression of the disease, compared with 26% of those in the placebo group.[10]

Diet: Some cruciferous vegetables contain compounds that decrease thyroid hormone production. Examples are brussels sprouts, cabbage, cauliflower, collard greens, mustard greens, turnip roots and greens, kale, radishes, and rutabagas.[9]

Iron and Vitamin B12: Researchers found significant deficiencies of iron and vitamin B12 in individuals with hyperthyroidism.[11] Supplementation to correct any deficiency would seem warranted.

Hypoglycemia/Low Blood Sugar

Hypoglycemia is not a disease in itself, but a condition characterized by an abnormally low level of blood glucose. That means a glucose level of 70 milligrams per deciliter (mg/dL) or less. Hypoglycemia is uncommon in patients not treated for diabetes and is most often related to medications that lower blood glucose levels in the treatment of diabetes mellitus. Other conditions such as alcoholism, severe sepsis, adrenal insufficiency, and panhypopituitarism,[1] as well as diet and medications (e.g., quinine, propranolol, high doses of aspirin) can also cause hypoglycemia. As blood glucose levels fall, a variety of symptoms and signs may ensue, including hunger, sweating, pallor, shakiness, clumsiness, weakness, trouble talking, confusion, loss of consciousness, and seizures, coma, or death. In severe hypoglycemia, the patient is unable to care for himself and requires emergency medical care.

CLINICAL CARE

Diet: If a patient is prone to low blood sugar, they should avoid excessive consumption of sugar and caffeine. Alcohol should also be avoided. A diet of frequent, small, high-protein, low-carbohydrate meals is often recommended. Having a light carbohydrate snack such as toast or biscuits before going to bed, may prevent blood sugar from dropping too low during sleep.[2]

Chromium: Eight female patients with symptoms of hypoglycemia were supplemented with 200 micrograms of chromic chloride for three months in a double-blind crossover experimental design study. Chromium supplementation alleviated the hypoglycemic symptoms and significantly raised the minimum serum glucose values observed two to four hours following a glucose load.[3]

Nicotinamide: Vitamin B3 was effective in normalizing blood sugar in 507 patients with alcoholism accompanied by hypoglycemia.[4]

First Aid Instructions: Anyone who has low blood sugar should first eat or drink 15 gm of a fast-acting carbohydrate, such as:

- three to four glucose tablets
- one tube of glucose gel
- four to six pieces of hard candy (not sugar-free)
- 1/2 cup fruit juice
- 1 cup skim milk
- 1/2 cup soft drink (not sugar-free)
- 1 tablespoon honey (under the tongue so it gets absorbed into the bloodstream faster)[5]

Treat the Cause: The underlying condition causing hypoglycemia must be well-managed to prevent recurrent episodes.[6]

Hypomagnesemia

Hypomagnesemia is a deficiency of magnesium in the blood. Low levels of serum magnesium are becoming more common because the modern diet contains lower amounts of magnesium. Typically, magnesium depletion results from both inadequate intake and impairment of renal or gut absorption. Also, alcohol, diarrhea, and certain drugs (e.g., loop diuretics such as furosemide) can cause increased excretion of magnesium.[1] Magnesium deficiency can cause a wide variety of features including hypocalcemia, hypokalemia, and cardiac and neurological problems. A chronic state of low magnesium has been associated with a number of chronic diseases including diabetes, hypertension, alcohol use, hyperparathyroidism (hypercalcemia), coronary heart disease, and osteoporosis.[2]

Clinical features of deficiency are often due to accompanying hypokalemia and hypocalcemia and include lethargy, tremor, muscle fasciculations, tetany (e.g., positive Chvostek's or Trousseau's sign), seizures (especially in children), heart arrhythmias, and cardiac arrest. Serum magnesium concentration may be normal even with decreased intracellular or bone magnesium stores.[1]

Arrhythmias caused by magnesium deficiency occur more frequently in patients withdrawing from alcohol, in long-term parenteral feeding, chronic diarrhea, short-bowel syndrome, surgical drainages of the gastrointestinal tract, and with anticoagulant binding drugs.[3]

REPLACEMENT THERAPY

Magnesium salts (e.g., magnesium gluconate 500–1,000 mg po tid) given for three to four days are indicated when magnesium deficiency is symptomatic or the magnesium concentration is persistently low (i.e., less than 1.25 mg/dL).[1]

Calcium may be used as an antagonist for temporary benefit.[4] Hypocalcemia, if present, must also be addressed.

Potassium: Patients with low magnesium often have low potassium levels as well.[5]

Hypothyroidism

Hypothyroidism, also called underactive thyroid or low thyroid, is a disorder of the endocrine system in which the thyroid gland is unable to produce adequate amounts of thyroid hormone. Primary hypothyroidism (due to thyroid gland destruction) accounts for >90% of cases. The most common cause is an autoimmune disorder known as Hashimoto's thyroiditis, but other causes include thyroidectomy, radioactive iodine treatment, and radiation. Also, medications such as amiodarone and lithium may also lead to an underactive thyroid.

Clinical symptoms are nonspecific and many individuals with normal thyroid function can have them as well. They include fatigue, constipation, weight gain, coarse dry hair, depression, hoarse voice, irregular menstruation, bradycardia (slow heart rate), hypercholesterolemia, and cold intolerance.[1] Hypothyroidism is far more common in women and the prevalence of mild hypothyroidism increases in the elderly (individuals older than 60). An underactive thyroid from any cause can contribute to high cholesterol, so individuals with an underactive thyroid should have their cholesterol checked regularly.

THERAPY STRATEGIES

Thiamine: In one case study, three patients who were affected by Hashimoto's thyroiditis were taking thyroid hormone. Each patient received thiamine oral (600 mg/day) or parenteral (100 mg/ml every four days). Treatment led to partial or complete regression of the associated fatigue within a few hours or days.[2]

Zinc: A significant decrease in the level of zinc in hypothyroidism patients compared to those of normal subjects has been observed.

Zinc and Selenium: Significant decreases in blood levels of zinc and selenium have been observed in patients with hypothyroidism. The clinical significance, if any, of these findings has yet to be determined.[3]

Selenium: Hashimoto's thyroiditis, also known as chronic lymphocytic thyroiditis, is the most common cause of hypothyroidism in the U.S. Research shows that taking 200 mcg of selenium daily along with thyroid hormone might decrease antibodies in the body that contribute to this condition. Selenium might also help improve mood and general feelings of well-being in people with this condition.[4]

Ichthyosis Vulgaris

Ichthyosis is rough, thickened, cracked, and dry "fish scale" skin which is an inherited or acquired skin disorder. There are many types of ichthyoses. The most common type, ichthyosis vulgaris, slows the skin's natural shedding process. This causes chronic, excessive buildup of the protein keratin in the outermost layer of the skin (stratum corneum). Symptoms can range from mild to severe. Ichthyosis may be congenital or have delayed onset. The disease usually first manifests in early childhood.

COSMETIC PRINCIPLES

Emollients: Petroleum jelly or mineral oil should be applied bid and especially after bathing.[1]

Moisturizers: Moisturizers or lubricating creams should be used while the skin is still moist from bathing. Moisturizers with urea, alpha hydroxy acids, or propylene glycol, that help keep skin moist, are good choices.[2] Helpful lotions and creams may include 50% propylene glycol in water, or equal parts of hydrophilic petrolatum and water, or cold cream and lactic and pyruvic hydroxy acids.[1]

Humidifier: A portable home humidifier or one attached to the furnace can be used to add moisture to the air inside the home.[2]

Exfoliation: Management includes the application of over-the-counter products containing urea, lactic acid, or topical glycolic acid (4%–10%) applied to the affected areas bid or a low concentration of salicylic acid (6%) gel twice daily to remove dead skin. Mild acidic compounds help skin shed its dead skin cells. Urea helps bind moisture to skin.[2] The skin may also be rubbed with a pumice stone.[3]

Baths: Saltwater baths may be helpful[3] as well as a non-soap cleanser because soap tends to exacerbate dryness.

Vitamin D supplementation is recommended for patients with severe forms of ichthyosis.[4] In a study of seven children with congenital ichthyosis, participants saw a dramatic and excellent clinical response with regard to skin scaling and stiffness after short-term high-dose vitamin D supplementation. All cases had severe vitamin D deficiency and secondary hyperparathyroidism. The children were given 60,000 IU of oral vitamin D3 daily for 10 days. Six out of seven responded with noticeable improvement by the fifth day of treatment and achieved further improvement thereafter.[5]

Vitamin B12 injections have been found to be helpful for some individuals with ichthyosis.[5,6,7,8,9]

Vitamin A: An older case study recommends vitamin A.[10] Vitamin A (retinoid) compounds are the standard medical treatment for ichthyosis.

Immune System Dysfunction/Immunodeficiency

The overall function of the immune system is to prevent or limit infection. An example of this principle is found in immune-compromised people, who are susceptible to a range of microbes that typically do not cause infection in healthy individuals. The immune system should be able to distinguish between normal, healthy cells and unhealthy cells by recognizing a variety of "danger" cues called danger-associated molecular patterns (DAMPs). When the immune system first recognizes these signals, it needs to respond to address the specific problem. If an adequate immune response cannot be achieved, then problems like an infection can arise.[1]

Immunodeficiency disorders inhibit or prevent the body from effectively fighting infections. There are primary (inborn errors) and secondary (acquired) types. Malnutrition, diabetes, severe burns, and chemotherapy or radiation are examples of acquired types of immune deficiencies. As a result of this disorder, patients are susceptible to frequent bacterial and viral infections and have more difficulties with recovery.

IMPROVING IMMUNE FUNCTION

Correct Nutritional Imbalances: Acquired immune dysfunctions may occur with deficiencies of iron, zinc, vitamins A and B12, pyridoxine, and folic acid, or with excesses of essential fatty acids and vitamin E.[2]

Immune system dysfunction can result from single-nutrient deficiencies or excesses, alone or in combination with generalized protein-energy malnutrition. Deficits or excesses of many trace elements and single nutrients thus have potential for causing immune dysfunctions in humans. Since nutritionally-induced immune dysfunction is generally reversible, it is important to recognize and identify clinical illnesses in which immunologic dysfunctions are due to nutritional origin. Correction of malnutrition should lead to prompt reversal of acquired immune dysfunctions.[2]

Zinc is known to have beneficial effects on the immune response. Supplemental zinc (220 mg zinc sulfate twice daily for a month) was administered to 15 subjects over 70 years of age. A significant improvement in the following immune parameters was observed in the treated group: (1) number of circulating T lymphocytes, (2) delayed skin hypersensitivity reactions to purified protein derivative, and (3) immunoglobulin G (IgG) antibody response to tetanus vaccine. The data suggest that the addition of zinc to the diet of older persons could be an effective and simple way to improve their immune function.[3]

Incontinence (Bowel)

Fecal or bowel incontinence is the loss of bowel control, causing a person to pass stool unintentionally and unexpectedly. Like urinary incontinence this is a highly distressing problem that has a significant negative impact on the quality of life. Severity can range from an infrequent involuntary passage of small amounts of stool to a total loss of bowel control.

Fecal incontinence can occur during a bout of diarrhea, but for some individuals, fecal incontinence is chronic or recurring. There are two types of bowel incontinence: (1) urge, where a sudden strong urge prevents getting to the toilet in time and (2) passive, where an individual is unaware of the need to defecate. Many different medical causes of incontinence exist.

CARE OPTIONS

Diet: If incontinence is associated with loose stools, ingesting 25–30 gm of fiber per day can optimize the consistency of the stool.[1] Fiber also helps prevent constipation which can cause incontinence.

Anti-diarrheal drugs such as kaolin, pectin, activated charcoal, loperamide hydrochloride (Imodium A-D), diphenoxylate, and atropine sulfate (Lomotil), as well as aluminum hydroxide, are often utilized to increase the viscosity of the stool. Bismuth agents (Pepto-Bismol) are also used for acute episodes of diarrhea due to their antisecretory, anti-inflammatory, and antibacterial effects.[1]

Bulk-forming agents such as psyllium (Metamucil), polycarbophil (FiberCon), and carboxmethycellulose (Citrucel) absorb water and increase stool bulk.[1]

Phenylephrine Cream: Preliminary studies evaluating the effect of phenylephrine on the anal sphincter demonstrated increased resting sphincter pressure with topical application of phenylephrine cream.[1] Overall, patients reported improvement when receiving the active drug rather than a placebo, and more cases receiving phenylephrine gel achieved full continence or improved their incontinence symptoms.[2]

Bowel Training and Exercises: Perineal, or Kegal, exercises, in which there are repeated contractions of the sphincters, perineal muscles, and buttocks can strengthen pelvic floor muscles and contribute to continence, particularly in mild cases.[3]

Chlorophyllin: Early case reports indicated that chlorophyllin (Derifil) doses of 100–200 mg/day were effective in reducing fecal odor in ostomy patients.[4,5] Oral doses of 100–300 mg/day in three divided doses have been used to control fecal and urinary odor.[6]

Phenylephrine Gel: Fifteen patients with radiation-induced fecal incontinence were treated with topical phenylephrine gel applied to the anus. The median length of treatment with phenylephrine gel was 28 days. Scores improved in 11 out of 15 patients, 4 out of 15 patients showed substantial improvements of seven or more points, and seven patients considered the gel helpful. Topical phenylephrine gel for the treatment of radiation-induced fecal incontinence has not been previously reported. This small, retrospective study suggests that it may help most patients and, in some, the improvement may be substantial.[7]

Incontinence (Urinary)

Urinary incontinence is the involuntary leakage of urine so that an individual urinates when they do not intend to. Control over the urinary sphincter is either lost or weakened. Urinary incontinence is more common in older individuals, especially women. It is a distressing problem that can have a profoundly negative impact on the quality of life.

There are several types of incontinence: (1) stress incontinence is leakage of urine from laughing, coughing, sneezing, exercising; (2) urge incontinence is involuntary leakage of urine from the bladder when a sudden strong need to urinate is felt; (3) overflow incontinence involves incomplete bladder emptying; (4) functional incontinence is a condition that impairs the ability to relieve oneself in time; and (5) mixed incontinence. The goals of treatment are to restore continence, reduce in the number of UI episodes, and prevent complications.[1] Incontinence can often be cured or controlled.

MANAGEMENT TECHNIQUES

Nonpharmacologic, nonsurgical treatment (e.g., lifestyle modifications, toilet scheduling every two hours while awake, and Kegel or pelvic floor muscle rehabilitation) is first-line treatment for UI.[2] This includes losing weight, quitting smoking, preventing constipation, and avoiding lifting heavy objects.[3] Consider utilizing pads and protective garments as a stop-gap measure.

Biofeedback can provide modest short-term improvements.[3]

Methionine produces ammonia-free urine by lowering the urinary pH. The lower pH also helps to prevent bacterial growth and the adherence of bacteria to the bladder wall, thus contributing to the healing of existing UTIs and the prevention of new ones.[4]

dl-Methionine, also known as racemethionine, 0.2 gm tid daily for seven days, reduced urinary odors and genital and perineal dermatitis in 10 mentally deteriorated elderly subjects, three of whom had a marked reduction in wetting.[5]

Diet: Clinical studies report that alcoholic beverages, caffeinated drinks, acidic foods and drinks (e.g., citrus fruits, coffee, tea, tomatoes, carbonated water, and spicy foods, as well as sugar, honey, and artificial sweeteners) should be avoided as they tend to irritate or otherwise stimulate the bladder.[6] All fluid intake should be reduced, especially in the evening several hours before bedtime.

Sacral nerve stimulation has been used as a second-line therapy for urge urinary incontinence since the 1980s.[7]

Infantile Colic

The term *colic* applies to any well-fed and otherwise healthy infant that cries more than three hours a day, more than three days a week, or for more than three weeks. Colic typically starts about two or three weeks of age for a full term infant and ends at about four months. A baby with colic often cries excessively at about the same time of day (usually in the late afternoon or evening). There are many different causes of excess crying in infants (e.g., a wet or dirty diaper, excessive gas, feeling cold, hunger, thirst, illness, or pain), but the cause of colic is unknown. The incidence of colic in breastfed and bottle-fed infants is similar.

RESEARCH RESULTS

White Noise: Provide white noise by running a white noise machine, a vacuum cleaner or clothes drier in a nearby room, or playing an audio of heartbeats or relaxing music to help calm the infant.[1]

Feeding: Bottle-feed the baby using a curved collapsible bag bottle and feed in an upright position to help reduce the intake of air.[1]

Formula: Parents can replace regular formula for a one-week trial with an extensive hydrolysate formula (Similac Alimentum, Nutramigen, Pregestimil, etc.) that has proteins broken down into smaller sizes.[1]

Maternal Diet: Mothers who are breastfeeding can try a diet that eliminates common food allergens, such as dairy, soy, eggs, nuts, wheat, and shellfish. They should also try to eliminate spicy and potentially irritating foods, such as cabbage, onions, raw vegetables, and caffeinated beverages.[2]

Probiotics: *Lactobacillus reuteri* was found to relieve colic symptoms in breastfed infants within one week of treatment.[3,4] In a more recent study, 50 exclusively breastfed colicky infants were randomly assigned to receive either *L. reuteri* or a placebo daily for 21 days.[5] A 50% reduction in crying time from baseline was noted in the *L. reuteri* group compared with the placebo group on day seven. The study concluded that *L. reuteri* at a dose of 108 colony-forming units per day improved symptoms of infantile colic and was well-tolerated and safe.

Herbal Teas: Feeding the baby herbal teas (150 mL per dose) containing mixtures of chamomile, vervain, licorice, fennel, and lemon balm, used up to three times a day, has been shown to decrease crying in colicky infants.[6]

Gripe Water: A product called "Gripe Water," which may include any of a variety of herbs and herbal oils, such as cardamom, chamomile, cinnamon, clove, dill, fennel, ginger, lemon balm, licorice, peppermint, and yarrow, is available online and in health food stores. This product is touted to provide relief from flatulence and indigestion.[6]

Gentle Manual Therapy: A systematic review was conducted of six randomized controlled trials (RCTs) to evaluate the effectiveness of manipulative therapies for infantile colic. The majority of the included trials indicated that infants receiving manipulative therapies had fewer hours of crying per day than infants who did not; this difference was statistically significant.[7] Crying time was reduced by an average of 72 minutes per day. This effect was sustained for studies with a low risk of selection bias and attrition bias. Combining all six RCTs suggested that manipulative therapies had a significant positive effect in treating infantile colic.

One randomized controlled trial was conducted in Denmark. One group of infants received spinal care for two weeks while the other was treated with the drug dimethicone. Between trial days four to seven, hours of crying were reduced by one hour in the dimethicone groups compared with 2.4 hours in the manipulation group. On days 8 through 11, crying was reduced by one hour for the dimethicone group, whereas crying in the manipulation group was reduced by 2.7 hours. From trial day five onward, the manipulation group did significantly better than the dimethicone group, which suggests that spinal manipulation is effective in relieving infantile colic.[8]

All things considered, obtaining manipulative therapy (osteopathic or chiropractic) resulted in fewer hours of daily crying with a safe track record of over 100 years of patient care. Osteopathic or chiropractic care should be a first-line treatment option.[9]

Fennel: Giving fennel seed oil (5–20 ml of 0.1% up to four times daily for one week) can relieve colic in infants 2–12 weeks old. For colic in breastfed infants, a specific multi-ingredient product containing 164 mg of fennel, 97 mg of lemon balm, and 178 mg of German chamomile (ColiMil) twice daily for a week can be used.[10]

Tea (Calma-Bebi, Bonomelli) containing fennel, chamomile, vervain, licorice, and balm-mint can also reduce colic severity in infants.[11]

Infections

***See also* Respiratory Infections**

An infection is the invasion of body tissues by a pathogenic agent (e.g., virus, fungus, parasite, or foreign bacterium). Infections can be localized or can spread through the blood and lymph to become systemic. They can be asymptomatic, or subclinical, or may have overt signs and symptoms. General local symptoms can be pus, redness, heat, soreness or swelling, foul odor, and fever. Systemic symptoms include fatigue, fever, aches, chills sweats, sore throat, nasal congestion, shortness of breath, stiff neck, urinary discomfort, diarrhea, or vomiting.

ADJUVANT CARE CONSIDERATIONS

Berberine: Berberine can be an effective adjunctive antimicrobial agent. A laboratory study found that berberine helped inhibit the growth of *Staphylococcus aureus* which can cause, among other things, sepsis, pneumonia, meningitis, and a range of skin conditions.[1]

Oregano oil contains high levels of carvacrol and thymol which have been shown to be effective in vitro against a range of gram positive and gram negative microorganisms, including *Staphylococcus aureus* and/or *Staphylococcus epidermidis, listeria, proteus, pseudomonas, salmonella*, and *clostridium* species.[2,3] Oregano has also inhibited aflatoxin production and prevented growth of *aspergillus*.[3] Thymol in oregano oil was found to be an effective treatment for common candida fungal infections.[4] Ingesting oregano oil supplements (e.g., 200 mg emulsified *O. vulgare* oil/day for six weeks) or rubbing the oil on the infected area can help make use of these antibacterial effects.[2] Applying diluted oregano oil to the skin may help protect cuts and scrapes on the skin as they heal.[1]

Phytoestrogens: To facilitate antibiotic actions, patients can increase their intake of phytoestrogens. Phytoestrogens, lignans (soybeans, beans, lentils), and isoflavones (cereals, fruits, and vegetables) are antiviral, anticarcinogenic, bactericidal, antifungal, and have been reported to have digitalis-like activity.[5]

Topical manuka honey inhibits approximately 60 kinds of bacteria. Laboratory studies demonstrated that the honey is also effective against methicillin-resistant *S. aureus* (MRSA), *β-haemolytic streptococci* and vancomycin-resistant *enterococci* (VRE).[6]

Echinacea: A study reported that the extract of *Echinacea purpurea* taken orally can kill many different kinds of bacteria, including *Streptococcus pyogenes* (*S. pyogenes*) which is responsible for strep throat, toxic shock syndrome, and the "flesh-eating disease" known as necrotizing fasciitis.[7]

Zinc is known to modulate antiviral and antibacterial immunity and regulate inflammatory response.[8] Recent studies have demonstrated that zinc supplementation can significantly reduce the morbidity and mortality of apparently well-nourished children and shorten the time to recovery from acute infectious diseases.[9] There are also indirect indications that zinc intake may be effective in the fight against coronavirus disease (e.g., COVID-19), but there is still insufficient data for recommendations.[10]

Infertility

An inability to conceive children or carry a pregnancy to term is referred to as infertility in both men and women. Infertility is further defined as not being able to conceive after one year or longer of unprotected sex. Because fertility in women is known to decline steadily with age, some providers diagnose the condition in women aged 35 years or older after six months of unprotected sex. Infertility problems are diagnosed in one in 10 American couples, yet half or more eventually bear a child.

MANAGEMENT GUIDES

For women, to improve the chances of getting pregnant, mayoclinic.org recommends:

- Quit smoking. Tobacco has multiple negative effects on fertility, not to mention the negative impact on general health and on the health of a fetus.
- Avoid alcohol and street drugs. These substances may impair the ability to conceive and to have a healthy pregnancy. Women who are trying to become pregnant should not drink alcohol or use recreational drugs, such as marijuana or cocaine.
- Limit caffeine. Women trying to get pregnant may want to limit caffeine intake. Medical professionals can provide guidance on the safe use of caffeine.
- Exercise moderately. Regular exercise is important but exercising so intensely that monthly periods are infrequent or absent has a negative effect on fertility.
- Avoid weight extremes. Being overweight or underweight can adversely affect hormone production and cause infertility.[1]

Inositol: As it presents a relevant role in ensuring oocyte fertility, inositol has been studied for its use in the management of polycystic ovaries. The use of 2,000 mg myo-inositol plus 200 μg folic acid bid is a safe and promising tool in the effective improvement of symptoms and infertility for patients with polycystic ovary syndrome (PCOS).[2]

Vitamin C (Ascorbic Acid): Supplementation with vitamin C increases progesterone levels in infertile women with luteal phase defect.[3]

Coenzyme Q10: A review and meta-analysis concluded that oral supplementation of CoQ10 resulted in an increase of clinical pregnancy when compared with a placebo or no treatment.[4]

For men, mayoclinic.org states that although most types of infertility are not preventable, these strategies may help:

- Avoid drug and tobacco use and excessive alcohol consumption.
- Avoid high temperatures (e.g., avoid hot tubs and steam baths).
- Avoid exposure to industrial or environmental toxins.
- Limit medications that may impact fertility, to include both prescription and non-prescription drugs.
- Exercise moderately. Regular exercise may improve sperm quality and increase the chances for achieving a pregnancy.[1]

L-carnitine is concentrated in the epididymis, where sperm mature and acquire their motility. Two uncontrolled trials of L-carnitine supplementation in more than 100 men diagnosed with decreased sperm motility found that oral L-carnitine supplementation (3 gm/day) for three to four months significantly improved sperm motility.[5,6] Carnitine has been shown to increase sperm count and to stimulate sperm motility in test tubes. Infertile men have been found to have lower carnitine concentrations in semen than fertile men.[6,7]

In one study, 100 men were given 3 gm/day of L-carnitine for four months. After treatment there was a significant increase in the proportion of sperm cells showing normal motility.[6,7]

Zinc is essential for male fertility and the treatment of male infertility. Zinc depletion in men is associated with reduced sperm count and motility and with impotence.[8]

Vitamin C has been utilized in the management of male infertility on empirical grounds, particularly in the presence of nonspecific seminal infections.[9] Vitamin C supplementation in men may improve sperm quality.[10,11,12]

Selenium deficiency is also associated with male infertility.[13]

Fish Oil: In a study involving 1,679 young men in Denmark, supplemental intake of ω-3 polyunsaturated fatty acid for three months has been found to be associated, in a dose response manner, with higher semen volume, total sperm count, larger testicular size, lower FSH and LH levels, and a higher free testosterone to LH ratio.[14]

Influenza

Influenza, aka the flu, is not the stomach flu. It is a respiratory illness caused by a virus that attacks the nose, throat, and lungs. Common symptoms can include fever, runny nose, sore throat, muscle pains, headache, cough, body aches, and fatigue. Not everyone with the flu gets a fever. The flu usually comes on suddenly and can cause mild to severe illness, and at times can lead to death. The CDC recommends getting the flu vaccine each year to help prevent this illness.

ADDITIONAL TREATMENT MEASURES

Sambucol, an herbal product that contains extracts of black elderberries (*Sambucus nigra L*) and raspberries (*Rubus idaeus L*) has been shown to inhibit the ability of the influenza virus to replicate. In one study, individuals suffering from the flu were given Sambucol. Ninety percent of the individuals receiving Sambucol became symptom-free within two to three days. In contrast, those in the placebo group did not recover for at least six days.[1] Sambucol one tablespoon (15 mL) by Nature's Way q.i.d. or lozenge (ViraBLOC) by HerbalScience containing 175 mg of elderberry extract q.i.d. for two days is recommended.[2]

N-Acetylcysteine (NAC): NAC has been in clinical use for more than 30 years as a mucolytic drug. A total of 262 subjects were given N-acetylcysteine 600 mg bid for the entire flu season. Only 25% of the NAC group who got the flu developed a symptomatic form. The non-NAC group had three times more symptomatic cases. Both local and systemic influenza symptoms were sharply and significantly reduced in the NAC group.[3]

Inosine Pranobex: A total of 463 subjects were randomly assigned to receive inosine pranobex or a placebo in a randomized, double-blind, multicenter study. The study results indicate the safety of inosine pranobex for the treatment of subjects with confirmed acute respiratory viral infections and confirm the efficacy of inosine pranobex versus a placebo in healthy non-obese subjects less than 50 years of age with clinically diagnosed influenza-like illnesses.[4]

Insect Stings and Bites (Prevention)

Most reactions to insect bites and stings are mild and cause little more than localized redness, itching, stinging, and a raised bump due to minor swelling. Bites or stings are rarely a cause for concern unless they cause an allergic reaction or become infected. A severe allergic reaction with difficulty breathing, dizziness, rapid heartbeat, hives, or swelling of the throat, eyelids, or lips requires immediate medical attention.

PREVENTIVE MEASURES

Precautions: To avoid attracting insects, individuals should not wear floral-patterned or dark clothing, choosing light-colored, smooth-finished clothing instead.[1] Scented soaps, perfumes, colognes, shampoos, and deodorants should be avoided.[2]

Essential oil of eucalyptus (*Eucalyptus globulus*) is a natural insect repellent. A homemade solution can be made by adding five drops of eucalyptus oil to one cup of water and dabbing it on the skin.[3]

Essential oil of citronella also discourages insects to land when placed on exposed skin.[3]

Calendula: A few dabs of calendula (*Calendula officinalis*) ointment on the face, arms, and legs may keep insects away and is also a commercially available product.[3]

Zinc supplements can alter body odor in a way that renders people less susceptible to being stung by bees or bitten by mosquitoes.[4]

Thiamine has also been used orally as an insect repellent, but there is a lack of adequate evidence to establish the efficacy of thiamine for this use.[5]

Insomnia

Insomnia is a common sleep disorder that makes it hard to fall asleep (sleep latency), hard to stay asleep, and/or hard to get back to sleep. Insomnia has also been associated with a higher risk of developing chronic diseases.[1] There are many possible psychological and medical causes of insomnia. Psychological causes can be bipolar disorder, depression, and anxiety or psychotic disorders. Some medical causes include chronic pain, chronic fatigue syndrome, congestive heart failure, angina, acid-reflux disease (GERD), chronic obstructive pulmonary disease, asthma, sleep apnea, Parkinson's and

Alzheimer's diseases, hormonal imbalances, hyperthyroidism, arthritis, brain lesions, tumors, and stroke.[1] Certain medications (e.g., corticosteroids, alpha or beta blockers, statins, ACE, or cholinesterase inhibitors) can also cause insomnia.

Prescription and over-the-counter sleep medications abound. Many patients who use such compounds report feeling drowsy, confused, or forgetful the next day. The benefits from prescription sleep aids are modest at best, increasing sleep time by approximately 20–30 minutes.[2]

TREATMENT MEASURES

Antihistamines: Many nonprescription sleep medications contain antihistamines that can make individuals drowsy, and are not intended for regular use. Diphenhydramine (Benadryl) and doxylamine (Unisom) are available over the counter for the treatment of insomnia, but they are recommended only for the treatment of pregnancy-related insomnia.[3]

Melatonin is a hormone released by the pineal gland. This hormone helps regulate sleep patterns. Low levels of melatonin can cause insomnia. Melatonin has little dependence potential, is not associated with habituation, and typically produces no hangover. There is no evidence of patients developing a tolerance to melatonin. Melatonin can provide meaningful improvements in sleep quality, morning alertness, and sleep onset latency.[4,5]

Melatonin capsules (0.3–10 mg) of the immediate release formulation should be administered in the evening (90 minutes before bedtime) to mimic the hormonal surge normally associated with the onset of darkness.[6,7,8] The dose may be repeated in 30 minutes up to a maximum of 10–20 mg.[9]

Melatonin is also used to help prevent and lessen sleep disturbances from jet lag. The recommended dosage is 5 mg/day for three days before departure and ending three days after departure.[10]

Valerian Root: Extracts from the root of valerian (*Valeriana officinalis*) are widely used for inducing sleep and improving sleep quality.[11] Valerian is considered safe by the U.S. Food and Drug Administration (FDA) and is gentler than synthetic drugs, such as benzodiazepines and barbiturates.[12] Recommended doses from previous studies ranged from 75 mg to 3,000 mg/day to improve sleep quality.[13] Valerian root, when used to treat insomnia, is recommended in dosages at 200–500 mg at bedtime.[14]

Glycine: Taking glycine (3 gm) before bedtime for two to four days improved subjective sleep quality and sleep latency.[15,16] Glycine before bedtime might also reduce feelings of tiredness the following day after a shortened night of sleep.[17]

Light Therapy: Delayed sleep phase syndrome (DSPS) is a form of insomnia in which patients prefer to sleep at hours that are much too late to be compatible with a conventional lifestyle; as a result, they usually wake up before sufficient sleep has been achieved. DSPS is due to an error in the timing system (body clock) that controls daily rhythms.[18]

Managing DSPS involves progressively delaying sleep times until they become correctly phased, then stabilizing them by a rigorous adherence to regular times of retiring. An hour or more of bright light (>2,500 lux) is recommended in the morning in addition to avoiding light at night.[18]

5-Hydroxytryptophan: For difficulty getting to sleep, L-tryptophan is effective in reducing sleep onset time on the first night of administration in doses ranging from 1–15 g. In more chronic, well-established sleep-onset insomnia or in more severe insomnias characterized by both sleep onset and sleep maintenance problems, repeated administration of low doses of L-tryptophan over time may be required for therapeutic improvement.[19]

Intermittent Claudication (IC)

Intermittent claudication causes aching, cramping, pain, and weakness most often in the calf on walking or other mild exercise and is relieved with rest. The term *claudication* comes from a Latin word meaning "to limp." This difficulty in walking is due to atherosclerosis, vasospasm, or arterial occlusion in the femoral artery. This restricts or blocks adequate blood flow and oxygen to the leg muscles. Intermittent claudication is the most common sign of peripheral artery disease (PAD).

The natural course of intermittent claudication is benign for the leg affected, with few patients ever requiring intervention or amputation. Only one in four patients with intermittent claudication will develop any deterioration in symptoms.[1] One serious potential complication of intermittent claudication is acute limb ischemia with signs of pain, pallor, pulselessness, paresthesia, and paralysis, which requires a rapid consultation with a vascular specialist. IC chiefly affects men over 70 and is associated with a significant increase in death from cardiovascular disease. The main treatment goal is to reduce the risk of death from cardiovascular disease by reducing platelet aggregation. Contributing disorders such as hypertension, diabetes, and hyperlipidemia need to be managed as aggressively as possible.[2]

MEDICAL MANAGEMENT OPTIONS

The first triad of treatments for claudication is to quit smoking, exercise more, and lose weight.

The second triad of treatments is to control diabetes, hypertension, and hyperlipidemia (e.g., diet, statins, and other lipid lowering agents).[1]

Aspirin reduces risk of serious vascular events in patients with PVD, with doses of 75–150 mg being as effective as higher doses.[2]

Magnesium: Individuals suffering from this problem have difficulty walking any great distance because pain in their legs forces them to stop before they have gone very far. In one study, 19 patients with intermittent claudication received 250 mg of magnesium hydroxide twice a day. After 60 days, walking distance had increased by an average of 82%.[3]

L-Carnitine: In a double-blind, placebo-controlled, dose-titration study, 1–3 gm/day of oral propionyl-L-carnitine for 24 weeks was well-tolerated and improved maximal walking distance in IC patients.[4]

In a randomized, placebo-controlled study of 495 patients with IC, 2 gm/day of propionyl-L-carnitine for 12 months significantly increased maximal walking distance and the distance walked prior to the onset of claudication in patients whose initial maximal walking distance was less than 250 meters.[5]

Supplemental forms of carnitine (e.g., L-carnitine and propionyl-L-carnitine) administered in conjunction with standard drug therapy appear to improve cardiac and skeletal muscle function during ischemia.[6]

Propionyl-L-carnitine, in particular, may benefit ischemic tissue by replenishing intermediates of energy metabolism or by increasing blood vessel dilation. Moreover, propionyl-L-carnitine has been reported to be a vasodilator.[6]

Several randomized controlled trials have found that oral supplementation with propionyl-L-carnitine improves exercise tolerance in some patients with intermittent claudication.[6]

In one study, 20 patients received 2 gm of carnitine twice a day. The average distance the patient could walk before developing pain was 76% greater during carnitine treatment than during the placebo period.[7,8]

Another study compared the efficacy of L-carnitine and propionyl-L-carnitine administered intravenously for the treatment of IC and concluded that propionyl-L-carnitine was more effective than L-carnitine when the same amount of carnitine was provided.[6]

Tocopherol: Doses of vitamin E (400–600 mg/day) have been reported to afford symptomatic improvement in intermittent claudication.[9] Five eligible studies regarding vitamin E were found with a total of 265, predominantly male, participants. The average age was 57 years. The follow-up varied from 12 weeks to 18 months. Five different doses of vitamin E were used, and four different physical outcomes were measured. All trials showed positive effects on one of their main outcomes. No serious adverse effects of vitamin E were reported.[10]

Policosanol is a dietary supplement made of medium-chain alcohols extracted from sugar cane. Policosanol has favorable effects on intermittent claudication, possibly due to its effects on platelet aggregation and endothelial function.

Clinical trials indicate that policosanol may have applications in the treatment of intermittent claudication.[11]

Padma 28: Because the arteries supplying blood to the legs are clogged, individuals with intermittent claudication are unable to walk very far without developing severe pain in their calf muscles. Patients with intermittent claudication received the herbal formula Padma 28 (760 mg twice daily) or a placebo for 16 weeks. Patients receiving Padma 28 were able to increase their walking distance by 115%. No side effects were reported.[12]

Inositol Hexaniacinate (INH): The use of niacin esters for the treatment of intermittent claudication secondary to atherosclerosis has been examined extensively. Significant improvement due to widening of blood vessels to improve blood flow has been reported by several investigators at INH dosages of 2 gm twice daily, typically for at least three months.[12,13] While arterial dilation may be a factor, it has been postulated that reduction in fibrinogen, improvement in blood viscosity, and resultant improvement in oxygen transport are involved in the therapeutic effects.[13,14,15,16,17,18]

EPA/DHA: Reducing platelet aggregation is the mainstay of medical treatment. A meta-analysis of 15 randomized controlled trials in humans confirmed that taking EPA/DHA (3 gm/day for four weeks) inhibits platelet aggregation, but does not increase the risk of clinically significant bleeds and may even reduce the risk of bleeding in the surgical setting.[19]

Irritable Bowel Syndrome (IBS)

Irritable bowel syndrome (IBS) is also known as spastic colon, irritable colon, mucous colitis, and spastic colitis. IBS is a functional GI disorder characterized by cramping, bloating, gas, pain in the abdomen, mucous in stools, and diarrhea or constipation, or both, in the absence of any structural abnormality.[1]

A diagnosis is made when these symptoms occur three or more times a month for at least three months duration. IBS is not an inflammatory bowel disease, although it does affect the large intestine. IBS does not cause physical signs of damage or disease in digestive tract tissues, nor does it increase the risk of colorectal cancer.[1] IBS is a complex condition whose pathophysiology is not well understood. Nonpharmacologic treatment options are the mainstay of therapy. The primary goal in treating IBS is symptom relief.

RESEARCH RESULTS

Gluten: Research shows that some people with IBS report improvement in diarrhea symptoms if they stop eating gluten (wheat, barley, and rye) even if they do not have celiac disease.[1]

Fiber supplementation may improve symptoms of constipation and diarrhea. Treatment should be individualized because some patients experience exacerbated bloating and distention with high-fiber diets. Polycarbophil compounds (e.g., Citrucel, FiberCon) may produce less flatulence than psyllium compounds (e.g., Metamucil).[2] Psyllium, however, can relieve chronic diarrhea and can be especially helpful for those with loose stools.[3]

The data regarding the effectiveness of fiber is controversial because 40%–70% of patients improve with a placebo. A Cochrane systematic review found no benefit of fiber/bulking agents on irritable bowel syndrome symptoms.[2]

Probiotics: A meta-analysis concluded that the probiotic *Bifidobacterium infantis* may help alleviate some symptoms of irritable bowel syndrome.[2]

Peppermint oil is a natural antispasmodic that relaxes smooth muscles in the intestines. Studies also show that, in people who have IBS with diarrhea, an enteric coated tablet (Colpermin) that slowly releases peppermint oil in the small intestine eases bloating, urgency, abdominal pain, and pain while passing stool.[1,4] In one study, IBS patients took Colpermin three to four times daily, 15 to 30 minutes before meals for one month. 79% experienced an alleviation in the severity of abdominal pain, 83% had less bloating, and 79% experienced less flatulence.[5] Other studies have confirmed the effectiveness of enteric coated peppermint oil (EPCO).[6,7]

Taking into account the currently available drug treatments for IBS, PO (1–2 capsules tid over two to four weeks) may be the drug of first choice in IBS patients with non-serious constipation or diarrhea to alleviate general symptoms and to improve quality of life.[8]

Palmitoylethanolamide (PEA), an endogenous fatty acid amide, is available as a supplement (PeaPure and PeaPlex) and as a cream (PEA cream). A European multicenter pilot study evaluated the effectiveness of PEA and polydatin in 54 patients with irritable bowel syndrome. Polydatin, also known as piceid, is a glucoside of resveratrol. This combination of PEA and piceid significantly improved the severity of abdominal pain when compared to a placebo.[9]

Vitamin D deficiency has been found to be strongly associated with many systemic disorders. One study found vitamin D deficiency in 82% of patients with IBS. The researchers concluded that the study showed vitamin D deficiency is highly prevalent in patients with IBS and the results seem to have therapeutic implications. Vitamin D supplementation could play a therapeutic role in the control of IBS.[10]

Licorice: Research indicates that a product containing slippery elm bark, lactulose, oat bran, and licorice root can reduce stomach pain and bloating, as well as improve bowel movements in patients with constipation that is related to IBS.[11]

Kidney Failure/Renal Insufficiency/ Chronic Kidney Disease (CKD)

Chronic kidney disease is the gradual progressive loss of kidney function persisting for more than three months. CKD is most commonly attributed to diabetes and hypertension and most patients with CKD are asymptomatic.[1] The number of patients with chronic kidney disease (CKD) is increasing.[2]

When the kidneys cannot sufficiently filter waste products (e.g., urea, sodium, etc.) from the blood, those toxic substances and excess fluids eventually build up, causing complications. When kidney function is less than 50% of normal, that is considered chronic renal or kidney failure. Common uremic symptoms include nausea, loss of appetite, dry itchy skin, blood in the urine, high blood pressure, shortness of breath, mental confusion, weight gain, cold intolerance, peripheral neuropathies, weakness, and fatigue.

Chronic kidney disease is typically identified through routine screening with serum chemistry profile and urine studies or as an incidental finding.[1]

Progression of CKD is associated with a number of serious complications, including increased incidence of cardiovascular disease, hyperlipidemia, hyperphosphatemia, low serum vitamin D, anemia, and hyperparathyroidism that can lead to hypercalcemia and altered bone morphology with reduced strength, higher risk of bone fractures, and development of vascular or other soft tissue calcifications.[3] Cardiovascular complications are the leading cause of mortality in patients with stage 5 disease.[2] Another complication of kidney disease is normocytic, normochromic anemia.

While anemia in CKD can result from multiple mechanisms (e.g., iron, folate, or vitamin B12 deficiency; gastrointestinal bleeding; severe hyperparathyroidism, systemic inflammation, and shortened red blood cell survival), decreased erythropoietin synthesis is the most important and specific etiology.[3] Treatment for chronic kidney disease focuses on addressing the primary cause (e.g., diabetes, hypertension, or glomerulonephritis) and potentially delaying progression of kidney damage while minimizing the development or severity of complications. Dialysis or a kidney transplant are the primary treatments in advanced (stage 5) CDK.

TREATMENT STRATEGIES

Traditional Medicine: The most important step in treating kidney disease is to control blood pressure.[4] Optimal management of CKD also includes cardiovascular risk reduction, treatment of albuminuria, avoidance of potential nephrotoxins, adjustments to drug dosing (e.g., antibiotics and oral hypoglycemic agents), and good management of diabetes.[1]

Vitamin D: Patients with kidney disease typically have low levels of vitamin D. Vitamin D is essential for healthy bones. Treatment with vitamin D3 is highly effective in increasing calcium absorption, promoting positive calcium and phosphorous balances, increasing serum calcium, reducing serum alkaline phosphatase, and improving skeletal x-ray and bony architecture.[5]

Sodium Bicarbonate: In a research project, 134 patients with advanced chronic kidney disease and low bicarbonate levels, a condition known as metabolic acidosis, were studied.[6] One group of these patients was treated with a small daily dose of sodium bicarbonate in tablet form in addition to their usual care. Oral sodium bicarbonate supplementation was given at a dosage of 1.82 gm/day. The results indicate that the rate of decline in kidney function was dramatically reduced in these patients. Overall, the decline was about two-thirds slower than in patients not given sodium bicarbonate.

Daily supplementation with sodium bicarbonate (baking soda) tablets or capsules slowed the progression rate of renal failure to end-stage renal disease (ESRD) and improved metabolic acidosis and nutritional status among patients with chronic kidney disease.

Coenzyme Q10: Treatment with CoQ10 reduced serum creatinine and blood urea nitrogen and increased creatinine clearance and urine output in patients with chronic renal failure. This treatment also decreased the need for dialysis in patients on chronic dialysis.[7]

Chitosan: Eighty individuals with chronic kidney failure on long-term hemodialysis were studied.[8] Half took chitosan (a natural poly-saccharide found in insects and shellfish) 1,450 milligrams, three times daily for 12 weeks; the other half were "controls." Those who took chitosan reduced serum cholesterol by 41% and increased mean serum hemoglobin. Significant reductions also were achieved in BUN (from 75–45 mm) and creatinine (from 1.001–0.875 mm). Appetite, sleep, and feelings of physical strength improved significantly in the treatment group. No significant side effects were seen.

Ascorbic Acid: Chronic kidney disease causes anemia with decreased hemoglobin. Approximately 65% of hemodialysis patients responded to treatment with 1,500 mg/wk of intravenous vitamin C over a 6-month period with almost a 2 gm/dL increase in hemoglobin concentration, together with a 2,500 IU/wk (30%) reduction in EPO dose.[9]

L-carnitine and many of its precursors are removed from the circulation during hemodialysis. Impaired L-carnitine synthesis by the kidneys may also contribute to the potential for carnitine deficiency in patients with end-stage renal disease undergoing hemodialysis.[10] The U.S. Food and Drug Administration (FDA) has approved the use of L-carnitine in hemodialysis patients for the prevention and treatment of carnitine deficiency. Carnitine depletion may lead to a number of conditions observed in dialysis patients, including muscle weakness and fatigue, plasma lipid abnormalities, and refractory anemia.[11] Carnitine administration has also been shown to be effective in many patients for the adjunctive treatment of anemia associated with chronic kidney disease.[12]

Turmeric: Clinical studies show that in more than 95% of kidney failure cases, kidney damage is caused by inflammation. Turmeric contains lots of curcumin which can help to block inflammation and thus stop progression of the illness or condition. Previous clinical studies also demonstrate that taking turmeric by mouth (1–3 gm) three times daily for eight weeks reduces itching in people with long-term kidney disease.[13]

NAC: Taking N-acetylcysteine by mouth can help prevent problems, such as heart attack and stroke, in people with serious kidney disease. The risk reduction can be as much as 40%.[14]

Amino Acid Supplements: Three mixtures containing varying proportions of threonine, tyrosine and ornithine, lysine, and histidine salts of branched-chain keto acids have been tested as dietary supplements to a 20–25 gm mixed-quality protein diet in patients with severe chronic uremia. Two of the three supplements improved the abnormalities of plasma amino acid concentrations, and slowed or arrested progression of renal insufficiency. The second supplement, which contained less threonine and lysine, led to subnormal plasma concentrations of these two amino acids and aggravated hypophosphatemia. The third supplement, which also contained a small amount of the hydroxy analogue of methionine, was the most effective in slowing the progression of the disease.[15]

For difficulty getting to sleep, L-tryptophan is effective in reducing sleep onset time on the first night of administration in doses ranging from 1–15 g. In more chronic, well-established sleep-onset insomnia or in more severe insomnias characterized by both sleep onset and sleep maintenance problems, repeated administration of low doses of L-tryptophan over time may be required for therapeutic improvement.[16]

Zinc Supplementation: Subnormal plasma zinc levels and decreased zinc concentration in hair and leucocytes, as well as increased plasma ammonia and ribonuclease activity in dialyzed and non-dialyzed uremic patients, indicate that zinc metabolism is abnormal in uremia and is not corrected by dialysis. Abnormalities of taste and sexual function improved significantly in patients receiving zinc supplements, but not in those on placebo therapy. These improvements in biochemical as well as clinical parameters confirm and add to earlier observations of improvement in taste and sexual function after zinc supplementation. Together, they suggest that zinc deficiency is a complicating feature of uremia and can be corrected by oral zinc acetate supplementation.[17]

Folic Acid: The vast majority of patients with serious kidney disease have high levels of homocysteine. High levels of homocysteine have been linked to heart disease and stroke. Taking folic acid lowers homocysteine levels in people with serious kidney disease.[18]

Citrate: Citrate preparations (e.g., potassium citrate) appear to be beneficial for preventing deterioration of renal function in the patients with CKD who have elevated levels of serum uric acid and who are also being treated with allopurinol.[19]

Diet: One study evaluated two levels of protein restriction in 840 patients, finding that a low-protein diet compared with usual protein intake resulted in slower GFR decline only after the initial four months.[1,20] Guidelines recommend that protein intake be reduced to less than 0.8 gm/kg per day.

Lower dietary acid loads (e.g., more fruits and vegetables and less meat, eggs, and cheese) may also help protect against kidney injury.[1,21,22] Low-sodium diets (generally <2 gm/day) are recommended for patients with hypertension, proteinuria, or fluid overload.[1,23]

Caffeine: In one study, individuals with the highest intake of caffeinated coffee had a 24% lower risk of dying from chronic kidney disease.[24]

Smoking cessation is encouraged to slow the progression of CKD and to reduce the risk of coronary vascular disease.

Calcium carbonate and calcium acetate (e.g., 365–500 mg with each meal) are used to restrict phosphate absorption in patients with hyperphosphatemia.[25]

Kidney Stones

Kidney stones, also known as nephrolithiasis or renal lithiasis, are deposits of minerals and salts that form inside the kidney. According to current estimates, kidney stones will develop in one out of ten people during their lifetime. The prevalence is highest among those aged 30–45 years. Once kidney stones develop, patients have a 50%–75% likelihood of developing another stone. When there is too much waste in too little liquid, waste material can come out of solution and form crystals. The crystals attract other elements that join together and harden to form a solid stone. The stone or stones tend to get larger unless passed out of the body in the urine.

The stone passing through the ureter can cause the sufferer to experience excruciating unilateral flank pain that can radiate to the same side of the back, abdomen, or groin. Some patients experience pain that comes in waves. Others may writhe in pain and frequently change positions in an effort to help pass the stone through the ureter and an attempt to ameliorate the pain. At other times, a stone may block the flow of urine and cause the kidney to swell and the ureter to spasm, which can also be very painful. In addition to pain, blood in the urine and nausea or vomiting can be present.

A CT scan is the most accurate imaging technique to confirm the diagnosis, but ultrasonography can also be used. Stones that are uncomplicated and 10 mm or less in diameter can usually be passed spontaneously in four to six weeks. The stones can be composed of calcium oxalate (most common and often associated with inadequate fluid intake), struvite (typically in response to an infection), uric acid (from lack of fluids or gout), or cystine (cystinuria). Prevention is paramount in addressing the formation of more kidney stones and is the main goal of treatment.

PREVENTION MEASURES

Diet: Sodium intake should be restricted (1,500–2,000 mg/24 h) to decrease urine calcium and reduce the risk of stone formation.[1] Increased sodium intake encourages stone growth by increasing kidney calcium and sodium excretion renal monosodium urates (which can act as nidus for stone growth) and decreasing urinary citrate excretion.

Magnesium is a known inhibitor of the formation of calcium oxalate crystals in the urine and was proposed for prophylactic treatment in kidney stone disease as early as the 17th and 18th centuries.[2] Magnesium oxide (400–500 mg/day) increases the solubility of calcium oxalate and thus decreases rates of stone recurrence.[3] Fifty-five patients with recurrent renal calcium stone disease without signs of magnesium deficiency were given 500 mg of magnesium hydroxide daily for up to four years. The authors concluded that magnesium treatment in renal calcium stone disease is effective with few side effects. No clinical signs of magnesium excess were observed.[2]

Potassium-Magnesium Citrate: Ettinger and colleagues have studied the effectiveness of potassium-magnesium citrate where 31 patients received 42 mEq of potassium, 21 mEq magnesium, and 63 mEq citrate in an attempt to prevent nephrolithiasis in patients with recurrent kidney stones.[4] At the end of three years, 64% of the placebo group had stones compared to 13% in the treatment group.[5] It would be wise to ask your pharmacist or physician for assistance with the dosing.

Pyridoxine and Magnesium: In one study, 149 patients with longstanding recurrent idiopathic calcium oxalate and mixed calcium oxalate/calcium phosphate renal stones each received 100 mg of magnesium oxide three times a day and 10 mg of pyridoxine (vitamin B6) once a day for 4.5–6 years. The mean rate of stone formation fell by 92.3% during the study. No significant side effects occurred.[6]

Rice Bran: In one study, 70 patients who had kidney stones and excessive urinary calcium excretion were treated with rice bran (1 gm twice a day) for up to three years. In almost all patients, there was a significant decrease in urinary calcium excretion, averaging about 30%.[7,8] Among patients who continued rice bran for at least one year, there was an 84% reduction in the formation of kidney stones.

Beer: In a Finnish study, beer consumption was strongly associated with a reduced risk of kidney stones; consumption of a daily glass or bottle of beer was estimated to reduce the risk by 40%. Stouts and porters are especially useful in preventing kidney stones due to their high hops content.[9]

Pyridoxine: The administration of physiologic or pharmacologic doses of vitamin B6 (10–500 mg/day) decreased oxalate production in a number of kidney stone patients. In a cohort study of 85,557 women with no history of kidney stones, findings support the hypothesis that high doses of vitamin B6 reduce the risk of kidney stone formation in women.[10]

Phytate, also known as IP-6 (inositol hexaphosphate), is a powerful agent for preventing calcifications and preventing kidney stones.[11] IP-6 has been studied as far back as the 1950s at Harvard where it was shown to reduce the frequency of calcium-based stones. This is a tremendous alternative to using hydrochlorothiazide in patients with hypercalciuria and is clearly without the potential side effects.[12]

Diet: Lemon juice increases urinary citrate and may prevent calcium stones. Whether one uses the recommended half cup of lemon juice per day straight up or diluted is a personal choice. Lemonade is another frequently recommended choice. Apple and cranberry juice contain oxalates associated with a higher risk of calcium oxalate stones and should be avoided.[12] A low-oxalate diet is advised to help avoid calcium oxalate stones.

Calcium: There is a substantial body of evidence, both from controlled trials and from observational studies, indicating that increased intake of calcium reduces the risk of kidney stones.[13,14] And decreased calcium consumption has been found to increase stone recurrence in many patients.[1]

For those at risk to calcium oxalate stones (e.g., patients with IBS), calcium carbonate or calcium acetate (e.g., 365–500 mg with each meal) can be used to restrict oxalate absorption to reduce the risk of recurrent kidney stones.[15]

General Advice: To prevent kidney stones, consider taking magnesium oxide, pyridoxine, citrate, and phytate. Some supplements are available that combine these substances. These include Renalstat (Rematech Nutrahealth), Kidney Support Formula (VRP), and Kidney Stone Formula (Bio Essence). This should help to minimize an individual's risk of recurrent kidney stones.[16]

URIC ACID STONES

General Advice: Uric acid stones require dietary manipulation, adequate fluid intake to optimize volumes, and manipulation of urinary pH.[16] (*See* Potassium Citrate *below.*)

Potassium Citrate: It is known that citrate preparations such as potassium citrate increase urine pH by accumulating HCO_3- in urine, and eliminate uric acid calculi by decomposing the uric acid crystal. The additional use of uric acid excretion stimulators with citrate preparations further reduces uric acid calculi in the kidney. Thus, citrate preparations appear to be beneficial for preventing deterioration of renal function in the patients with CKD who also have elevated levels of serum uric acid and are treated with allopurinol.[17]

Low urine citrate (<300 mg/24 h; a crystallization inhibitor) or a lower urine pH (<6.5 for uric acid stones) can both be managed with potassium citrate (e.g., 20–30 mEq twice daily).[18]

Lead Poisoning

Lead is a poisonous heavy metal that human bodies cannot use. If lead levels build up over months or years in the body, it causes lead poisoning. Even small amounts of lead can cause serious health problems. Signs and symptoms usually do not appear until dangerous levels of lead are present. Lead poisoning can permanently damage a child's brain, and most children do not usually show other symptoms of lead poisoning.[1] Symptoms and signs that can be present include muscle and joint pain, headaches, memory and concentration problems, nerve disorders, anemia (hypochromic and microcytic with basophilic stippling), constipation, cramps, gingival lead lines, and slowed growth. Lead-based paint, lead-contaminated water, or dust from older buildings are the most common sources of lead poisoning in children.

CONSERVATIVE MEASURES

Ascorbic Acid: As an adjunct to chelation therapy, vitamin C should be used to help prevent lead from being absorbed.[1] A recent study published by the Journal of the American Medical Association found that subjects with high levels of vitamin C intake (e.g., 1,000 mg/day) had less measurable lead in their blood stream than subjects with low levels of vitamin C intake. Children with the higher vitamin C intake were 89% less likely to have elevated blood lead levels.[2]

Mineral deficiencies appear to have some of the most profound effects on lead toxicity, since the consequences can be exaggerated by diets low in calcium, phosphorus, iron, zinc, and, in some cases, copper.[3] Epidemiological surveys have suggested a negative correlation between the poor nutritional status of children with regard to calcium and the concentration of lead in blood.[3]

Iron sulfate supplementation lowered blood lead levels in affected children.[4,5]

Sodium Iron EDTA: A team of researchers recommended using sodium iron EDTA to fortify foodstuffs and lower blood lead concentrations. EDTA, which stands for ethylene diamine tetraacetic acid, forms stable complexes with iron, aiding its uptake into the bloodstream. The researchers concluded that sodium iron EDTA was more effective than iron sulfate in reducing the level of lead in the bloodstream.[6]

Vitamin B1 has been reported to decrease lead (Pb) levels in the liver, kidneys, bone, and blood in animal studies.[4] Vitamin B1 influences the absorption of Pb and its pyrimidine ring may cause an increase in Pb excretion and the alleviation of its toxicity.[7]

Vitamin B6 has also been found to be effective in reducing accumulation of Pb in tissues and in reducing inhibition of ALAD activity from higher blood lead levels.[7]

Vitamins C and E: Vitamin C (1 gm/day) and E (400 IU/day) reduced lipid peroxidation in erythrocytes to lower levels compared to non-lead exposed workers.[7] Another study reported vitamin E to be very effective against lead toxicity.[8]

Probiotics: Research has shown that two lactobacilli strains (*L. plantarum* and *L. rhamnosus*) exhibit protective effects against lead toxicity in mice.[7]

Leber's Hereditary Optic Neuropathy (LHON)/ Leber's Optic Atrophy (LOA)

LHON is an inherited mitochondrial disorder that affects men (60%–90%) more than women and leads to painless subacute loss of central vision. The condition usually begins in an individual's teens or twenties. Loss of visual acuity (blurring or clouding) and color vision are usually the first symptoms of LHON. The condition mainly affects central vision and significantly interferes with reading, writing, driving, and recognizing faces and colors, as well as doing close-up work (e.g., reading, cooking, or fixing things). Even if symptoms start in one eye, both eyes are eventually affected. Although central vision improves in a small percentage of cases, no generally accepted measures have been shown either to prevent or delay the onset of blindness.[1]

COMMON SENSE CARE STRATEGIES

Avoidance of Alcohol and Nicotine: For general health reasons, it would be wise even for unaffected LHON carriers to moderate their alcohol intake and to stop smoking. It has been reported that in many cases of LHON the severity of the disease is related to smoking tobacco products.[2]

General Advice: Treatment of LHON is limited to symptomatic therapy and nutritional supplements.[3]

Idebenone: Taking idebenone can improve vision in people with early stage Leber's disease.[4] One small, non-randomized trial reported that oral administration of a quinone analogue (idebedone) and vitamin supplementation with vitamins B12 and C helped with visual recovery.[5,6]

Cyanocobalamin and Hydroxycobalamin: In two patients, hydroxocobalamin, a synthetic, injectable form of vitamin B12, was found to be superior to cyanocobalamin (a manufactured form of vitamin B12) in the treatment LHON. The dose was 1 mg twice weekly in one subject and 1 mg weekly in the other subject. Visual acuity in both eyes improved.[7]

Tocopherol: The antioxidant α-tocotrienol-quinone (EPI-743), a vitamin E derivative, has also shown promising early results. A small open-label study of five patients with acute LHON showed that early treatment with EPI-743 arrested disease progression in four out of five of the LHON-patients.[8]

Leigh Syndrome (Encephalopathy)

Leigh syndrome (LS) is a severe genetic neurodegenerative disease that usually becomes apparent between the ages of three months and two years. It is characterized by the degeneration of the central nervous system (i.e., brain, spinal cord, and optic nerve). The first signs of Leigh syndrome in infancy are usually vomiting, diarrhea, and difficulty swallowing (dysphagia). LS results in a failure to grow and gain weight (failure to thrive). Hypotonia, dystonia, and ataxia develop, making movements difficult. Leigh's typically results in death within two to three years, usually due to respiratory failure. A small number of individuals do not develop symptoms until adulthood or have symptoms that worsen more gradually.[1]

THERAPY CHOICES

Thiamine: The most common treatment for Leigh syndrome is the administration of thiamine (vitamin B1) 100 mg tid or thiamine derivatives. Some people with this disorder may experience a temporary symptomatic improvement or a modest slowing of the progression of the disease.[2,3]

Diet: In those patients with Leigh syndrome who also have a deficiency of pyruvate dehydrogenase enzyme complex, a high-fat, low-carbohydrate diet may be recommended.[3]

Biotin: Specific therapy via biotin administration is appropriate for three forms of Leigh-like syndrome:

- biotin-thiamine-responsive basal ganglia disease
- biotinidase deficiency
- coenzyme Q10 deficiency due to PDSS2 mutation[4]

Riboflavin and coenzyme Q10 are often recommended.[4]

Biotin and Thiamine: One study recommended that every patient with suspected LS obtain high-dose biotin (10–20 mg/kg) and thiamine (100–300 mg) treatments immediately.[5] A patient with Leigh's whose brain MRI revealed fairly symmetrical, bilateral signal changes with swelling in the caudate nuclei and putamen was treated with a dose of thiamine 150 mg and biotin 10 mg with positive results.[6]

Leiner Disease

Leiner disease, also known as erythroderma desquamativum, is a systemic skin disease that occurs in infants. It is more common in breast-fed infants and females than males. Leiner disease resembles severe seborrheic dermatitis. The disorder may be present at birth but more commonly develops within the first few months of life. The condition usually starts off as a scaly rash (exfoliative dermatitis) on the scalp, face, or neck and chest areas. The rash spreads rapidly to other parts of the body. The affected areas are bright red (erythroderma) and may look swollen. Infants appear uncomfortable but do not itch. Other symptoms may include intractable diarrhea, recurrent infections, and failure to thrive.[1] The cause of Leiner disease remains unknown.

TREATMENT STRATEGY

Biotin: Treatment with 2–4 mg/day of biotin for two to three weeks has been shown to significantly improve the condition.[2]

Leprosy

Leprosy, also known as Hansen's disease, is a chronic infection of skin and peripheral nerves caused by *Mycobacterium leprae.* The main symptom of leprosy is disfiguring pale-colored skin sores, lumps, or bumps that do not go away after several weeks or months. If left untreated, signs of advanced leprosy can develop, which include crippling of hands and feet, shortening of toes and fingers due to reabsorption, a marked flattening of the nose, loss of eyebrows, and blindness.

THERAPEUTIC APPROACHES

Zinc: The addition of oral zinc to antileprosy treatment has been shown to improve therapeutic outcome. Rapid clinical improvement in leprosy lesions (erythema nodosum leprosum) has been reported with oral zinc in addition to multiple drug treatment.[1]

Leukemia

Leukemia is cancer of the early blood-forming cells (lymphoid cells and myeloid cells). Most often, leukemia is a cancer of the white blood cells causing a rise in the number of white blood cells that end up being too numerous and do not work properly. Some leukemias, however, can start in other blood cell types. People with leukemia are at significantly increased risk for developing infections, anemia, and bleeding. Other symptoms and signs include easy bruising, weight loss, night sweats, and unexplained fevers.[1] Leukemia can affect children, but affects adults more often. Nothing can be done to prevent leukemia.

ALTERNATE TREATMENT OPTIONS

Ascorbic Acid: Since the 1970s, researchers have taken an interest in high-dose intravenous vitamin C and its therapeutic potential for treating cancer. New research shows how vitamin C might stop leukemic stem cells from multiplying, and thus block some forms of blood cancer from advancing.[1] Intravenous treatment with vitamin C promoted DNA demethylation, which "tells" leukemic stem cells to mature and die as they are supposed to.[2,3,4]

Para-Aminobenzoic Acid (PABA) and its metallic salts are used in the treatment of diseases such as leukemia[5,6] and lymphoblastoma cutis.[7] A typical therapeutic dosage is 300–400 mg/day. Side effects have been noted in doses above 8,000 mg/day.[8]

Leukoplakia

Leukoplakia is a precancerous condition that causes thickened white or gray patches to develop on the gums, mucosa (inside of the cheek), or on the tongue. A biopsy is often obtained for diagnosis. The patch or patches are typically painless and form as a result of chronic irritation (e.g., from smoking, a rough tooth surface, or poorly fitting dentures).

MANAGEMENT

Removing the source of the irritation such as smoking, etc., is the primary treatment.

Lycopene: Preliminary evidence suggests a significant clinical response with use of lycopene for oral leukoplakia.[1] A typical oral dose is 13–75 mg/day.

Liver Disease—Alcoholic Hepatitis/Cirrhosis

A liver disease is any disturbance of liver function that causes illness. Liver disease can present as a spectrum of clinical conditions that ranges from asymptomatic disease to end-stage liver disease.[1] The two most common chronic liver diseases are viral hepatitis (*see* Hepatitis) and cirrhosis. In cirrhosis, liver cells are replaced with fibrotic tissue. The term *cirrhosis* is derived from the Greek "kirrhos" meaning orange-colored, and refers to the yellow-orange hue of the liver seen by the pathologist or surgeon.[2] Cirrhosis is the twelfth most common cause of death in the U.S. and the fourth most frequent cause in the 45–54 year age group.

Cirrhosis can result from any cause of chronic liver inflammation, but is primarily due to alcoholic hepatitis, NASH, or the hepatitis C virus.[3] The spectrum of alcoholic liver disease encompasses several conditions so that a single patient may be affected by fatty liver, and/or alcoholic hepatitis, and/or alcoholic cirrhosis. Symptoms of liver toxicity are right upper abdominal pain, jaundice (yellowing of the skin and whites of the eyes), itching, fatigue, loss of appetite, weight loss, and dark or tea-colored urine. Alcoholic hepatitis can lead to scarring, or cirrhosis, of the liver and ultimately liver failure.

Complications of cirrhosis include portal hypertension (due to increased resistance to blood flow with rupture of esophageal varices), encephalopathy, hepatorenal syndrome, and hepatopulmonary syndrome. Tobacco smoking and certain drugs may also contribute to cirrhosis.[4]

NUTRITIONAL SUPPORT

Alcohol: Abstinence counseling is recommended. The progression of cirrhosis secondary to alcohol abuse can be interrupted by abstinence. Therefore, it is of the utmost importance to avoid alcohol.[5]

Medical Nutrition: Medical management for alcoholic hepatitis should include a high-protein diet supplemented with B vitamins, including B1 and folic acid. Fat-soluble vitamins should be administered as well. Vitamin deficiencies are common among people who consume excessive amounts of alcohol, even in the absence of liver disease. Deficits of vitamins A, B1 (thiamine), B6 (pyridoxine), and folic acid are of particular concern, as they not only are common but may exacerbate the detrimental effects of alcohol.[6] In alcoholic hepatitis, treatment with folic acid is frequently associated with dramatic improvement.[7]

Illegal Drugs: Avoidance of illegal drugs is also critical to reducing damage and promoting recovery.[5]

Vitamin D: An association between low concentrations of vitamin D and occurrence as well as severity of chronic liver disease (CLD) has been well-established.[8] Vitamin D3 is responsible for reduced levels of infectious amounts of hepatitis C virus. It is known that vitamin D deficiency causes an increase in fibrosis and inflammation in the liver.[8] Epidemiological evidence also shows a correlation between the status of vitamin D and different forms of liver cancer.

The anti-inflammatory and immunoregulatory properties of vitamin D make its analogs a good choice for the prevention and treatment of liver disorders and cancer.[8]

Vitamin K: Nutritional deficiency is common with cirrhosis, especially in individuals with coexisting biliary disease. This leads to a reduction in bile production and flow, resulting in decreased intraluminal concentrations of biliary salts. The end-result is decreased absorption of fat-soluble vitamins, including vitamin K.[9] Vitamin K is often administered in the treatment of coagulopathies (prolonged prothrombin time) secondary to parenchymal liver disease.

Sodium Restriction: Sodium restriction (less than 2 gm/day) is indicated when ascites and/or edema is present.

L-Carnitine: Giving L-carnitine intravenously (by IV) can prevent severe liver toxicity and side effects caused by accidental or intentional overdose of valproic acid (Depacon, Depakene, Depakote, VPA).[10]

NAC: N-acetylcysteine has been used to prevent liver damage due to excessive alcohol consumption.[11]

Selenium and Zinc: Low levels of both zinc and selenium are associated with increased damage to the liver and are low in alcoholic cirrhosis.[12,13] Studies regarding the possible therapeutic effect of zinc and selenium supplementation are worth pursuing.[13]

In one study, the administration of vitamin E, together with selenium and zinc, resulted in a greater decrease in bilirubin and in a lower one-month mortality in patients with alcoholic hepatitis.[14]

Silymarin is an extract of milk thistle. There is substantial evidence suggesting that silymarin treatment improves hepatic diseases.[15] Four of six studies regarding milk thistle and chronic alcoholic liver disease reported significant improvement in at least one measurement of liver function (i.e., aminotransferases, albumin, and/or malondialdehyde) or histologic findings.[16] A clinical study conducted in 170 cirrhosis patients treated with 140 mg of silymarin three times daily for 41 months showed significant improvement.[17]

Liver Disease—Viral Hepatitis

Hepatitis refers to inflammation of liver cells and damage to the liver. It encompasses a broad range of clinico-pathologic conditions resulting from viral, toxic (e.g., excessive alcohol, drugs, chemicals), or immune-mediated damage to the liver. There are five common types of hepatitis caused by viruses (A, B, C, D, and E), but the most common are A, B, and C. Each type has different characteristics and transmission happens in different ways, but the symptoms tend to be similar.[1]

Hepatitis A is the most common cause of viral hepatitis worldwide and is characterized by the abrupt onset of fever, abdominal pain, malaise, jaundice, anorexia, and nausea in older children and adults. However, a number of individuals with hepatitis A, B, or C have no symptoms at all. Hepatitis B or C can have an insidious onset and symptoms may be absent or mild but can also include jaundice, fever, fatigue, anorexia, nausea, dark urine, and abdominal discomfort. Hepatitis B is 100 times more contagious than HIV and is spread from contact with bodily fluids.[2] Hepatitis can be self-limiting or can progress to fibrosis (scarring), cirrhosis, or liver cancer.

MANAGEMENT

Milk thistle (silymarin) has three active flavonoid components: silybin, silydianin, and silychristine. Silybin has the greatest degree of biologic activity and standard silymarin extracts contain 70% silybin.[1] Silymaryin appears to have antioxidant and toxin-reducing properties in the liver and has been shown to reduce liver fibrosis and enhance liver regeneration in animal studies.[3]

SNMC (Stronger Neominophagen C): A typical neominophagen C formulation contains 200 mg of glycyrrhizin (a major component of licorice root), 100 mg of cysteine, and 2,000 mg of glycine in 100 cc of saline for the treatment of chronic hepatitis. The reported beneficial effects of glycyrrhizin on liver tissue include:

- Stabilization of hepatic cellular membranes.
- Inhibition of production of PGE2.
- Augmentation of the effects of interferon.[1]

Most SNMC studies have administered daily IV injections; however, more recent studies suggest that an oral form may be equally effective.

Oral thymus preparations include components such as bovine thymopoeitin and thymic humoral factor. They have been used to treat hepatitis with some promising results, but the small sample size is a problem.[1,4]

Vitamin B12 and Folic Acid: Eighty-eight patients with acute viral hepatitis received either conventional treatment (a high-protein diet and bed rest) or conventional treatment plus vitamin B12 injections. Patients treated with vitamin B12 were also given folic acid tablets (5 mg three times a day for 10 days). Those receiving the vitamins had a more rapid return of appetite, faster improvement in liver function, and a reduction in duration of illness.[5]

Taurine: Previous clinical studies demonstrate that taking 1.5–4 gm of taurine daily for up to three months improves liver function in patients with hepatitis.[6]

Low Birth Weight Infants

Premature infants born with a birth weight less than 2,500 gm or 5.5 lbs are defined as low birth weight (LBW) infants. LBW infants are more likely to die within the first 28 days of life and are at substantially higher risk for increased morbidity and rehospitalization than children born at normal birth weights.[1] LBW babies are at risk for respiratory distress syndrome, intraventricular hemorrhage, patent ductus arteriosus, retinopathy of immaturity, exaggerated hyperbilirubinemia, and necrotizing enterocolitis. Low birth weight infants are also at increased risk for behavioral and emotional problems.[2] The rates of low birth weight deliveries in the U.S. continue to be high.

IMPROVING FETAL OUTCOMES

Smoking, alcohol, or recreational drug use should be avoided.[3]

Vitamin A: A study of 807 extremely low birth weight infants (weighing less than 2.5 lbs and requiring respiratory support within 24 hours of birth) received intramuscular injections of vitamin A (5,000 IU) three days a week for four weeks.[3] By 36 weeks, the overall incidence of complications, namely chronic lung disease or death, were significantly lower in the vitamin A group (55%), compared with the control group (62%).[4]

Vitamin E: Low birth weight infants are born with low serum and tissue concentrations of vitamin E. When these infants are fed a diet unusually rich in polyunsaturated fatty acids and inadequate in vitamin E, a hemolytic anemia will develop by four to six weeks of age, particularly if iron is also present in the diet. The anemia is often associated with morphologic alterations of the erythrocytes, thrombocytosis, and edema of the tops of the feet and the pretibial area. Treatment with vitamin E produces a prompt increase in hemoglobin level, a decrease in the elevated reticulocyte count, a normalization of the red cell life span, and a disappearance of the thrombocytosis and edema. Modifications of infant formulas have all but eliminated vitamin E deficiency in preterm infants.[5]

Folic Acid: Folic acid plays a major role in preventing birth defects or health problems in infants. Four hundred micrograms of folic acid daily, usually starting before conception, can reduce the chances of a baby being born with low birth weight. For mothers who smoke, taking 4 mg of folic acid per day resulted in a 31% lower risk of the fetus being small for gestational age.[6] No adverse effects were associated with higher-dose folic acid.[6]

Lupus (Discoid)

Discoid lupus is an autoimmune disorder that affects the skin, causing thick, scaly, coin-shaped bumps or a rash with raised borders, ranging in color from red to purple on areas of the body that are exposed to sunlight.[1] The scalp, ears, cheeks, and nose are the most common sites. Scarring and hair loss are common complications. Treatment is directed at preventing flares, improving appearance, and preventing scarring.

MANAGEMENT TECHNIQUES

Sun blocks are essential to treatment.

Topical corticosteroids effectively reduce inflammatory symptoms in all types of CLE.

Vitamin E: Since vitamin E is a physiologic stabilizer of cellular and lysosomal membranes, and since some autoimmune diseases respond to vitamin E, one researcher suggested that a relative deficiency of vitamin E damages lysosomal membranes and may initiate an autoimmune process such as in lupus. Vitamin E, when properly administered in adequate doses, is a safe and effective treatment for chronic discoid lupus erythematosus.[2] A case report of two patients indicated that a topical formula containing vitamin E improves the health of skin in people with discoid lupus erythematosus.[3]

Lupus (Systemic Lupus Erythematosus)

Systemic lupus erythematosus is a multisytem disease that primarily affects women of childbearing age.[1] The word "lupus" is Latin for "wolf." The disease is called lupus because a distinctive cheek rash in a percentage of patients can resemble the markings on a wolf's face.

Systemic lupus erythematosus (SLE) is a chronic inflammatory and systemic autoimmune disease where the body's immune system attacks its own tissues and organs. Inflammation caused by lupus can affect many different body systems including joints, skin, kidneys, blood cells, brain, nerves (neuropathies), heart, and lungs. The most common nervous system manifestation is intractable headaches.[2] Organ involvement can range from mild to potentially life threatening. Connective tissue diseases like SLE are associated with early and accelerated atherosclerosis, also known as early vascular aging. The disease is not contagious. The majority of lupus patients are female and the disease often develops between the ages of 15 and 35, but can occur at any age. The disease affects African Americans and Asians to a greater extent than other races.

Nonspecific lupus symptoms and signs include fatigue, swollen and painful joints, weight loss, fever, and rash. Lupus has been called "the great imitator" because symptoms are often like those of rheumatoid arthritis, blood disorders, fibromyalgia, diabetes, thyroid problems, Lyme disease, and a number of heart, lung, muscle, and bone diseases.[3] Two-thirds of individuals with lupus have increased sensitivity to ultraviolet rays, either from sunlight or from artificial inside light, such as fluorescent light—or both. Lupus typically follows a pattern of periodic flare-ups alternating with periods of remissions. Infections are the leading cause of morbidity and mortality in individuals with SLE.

TREATMENT PROTOCOLS

Conservative therapy alone is warranted if the patient's manifestations are mild. This includes obtaining adequate sleep and avoiding fatigue, as mild disease exacerbations may subside after a few days of bed rest.[4]

Cigarette smoke and excessive exposure to direct sunlight should be avoided. Wearing a SPF 30 sunscreen or higher is often recommended.

Alcohol: There is a link between moderate alcohol intake and a reduced risk of SLE which has not been explained.[5]

Healthy Diet: A healthy diet is important in general, but perhaps even more so for the individuals who suffer from systemic lupus erythematosus (SLE).[6] Consuming adequate amounts of the right nutrients, and limiting others, can help relieve symptoms and improve outcomes.[6]

Complementary Therapies: In a review of complementary therapies for lupus, scientists noted that the following have shown promise in the treatment of systemic lupus erythematosus (SLE):[5]

- Vitamin D (*see below*)
- Omega-3 fatty acids
- N-acetylcysteine
- Turmeric

NSAIDs may be used to alleviate musculoskeletal pain, swelling, and aches.

Medications to Avoid: A number of medications (e.g., Rozerem, Bactrim, Septra, and melatonin) can trigger symptoms and should be avoided if possible. At least 80 medications can cause drug-induced lupus erythematosus flare-ups.[7]

DHEA: Twenty-eight women with mild to moderate systemic lupus erythematous (SLE) received the adrenal hormone DHEA (200 mg/day) or a placebo for three months in a double-blind study. In patients receiving DHEA, the severity of the disease and the requirement for prednisone (a cortisone-like drug) decreased. DHEA also appeared to have a beneficial effect on overall well-being, fatigue, and energy levels.[8] Dehydroepiandrosterone (DHEA) may help with fatigue and muscle pain.[9] DHEA is also effective in treating some of the symptoms of mild to moderate lupus, including hair loss (alopecia), joint pain, fatigue, and cognitive dysfunction (e.g., difficulty thinking, memory loss, distractibility, difficulty in multitasking).[10]

Vitamins A and E: Lupus is often associated with low levels of vitamins A and E.[9]

In one study, 12 women among 36 outpatients with SLE received vitamin E (150–300 mg/day) together with prednisolone (PSL). The study suggested that vitamin E can suppress autoantibody production via a mechanism independent of antioxidant activity.[11]

Fish Oil: Fish oil supplements contain omega-3 fatty acids that may be beneficial for individuals with lupus. Preliminary studies have found some promise, although additional studies are necessary.[12]

Para-Aminobenzoic Acid (PABA): PABA has been used to treat SLE.[12] PABA and its metallic salts have also been used in the treatment of such diseases as dermatomyositis, the rickettsial diseases, dermatitis herpetiformis, scrub and murine typhus fevers, rheumatic fever, leukemia, and vitiligo.[13,14] Most of these studies are old and new research would be beneficial.[15,16] A typical therapeutic dosage is 300–400 mg/day. Side effects have been noted in doses above 8,000 mg/day.[17]

Vitamin D: Inadequate levels of vitamin D has been reported in patients with SLE.[18] In one study, 67% of lupus patients were deficient in vitamin D. Research suggests that patients with lupus can benefit from supplemental vitamin D. Any existing vitamin D deficiency can be corrected by prescribing 50,000 IU capsule of vitamin D2 weekly for eight weeks, followed by either 50,000 IU of vitamin D2 every two to four weeks, or daily doses of 1,000 IU to 2,000 IU of vitamin D3.[19] Vitamin D supplementation with regular monitoring should be considered as part of SLE management plans.[18]

Macular Degeneration/ Age Related Macular Degeneration (AMD)

Macular degeneration is an eye condition which may result in blurred or dark areas, or loss of vision in the center of the visual field. There are two types of AMD. In the more aggressive wet type (15% of cases), pathologic angiogenesis occurs which is the formation of fragile new blood vessels where they do not belong, under the macula, a small spot in the center of the retina at the back of the eye. These blood vessels break and bleed easily. The ensuing macular damage leads to the loss of central vision.[1] In the dry type of AMD (85% of cases), small yellow deposits (drusen) slowly accumulate under the macula, also causing loss of central vision. As a result, driving and recognizing faces and colors as well as doing close-up work (e.g., reading, writing, cooking, or fixing things) are seriously compromised.

Macular degeneration is the leading cause of vision loss among people 50 years and older, more than cataracts and glaucoma combined. AMD is more likely to occur after age 60. AMD is an incurable eye disease, but it is treatable. There are three stages of AMD. The early stage has no symptoms and no treatment exists. The intermediate stage usually has no symptoms, but some vision loss may occur. At this stage, nutritional supplements can slow the progression of the disease. In late-stage AMD, vision loss is definitely present.

PREVENTIVE MEASURES

Nicotine: Smokers are up to four times more likely than non-smokers to have macular degeneration, so patients should try to stop or cut down on smoking. Cessation counseling may be appropriate.

Glutathione and Vitamin E: Chemical damage to the retinal cells may be prevented with glutathione and vitamin E.[2]

Lutein is an antioxidant found in fruits and vegetables. A group of patients with AMD were given lutein (10 mg/day) plus antioxidants, minerals, and other nutrients, or a placebo, for 12 months. Supplementation with lutein in a dosage of 10 mg/day in men with age-related macular degeneration resulted in improved visual acuity. Antioxidants, however, were found to be of no benefit.[3]

Taking vitamin C, vitamin E, beta-carotene, and zinc helps prevent AMD from becoming worse in people at high risk for developing advanced AMD.[4]

The Age-Related Eye Disease Study (AREDS), led by NIH's National Eye Institute, showed that daily high doses of vitamins C and E, beta-carotene, and the minerals zinc and copper, called the AREDS formulation, can help slow the progression to advanced age-related macular degeneration (AMD), a blinding eye disease.[5,6] The AREDS2 formula, together with lutein and zeaxanthin, may help slow or stop AMD. The following daily supplementation is recommended based on AREDS and AREDS2 research:

- 500 mg of vitamin C
- 400 international units of vitamin E
- 80 mg zinc as zinc oxide
- 2 mg copper as cupric oxide
- 10 mg lutein and 2 mg zeaxanthin[3]

Coenzyme Q10, acetyl-L-carnitine, and omega-3 fatty acids (Phototrop) by mouth can improve vision in patients with age-related vision loss.[7]

Sunglasses: Helping to protect damaged eyes by wearing sunglasses with 100% UV absorption is important.[8]

Resveratrol: The development of new blood vessels in the choroid layer of the eye (choroidal neovascularization) is a critical step in the pathogenesis of age-related macular degeneration (AMD). In animal studies, resveratrol suppressed development of these blood vessels.[9] Three case studies in patients with age-related macular degeneration demonstrated dramatic anatomic retinal restoration and visual improvement subsequent to daily administration of a resveratrol-based nutritional supplement. A typical daily dose of resveratrol for a 150 pound person is 450 mg.

Pyridoxine deficiency has been identified in two observational studies in AMD populations. Folate deficiency has been identified in one of the studies. The B vitamins, in general, are important for nerve conduction, and the methylators (B4, B6, and B12) reduce homocysteine levels. Christen et al. reported a reduction in AMD development in 5,205 women observed for 7.3 years who were given daily supplementation consisting of 2,500 mcg B9 (folate), 500 mg B6 (pyridoxine), and 1,000 mcg B12 (cyanocobalamin).[10]

Maple Syrup Urine Disease (MSUD)

Maple syrup urine disease is an inherited disorder that affects branched-chain amino acids. It is one type of organic acidemia. The condition gets its name from the distinctive sweet odor that emanates from an affected infant's urine. This disorder is characterized by mild intellectual disability and neurologic symptoms. Initially, nonspecific symptoms such as lethargy, irritability, and poor feeding are indicative of increasing neurological dysfunction. Soon thereafter, these symptoms are followed by focal neurological signs such as abnormal movements and increasing spasticity. Convulsions and deepening coma develop soon after the appearance of focal signs.[1] If untreated, progressive brain damage is inevitable and death ensues usually within weeks or months.[1] Newborn screening for MSUD is performed throughout the U.S. to allow for rapid diagnosis.

MANAGEMENT TECHNIQUES

Diet: The disorder can be successfully managed through a specialized protein-restrictive diet that limits the amount of branched-chain amino acids (leucine, isoleucine, and valine) taken in. It is particularly important to limit the amount of leucine in the diet. The three amino acids are added to the diet separately in small amounts so that affected individuals can grow and develop normally.[2]

Thiamine: A number of physicians recommend a clinical trial of thiamine therapy to determine whether an affected individual is thiamine-responsive.[2,3] Thiamine dosages used to treat MSUD range from 10–100 mg each day.[4]

Measles/Rubeola

Measles is an acute and highly contagious respiratory illness caused by the rubeola virus. Symptoms start about 7-10 days after an individual is infected. It starts with fever, runny nose, cough, red eyes, and sore throat. Those are followed by a red, mostly flat rash that starts on the face and then spreads over the body. Koplik's spots may form inside the mouth two or three days after the start of symptoms. Measles can be very unpleasant and can sometimes lead to ear infections or diarrhea, or more serious complications such as pneumonia or encephalitis. Pneumonia is the most common cause of death from measles in young children.[1] Measles can also cause pregnant women to give birth prematurely.[1]

REDUCING INFECTIONS, COMPLICATIONS, AND DEATHS

General Measures: There is no specific antiviral therapy for measles. Treatment, therefore, is primarily supportive with control of fever and prevention and correction of dehydration.[2]

Isolation: To reduce the spread of the disease, isolate affected individuals from others, particularly unimmunized children, for at least four days after the appearance of the rash.

Vitamin A: Children with measles or malnutrition are at very high risk of vitamin A deficiency.[3] Taking vitamin A by mouth reduces the risk of complications and death in children with measles and vitamin A deficiency,[4] so high-dose supplements should be part of their treatment. In a Cochrane review, children under two years of age with severe measles received 200,000 IUs of vitamin A for two consecutive days. This lowered the number of deaths from pneumonia-specific mortality.[5] For children with severe measles, the CDC endorses age-specific daily doses of: 50,000 IU for infants younger than 6 months of age, 100,000 IU for infants 6-11 months of age, and 200,000 IU for children 12 months of age and older.[6]

Melanoma

Melanoma, also known as malignant melanoma, is a cancer of melanocytes in the bottom layer (stratum basale) of the skin's epidermis. It is the most serious and highly aggressive form of skin cancer because of its ability to rapidly spread to other organs. This type of skin cancer can develop in an existing mole or look like a new mole on the skin. Suspicious moles usually present with asymmetry, border irregularity, color changes, and a diameter of more than 6 mm (about the size of a pencil eraser). Early surgical intervention remains the most successful therapy for melanoma. Despite progress, results of pharmacological therapies are still disappointing.[1]

LOWERING RISKS

Coenzyme Q10: A three-year trial contemplating uninterrupted treatment with low-dose recombinant interferon alpha-2b administered twice daily and coenzyme Q10 (400 mg/day) was conducted in patients with stage I and II melanoma and surgically removed lesions. Treatment efficacy was evaluated as incidence of recurrences at five years. Significantly different rates of disease progression were observed in the interferon plus CoQ10 group. Long-term administration of an optimized dose of recombinant interferon alpha-2b in combination with CoQ10 significantly decreased rates of recurrence and had negligible adverse effects. CoQ10 supplemented patients were 10–13 times less likely to develop metastasis.[1]

Aspirin: A recent observational study and a meta-analysis indicate that low-dose aspirin may have a preventive effect on melanoma as well as basal and squamous cell cancers.[2,3]

Vitamin A deficiency is accompanied by morphologic changes in the epithelial cells and is characterized by metaplasia and hyperkeratosis.[4]

Researchers analyzed melanoma risk among 69,635 people. Study participants were aged 62 on average. The researchers found that those participants who took vitamin A via supplements were about 40% less likely to develop melanoma than those who did not.[5]

Ketogenic Diet: A ketogenic diet has been of interest in oncology research as an adjunctive therapy. The hypothesis is that because cancer cells cannot metabolize ketones but normal cells can (Warburg effect), a ketogenic diet can aid in the treatment of malignant disease.[6] Further studies are needed.

Selenium supplementation to slow the progression of pre-existing skin neoplasms has been reported to also lower all-cause mortality in patients with skin cancer.[7]

Melasma/Chloasma

Melasma is a common skin problem that causes a patch or patches of tan or dark (hypermelanosis) discolored skin that is difficult to treat. It typically appears on the upper cheeks, upper lip, forehead, and chin of women 20–50 years of age. Although it can affect anyone, melasma is particularly common in women, especially pregnant women and those who are taking oral or patch contraceptives or hormone replacement therapy (HRT) medications.

COSMETIC APPROACHES

Zinc Sulfate or Ascorbic Acid: Twenty melasma patients between the ages of 25 and 54 were studied. Patients received treatment with either 10% zinc sulfate or 10% L-ascorbic acid applied once daily. After two months of treatment there was significant improvement of melasma with both treatments. Minimal side effects were found with zinc sulfate.[1]

Niacinamide 4% is an effective topical agent when used daily for eight weeks for the treatment of melasma, as assessed by objective methods and clinical evaluation. Results indicate that 4% niacinamide was effective in approximate 40% of patients, showing outstanding clinical results.[2]

Emblica: Limited clinical studies have been conducted using emblica extracts in combination with other agents in skin-lightening creams as an alternative to hydroquinone.[3] Some research suggests that applying a cream containing emblica and belides twice daily for 60 days is effective for lightening skin in people with skin discolorations.[4]

Memory Loss/Forgetfulness

It is common to worry about becoming forgetful. Everyone forgets things at times, whether it is occasional mild forgetfulness (e.g., a person's name or where the car keys were last seen) or a more persistent loss of memory. With increasing age, it is rational to be concerned that short-term problems may be the start of long-term mental decline. Short-term memory loss is an unusual degree of forgetfulness due to the process of losing the ability to store and remember information. An example is when a person can remember incidents from 20 years ago clearly, but is fuzzy on the details of things that happened recently.

Causes for short-term memory problems include normal aging, different medical conditions, medications (e.g., antidepressants, anti-anxiety meds, muscle relaxants, tranquilizers, sleeping pills, and pain medications), mild cognitive impairment, and dementia. Most medical conditions causing short-term memory loss can be improved with treatment.

ANCILLARY MANAGEMENT METHODS

Deficiencies specifically in vitamin B1 and B12 can adversely affect memory.[1]

Choline is a vitamin-like essential nutrient and is a precursor and necessary building block for the production of two vital components of the nervous system: (1) acetylcholine (a vital neurotransmitter) and (2) sphingomyelin (which is required for nerve cell protection).

An Italian study examined 349 patients older than 64 years who had memory complaints and evidence of vascular lesions, but did not have probable Alzheimer's disease. Results showed that the participants who received citicoline (500 mg bid) had significantly better memory scores.[2]

In other studies, older individuals with vascular diseases were given therapeutic doses of citicoline orally (e.g., 500–2,000 mg/day in two divided doses), by intramuscular injection, or by intravenous infusion. This resulted in improvements in cognitive, emotional, and behavioral functions.[3,4,5,6]

CDP-choline (citicoline) and choline salts, such as choline chloride and choline bitartrate, are available as supplements.[7]

A cross-sectional data analysis of a subgroup of 1,391 volunteers between the ages of 36 and 83 from the large Framingham Heart Study Offspring cohort indicates that dietary choline intake was positively associated with specific cognitive functions, namely verbal memory and visual memory.[8]

Another cross-sectional study of 2,195 individuals between the ages of 70 and 74 found high plasma concentrations of free choline to be significantly associated with a better performance on cognitive tests assessing sensory motor speed, perceptual speed, executive function, and global cognition.[9]

Acetyl-L-Carnitine: In one study, 279 individuals with mild to moderately severe mental decline received 1,500 mg/day of acetyl-l-carnitine and a placebo, during two separate treatment periods. Compared with the placebo, acetyl-l-carnitine significantly improved cognitive function, emotional status, and behavior.[10]

Ginkgo Biloba: Significant improvements were noted in short-term memory, vigilance, and mood with 120 mg/day of ginkgo biloba.[11,12,13]

Glycine: Previous studies demonstrate that taking glycine by mouth can improve memory and mental performance.[14]

Flavonoids: Evidence suggests that flavonoids (600 mg/day of flavones, flavanones, or anthocyanins) are powerhouses when it comes to preventing thinking skills from declining as a result of aging.[15] In one study, 215 men and women aged 60–70 years in a 6-month clinical trial received a placebo or 600 mg/day of a polyphenol-rich grape and blueberry extract that contained 258 mg of flavonoids. In one group cognitive age estimated from baseline test results improved by nearly 14 years compared with about 5½ years in the placebo group.[16,17]

Diet: Research findings suggest that certain diets, especially those containing the flavonol kaempferol (e.g., in grapes, strawberries, tomatoes, broccoli, tea, and ginkgo biloba leaves), can slow aging related cognitive decline.[18]

Pycnogenol: In a university study, 38 participants were supplemented pycnogenol 50 mg/twice daily. After 12 months, the subjects, aged 55–70, had significantly better memory, attention span, daily decision making, and sociability.[19]

Meningitis

Meningitis is an inflammation of the three membranes (meninges) that surround the brain and spinal cord. Bacterial or viral infections in the cerebrospinal fluid within the subarachnoid space typically cause the inflammation and swelling. The disorder is characterized by intense headache and fever, sensitivity to light, and muscular rigidity (stiff neck), leading in severe cases to convulsions, delirium, and death.

Viral meningitis is more common than bacterial meningitis. Viral meningitis primarily affects babies and young children. Most individuals will make a full recovery from viral meningitis, but full recovery can be slow.[1]

Bacterial meningitis is very serious. While most patients recover, death can occur in as little as a few hours and permanent disabilities (such as brain damage, hearing loss, and learning disabilities) can result from the infection.[1]

ADJUVANT CARE

Gamma-Aminobutyric Acid (GABA): In one study, children with febrile convulsions and acute meningitis had significantly decreased GABA concentrations in the cerebrospinal fluid. This study supports the concept that low GABAergic activity within the CNS may be one cause for increased seizure frequency.[2]

Previous studies demonstrate that taking GABA (0.5–1.5 gm of Aminalon) reduces the development of symptoms after recovery and prevents the development of other serious conditions in children with meningitis who are between seven months to 16 years old.[3,4]

Menkes Kinky Hair Syndrome

Also known as Menkes syndrome or Menkes disease, this is an inherited disorder that leads to a copper deficiency. Characteristic findings include kinky hair, growth failure, and deterioration of the nervous system with seizures, poor head control, and reduced muscle tone. Most children with Menkes have severe symptoms that lead to death at an early age.[1]

ADDRESSING COPPER DEFICIENCY

Copper: The most common treatment for Menkes disease is copper replacement therapy via injection (e.g., copper chloride and L-histidine solutions of 350–500 mcg/day, or qod, injected intravenously or subcutaneously to increase the serum and cerebrospinal fluid copper levels to the normal range after six weeks) therapy.[2] Newborns and fetuses treated in utero with copper histidine may avoid neurologic symptoms.[2] Treatment with daily copper injections may improve the outcome in Menkes disease if it begins within days after birth.[3]

Menorrhagia

Menorrhagia is the medical term for menstrual periods with abnormally heavy (passing clots the size of a quarter or larger or needing to change a tampon or pad after less than two hours)[1] or prolonged (more than seven days) bleeding that is often accompanied by severe pelvic pain. It is one of the most common gynecologic complaints. If the condition becomes chronic, anemia from recurrent excessive blood loss may result. Low hemoglobin levels reduce the blood's capacity to carry oxygen, leading to extreme tiredness, fatigue, unusual weakness, and shortness of breath.

There are many different possible medical causes with anovulation being the most common cause of heavy menstrual bleeding. In half of the women diagnosed, an underlying cause of heavy cyclic bleeding cannot be identified, but menorrhagia can be a sign of a serious problem.[2]

PALLIATIVE MEASURES

NSAIDs: Non-steroidal anti-inflammatory drugs (NSAIDs) are firstline treatments for menorrhagia associated with ovulatory cycles. Their use is associated with a significant reduction in menstrual blood loss. A 20% to 50% reduction in blood loss has been observed in 75% of treated women.[3] Both naproxen (500 mg loading dose, then 750 mg/day for five days[4]) and ibuprofen (600–800 mg/day starting on the first day of bleeding then daily until menstruation stops[5]) were effective in significantly reducing menstrual blood loss.[6]

Iron Therapy: Several studies have shown that iron therapy often improves menorrhagia in women diagnosed with iron deficiency.[7,8,9]

Ascorbic Acid: Administering vitamin C along with iron can increase how much iron the body absorbs in adults and children.[10] This can help prevent or minimize iron deficiency anemia due to blood loss.

Vitamin A (25,000 IU twice daily for 15 days) has been shown to increase the level of estradiol (a form of estrogen) in women with heavy menstruation. Menstruation returned to normal in 57.5% of these women and there was substantial improvement in an additional 35% (for a total of 92.5% cured or improved).[11]

Yarrow (e.g., 4.5 gm/day) reduces pain and heavy bleeding resulting from menstrual irregularities and helps to regulate the menstrual cycle.[12]

Vitamin E (400–800 IU) for two days before and for three days after bleeding begins decreased pain severity and duration, and reduced menstrual blood loss.[13]

Methylmalonic Acidemia

Methylmalonic acidemia is an inherited disorder in which the body is unable to properly process certain proteins and lipids. The result is a buildup of a substance called methylmalonic acid in the blood.[1] The effects of methylmalonic acidemia usually appear in early infancy. Affected infants may experience vomiting, dehydration, weak muscle tone (hypotonia), developmental delay, excessive tiredness (lethargy), an enlarged liver (hepatomegaly), seizures, and/or failure to gain weight and grow at the expected rate (failure to thrive). Long-term complications include feeding problems, intellectual disability, chronic kidney disease, and inflammation of the pancreas (pancreatitis).[1] Without treatment, this disorder can lead to coma and death.

CLINICAL CONSIDERATIONS

Diet: Treatment includes carnitine supplements[2] and a low-protein diet, as well as the avoidance of the amino acids isoleucine, valine, threonine, and methionine.[3]

Vitamin B12: Massive doses of vitamin B12 are indicated in B12-responsive variants. In the disorders of cobalamin metabolism, the administration of intramuscular and/or oral hydroxycobalamin may correct the defect and restore normal metabolism.[3]

Migraine

Migraine is a long-term, disabling neurologic disease that has a severe negative impact on affected individuals and is the third most prevalent illness in the world, affecting 12% of the population. Severe recurring throbbing or pounding headaches with photophobia, phonophobia, nausea, or vomiting are likely to be migraines. The pain can be debilitating and last from several hours to several days in duration.

Migraine sufferers have a higher incidence of heart disease, allergies/hay fever, asthma, and depression.[1] Repeated attacks with unusually severe headache pain intensity are associated with an increased risk of gastric ulcer/GI bleeding, vitamin D deficiency, and diabetes.[2] Some patients get a warning symptom (aura) before the start of the migraine headache.

Migraine is a primary headache disorder whose specific cause is not known. The goals of treatment are to have fewer headaches that do not last as long or hurt as much. Migraine triggers can include certain foods or smells, bright or fluorescent lights, alcohol (especially wine), stress, oversleeping, and passive motion (i.e., travel sickness) especially trips lasting over 45 minutes.

For adult migraines, medications such as antidepressants, antiepileptics, antihypertensive agents, and calcium channel blockers are often used with varying degrees of success. Unfortunately, researchers found that these same medications in children yielded only short-term signs of efficacy over a placebo, with no benefit lasting more than six months.[3]

TREATMENT AND PREVENTION STRATEGIES

Migraine Headache Treatments

Analgesics: The combination of acetaminophen, aspirin, and caffeine (e.g., Excedrin Migraine) is approved in the U.S. for relieving migraine pain. Medication needs to be taken early in the attack and possibly with an antacid to help avoid stomach upset. Ibuprofen 200–800 mg can be taken every six hours. Naproxen sodium (Aleve) 525–825 mg or acetaminophen (Tylenol) 1,000 mg at onset or aspirin 500–1,000 mg every six hours are other options.[4]

Magnesium injections have also been reported to abort acute attacks of migraine. Forty patients suffering a migraine received intravenous magnesium sulfate (1 gm over five minutes). Within 15 minutes, pain was relieved by at least 50% in 35 of the 40 patients (87.5%), with complete relief occurring in nine cases (22.5%).[5]

Oral magnesium for acute pain is generally absorbed too slowly to give significant pain relief from headaches. Migralex was developed to dissolve and absorb quickly for better pain relief from a magnesium tablet. It can deliver magnesium (along with aspirin) to the brain within 15–30 minutes.[6]

Magnesium Plus: A combination of magnesium, calcium, B-vitamins, and vitamin C given intravenously is reported to relieve a migraine attack within one or two minutes.[7]

Folic Acid: Thirty-one patients suffering an acute migraine were given 15 mg of folic acid by slow intravenous infusion. In 60% of the patients, the headache disappeared within an hour of receiving the injection. Of the remainder, all but three patients experienced marked relief of pain.[8]

Ginger has long been recommended as an effective home remedy for the acute treatment of migraine, relieving both headache pain and the associated nausea. Meta-analysis of three randomized controlled studies (RCTs) revealed that ginger powder (e.g., 400–500 mg) at the onset of migraine significantly reduced pain, nausea, and vomiting after two hours.[9]

Migraine Prevention Measures

Headache Triggers: One standard method toward achieving fewer headaches is to eliminate as many known headache triggers (e.g., skipping meals, oversleeping, caffeine withdrawal, drinking red wine, pungent odors, certain foods, etc.) as possible.

Oral Magnesium: One doctor has reported that magnesium supplements (e.g., 200–400 mg/day) prevented migraines in about 80% of 3,000 patients.[10] In a double-blind study, 20 women with migraines occurring around the time of menstruation received 360 mg/day of magnesium or a placebo. The treatments were given for two months, starting on the 15th day of each cycle and continuing until menstruation. Magnesium treatment reduced the frequency as well as the duration and severity of migraines.[11] Magnesium is also an adjunct treatment for photophobia (sensitivity to light).[12]

In a second study, patients received oral 600 mg (24 mmol) magnesium (trimagnesium dicitrate) daily for 12 weeks, which reduced the frequency of migraine attacks. The number of days with migraine and the drug consumption for symptomatic treatment per patient also decreased significantly in the magnesium group. High-dose oral magnesium appears to be effective in migraine prophylaxis.[13]

In yet another study, 41% of 32 patients with an acute migraine had low serum magnesium.[14]

Diet: More than 90% of all teenage headaches were reported to disappear within two weeks if individuals totally eliminated refined carbohydrates from their diet.[15] A diet high in omega-3 fatty acids and low in omega-6 fatty acids was shown in a systematic review to reduce the duration of migraine, but not the frequency or severity.[16]

Coenzyme Q10 supplements are reported to decrease the frequency and duration of migraines.[17] The recommended dose is 100–1,200 mg/day.[18]

Riboflavin: In a randomized trial in 55 adults with migraine, 400 mg/day riboflavin reduced the frequency of migraine attacks by two per month compared to a placebo.[19] In a retrospective study, 41 children (mean age 13 years) in Italy who took 200 or 400 mg/day of riboflavin for three to six months experienced a significant reduction in the frequency and intensity of migraine headaches.[20] High doses of riboflavin (vitamin B2) helps prevent migraines and reduce the frequency of headaches.[20] For migraine headaches, the most common dose is 400 mg of riboflavin daily for at least three months.

In another study involving 90 children with migraines, patients were randomized into three groups (200 mg of riboflavin a day, 100 mg of riboflavin a day, or a placebo) after observation during a one-month baseline period.[21] There was a significant reduction in migraine frequency and duration in patients receiving 200 mg of riboflavin daily, compared with a placebo.

For migraine prophylaxis, riboflavin (400 mg/day for 12 months) resulted in marked reduction in frequency, duration, and severity of migraines not statistically different from taking valproate 500 mg/day.[22]

Alpha-Lipoic Acid: In a small RCT, subjects received 600 mg of alpha lipoic (thioctic) acid daily for three months. Within-group analyses also showed a significant reduction in attack frequency, headache days, and headache severity in the treatment group.[23]

Riboflavin Plus: A specific product (Dolovent; Linpharma Inc., Oldsmar, FL) dosed at two capsules in morning and two capsules in the evening for three months has also been studied and found to be beneficial. This dose provides a total of 400 mg of riboflavin, 600 mg of magnesium, and 150 mg of CoQ10 per day.[24]

Spinal Manipulative Therapy (SMT): Manipulative treatment is effective in reducing the frequency of migraines, severity of pain, disability, and the amount of drugs used to treat migraines. SMT is also effective in improving quality life in migraine patients.[25]

In another study, manipulation also demonstrated superiority in complete cure, reducing frequency of attacks (40% reduction), mean duration of headache, intensity of pain (43% reduction), and mean disability.[26] In a follow-up study, a further 19% improvement in migraine patients from the previous study was reported.[27]

Occipital nerve blocks for select patients, especially those with chronic migraines, can prove a more effective means of suppressing chronic headache than any oral medication.[28]

Vitamin B12: Recently, the role of vitamin B12 as a possible treatment option for chronic migraine management has been investigated and shown to be promising.[29]

Butterbur (*Petasites hybridus*) root extract contains petasin and isopetasin, which have vasodilation properties and reduce inflammation. A dosage of 50–75 mg/day in two divided doses in children 6–9 years and 50–75 mg twice daily for four months in adults for four months has been shown to reduce migraines.[30,31]

Ginger: In one RCT, ginger (e.g., 500–1,000 mg/day) was found to be more effective than placebo in bringing a ≥50% reduction in the frequency of monthly migraine episodes.[9]

Green Light Therapy: In a small study at the University of Arizona, patients with episodic and chronic migraines were exposed to green light therapy (intensity of between 4 and 100 lux). Exposure to green light emitting diodes (GLED) was for 1-2 hours per day for 10 weeks. This reduced headache days from 7.9–2.4 days in the episodic migraine group and from 22.3–9.4 days in the chronic migraine group.[32]

L-Tryptophan: Research has found that low dietary L-tryptophan and low plasma levels of serotonin are implicated in migraine pathogenesis.[33] Some studies show that tryptophan supplementation might be as beneficial as prescription drugs for adults.[34] In one study, tryptophan (9 gm/day) completely prevented migraine in three of five patients and reduced the frequency of migraine in a fourth.[35] In a second study, tryptophan 500 mg every six hours for three months helped four of eight migraine patients.[36] L-tryptophan or 5-HTP (e.g., 8–12 gm/day) as an adjuvant therapy has been recommended for refractory migraine patients[37] and may lessen the susceptibility to more severe headaches, nausea, and sensitivity to light.[38]

Miscarriages (Habitual and Unexplained Losses)

A miscarriage is the loss of a fetus before the twentieth week of pregnancy. The etiology of recurrent spontaneous abortions in otherwise healthy women remains unknown in about half of all cases. Recurrent pregnancy loss is defined as the loss (miscarriage) of three or more consecutive pregnancies. According to the March of Dimes, as many as 50% of all pregnancies and almost 20% of all recognized pregnancies end in miscarriage.

It is scientifically undetermined whether bed rest, lifestyle adaptation (smoking cessation, reduction of alcohol consumption, and weight loss), low-dose aspirin (75–81 mg/day), human chorionic gonadotropin therapy, trophoblastic membrane infusion, or vitamin supplementation increases the likelihood of a successful pregnancy in women with unexplained, recurrent miscarriage.[1]

MINIMIZING RISKS AND PREVENTING MISCARRIAGES

Prenatal vitamins contain recommended amounts of folic acid, iron, calcium, and other vitamins to help the baby properly develop, which helps to prevent miscarriages.

Nicotinamide: An Australian study traced the cause of a number of abnormal embryonic developments to a deficiency in nicotinamide adenine dinucleotide (NAD). The researchers point out that there might be a relatively simple solution. NAD deficiency can be cured and miscarriages and birth defects may be prevented by taking niacin, also known as vitamin B3, (RDA 18 mg/day), available as a dietary supplement.[2]

B Vitamins: According to an existing study, a significant number of expectant mothers tend to have a vitamin B3 deficiency (as well as deficiencies in vitamins B1, B6, B12, and A) during the first trimester of pregnancy, despite taking supplements.[3] This is particularly important because organ development in the womb begins at that time. This may mean that some pregnant women require an even higher vitamin B3 intake than the quantities obtainable through current prenatal vitamin supplements.

Folate and Vitamin B12: Hyperhomocysteinemia has been described as a risk factor for unexplained recurrent pregnancy loss. Increased levels of homocysteine may be due to inadequate dietary intake of folate and vitamin B12.[4]

Niacin and B12: Daily increases in supplementation of both niacin and vitamin B12 seems warranted in cases of unexplained pregnancy losses to inhibit the likelihood of future losses.[4]

Mitral Valve Prolapse

The mitral valve connects the left atrium with the left ventricle of the heart. Prolapse means the valve bulges back into the atrium when the stronger ventricle contracts.

Mitral valve prolapse, or a leaky valve, causes a systolic heart murmur (click murmur) heard on auscultation. Many patients with mitral valve prolapse have no symptoms. Mitral valve prolapse usually is asymptomatic, nonprogressive, and benign.[1] When symptoms are present, they can include palpitations, anxiety, rapid heart rate, shortness of breath, and weakness, but it is uncertain if the prolapse is the actual cause of these symptoms. Mitral valve prolapse does not increase the risk of heart attack, death, or other heart problems.[2] Most cases of mitral valve prolapse are not serious and only need to be monitored.

SYMPTOMATIC TREATMENT

Magnesium: Clinical symptoms of weakness, chest pain, dyspnea, palpitations, and anxiety were significantly reduced by magnesium supplementation (5 mg/kg/day for five weeks).[2] For disease of heart valves including mitral valve prolapse, 1,200–1,800 mg of magnesium carbonate taken daily for five weeks has also been used with success.[3]

Carnitine: A 44-year-old man with mitral valve prolapse and a five-year history of all the above symptoms was found to have unusually low levels of carnitine.[4] He was given one gm of carnitine, three times a day, and after four months all of his symptoms disappeared, and his heart rate fell from 115 to 70 beats per minute. In four other randomly selected patients with mitral valve prolapse, low levels of carnitine were found in each case.[4,5]

Morning Sickness/Nausea of Pregnancy/ Hyperemesis Gravidarum

Nausea is a general term describing a queasy stomach, with or without the feeling that vomiting is likely to occur. Nausea and vomiting are a common symptom and sign that can be caused by a number of different conditions. The nausea and vomiting of pregnancy (morning sickness) typically begin about the fourth to sixth week and often end about the twelfth week. Morning sickness can last longer though. Nausea is often worse in the morning and tends to ease up during the day, but can occur any time of day. For some individuals, the nausea is present throughout the day. Hyperemesis gravidarum is a severe form of morning sickness.

MANAGEMENT CHOICES

Diet: Eating dry toast or a plain biscuit in the morning 20 minutes prior to getting out of bed may help because it prevents moving around on an empty stomach.[1] Eating bland foods, as for example the "BRATT" diet (bananas, rice, applesauce, toast, and tea) which is low in fat and easy to digest, can be helpful.[1] Salty foods (e.g., salted crackers, pretzels, potato chips) are usually tolerated early in the morning, and sour and tart liquids (e.g., lemonade) are often tolerated better than plain water.[2] Day-old unsalted popcorn is an inexpensive way to combat nausea caused by pregnancy or motion sickness. Ideally, the patient should eat popcorn one hour before or two hours after ingesting fluids.[3] Taking small, frequent meals is typically better than eating three large meals.

Fluids: Fluid intake should be increased. Clear fluids are easy for the stomach to absorb and include water, sports drinks, clear broths, popsicles, and Jell-O. Taking small sips of broth is recommended.[1]

Ginger is a popular alternative treatment for morning sickness.[4,5] Ginger ale made with real ginger, ginger tea made from fresh grated ginger, ginger capsules, and ginger candies are often well-tolerated.[1] One European study demonstrated that ginger powder (1 gm/day) was more effective than a placebo in reducing the symptoms of hyperemesis gravidarum.[6]

General Considerations: Taking a multivitamin and avoiding bothersome smells can be helpful as well.

Medications can be given to treat nausea and vomiting during pregnancy:

- **Vitamin B6 (pyridoxine)** is effective in relieving the severity of nausea in early pregnancy.[7] The American Congress of Obstetrics and Gynecology (ACOG) recommends monotherapy with 10–25 mg of vitamin B6 three or four times a day to treat nausea and vomiting in pregnancy.[8]
- **Doxylamine** (25 mg aka Unisom tid), an over-the-counter sleep medication, is safe to take at night if vitamin B6 alone does not relieve symptoms.[5] A prescription drug that combines vitamin B6 and doxylamine (Diclectin) is also available. Both drugs, taken alone or together, have been found to be safe to take during pregnancy and have no harmful effects on the baby.[9]
- **Thiamine:** Severe nausea and vomiting of pregnancy (hyperemesis gravidarum) can lead to vitamin B1 (thiamine) deficiency and Wernicke's encephalopathy in women. Vitamin B1 replacement is needed for all women with vomiting that lasts for more than three weeks. Prophylaxis with multivitamins and therapy with B6, with or without doxylamine, are safe and effective therapies for nausea and vomiting of pregnancy.[4]

Peppermint: Some women find relief from sipping peppermint tea or sucking peppermint candies, especially after eating.[10]

Aromatherapy: One hundred pregnant women with nausea and vomiting participated in a randomized clinical trial. The study concluded that lemon inhalation aromatherapy at the first sign of nausea can be effective in reducing nausea and vomiting of pregnancy.[11]

Morphea

Morphea, also known as localized scleroderma, causes painless reddened single or multiple patches of skin that gradually become white or yellow. The patches eventually thicken into firm, oval-shaped discolored plaques (due to excessive collagen deposition). Over time the patches may become hard, dry, and smooth.[1] It is noncontagious and is more likely to occur in women. Plaques most often occur on the abdomen, chest, and back, but can appear on the face, arms, or legs. There are several types of morphea. The lesions tend to disappear on their own, but this may take years. Therapy aimed at reducing inflammatory activity in the early stages of the disease is more successful than attempts to decrease sclerosis in well-established lesions.

COSMETIC CONSIDERATIONS

Vitamin D Cream: A topical vitamin D cream may help to treat morphea.[2,3]

Oral Vitamin E: Good results have been reported with oral vitamin E (300–1,600 IU/day).[4]

Motion Sickness/Travel Sickness/Car Sickness

Motion sickness is a common problem for people travelling by boat, car, train, or airplane. It is the sick feeling one gets when in motion but not in control of that motion (e.g., on an amusement park ride or as a passenger on a long car ride). The feeling builds from uneasiness to nausea, dizziness, possibly sweating, and vomiting. A headache may ensue for migraine sufferers.

SCIENTIFIC RESEARCH

OTC Products: Prevention is the key, so meclizine (Bonine, Antivert) or Ranitidine (Zantac) may be used in the evening before travel to obtain adequate blood levels. Meclizine is often used in a dosage of 25 mg every six hours. Two doses are to be taken the night before travel and the regimen should be continued throughout the actual travel time.[1] If not taken the night before, meclizine 50 mg can be taken orally one hour before departure.[2] Ranitidine 150 mg should be taken at bedtime the night before travel and again in the morning.[1] Recently, the FDA alerted the public that the drug ranitidine (Zantac) can contain a cancer-causing impurity called N-nitrosodimethylamine (NDMA). No recall of the drug has been issued.

GABA: GABA works by blocking brain signals (neurotransmissions). Some research shows that taking gamma-aminobutyric-acid (e.g., 0.5 gm of Aminalon) before anticipating motion sickness or three times daily for four days slows the onset of motion sickness and reduces symptoms such as chills, cold sweats, and pale skin.[3]

Dimenhydrinate (Dramamine) and cyclizine (Cyclivert) are commonly used medications for motion sickness.[4]

Diphenhydramine (Benadryl, Compoz Nightime Sleep Aid, Unisom Sleep Gels, etc.): To prevent motion sickness as a passenger, taking a dose 30 minutes before starting an activity such as travel may help.[5] Diphenhydramine may have a greater impact on poor driving than alcohol and should be avoided in that circumstance.

Multiple Sclerosis

Multiple sclerosis (MS) is a lifelong central nervous system disease. Most patients with MS are females diagnosed between the ages of 20 and 40. In this disease, myelin, a material that covers and insulates nerves in the brain and the spinal cord, is damaged. This interrupts proper communication and signaling between the affected nerves. The result is often a sudden loss of function followed by some recovery and a relatively stable period. However, the course of the disease is marked by recurrent relapses.

Weakness or clumsiness of a leg or hand or visual disturbances may be an early presenting symptom. Also, paresthesias on the trunk, in one or more extremities, or one side of the face may present as the first symptoms. There is no cure for MS and patients deteriorate over time, losing their ability to function. Life-span is shortened only in severe cases.[1]

MEDICAL RATIONALES FOR CARE

Lifestyle: Because a small rise in body temperature (about 0.5°F) can worsen symptoms, hot weather, vigorous exercise, hot showers, and heavy meals should be avoided. Smoking should also be eliminated since recent research has linked smoking after clinical onset to a worsening of long-term cognitive function and neuronal integrity.[2]

Vitamin D: Higher vitamin D levels suggested a beneficial effect on the course of MS disease activity. Also, supplemental intake of vitamin D was found to reduce exacerbation risk in relapsing-remitting MS.[3]

The medical rationale for treating MS with vitamin D is that metabolites of the vitamin function as paracrine immune modulators, decreasing the proliferation of proinflammatory T lymphocytes and decreasing the production of cytokines, both of which contribute to the pathogenesis of MS.[4]

A deficiency of vitamin D has been proposed to be a potential risk factor for MS, autism, and schizophrenia. Along those same lines, a deficiency in vitamin D has been linked to both early and long-term cognitive impairment and diminished neuronal integrity in MS.[2]

In a study of patients with MS undergoing interferon-β treatment, taking high-dose oral vitamin D3 supplementation was found to reduce new combined unique active lesions and T1 hypointense lesions.[3]

Studies at the University of Oxford and the New Jersey Medical School suggest that maintaining adequate levels of vitamin D may have a protective effect and lower the risk of developing multiple sclerosis.[5]

Another study conducted at Maastricht University in the Netherlands in addition to others indicated that, in patients who already have MS, vitamin D may lessen the frequency and severity of their symptoms.[6]

Taking a dose of vitamin D3 (up to 10,400 IUs/day) is safe for patients with MS and may help regulate the body's hyperactive immune response according to a pilot study published by Johns Hopkins physicians.[7]

Biotin: Several studies have found that high doses of biotin can reduce symptoms in patients with progressive MS. Individuals who took these high doses of biotin did not develop any significant adverse reactions.[7] A pilot study in 23 patients with progressive MS tested the use of high doses of biotin (100–600 mg/day). Over 90% of participants had some degree of clinical improvement.[8] Research also shows that taking high doses of biotin might improve vision and reduce partial paralysis in some people with multiple sclerosis.[9] At least two studies are currently underway to test the effect of 300 mg of biotin per day on patients with MS.[10,11]

Padma 28 is a Tibetan herbal formula that contains a mixture of 22 herbs. In one study, 100 patients with chronic progressive multiple sclerosis were randomly assigned to receive six tablets per day of Padma 28; 44% of those receiving Padma 28 noticed improvements in their general condition, increased muscular strength, or fewer neurologic problems.[12,13]

Glucosamine: Previous clinical studies demonstrate that taking 1,000 mg of glucosamine sulfate by mouth daily for six months might reduce the relapse of multiple sclerosis.[14]

Vitamin B12: A retrospective single center study demonstrated that multiple sclerosis patients with low B12 levels have increased disability. Supplementation would seem worthwhile.[15]

Muscle Cramps/Leg Cramps

Leg cramps, or charley horses, involve a sudden, painful, and involuntary localized contraction of an entire muscle group, individual muscle, or select muscle fibers.[1] Generally, the cramp can last from a few seconds to several minutes. It is a common problem that often affects the feet, calves, or thigh muscles. Leg cramps are a clinical diagnosis. A magnesium, calcium, or potassium imbalance can cause lower extremity muscle cramps.[2] Heat-associated muscle cramping is often seen during sports and rigorous exercise or physical activity.[1]

METHODS OF MANAGEMENT

Magnesium supplements can help reduce muscle cramps. In one study, taking 365 mg/day of magnesium was significantly more effective than the placebo in relieving leg cramps. The severity of the cramps decreased by more than 70%.[3]

For leg cramps in pregnancy, magnesium lactate or citrate 5 mmol in the morning and 10 mmol in the evening are recommended.[4]

Magnesium glucoheptonate or magnesium gluconate are oral magnesium supplements that appear to work best for muscle cramps.[5]

Calcium (2,000 mg/day) is recommended for the treatment of leg cramps.[6] Calcium also appears to be effective in relieving leg cramps in pregnancy.[7]

Both magnesium and calcium appear to offer safe and effective symptom management of leg cramps, although their efficacy has not been definitively established in large clinical trials.

Nicotinic Acid: If leg cramps are associated with impaired peripheral circulation, niacin (nicotinic acid) is suggested to reduce the cramps.[8]

Potassium citrate or gluconate (up to 4,700 mg/day in adults) may be helpful.[9]

Multivitamins: Adding multivitamins with magnesium and zinc is another option.[10]

Vitamin B12 can be recommended for some patients.[11]

Quinine: The FDA warns against quinine for muscle cramps.[12]

Acetic Acid: Anecdotal evidence suggests that ingesting small volumes (2.5 ounces) of pickle juice, which contains acetic acid, relieves muscle cramps within 35 seconds of ingestion. A study found that pickle juice inhibited electrically induced muscle cramps in hypohydrated humans.[13] Acetic acid may also be why apple cider vinegar has a reputation for relieving leg cramps.

Vitamin B Complex: In a Class II study of 28 patients, treatment with a combination of B vitamins three times daily was associated with remission of leg cramps in 86% of those patients.[14]

Water/Sports Drinks: For heat associated muscle cramps, sufferers should drink water and have a snack or electrolyte replacement liquids (e.g., sports drinks) every 15-20 minutes. Avoid salt tablets.[15]

Muscle Cramps/Night (Nocturnal) Cramps

Up to 60% of adults report that they have had nocturnal leg cramps.[1] Most of the time, it is not possible to identify an apparent cause for night-time leg cramps or charley horses. Most often, muscle cramps involve a calf, foot, or thigh. Nocturnal leg cramps are quite painful and can leave the muscle tender for up to a day or so. Cramps can be caused by low blood mineral levels of calcium, potassium, or magnesium.[2,3] Deficiencies of certain vitamins, including thiamine (B1), pantothenic acid (B5), and pyridoxine (B6), can also cause muscle cramps.[3] Medications strongly associated with causing leg cramps include intravenous iron sucrose, conjugated estrogens, raloxifene, naproxen, and teriparatide.[1]

No prescription medication is recommended for muscle cramps.[4]

RESEARCH ANALYSIS

Stretching calves and hamstrings at bedtime reduced the frequency of cramps after six weeks.[5]

Calcium plays an essential role in muscle contraction. Low blood levels of calcium directly increase the excitability of both the nerve endings and the muscles they stimulate.[6] Muscle aches, cramps, and spasms are the earliest signs of a calcium deficiency.[7] Cramps are also seen in circumstances that decrease the availability of calcium or magnesium in body fluids, such as taking diuretics, parathyroid gland dysfunction, excess vomiting, or inadequate calcium absorption.[6]

In a study with 42 pregnant women with leg cramps, 21 patients were treated with 1 gm calcium orally twice daily for two weeks. The group that received calcium experienced good clinical improvement.[8]

In another study, six randomized controlled studies were reviewed in which a total of 390 women with leg cramps received either magnesium, calcium, or a placebo. A greater proportion of women receiving calcium experienced no leg cramps after treatment compared to women who did not receive any treatment.[9] Adults over 51 should take 2,000 mg/day of calcium.[10]

Magnesium is also recommended for preventing nocturnal leg cramps.[11]

Vitamin E: Doses of vitamin E (400–600 mg/day) have been reported to afford symptomatic improvement in night cramps.[12] Vitamin E (d-α-tocopheryl acetate) in doses of 300–400 IU/day was also reported to be more effective than quinine, a drug that was commonly prescribed for nocturnal leg cramps but is no longer recommended. In addition, vitamin E is safer than quinine.[13]

Gabapentin (Neurontin): In a limited population of 30 patients, a study found that a dose of 600 mg/day of the prescription medication gabapentin reduced the frequency and severity of muscle cramps within two weeks, and gabapentin maintained 100% efficacy in relieving muscle cramps at three months. The therapeutic effect persisted for six months.[13] Results suggest that a gabapentin dose of 600–1,200 mg/day would be helpful in the treatment of muscular cramps.[14]

Vitamin B complex represents a potentially effective non-prescription treatment that is recommended as a preventative measure for night cramps.[1,15]

Quinine: The FDA warns against quinine for muscle cramps because of its potential toxicity.[16]

Muscle Pain (Myalgia)

Myalgia, or muscle pain, is a symptom of many different diseases and disorders. Muscle pain can be localized (e.g., injury, overuse) or throughout the body (e.g., infections, illness, or side effects from medications such as anticonvulsants, antibiotics, anticancer agents, statins, and diuretics).

Muscle pain has been associated with several mineral metabolism abnormalities such as selenium (Se) deficiency[1] and magnesium (Mg) deficiency.[2,3,4]

PALLIATIVE MEASURES

Selenium and Magnesium: Patients with myalgia or myotonia have been successfully treated with selenium and/or magnesium.[1,2,3,4]

Taurine: Previous clinical studies indicate that taking 2 gm of taurine together with branched chain amino acids (BCAAs) three times daily for two weeks reduces muscle soreness in healthy people who do not exercise regularly.[5]

Vitamin D: Vitamin D deficiency is associated with symptoms of myalgia that resemble those caused by statins.[6]

In uncontrolled studies, some authors have used vitamin D2 supplements (from 50,000 units to 100,000 units per week) in statin-treated patients with muscle symptoms and low vitamin D levels and reported resolution of myalgia in about 90% of patients.[6]

Muscle Performance and Damage (Related to Exercise)

Skeletal muscle comprises the largest organ system in the human body. Exercise-induced muscle injury most frequently occurs after unaccustomed exercise. The damage is characterized by ultrastructural alterations in muscle tissue, clinical signs, and symptoms (e.g., reduced muscle strength and range of motion, increased muscle soreness and swelling). Fortunately, muscle pain from overuse and most injuries is self-limited.

ENHANCING PERFORMANCE

Creatine is an amino acid that has been shown to improve burst performance in skeletal muscle. This is thought to be due to its enhancement of muscle phosphocreatine stores, which results in faster adenosine triphosphate (ATP) regeneration.[1]

Vitamin D: A systematic review revealed that supplemental vitamin D at daily doses of 800–1,000 IU consistently had beneficial effects on muscle strength and balance.[2]

Proximal muscle weakness impairs reaching upward (e.g., combing hair, lifting objects over the head), ascending stairs, or getting up from a sitting position.[3] The main causes are myopathies, alcohol use, and steroids, but vitamin D deficiency also causes this disorder.[4]

DAMAGE PREVENTION INTERVENTIONS

Methylsulfonylmethane (MSM): Research shows that taking MSM (e.g., 1,000–2,000 mg/day or in divided doses) daily beginning 10 days before a 14 km running exercise can help reduce muscle damage.[5]

Cherry Juice: Data shows efficacy for a tart cherry juice blend (CherryPharm, Inc.) in decreasing some of the symptoms of exercise-induced muscle damage. Most notably, strength loss averaged over the four days after eccentric exercise was 22% with the placebo but only 4% with the cherry juice.[6]

Ascorbic Acid: Vitamin C (3,000 mg/day for three days prior to strenuous exercise) abated pain from delayed-onset muscle soreness by 25%–44%.[7] Another study also found decreased muscle pain with 1,000 mg of ascorbic acid taken 90 minutes prior to exercise.[8] Even smaller amounts of vitamin C prior to exercise had a positive effect.[9]

Vitamins C & E: Especially for female athletes, supplementation with vitamins C and E can help to reduce muscle damage markers induced by prolonged and intense exercise.[10]

MUSCLE REPAIR

Protein supplements are used by some athletes to enhance muscle repair and growth.[1]

Myasthenia Gravis

The term *myasthenia gravis* literally means "grave or serious muscle weakness."

Myasthenia gravis is an autoimmune disorder in which the body's own antibodies block the transmission of nerve impulses to muscles, causing varying degrees of voluntary muscle weakness and muscles that tire easily. The muscles that control eye and eyelid movement, facial expression, chewing, talking, and swallowing are most often involved in the disorder.[1] A variable combination of legs, arms, or respiratory weakness can also occur. Myasthenia gravis in 15%–20% of cases can cause respiratory failure, which can be fatal and requires immediate emergency medical care.

The hallmark of myasthenia gravis is fluctuating muscle weakness that worsens after periods of activity and improves after periods of rest.[1] It most commonly affects young adult women under 40 and men over 60. However, it can occur at any age, including during childhood.[1] The disorder is painless. Some cases of myasthenia gravis may go into remission, either temporarily or permanently, and muscle weakness may disappear completely so that medications can be discontinued. Thymectomy is one of the main medical treatment methods for myasthenia gravis. Stable, long-lasting remissions are the goal of treatment.[1]

TREATMENTS

Vitamin D has been shown to be related to autoimmune diseases, such as multiple sclerosis and psoriasis. A case report of a patient with severe and refractory myasthenia gravis (MG) outlined the patient's experience during "high-dose vitamin D treatment." A large-dose treatment (80,000–120,000 IU/day) was carried out by a medical center in Brazil, and the patient had her first complete remission with this type of treatment after achieving increased vitamin D serum levels (400–700 ng/mL). The patient was also on a calcium-restricted diet to prevent hypercalcemia. More studies are needed to validate this approach.[2]

Huperzine A: Huperzine A acts as a cholinesterase inhibitor. Previous clinical studies demonstrate that giving huperzine A intramuscularly for 10 days may prevent muscle weakness in patients with myasthenia gravis and may have equal or longer lasting effects compared to intramuscular neostigmine.[3]

Myocardial Infarction/Heart Attack

Myocardial infarction (MI), or heart attack, means necrosis, or death, of a portion of the heart muscle. An MI is a life threatening medical emergency. Two main coronary arteries and their branches supply blood and oxygen to the heart. If any of those arteries becomes significantly or completely blocked off, then an inadequate amount of blood is getting through to the heart muscle. This cardiac ischemia results in a shortage of oxygen. If ischemia continues long enough, that portion of the myocardium that lacks oxygen starts to die. Irreversible damage begins to occur within 30 minutes of the blockage. The most common symptom is chest pain. The pain may also affect the arm, neck, jaw, or shoulder.

Shortness of breath with exertion, nausea, sweating, or clammy skin are also common symptoms.

Major modifiable risk factors for a heart attack include:

- Smoking
- High blood pressure
- High blood cholesterol
- Overweight and obesity
- An unhealthy diet (for example, a diet high in saturated fat, trans fat, cholesterol, and sodium)
- Lack of routine physical activity
- High blood sugar due to diabetes[1]

The most common complications of a heart attack are heart failure, cardiogenic shock, arrythmias including ventricular fibrillation, and sudden death. According to the American Heart Association, an abrupt loss of heart function, or sudden cardiac arrest, resulting from an MI-induced arrhythmia is the most common cause of death in the U.S.

LOWERING RISKS AND SEQUELAE

D-Alpha Tocopherol: Researchers at Cambridge University in England reported that patients who had been diagnosed with coronary arteriosclerosis could lower their risk of having a heart attack by 77% by supplementing with 400 IU to 800 IU/day of the natural (d-alpha tocopherol) form of vitamin E.[2]

Two landmark studies published in the New England Journal of Medicine followed a total of 125,000 men and women health care professionals. It was found that those who supplement with at least 100 IU of vitamin E daily reduced their risk of heart disease by 59%–66%.[3,4]

Results of several large observational studies in both men and women have suggested an inverse relationship between vitamin E consumption and risk of myocardial infarction or death from heart disease. In two of the studies, individuals who consumed more than 7 mg/day of dietary vitamin E were 35% less likely to die from heart disease.[5,6]

L-Carnitine: One meta-analysis of 13 controlled trials including more than 3,600 patients showed that L-carnitine supplementation (2–3 gm/day) led to a 27% reduction in all-cause mortality, a 65% reduction in ventricular arrhythmias, and a 40% reduction in angina symptoms in patients after a myocardial infarction.[7] Following an acute myocardial infarction, prompt L-carnitine administration and subsequent maintenance therapy also attenuates progressive left ventricular dilatation.[8]

In one trial, half of 160 men and women diagnosed with a recent MI were randomly assigned to receive 4 gm/day of oral L-carnitine in addition to standard pharmacological treatment. After one year of treatment, mortality was significantly lower in the L-carnitine supplemented group compared to the control group (1.2% vs. 12.5%), and angina attacks were less frequent.[9]

L-carnitine supplementation also prevented ventricular enlargement and dysfunction, reduced the infarct size and cardiac biomarkers, and diminished the total number of cardiac events, including cardiac deaths and nonfatal infarction.[10,11]

Vitamin D: Low serum vitamin D3 levels were highly associated with heart attack, stroke, heart failure, coronary artery disease, and incident death.[12]

Most importantly, studies show that treatment with vitamin D3 can significantly reverse the damage to the cardiovascular system caused by several diseases, including hypertension, atherosclerosis, and diabetes, while also reducing the risk of heart attack.[13]

A team at the Westmead Institute for Medical Research found that vitamin D prevented excessive scarring and thickening of heart tissue following a heart attack, which may help reduce the risk of heart failure.[14]

Another study found that a short course of treatment with vitamin D (4,000 IU for five days) effectively attenuated the increase in circulating levels of inflammatory cytokines after an acute coronary event.[15]

EPA/DHA: Secondary prevention fish oil studies demonstrate a significant reduction in MI.[16]

Niacin: Several well-designed, randomized, placebo-controlled studies show that niacin prevents cardiovascular disease and death.[17] Niacin was the first drug to show efficacy in reduction of both major cardiovascular events and mortality in patients with prior myocardial infarction.[18] The Coronary Drug Project was the first clinical study to show the benefits of niacin in patients with a history of myocardial infarction.[19] It reduced the incidence of nonfatal re-infarction by 27% in the initial five-year follow-up period and was associated with a significant decrease of 9% in all-cause mortality at the 15-year follow-up.[19]

In previous studies, niacin therapy led to clinically significant relative risk reductions in clinical events and either stabilization or modest regression of atherosclerosis.[17,20]

Bromelain: A drastic reduction in the incidence of coronary infarct was seen after administration of potassium and magnesium orotate along with 120–400 mg of bromelain per day.[21]

Aspirin: In addition to seeking medical help immediately, anyone (without a severe aspirin sensitivity) experiencing an acute coronary syndrome (chest pain and shortness of breath with nausea or vomiting, etc.) and not already taking aspirin, should chew and swallow a nonenteric coated 162–325 mg aspirin. This should be followed by 100–150 mg/day. This has been shown in large clinical trials to improve short- and long-term outcomes by 20%–30%.[22]

PREVENTING MORE HEART ATTACKS

Lifestyle Modifications: *Medicine.net* recommends weight reduction and maintenance, regular exercise, and no smoking.[23]

Folic Acid: *Medicine.net* recommends taking EPA/DHA and multivitamins with an increased amount of folic acid.[23]

Aspirin: The benefit of daily low-dose aspirin for primary prevention of nonfatal myocardial infarction (MI) has been shown in multiple randomized controlled trials.[24,25,26] Currently, low-dose aspirin is recommended for individuals with a higher risk of CVD, ages 40–70, who are not at increased risk of bleeding.[27]

Myocarditis

Myocarditis is an inflammation of the myocardium, often the result of an infective process (virus, bacterium, fungus, or parasite) leading to degeneration or death of heart muscle cells and dilated cardiomyopathy. Myocarditis continues to be a significant cause of morbidity and mortality in the pediatric population and is the most common cause of cardiac failure in an otherwise healthy child. The disorder typically has an acute onset of effort dyspnea and fatigability due to elevated left ventricular pressure and low cardiac output resulting from dilated congestive cardiomyopathy secondary to an infection.[1] Other symptoms may include chest pain and fast or irregular heart beat.

Myocarditis can result in a range of outcomes from mild to rapidly progressing fatal disease. In mild cases, myocarditis presents briefly and often improves on its own with or without treatment, leading to a complete recovery. If myocarditis worsens, the heart weakens and signs and symptoms of heart failure (e.g., fatigue, trouble breathing, and swelling of the feet and ankles) usually follow. Treatment is symptomatic since there is no cure at present.

ANCILLARY MEDICAL MANAGEMENT

L-Carnitine: L-carnitine is employed in the treatment of myocarditis as it is known to prevent apoptosis (programmed cell death) of muscle cells and plays a role in managing CHF associated myopathies.[2] L-carnitine (100 mg/kg/day for four days) by mouth appears to reduce the risk of death from severe myocarditis.[3,4]

Nails—Beau's Lines/Onychorrhexis

Beau's lines are horizontal (transverse) white bands comprised of depressions, or indentations, in the nail plate. They run parallel to the white, moon-shaped portion of the nail bed (lunula) seen at the nail's origin. The lines, or ridges, grow out with the nails. Causes can include trauma, pemphigus, chronic infection, malignancy, malnutrition, collagen disease, and Raynaud's disease. Trauma typically affects one or two nails. Systemic illnesses can affect all 20 nails.[1] Onychorrhexis causes longitudinal ridges to form on thin brittle nails. The cause can be medical (e.g., arteriosclerosis, thyroid disease, lack of iron, folic acid, protein, etc.)[2] or environmental (e.g., strong soaps, water exposure, nail polish remover, etc.). If the cause is a deficiency or medical condition, then both fingernails and toenails should be affected. Otherwise, consider environmental factors.

TREATMENT

Zinc Therapy: Researchers have proposed severe zinc deficiency as a cause of Beau's lines in fingernails and toenails.[3,4,5] Zinc deficiency is also associated with brittle nails[6] and onychorrhexis.[7] Oral zinc therapy is initially given in doses of 150 mg/day. Long-term high zinc doses may interfere with copper metabolism and are only indicated for acrodermatitis enteropathica.[8,9]

Nails—Brittle Nail Syndrome/Onychoschizia

Idiopathic brittle nail syndrome is the most common cause of brittle nails and is almost exclusively seen in the fingernails.[1] Basically, brittle nails are divided into (1) dry and brittle nails from too little moisture or (2) soft and brittle nails often from too much moisture. Brittle nails can also be caused by medical conditions such as hypothyroidism or anemia (e.g., iron deficiency).[2]

Onychoschizia, or lamellar dystrophy, is splitting of the fingernails at the tip. The nails are typically soft, thin and brittle, easily cracking, chipping, and splitting horizontally at the tip. Onychoschizia is more common in women and children.[3]

MANAGEMENT MEASURES

Avoidance of Prolonged Contact with Water: To help prevent nail splitting, fingernails should be kept dry. Repeated or prolonged contact with water can contribute to split fingernails.[4]

Biotin: Taking biotin (2.5 mg/day) orally for 6 to 16 months can increase the thickness of fingernails and toenails in individuals with brittle nails.[5] In one study, eight people with brittle nails were given 2.5 mg of biotin per day for 6 to 15 months. Nail thickness improved by 25% in all eight participants. Nail splitting was also reduced.[6]

In another study, patients with splitting fingernails were treated with 2,500 mg/day of biotin. Of the 35 patients who answered a follow-up questionnaire, 63% reported improvements in the strength of their nails. Results were noticeable after one to four months of treatment, with the average being two months.[4,7]

Alpha-Hydroxy Acids or Lanolin: For brittle nails, it can be beneficial to apply lotions containing alpha-hydroxy acids or lanolin (e.g., Elon by the Dartmouth Co.) to the nails after soaking them in warm water for five minutes.[8]

Nail polish with nylon fibers applied once a week can often help soft and splitting nails.[8]

Nail Hardeners: A variety of commercial nail hardeners are available and should be used as directed.

Calcium: Soft nails have also been reported with low serum calcium, so supplemental calcium may be of benefit.[9]

Zinc deficiency can also cause thin and brittle nails that break easily. The National Institutes of Health considers 40 mg of elemental zinc a day to be the upper limit dose for adults. For example, approximately 23% of zinc sulfate consists of elemental zinc; thus, 220 mg of zinc sulfate contains 50 mg of elemental zinc.[10,11]

Iron: Correct iron deficiency if present.

Nails—Brown-Gray Discoloration

A brown-gray discoloration of the fingernails or toenails can be associated with vitamin B12 deficiency.[1,2]

TREATMENT METHOD

Vitamin B12 supplementation in the wake of a deficiency normalizes the discoloration.

Nails—Fungal Infection/Onychomycosis

Onychomycosis is a fungal infection that gets in through cracks in the nail or cuts in the skin. It begins as a white or yellow spot under the tip of the fingernail or toenail, although toenails are affected 10 times more often than fingernails. As the fungal infection goes deeper, nail fungus may cause the nail to discolor, thicken, and crumble at the edge. The most effective treatments for onychomycosis are systemic antifungals such as terbinafine (Lamisil) which is 76% effective. Treatment (250 mg/day) may be required for 6-12 weeks. Treatment ends before clinical improvement is seen. Fingernails typically require six months to see clearance and toenails require 18 months.[1,2]

TREATMENT OPTIONS

Tea Tree Oil: Sixty-four patients with fungal infections of the toenails applied 100% tea tree oil to the affected nail(s) twice daily for six months.[3] By clinical assessment, there was partial or full resolution of the problem in 60% of the patients.

Anti-Fungals: There are several safe, natural anti-fungals, but getting them beneath the toenail(s) in a sufficient concentration to do the job is challenging. Three of the most effective natural anti-fungals are oregano oil, tea-tree oil, and saturated solution of potassium iodide (SSKI). The oregano oil is rubbed on each nail and on the adjacent tissue and DMSO is applied to the same areas immediately afterward. The DMSO "carries" the oregano oil right through the nail, where it can start to work against the fungus.[4]

Nails—Koilonychia

Koilonychia is a flat and spoon-shaped nail plate associated with iron deficiency anemia.

A central nail plate ridge can arise from iron deficiency, folic acid deficiency, or protein deficiency.[1] SLE, hemochromatosis, and Raynaud's disease can also cause koilonychia.

NUTRITIONAL MANAGEMENT

Iron Deficiency: Correction of deficiencies including iron deficiency anemia can help eliminate this abnormal nail shape.[2]

Nails—Paronychia/Infection

Paronychia, or an ingrown nail, is caused by the introduction of bacteria into the nail fold, which can cause cellulitis and/or abscess formation. Generally, nail grooming behaviors, nail biting, and wet work are the causes of acute or chronic paronychia.[1] Typically, there is pain, redness, and swelling around the base or sides of the nail.

MEDICAL TREATMENT

Wet Work: Avoid excessive or regular exposure to water and dry hands meticulously after washing them.[2]

Soaks: Early paronychia without purulence may be managed with warm-water soaks four times a day with or without oral antibiotics.[3] For paronychia treatment, including for pseudomonas infection, also known as green nail syndrome, 1% acetic acid (white vinegar) soaks for 2-3 weeks is often curative. Burow (aluminum acetate) solution combined with warm soaks has also been used for years as a topical treatment.[4]

New Skin Antiseptic: Spraying the nail bed three or four times a day with New Skin Antiseptic, an over-the-counter liquid bandage, greatly speeds the elimination of infection and decreases the likelihood of recurrence.[5]

Nails—Transverse Leukonychia/Mees' Lines

Transverse leukonychia, or Mees' lines, causes spots or horizontal whitish bands (running parallel with the lunula) of discoloration on the nails. There are many different medical causes of Mees' lines including calcium, zinc, or iron deficiency; toxicity (arsenic, carbon monoxide, thallium, chemotherapy) psoriasis; renal failure; cardiac failure or MI; childbirth; pellagra; and others.[1] Mees' lines are indicative of systemic pathology and can serve as a useful clinical guide.[2]

NUTRITIONAL CARE

Calcium: The horizonal white lines of transverse leukonychia can be associated with severe hypocalcemia and good response has been reported to treatment with calcium. Other nail changes reported to be associated with hypocalcemia include brittle nails with onychorrhexis and longitudinal striations.[3,4] Soft nails have also been reported with low serum calcium.[5]

Nails—Yellow Nail Syndrome

The yellow nail syndrome includes thickened, slow growing, opaque yellowish-to-greenish nails with exaggerated curvature. Causes include RA, nephrotic syndrome, thyroiditis, TB, lymphedema, and chronic respiratory disorders such as chronic bronchitis, bronchiectasis, pleural effusions, and chronic sinusitis.[1]

TREATMENT MODALITY

Vitamin E in an oral dosage of 1,000–1,200 IU once a day for a period of six months is an effective treatment for yellow nail syndrome especially when combined with triazole antifungals.[2]

Oral zinc sulfate supplementation (300 mg/day) helped to lessen the severity of yellow nail syndrome after eight months.[3]

Necrolytic Migratory Erythema

Necrolytic migratory erythema (NME) is a red, blistering rash that spreads across the skin. It particularly affects the skin around the mouth and distal extremities, but may also be found on the lower abdomen, buttocks, perineum, and groin. The dermatosis is usually associated with the glucagonoma syndrome,[1] which is due to a slow-growing cancerous tumor located in the alpha cells of the pancreas. NME has also been associated with intestinal malabsorption disorders, hepatic cirrhosis, chronic pancreatitis, inflammatory bowel disease, and non-pancreatic malignancies.[2]

COSMETIC CARE

Zinc: It has been observed that patients of NME have low serum zinc levels and the most consistent improvement is noted with zinc sulfate 440 mg/day.[3] Even in patients with normal serum zinc levels, zinc supplementation leads to clinical improvement of NME.[4]

Amino Acids/EFAs: Supplementation with zinc, amino acids, and essential fatty acids appears to be beneficial in some cases.[5,6]

Neural Tube Defects (NTDs)

During the embryo's development, a structure called the neural tube will later become the spinal cord, brain, and spinal column. Neural tube defects (NTDs) are a group of birth defects in which an opening in the spine or cranium from the first month of development remains open. This results in a hole somewhere over the spine (spina bifida) or anencephaly in a developing fetus.[1] Many affected individuals do not survive. Females are more likely to be affected by NTDs than males. These defects occur in the first month of pregnancy, before a woman even suspects or knows that she is pregnant.

PREVENTION

Folic Acid: Years ago, no one knew what caused these birth defects, which occur when the early development of tissues that eventually become the spinal cord, the tissues that surround it, or the brain goes awry. British researchers found that mothers of children with spina bifida had low vitamin levels.[2] Eventually, two large trials in which women were randomly assigned to take folic acid (the form of folate added to multivitamins or fortified foods) or a placebo showed that getting too little folate increased a woman's chances of having a baby with spina bifida or anencephaly and that getting enough folate could greatly reduce the incidence of these birth defects.[3,4]

The timing of folate supplementation is critical. For folate to be effective, it must be taken in the first few weeks after conception, often before a woman knows she is pregnant. Because about half of all pregnancies are unplanned, it is recommended that any woman who could get pregnant take 400 micrograms (mcg) of folic acid daily, starting before conception and continuing for the first 12 weeks of pregnancy.[5]

Enough folate, at least 400 mcg/day, isn't always easy to get from food that is not fortified. This is why women of childbearing age are urged to take extra folic acid as a supplement. That is also why the U.S. Food and Drug Administration now requires that folic acid be added to most enriched breads, flour, cornmeal, pastas, rice, and other grain products, along with the iron and other micronutrients that have been added for years.[6,7]

If women have an increased risk of a pregnancy affected by a neural tube defect, they are advised to take a higher dose (5 mg) of folic acid each day until they are 12 weeks pregnant.[8]

Choline: Some research indicates that women who consume a lot of choline in their diet around the time of conception lower their risk of having babies with a neural tube defect compared to women with lower intake of choline.[9]

Nitroglycerine

Nitroglycerin is a prescription drug used to help treat sudden chest pain (angina) in patients with certain heart conditions (e.g., coronary heart disease). Nitroglycerin works primarily via venous dilation to lower blood pressure, but it also dilates the coronary arteries, contributing to the relief of angina.

PROLONGING NITROGLYCERINE'S EFFECTS

Ascorbic Acid: In patients who take medicines for chest pain, including nitroglycerine, the body develops a tolerance and the medicines stop working as well.[1] One study found that coadministration of vitamin C (1,000–1,500 mg/day) and glyceroltrinitrate (GTN) fully maintained the GTN-induced changes in the orthostatic blood pressure. This finding demonstrates that dietary supplementation with vitamin C helps nitroglycerine to work longer.[1,2]

Nonalcoholic Fatty Liver Disease (NAFLD)

NAFLD is one of the most common liver diseases globally. Generally, fatty liver disease means there is extra fat in the liver, even in people who drink little or no alcohol. If more than 5%–10% of the liver's weight is fat, it is called a fatty liver. Even though there is extra fat, there is not necessarily any inflammation in the liver or damage to the cells. However, nonalcoholic fatty liver disease (NAFLD) can consist of a spectrum of conditions ranging from a simple fatty infiltration to steatohepatitis, fibrosis, and cirrhosis. NAFLD is histologically similar to alcoholic liver disease.[1] Conditions such as alcohol abuse, type 2 diabetes, hypertension, high triglycerides, low HDL levels, and obesity are often associated with fatty liver disease. NAFLD is estimated to progress to a more severe condition called nonalcoholic steatohepatitis (NASH) in about one-third of NAFLD patients. It also increases the risk of cirrhosis and liver cancer.[2]

CLINICAL APPROACHES

Choline: Men and women fed (IV) with solutions that contained adequate methionine and folate but lacked choline have been found to develop a condition called nonalcoholic fatty liver disease (NAFLD) and signs of liver damage that resolved when choline was provided. Choline supplementation is recommended.[3] CDP-choline (citicoline) and choline salts, such as choline chloride and choline bitartrate, are available as supplements. Phosphatidylcholine supplements also provide choline, but in smaller amounts than those mentioned above.[4,5]

Weight Loss: Weight loss is one of the best treatments for NAFLD. Weight loss helps reduce fat, inflammation, and scarring in the liver.[6]

Diet: New evidence indicates that a Mediterranean diet (rich in monounsaturated fatty acids) may be more beneficial than a low-fat diet.[6]

Coffee: Large cohort studies suggest that drinking coffee appears to decrease the risk of having fatty liver disease.[7]

Silymarin: In one study, the researchers evaluated the effects a mixture of silybum marianum (silymarin), vitamin B12, and vitamin E (Epaclin 3.5 gm bid for six months) on NAFLD patients. The researchers concluded that silymarin appears to be effective in reducing the biochemical, inflammatory, and ultrasonic indices of hepatic steatosis in NAFLD.[1]

Tocopherol: There is currently no established treatment for NAFLD and NASH. In one study, a total of 247 nondiabetic subjects with NASH were randomized to receive 30 mg/day of pioglitazone (an insulin-sensitizing drug), 800 IU/day (536 mg/day) of vitamin E, or a placebo for 96 weeks. Only vitamin E supplementation significantly increased the overall rate of improvement in histological abnormalities that characterize NASH on liver biopsies (i.e., hepatocellular ballooning, steatosis, and lobular inflammation).[8]

In 173 children with NAFLD between the ages of 8 and 17, vitamin E supplementation significantly improved the overall disease activity score (this score is used to quantify the severity of the disease). In addition, a recent meta-analysis of another six trials found that vitamin E (400–800 mg/day) significantly lowered circulating aminotransferase concentrations in NAFLD and NASH patients, suggesting liver function improvements.[9,10]

Choline: An intervention study in 57 healthy adults who were fed choline-deficient diets under controlled conditions found that 77% of men, 80% of postmenopausal women, and 44% of premenopausal women developed fatty liver, liver damage, and/or muscle damage. These signs of organ dysfunction resolved upon choline reintroduction in the diet.[11] The highest versus lowest quintile of choline intake (412 mg/day vs. 179 mg/day) was associated with a 28% lower risk of fatty liver disease in normal-weight women.[12]

Vitamin D: A meta-analysis of approximately 5,000 NAFLD cases and 8,000 controls showed that, on average, NAFLD patients exhibited lower levels of vitamin D3 as compared to the controls, showing that a lack of this vitamin could be a part of the pathogenesis of NAFLD.[13]

L-Carnitine: Patients with underlying liver disease (e.g., nonalcoholic fatty liver disease from obesity) do not produce adequate levels of L-carnitine.[14]

Licorice: Some research suggests that taking 2 grams of licorice root extract daily for two months reduces test markers of liver injury in individuals with NAFLD.[15]

Turmeric: Research demonstrates that turmeric extract (curcumin) reduces markers of liver injury in people who have liver disease not caused by alcohol. Taking curcumin (70 mg/day for eight weeks) resulted in a 78.9% reduction in liver fat content.[16] There were also significant reductions in body mass index and serum levels of total cholesterol, low-density lipoprotein cholesterol, triglycerides, aspartate aminotransferase, alanine aminotransferase, glucose, and glycated hemoglobin compared with the placebo group.[16]

Curcumin can also be an effective therapy to treat and prevent liver fibrosis associated with non-alcoholic steatohepatitis (NASH).[17]

Alcohol Abstinence: Although not scientifically verified, abstaining from alcohol is a likely target for nonalcoholic liver disease control.[18]

Resveratrol: In a double-blind, randomized, placebo-controlled Chinese trial, resveratrol 600 mg/day for three months significantly decreased liver enzymes (ALT, AST), glucose, insulin resistance, LDL-cholesterol, and total cholesterol.[19]

Obsessive-Compulsive Disorder

Obsessive-compulsive disorder (OCD) affects adults, adolescents, and children all over the world. It is a common, chronic, long-lasting disorder in which an individual has uncontrollable, recurring thoughts, urges, or mental images (obsessions) that cause anxiety (e.g., needing to have things symmetrical and in perfect order).[1] This is coupled with behaviors (compulsions) such as ordering or arranging things in a particular fashion. Sufferers feel compelled to repeat those behaviors over and over in an effort to relieve their anxiety.[1] Symptoms often first appear in teens or young adults. OCD symptoms can interfere with all aspects of life, such as work, school, and personal relationships.[1]

RESEARCH RESULTS

Inositol: High-dose myo-inositol (mI) (12–18 gm/day) has been shown to be clinically effective in the treatment of obsessive-compulsive disorder, as well as panic disorder and depression.[2] Inositol should not be combined with SSRIs.

L-Tryptophan: The amino acid tryptophan, which is a precursor to serotonin, increases serotonin levels and helps treat OCD.[3]

St. John's Wort: Two double-blind, placebo-controlled studies were performed that compared the effects of a 900 mg/day dose of St. John's wort extract to 20 mg/day doses of Paxil or Prozac, commonly used to treat OCD. Those who took the St. John's wort supplement showed a 57% decrease in OCD symptoms and were 47% less likely to exhibit side effects.[4] In comparison to patients taking Fluoxetine, consumption of the St. John's wort extract reduced 48% of OCD patients' symptoms.[5]

Glycine: In one case study, an individual's symptoms was so severe that it caused him to be homebound without social contacts. Treatment with glycine over the course of five years led to robust reduction of OCD/BDD signs and symptoms, except for partial relapses during treatment cessation. Target doses of glycine varied from 50–66 gm/day (0.6–0.8 gm of glycine per kilogram of body weight) off and on over the five years. After treatment, he resumed his education and social life and there was evidence to suggest improved cognition as well.[6]

Olivopontocerebellar Atrophy (OA)/Multiple System Atrophy

Olivopontocerebellar atrophy is progressive degeneration of the neurons deep in the brain just above the spinal cord (olivopontocerebellar pathway that connects the inferior olive, pons, and cerebellum). OA is characterized by progressive balance problems (disequilibrium), impairment of the ability to coordinate voluntary movements (cerebellar ataxia), and difficulty speaking or slurred speech (dysarthria).[1] No specific treatment exists for individuals with OA. Treatment is symptomatic and supportive.[1]

CARE CONSIDERATIONS

Idebenone: Many patients are interested in alternative therapies and express a desire to pursue treatment with nonprescription medications. Antioxidants are one treatment approach tested in ataxia patients. Patients given idebenone 5 mg/kg per day for 12 months showed improvement for fine motor skills and eye movements. Patients with milder disease states and a lower number of triplet repeats also showed improvements in kinetic and gait function. Serum idebenone levels correlated negatively with the number of repeats, suggesting that more-affected individuals may need higher doses to achieve benefit.[2]

Diet: Affected individuals should take steps to raise the blood pressure by adding a little salt to the diet and drinking more fluids. Salt and fluids can increase blood volume and raise the blood pressure. Coffee and other caffeinated fluids can also raise blood pressure.[3]

Sleeping: Some patients may want to elevate the head of the bed. Raising the head to about a 30-degree angle will increase blood pressure during sleep. Individuals should also get up slowly from a reclining position.[3]

Leucine: One study found that 10 gm of leucine per day helped to treat olivopontocerebellar atrophy symptoms.[4]

Gamma-Aminobutyric Acid: GABA in the CSF of patients with olivopontocerebellar atrophy and Parkinson's was quite low compared with controls.[5] Two concerns with oral GABA supplementation are whether adequate amounts could be delivered to the brain and whether it would be quickly broken down if it did. Further research is needed in this area.

Operative Nutritional Status (Preoperative and Postoperative)

Preoperative and postoperative health status has many subparts, including nutritional status. The nutritional and immune status of surgical patients are important for preoperative management and postoperative recovery. A preoperative patient's nutritional condition reflects not only his or her health status, but also, indirectly, the patient's immune status. Thus, preoperative nutrition status influences a patient's tolerance to surgical stress, postoperative physical recovery, local wound healing, and surgical infection rates.[1]

Depletion of body protein, for example, is associated with prolonged convalescence, poor healing of wounds, increased susceptibility to infection, anemia, edema, impaired gastrointestinal motility, and skeletal muscle weakness.[1] Following cardiac surgery, a low level of serum albumin is associated with renal complications, since hypoalbuminemia is a reliable predictor of renal failure.[2] Malnutrition is an abnormal state that can be detected and corrected in most cases.

IMPROVING OUTCOMES

General Advice: For patients with significant under nourishment or at risk of developing malnourishment (e.g., ICU patients, head and neck or esophageal cancer patients), consult hospital dieticians for nutritional assessment and guidance regarding supplemental nutrition.[3]

Ascorbic Acid: Ascorbic acid plays an important role in the preoperative and postoperative nutrition of surgical patients.[4] During and after surgery, vitamin C levels in the body are measurably decreased and replacement above the normal dietary recommendations is necessary to correct this.[5] To enhance wound healing, doses of 300–500 mg/day for a week to 10 days, both preoperatively and postoperatively, are generally considered adequate, although considerably larger amounts have been recommended.[6] The authors of one study administered daily doses of 500–3,000 mg.[7] Studies have shown that this vitamin can help speed the healing process of wounds and that high doses of vitamin C enhance healing.[4] Postoperatively, vitamin C is recommended, not only to augment normal healing, but also to guard against suboptimal healing.[8]

A Finnish study found that oral administration of supplemental vitamin C after heart surgery could slash the risk of AF by up to 73% in high-risk patients, without adding side effects. Furthermore, the researchers reported that intravenous administration of vitamin C significantly reduced the length of hospital stay.[9]

Taking vitamin C after surgery or injury to the arm or leg helps prevent complex regional pain syndrome from developing.[10]

In a separate study, high-dose vitamin C infusion decreased postoperative pain during the first 24 hours and reduced morphine consumption in the early postoperative period.[11]

Cirrhosis: Patients with cirrhosis often have hypokalemia and alkalosis. These conditions should be corrected preoperatively to minimize the risks of cardiac arrhythmias and to limit encephalopathy.[12]

Vitamin D: A new study indicates that many patients undergoing spine surgery have low levels of vitamin D, which may delay their recovery. Vitamin D helps with calcium absorption, and patients with a deficiency can have difficulty producing new bone, which can, in turn, interfere with healing following orthopedic surgery.[13]

Bromelain: Previous studies demonstrate that taking bromelain by mouth decreases pain and postsurgical inflammation and swelling after surgery. Also, taking a product containing bromelain and other ingredients (Tenosan, Agave) is reported to decrease shoulder pain after surgery.[14,15] Trials indicate that bromelain might be effective in reducing swelling, bruising, and pain in women having episiotomy. Participants who were given 40 mg of bromelain four times daily for three days, beginning four hours after delivery, showed a statistically significant decrease in edema, inflammation, and pain.[16] Bromelain has been approved by the German Commission E for postsurgical and/or post-traumatic edema.[17]

Glutamine: Administering glutamine through a feeding tube ostensibly reduces infections and complications, shortens hospital stays, and improves wound healing in people with severe burns but without lung injury.[18]

In addition, giving glutamine along with nutrition intravenously after a bone marrow transplant decreases the risk of infection and improves recovery compared to intravenous nutrition alone.[19]

Optic Neuritis/Retrobulbar Neuropathy

The term *optic neuritis* (ON) refers to inflammation of the optic nerve. The most common symptoms of ON include unilateral painful vision loss, ranging from blurring of vision to complete blindness in one eye, pain on eye movement, loss of color vision (where colors are less vivid), and seeing flashing or flickering lights.

The disorder occurs mostly in young healthy females and people who live in high latitudes. Multiple sclerosis is the most common cause of demyelinating ON. Other causes include neurological disorders, nutritional deficiencies, and toxins (i.e., ethambutol, amiodarone, methanol, ethanol, and tobacco).

Corticosteroids are the main medical treatment for ON.[1] Recovery of visual functions in ON is observed spontaneously over 2–3 weeks in more than 80% of patients without treatment. Vision tends to stabilize over the following months or continues to improve up to one full year, although long-term defects in visual functions are possible.[2]

RECOVERY PROTOCOLS FOR OPTIC NEUROPATHY

Nutritional Deficiencies of thiamine (B1), riboflavin (B2), folate, B12, and B6 have all been associated with optic neuropathy.[3] Patients who follow high protein, ketogenic, and low-carbohydrate diets are at risk for developing thiamine deficiency. Similarly, patients who have undergone gastrointestinal surgery may develop optic neuropathy due to interference with the absorption of vitamin B12.[3]

Caveats: For optic neuropathy due to B12 deficiency, incomplete treatment of vitamin B12 deficiency with oral B12 supplementation coupled with oral folic acid can aggravate neurological impairment secondary to vitamin B12 deficiency if the B12 deficiency is not corrected first.[3] No current treatment can restore lost function from a damaged optic nerve in optic neuritis.[4]

RECOVERY PROTOCOLS FOR OPTIC NEURITIS

General Measures: Good nutrition and hydration, avoidance of tobacco, and refraining from vigorous exercise or over-heating are often recommended during the acute phase of optic neuritis.[5]

B Vitamins: Partial or complete recovery is possible when B vitamins and a nutritious diet are supplemented.[6]

Vitamin B12: Vitamin B12 intramuscularly or subcutaneously is considered medically necessary for retrobulbar neuritis.[5] B12 deficiency has traditionally been treated with intramuscular injections at a dosage of 1 mg weekly for eight weeks followed by 1 mg monthly for life or until the underlying etiology is eliminated.[2,7] It is also considered medically necessary for retrobulbar neuritis associated with heavy smoking.[8]

Osteitis Fibrosa Cystica

Osteitis fibrosa cystica (OFC), also known as Von Recklinghausen's disease, is a serious skeletal disorder and a complication of primary or secondary hyperparathyroidism. As a result, osteoclasts are activated to resorb bone. This results in fibrous tissue replacing calcified supporting structures. The loss of bone mass causes bone pain and susceptibility to fractures, especially in the arms, legs, or spine. Ultimately, sites of increased bone activity (i.e., phalanges, skull bones, ends of long bones, and trabecular bones of the vertebrae) are softened, weakened, and deformed.[1] Advanced OFC results in lytic lesions due to defective remodeling called brown tumors, which are more severe in young adults. Persistent hypercalcemia and an elevated serum parathyroid hormone (PTH) level help confirm the diagnosis of primary hyperparathyroidism. Whenever possible, the underlying cause of secondary hyperparathyroidism should be removed.

NUTRITIONAL SUPPORT

Vitamin D and Calcium: The goal of medical management is to normalize calcium levels. Therefore, supplementation of vitamin D and calcium is necessary.[2]

Regardless of the clinical severity of primary hyperparathyroidism, the disease is generally more severe in those with concomitant vitamin D deficiency. Second, vitamin D deficiency and insufficiency seem to be more prevalent in patients with primary hyperparathyroidism than in geographically matched populations.[3] In some cases, correction of vitamin D deficiency may be accomplished without worsening the underlying hypercalcemia. Vitamin D-deficient patients undergoing parathyroidectomy are also at increased risk of postoperative hypocalcemia and "hungry bone syndrome," which underscores the importance of preoperative assessment of vitamin D status in all patients with primary hyperparathyroidism.[3] Taking vitamin D3 by mouth lowers parathyroid hormone levels and bone loss in women with hyperparathyroidism.[4]

Osteoarthritis (OA)

Osteoarthritis, also known as degenerative joint disease, is the most common form of arthritis and is the leading cause of disability wordwide. Osteoarthritis is characterized by deterioration of articular cartilage (becoming soft, thin, and frayed) with formation of reactive new bone (osteophytes or bone spurs), pain, limitation of motion, joint deformity, and disability. This chronic joint condition is often referred to as a noninflammatory type of arthritis because it lacks inflammatory features, such as warm or swollen joints. However, OA is not a simple "wear and tear" process as previously thought, but a true inflammatory disease according to the American College of Rheumatology (ACR). OA can occur in people of all ages, but is most common in people older than 65. Risk factors include increasing age, obesity, previous joint injury, genetics, and overuse of the joint.

The breakdown of protective cartilage in the joints, joint lining, and underlying bone causes pain and stiffness with restricted motion. Pain tends to subside with rest while stiffness is typically worse after prolonged rest (i.e., waking up in the morning). Some patients with OA have no pain or minimal pain. Symptoms can be intermittent, and many times do not correlate to the x-ray findings. OA most frequently occurs in the hands, fingers, hips, knees, and spine (especially neck and lower back). Grating or grinding sensations on joint movement are common.

The goals of treatment are to reduce pain and improve function. Current treatments only address symptoms and pain, and only one-third of patients are satisfied with the treatments they receive.[1] The goals of OA management are to minimize pain, optimize function, and tailor care to the individual's needs, goals, and values.[2]

CLINICAL CARE OPTIONS

Nonpharmacologic interventions such as patient education, heat and cold, judicious exercises (caution: no exercises during an acute painful episode), and joint protection are the mainstays of OA management and should be tried first.[2]

Lifestyle: Weight reduction and avoiding activities that are stressful to the affected joints are recommended.

Over-the-Counter Interventions: Topical nonsteroidal anti-inflammatory drugs are often recommended (e.g., diclofenac sodium gel, 1%) followed by oral forms if results are inadequate. Nonsteroidal anti-inflammatory drugs (NSAIDs) are the first-line pharmacologic treatment for OA. In attempting to alleviate pain from OA, oral acetaminophen (Tylenol) was found to be no more effective than a placebo.[3] Diclofenac sodium (Voltaren Arthritis Pain) 50 mg 2–3 times a day was found to be more effective than ibuprofen.[4] Nonetheless, ibuprofen (Motrin, Advil) 2,400 mg/day has been shown to have good treatment effect.[3] Naproxen (Aleve) 750–1,000 mg/day was somewhat less effective than ibuprofen but did reduce resting pain, movement pain, and night pain.[3,5] Aspirin (plain, buffered, or enteric-coated at 325–650 mg every 4–6 hours) can be also used to help alleviate pain.[6]

Ascorbic Acid: Taking vitamin C from dietary sources or from calcium ascorbate supplements helps prevent cartilage loss and worsening of symptoms in people with osteoarthritis.[7,8]

Vitamin D and Calcium: Published research suggests that low intake and low blood levels of vitamin D are associated with an increased risk for progression of osteoarthritis.[9] All individuals should have a balanced diet with adequate daily intake of calcium and vitamin D. Calcium carbonate is the salt of choice because it contains the highest concentration of elemental calcium (40%) and is least expensive.[10]

Vitamin B12: Twenty-six elderly individuals with osteoarthritis of the hands received 6.4 mg/day of folic acid plus 20 mcg/day of Vitamin B12. Grip strength improved and pain was reduced.[11]

S-Adenosylmethionine (SAMe): Osteoarthritis results from progressive catabolic loss of cartilage proteoglycans. Standard drug therapy is only of palliative benefit and may be rate-limiting for proteoglycan productions. By mechanisms that are still unclear, SAMe also promotes production of cartilage proteoglycans and is therapeutically beneficial in osteoarthritis in well-tolerated oral doses.

Glucosamine Sulfate: Double-blind studies dating from the early 1980s demonstrate that oral glucosamine sulfate (500 mg tid) decreased pain and improved mobility in osteoarthritis, without side effects.[12,13] Glucosamine is contraindicated in shellfish allergy.

B vitamins have been shown to increase the analgesic effects of diclofenac in the treatment of osteoarthritis.[14,15]

Vitamin E: A six-week treatment with high-dose vitamin E was compared with a placebo. Physician-assessed global effectiveness significantly favored vitamin E, and three pain parameters indicated significantly earlier and greater pain reduction with vitamin E compared with a placebo. Consumption of analgesics was reduced by 50% in the vitamin E group and by 25% in the placebo group.[15]

Treatment with vitamin E and vitamin A were compared in patients with radiologically confirmed spondylosis who had not responded to conventional treatment. After a preliminary single-blind trial, a subsequent double-blind RCT in 20 patients after three weeks found that pain intensity was reported as "completely relieved" in all patients treated with vitamin E (100 mg/day).[16]

Bromelain: A combination of bromelain, trypsin, and rutin was compared to diclofenac in 103 patients with osteoarthritis of the knee.[17] After six weeks, both treatments resulted in significant and similar reduction in the pain and inflammation.[18] Bromelain is a food supplement that may provide an alternative treatment to nonsteroidal anti-inflammatory drugs (NSAIDs).[18]

Non-Drug Treatments: In acute painful spinal arthritis, the following are some non-pharmacological treatments: light massage to paraspinal muscles improves tone, circulation, and elasticity; cervical traction in the position of maximum comfort to neck (5–10 pounds) for 10–15 minutes; ultrasonic exposure on painful trigger points in cervical and shoulder muscles; interferential therapy (IFT) for acute neck and back pain; removable soft cervical collar/back corset/back belt for symptomatic relief.[19]

Spinal Manipulation: The Arthritis Foundation has recognized spinal manipulation as beneficial for spinal arthritis and recommends chiropractic care for spinal pain, stiffness, and limited motion.[20] The American College of Physicians also recommends spinal manipulation, especially for low-back pain.[21] Published research in the *British Medical Journal* by a rheumatologist summarized that the best treatment for cervical spondylosis, or neck arthritis, includes exercise and spinal manipulation.[22]

Osteoarthritis (Knee and Hip)

Osteoarthritis (OA) is likely to affect the joints that bear most of the weight, such as the knees and hips. (*See also* "Osteoarthritis" *above.*) Osteoarthritis of the knee or hip is common and can result in severe joint pain and disability. With hip OA, at times, the pain may be felt in the groin, inner thigh, buttocks, or even the knees. As a result of this condition, several hundred thousand people each year in the U.S. undergo total joint replacement. Nonetheless, many patients with osteoarthritis of the knee or hip can be managed without surgery. Weight management is crucial for long-term care of knee and hip arthritis.

PALLIATIVE CARE

Intensive weight loss of 20% can help reduce painful knee arthritis in people who are overweight or obese.[1]

Over-the-Counter Pain Medicines: Acetaminophen (Tylenol) is a preferred first-line treatment; it may be less effective than oral nonsteroidal anti-inflammatory drugs (NSAIDs) but has less risk of serious gastrointestinal (GI) and cardiovascular events.[2] NSAIDs (aspirin, ibuprofen, naproxen, and diclofenac) or topical rubs (e.g., diclofenac or capsaicin) from the drugstore can also be used to help minimize hip and knee pain.

Vitamin D: One study involving 556 patients with an average age of 70 found that the risk of progression of osteoarthritis of the knee for participants who had low vitamin D intake and blood levels was three times over that of patients without these deficiencies. Low blood levels of vitamin D also correlated with loss of cartilage and degenerative bony spur formation.[3]

Men with vitamin D deficiencies are twice as likely to have prevalent radiographic hip OA, and therefore vitamin D therapy to augment skeletal health in elderly men is warranted.[4]

Vitamin D should be taken at doses of 800–1,000 IU/day.

S-Adenosyl-L-Methionine (SAMe) is a naturally occurring intermediate of methionine metabolism. In one study, researchers compared 400 mg of SAMe dosed three times a day to 400 mg of ibuprofen also dosed three times a day in 150 patients who suffered from hip and/or knee osteoarthritis.[5] The researchers found that SAMe was more effective at increasing range of motion as well as decreasing pain and spasm than ibuprofen. The gastric side effects typical with ibuprofen were not exhibited. SAMe was also studied against other anti-inflammatory medications such as naproxen sodium and indomethacin.[6] SAMe was just as effective as non-steroidal anti-inflammatories in all of these studies but without gastric side effects.[5] Another study found SAMe (600 mg bid) had a slower onset of action but was as effective as celecoxib in the management of symptoms of knee osteoarthritis.[7]

Glucosamine: Most research shows that taking glucosamine sulfate can provide pain relief for individuals with osteoarthritis, especially those with osteoarthritis of the knees.[8] Data from double-blind studies showed glucosamine was superior to ibuprofen in patients with osteoarthritis of the knee.[9]

Methylsulfonylmethane (MSM): One preliminary study suggested that taking 6,000 mg of MSM improved pain and function without side effects in people with OA of the knee. Some preparations combine MSM with glucosamine to treat OA. One study suggests that this approach might help but more research is needed.[10]

Chondroitin sulfate (e.g., 200–800 mg/day) can slow disease progression and reduce symptoms in patients with osteoarthritis of the knee.[11,12] Pharmaceutical-grade chondroitin sulfate, manufactured by IBSA, is approved in Europe for the treatment of OA and has been shown to be effective for both hand and knee pain.[13]

Osteogenesis Imperfecta (OI)

Osteogenesis imperfecta (OI) means imperfect bone formation and is also known as brittle bone disease. OI is a genetic disorder characterized by bones that break easily, often from little or no apparent trauma. There are eight recognized forms of OI.[1] OI can cause weak muscles, brittle teeth, a curved spine, and hearing loss. With a curved spine there is limited space for the lungs, which are already compromised from lack of collagen, to properly expand.[1] Patients with OI are more vulnerable to lung problems, including asthma and pneumonia. In fact, respiratory failure is the most common cause of death in patients with OI.[2] Because OI is a genetic disorder of collagen (abnormal type 1 collagen), and not a calcium or nutrient deficiency, there are no foods or supplements that can cure OI.[3]

ADJUVANT MANAGEMENT CHOICES

Exercise: Patients with osteogenesis imperfecta are encouraged to exercise using swimming and water therapy as much as possible to promote muscle and bone strength, which can help prevent fractures.

Fiber: Pelvic asymmetry, seen in people with more severe OI, is associated with a tendency to have constipation. A high-fiber diet, drinking plenty of water and other fluids, and physical activity may help remedy this problem.[3]

Calcium does not improve the basic collagen defects that cause OI. Nonetheless, nearly all patients with OI have osteoporosis because they do not develop appropriate bone mass.[4]

Therefore, individuals with OI should get adequate calcium in their diets to develop peak bone mass and to prevent more bone loss. Bone loss, or osteoporosis, from any cause (calcium-related, inactivity-related, age-related) makes OI bones even more fragile. The National Academy of Sciences developed the following Recommended Daily Allowances for calcium:

Young children (1-3)	700 mg/day
Older children (4–8)	1,000 mg/day
Preteens/adolescents (9–18)	1,300 mg/day
Men and women (19–50)	1,000 mg/day
Men and women (50+)	1,200 mg/day

These guidelines were developed for people of average height and weight.[3,4]

Vitamin D: Clinical studies demonstrate that low levels of vitamin D contribute to osteoporosis/bone loss and may contribute to chronic pain. Most of the vitamin D in our bodies is made from sunlight absorbed through the skin. The latest research supports the following guidelines for vitamin D for people with OI. *See also* Vitamin D Research in the Resources section for more information.[4,5]

Suggested Vitamin D-3 Intake for People with OI

Weight	IU/day
50 lbs. (20 kg)	600–800
90 lbs. (40 kg)	1,100–1,600
110 lbs. (50 kg)	1,200–2,00
150 lbs. (70 kg) and above	2,000–2,800[3]

Ascorbic Acid: Collagen is the most abundant protein in the body and is the main fibrous component of bone. Ascorbic acid is one cofactor in the hydroxylation of proline to form hydroxyproline before incorporation into the collagen molecule. In the year preceding the start of a study, at least 25 fractures occurred among patients. In contrast, eight fractures occurred after supplementation with 1 gm/day of ascorbic acid. The decrease in the incidence of fractures provided clinical evidence of the formation of more stable bone collagen and decreased bone fragility. It was concluded that ascorbic acid treatment of patients with osteogenesis imperfecta is beneficial.[6,7]

Osteomalacia

Osteomalacia is defective mineralization that keeps bones from hardening as they should, resulting in softening and weakening of bones, leading to fractures. In other words, bones are breaking down faster than they can be rebuilt. Most often, osteomalacia is due to a deficiency of vitamin D. (*See* "Common causes of osteomalacia" *below.*) Osteomalacia is a common metabolic bone disease among the elderly that can be associated with osteoporosis. Only adults get osteomalacia. When the same condition happens in children, it is called rickets.

Patients with osteomalacia often present with weakened bones that easily fracture and diffuse pain that may be misdiagnosed as fibromyalgia.[1] Additional symptoms can include nonspecific musculoskeletal pain, muscle weakness, bone and hip pain, and difficulty walking (e.g., a waddling gait). Pain is especially likely to occur in the hips and spread to the lower back, legs, pelvis, or ribs.

Common causes of osteomalacia are:

1. Vitamin D deficiency (e.g., from lack of sunshine plus inadequate intake). Also, if the body cannot absorb fats properly, they are passed directly out of the body in the stool (steatorrhea). As a result, vitamin D, which is a fat-soluble vitamin, and calcium are poorly absorbed.
2. The kidneys do not function properly (tubular acidosis), causing metabolic acidosis. The increased acid helps to dissolve the skeleton.
3. Digestive organs do not adequately function for proper absorption of calcium.[2]
4. Chronic liver disease that interferes with vitamin D metabolism.
5. Deficient intake of calcium or lack of phosphate.[3]

On x-rays, demineralized bands known as pseudofractures, or Looser lines, can be observed. Common sites for Looser zones include the scapula, pubic rami, and proximal femurs medially.[2]

THERAPEUTIC OPTIONS

Vitamin D: Osteomalacia is most often caused by not getting enough vitamin D.[4,5]

Treatment for osteomalacia involves providing enough vitamin D and calcium because both are required to harden and strengthen (mineralize) bones.[6] Sometimes phosphate supplements may be needed as well.[7]

Dietary vitamin D deficiency can initially be treated with vitamin D2 (50,000 International Units [IU] by mouth weekly for eight weeks to replete body stores, followed by long-term therapy 400–1,000 IU/day).[8]

Calcium: Individuals with malabsorption or poor nutrition should receive calcium supplementation. Usually 1–1.5 gm/day of oral elemental calcium is a reasonable initial dose. Frequent small doses (e.g., three times a day) are more effective and tolerable than fewer larger ones. The absorbability of calcium supplements is enhanced with meals. Calcium preparations such as calcium carbonate (40% calcium as in Os-Cal or the equivalent) can be used. Some patients with adverse gastrointestinal side effects with the above preparations prefer using chocolate- or coffee-flavored formulations known as Viactiv (500 mg calcium per tablet). PPIs or H2 blocking drugs do not impair calcium carbonate absorption.[7]

Phosphorus and Vitamin D3: If phosphorous replacement is required, the therapy for chronic hypophosphatemia is aimed at maintaining normal concentration of serum phosphorus without inducing secondary hyperparathyroidism or nephrocalcinosis. Divided doses of phosphorus supplements 1–3 gm/day and D3 (50,000 IU 3x/week for 10 weeks and 3x/month thereafter) may be used to increase the absorption of phosphorus.[9]

Osteoporosis

Osteoporosis is the most common bone disease and is characterized by painless bone loss (low bone density). It results from a decline in normal bone architecture due to decreased mineralization and decreased bone strength that lead to increased risk of fractures.[1] Osteoporosis is known colloquially as "thinning bones" or the "silent disease" because it has no symptoms initially. The disorder affects both males and females, but it is most likely to occur in women with low body weight after menopause because of the sudden decrease in estrogen.[2] Smoking and poor diet also increase the risk of acquiring osteoporosis.

The loss of bony material, or mass, leads to structural deterioration of bone tissue. Both increased osteoclastic activity and decreased osteoblastic activity contribute to the development of osteoporosis. There is mainly the loss of trabecular bone tissue, as opposed to cortical bone such as in the cranium. This loss of tissue substance thins the framework inside bone, resulting in a weaker honeycomb-like structure that is brittle and fragile. Once that occurs, even mild stress such as bending or coughing can cause a fracture. Fractures, especially in the hip, spine (crush fractures), and wrist, are the most common and most serious complication from osteoporosis. If an osteoporotic fracture has occurred, a diagnosis of severe osteoporosis is required.

Chronic pain and depression are not uncommon accompanying symptoms. Decreased bone mass can also weaken spinal vertebrae to the extent that there is lost height and the development of a kyphosis, or dowager's hump, which is an abnormal curving and twisting of the thoracic spine that gives a hunched-over appearance. Osteoporosis may significantly limit mobility and may require long-term nursing home care. The goals in treating osteoporosis include lowering the risk of fractures and preventing disabilities related to osteoporosis.

HELPING TO PREVENT FURTHER BONE LOSS

Exercise: Weight-bearing aerobic and strengthening exercises can decrease risk of falls and fractures by improving muscle strength, coordination, balance, and mobility.[1]

Tobacco Products: Smoking and a poor diet increase the risk of getting osteoporosis.[3] Anyone with osteoporosis should avoid nicotine because smoking cessation helps optimize peak bone mass, minimize bone loss, and ultimately reduce fracture risk.

Diet: For prevention and treatment of osteoporosis, the diet should be adequate in protein, total calories, and extra calcium, magnesium, and vitamin D as set forth below.[3] The diet should also be low in refined sugar, caffeine, and alcohol.[1]

General preventive measures also comprise exercise and fall prevention techniques.

Calcium: Calcium and vitamin D supplementation increases bone mineral density, and the combination decreases the risk of hip and vertebral fractures. Men and women with osteoporosis need 1,000–1,200 milligrams of calcium a day.[4]

Calcium is also recommended to help prevent osteoporosis. Calcium carbonate supplements dissolve better in an acid environment, so they should be taken with a meal. Calcium citrate supplements can be taken any time because they do not need acid to dissolve. For this reason, individuals who might have problems absorbing medications (e.g., those taking PPIs) could consider using calcium citrate (e.g., Citrical) instead of calcium carbonate to increase absorption. The higher the individual calcium dose, the less it is absorbed. For the maximum absorption, no more than 500 mg of calcium should be taken in a single dose with the next dose at least four hours later.[5]

Vitamin D: Vitamin D supplementation decreases vertebral and nonvertebral fractures in older men and women living independently.[6] Vitamin D increases calcium and phosphorus absorption in the intestines and is essential for the development and maintenance of bone. Vitamin D deficiency results in low serum calcium and phosphorus. That is why this important vitamin is recommended to prevent osteoporosis. A good starting point for adults is 800–1,000 international units (IU) a day although up to 4,000 IU vitamin D/day is considered safe.[7,8,9,10]

Magnesium deficiency directly contributes to osteoporosis. Magnesium is involved in bone formation and influences the activities of osteoblasts and osteoclasts. Magnesium also affects the concentrations of both parathyroid hormone and the active form of vitamin D, which are major regulators of bone homeostasis.

One study found that 290 mg/day elemental magnesium (as magnesium citrate) for 30 days in 20 postmenopausal women with osteoporosis suppressed bone turnover even on a short-term basis compared with a placebo, suggesting that bone loss decreased.[11,12]

Magnesium deficiency was found in 16 of 19 women with osteoporosis and was associated with abnormal bone-mineral crystals.[13] In a recent study, 31 postmenopausal women took 250–750 mg/day of magnesium for two years. Bone density increased in 75% of these women by 1%–8%.[14]

For osteoporosis, 300–1,800 mg/day of magnesium hydroxide for six months, followed by 600 mg/day of magnesium hydroxide for 18 months, has been employed.[15] Magnesium citrate 1,830 mg/day for 30 days has also been used. In addition to estrogen, 600 mg of magnesium plus 500 mg of calcium and a daily multivitamin supplement for one year helps manage osteoporosis.[16]

Copper: Osteoporosis is a consequence of copper deficiency.[17] Women who took 3 mg of copper per day lost an average of 0.64% of their bone density, whereas those who took the placebo lost 10 times more (6.2%) bone density.[18]

Boron: A boron supplement of 3 mg/day significantly reduced the urinary excretion of calcium and magnesium. Boron supplementation markedly elevated the serum concentrations of 17 beta-estradiol and testosterone.[19] The findings suggest that the addition of a boron supplement with an amount of boron commonly found in diets high in fruits and vegetables induces changes in postmenopausal women consistent with the prevention of calcium loss and bone demineralization.

Soy protein appears to have an effect that is similar to estrogen on bone tissue. Ipriflavone is a product made in a laboratory from one of the isoflavones found in soy. When combined with calcium, ipriflavone 600 mg/day appears to prevent bone loss and reduce pain associated with compression fractures in the spine.[20]

Ipriflavone: Taking ipriflavone in combination with 1,000 mg of calcium daily can prevent loss of bone mineral density (BMD) in postmenopausal women with osteoporosis or low bone strength.[21]

Ipriflavone can also significantly reduce pain due to osteoporosis and is as effective as inhaling a medication called calcitonin.[21]

Manganese: Taking manganese by mouth in combination with calcium, zinc, and copper helps reduce spinal bone loss in older women. Also, taking a specific product containing manganese, calcium, vitamin D, magnesium, zinc, copper, and boron for one year is reported to improve bone mass in women with weak bones.[22]

Otitis Externa/Swimmer's Ear

Acute diffuse otitis externa is inflammation of the external ear canal. Typically, only one ear is affected, and it can last up to three weeks. Symptoms may include pain, itchiness, drainage of liquid or pus, and temporary hearing loss. Most cases are caused by bacterial (gram negative rods) infection. Such infections are common especially in the summertime and associated with water activities. Moisture provides an ideal environment for bacterial growth. With treatment, symptoms usually clear up in a few days. Necrotizing otitis externa is a life-threatening complication of otitis externa especially in elderly patients with diabetes.[1]

TREATMENT MEASURES

Pain is treated with oral analgesics; usually an NSAID or acetaminophen is adequate.[2]

Acetic Acid: Acidification of the ear canal with a topical solution of 2% acetic acid (VoSol) combined with hydrocortisone (VoSol HC Otic) for inflammation is an effective treatment in most cases.[3] Acetic acid is known for its antimicrobial effect on bacteria. Acetic acid is present in vinegar in a 3%–5% concentration. Vinegar has been used in medicine for thousands of years.[1,4] To promote continuous contact, a soft cotton gauze plug (ear wick) can be inserted into the ear canal. The wick is then saturated with the acetic acid solution. Patients should keep the wick in for the first 24 hours and keep it moist by adding 3–5 drops of the solution every 4–6 hours. After 24 hours the wick can be removed, but the patient should continue to instill five drops of (2%)

acetic acid otic solution three or four times daily thereafter for five to seven days or as long as needed. In pediatric patients, 3–4 drops may be sufficient due to the smaller capacity of the ear canal.[1,5]

Neomycin otic ear drop solutions and suspensions with polymyxin B-hydrocortisone (Cortisporin) or with hydrocortisone-thonzonium (Coly-Mycin S) are used to treat bacterial otitis externa.[3]

Combining acetic acid with an astringent such as alcohol drops (e.g., Swim Ear) can also be effective, but many physicians feel that the combination is too irritating and therefore prefer to use a Burow's solution (Star-Otic) as an astringent.[3] A multitude of ear drops with an astringent are available over-the-counter. Ask your pharmacist for guidance.

Otitis Media

Acute otitis media is a type of ear infection in the middle ear space behind the eardrum, or tympanic membrane. Pain is the major symptom of acute otitis media. It primarily occurs in children 6–36 months old, but adults can also be affected. About three out of four children have at least one episode of otitis media by the time they are three years old. Otitis media, whether acute, with effusion, chronic suppurative, or adhesive, is the most common cause of earaches.[1] Earaches can be debilitating, but do not always warrant antibiotics. Otitis media with fluid (effusion) does not respond to antibiotics.[1] When antibiotics are prescribed, high-dose amoxicillin is most often recommended, but antibiotics do not decrease ear pain.[2]

LESSENING EAR PAIN

Warm Washcloth: A warm, moist washcloth can be applied over the ear.[3]

OTC Eardrops: Over-the-counter eardrops (e.g., Hyland's Earache Drops, Similasan) may be used to lessen pain.[3] A Cochrane study found that naturopathic herbal ear drops in 274 patients were more effective than anaesthetic drops. There were statistically significant differences at instillation of the drops, or 15 to 30 minutes after the instillation on one to three days after diagnosis, always favouring the naturopathic drops.[4]

Pain Relievers: OTC oral pain relievers such as acetaminophen (Tylenol), ibuprofen (Advil, Motrin), or naproxen (Naprosyn) can be used as instructed.[3]

Calendula: Previous clinical studies demonstrate that applying a specific product (Otikon Otic Solution) that contains mullein, garlic, calendula, and St. John's wort to the ear for three days reduces ear pain in children and teenagers with ear infections.[3,5]

Chiropractic Care: One study found that 93% of 46 child participants with symptoms of ear infections improved following chiropractic adjustments, and 43% improved after only one or two sessions.[6]

Tea Tree Oil and Olive Oil: Tea tree oil has antiseptic, antifungal, and anti-inflammatory properties. A couple of warmed tea tree oil drops in the ear per day may ease earache. Tea tree oil should be diluted (3–5 drops) in olive oil or sweet almond oil.[7] The American Academy of Pediatrics states that a couple drops of warmed olive oil is safe and moderately effective.[7]

Otosclerosis

Otosclerosis or otospongiosis is an abnormal overgrowth of spongy bone tissue that forms around the innermost bone in the middle ear known as the stapes, or stirrup, and basically locks it in place. This can result in hearing loss, especially of low pitched sounds, or not being able to hear a whisper. Some patients may also experience balance problems or tinnitus. Middle-aged Caucasian women are most at risk.

FOR ADULT OTOSCLEROSIS

Sodium fluoride reduces enzyme levels in the perilymph of patients with otosclerosis and inhibits trypsin. It could also increase mineralization and stabilization of otospongiotic lesions and halt the otosclerotic process.[1]

One study found that the use of sodium fluoride (e.g., 20 mg twice daily for six months) in otosclerosis patients resulted in a reduced incidence of deterioration in hearing after two years of treatment. Several case-control series have described a hearing benefit in the group treated with sodium fluoride.[2]

In another study, sodium fluoride therapy (Fluoritab, Luride, Pediaflor) was successful for 79% of the patients who were losing their hearing at a rate of 5 dB or more per year at one or more of the speech frequencies. The finding that patients with more rapid rates of progression responded most favorably to sodium fluoride therapy suggests that patients with the most active otospongiotic processes will be the most responsive to treatment.[3]

Calcium (500–2,000 mg/day) **and Vitamin D** replacement therapy (400–800 IU/day) resulted in significant hearing improvement in 3 of 16 patients in a prospective study; these data support a causal correlation. Vitamin D deficiency is probably a factor in the etiology of some cases of otosclerosis and is important since the deafness resulting from cochlear involvement may be reversible.[4] These treatments, if unable to reverse hearing loss, may at least slow the rate of hearing loss.[5]

Surgery: A stapedectomy, which involves replacement of the fixed stapes with a prosthesis, is highly successful in correcting the conductive component of the hearing loss.

FOR PEDIATRIC OTOSCLEROSIS

Vitamin D stimulates calcium and phosphate absorption from the small intestine and promotes calcium release from bone into blood.[6]

Calcium carbonate (Oyster Cal) can be used in combination with vitamin D and sodium fluoride.[6]

Overweight/Obesity

The disease is complex, chronic, and progressive.[1] Since 1980, people's weight in the U.S. has been increasing at an alarming rate.[2] The worldwide prevalence of obesity has nearly tripled between 1975 and 2016. Over 40% of U.S. adults are classified as having have obesity.[1] Obesity has now reached epidemic proportions.[3] Obesity is the second-leading modifiable cause of death in the U.S., trailing only deaths related to smoking. Many factors contribute to being overweight. In order to lose weight, individuals typically must burn more calories than they consume, but this is often easier said than done.

Obesity, in general terms, is an accumulation of body fat, typically 20% or more over an individual's ideal body weight. Genetics makes a significant contribution to body weight.[1] The vast majority of people with acid reflux have obesity, as do those with nonalcoholic fatty liver disease. The following complications are associated with the medical problem of excess weight: heart disease (especially CAD), osteoarthritis, stroke, some types of cancer, diabetes, gallstones, hyperlipidemia, hypertension, kidney disease, and respiratory problems (e.g., sleep apnea). Diets, supplements, medications, and surgeries are available as treatments.[4]

Regarding diets, a great variety and number of diet plans are available. Most weight-loss diets are usually short-term solutions doomed to failure. That is because dieting is uncomfortable, boring, abnormal, and unsustainable as a way of life. The lost weight is typically regained, plus a bit more. Nonetheless, to treat excess weight, a diet plan yielding reduction of 5%–10% of initial body weight is the minimal initial goal because this correlates with improvement in comorbidities.[5]

Bariatric surgery is the gold standard in terms of obesity treatment, but not all patients are good candidates. Phentermine (3.75 mg) plus topirimate (23 mg) is the most prescribed short-term obesity medication.[1] Semaglutide (2.4 mg) shows great promise as a long-term treatment.

AIDS IN WEIGHT LOSS

Diets: It is important to adhere to a low-carbohydrate reduced-calorie diet (e.g., 1,200–1,500 kcal/day for women and 1,500–1,800 kcal/day for men). The diet should have fewer sodas and sugary drinks (i.e., liquid candy)[6] and also be high in fiber and whole grains.[5] Also, different types of intermittent fasting reduce body weight and reduce diabetes parameters such as fasting glucose, fasting insulin, insulin resistance index, and HbA1c.[7]

Exercise: At least 150 minutes of physical activity/week is recommended.[5]

Pantothenic Acid: Taking large doses of B5, or pantothenic acid, may be the answer for some overweight individuals. 100 patients attempting to lose weight were prescribed a 1,000-calorie diet, plus 10 gm/day of pantothenic acid (2.5 gm four times a day).

The dieters did not experience hunger or weakness and all of them were able to carry on their daily routines without problems.[8]

Hydroxycitric Acid and Chromium: In a double-blind study, researchers found that taking 500 mg of hydroxycitric acid (Citrin), an extract from garcinia cambogia, and 100 mcg of chromium picolinate three times a day, approximately one half-hour before meals was both safe and effective. Subjects reported decreased appetite, fewer cravings for sweets, and increased energy. Individuals taking the supplement lost an average of 11 pounds in eight weeks compared to a four-pound average loss for those taking a placebo.[9,10,11,12] Patients were also put on a "smart choice" eating program, which is a low-fat, low-sugar, low-sodium version of three meals per day, and also participated in a sensible daily exercise program.

Ancillary Methods: Many significantly overweight individuals need digestive enzymes, lipolytic agents (choline, inositol), metabolic correctors, and nutritional supplements.[13]

Alpha-Lipoic Acid: Previous clinical studies demonstrate that taking alpha-lipoic acid for 8 to 48 weeks can reduce body weight in people who are overweight.[14]

Glutamate and GABA: Appetite is regulated by a coordinated interplay between the gut, adipose tissue, and the brain. A primary site for the regulation of appetite is the hypothalamus. GABA (γ-aminobutyric acid) is the main inhibitory neurotransmitter in the central nervous system, while glutamic acid is the most common excitatory neurotransmitter in the central nervous system. Glutamate and GABA dominate synaptic transmission in the hypothalamus.[15] Unfortunately, well-done studies are lacking on their impact upon weight gain or loss.

Aloe Vera: Clinical studies indicate that taking a specific aloe product (Aloe QDM complex) containing 147 mg of aloe gel twice daily for eight weeks reduced body weight and fat mass in overweight or obese people with diabetes or prediabetes.[16]

Ketogenic Diet: In a recent eight-week randomized trial including 34 obese men and women ages 60 through 75, those who ate a ketogenic diet lost 9.7% of their body fat, while those on a low-fat diet lost just 2.1%. The ketogenic dieters also lost three times more visceral adipose tissue than the low-fat dieters.[17] Individuals on a ketogenic or low carbohydrate regimen should supplement their diet with B vitamins.[18]

Berberine: One study reported that individuals who took 750 mg of barberry (which contains high concentrations of berberine) twice a day for three months had a significant decrease in weight.[19]

GABA: In a Korean study, participants received either GABA or a placebo and abstained from exercise for eight weeks. GABA (gamma aminobutyric acid) supplements caused a reduction in body fat and triglyceride levels while increasing lean muscle mass. Dosing levels are not well documented but supplements are available (e.g., 500–750 mg once or twice/day).[20]

Psyllium (psyllium seed, Metamucil) is the seed of the plantain plant that is rich in a spongy fiber called mucilage. When psyllium comes in contact with water, its mucilage absorbs the fluid and expands substantially. In the stomach, psyllium expansion can produce feelings of fullness.[21]

Hot spicy herbs such as red pepper and mustard (one teaspoon with each meal) give foods a spicy heat and increase the basal metabolic rate so that calories burn faster. Hot herbs also stimulate thirst, so more liquids are consumed instead of food.[21]

Medium-Chain Triglycerides (MCTs): It is well established that consumption of medium-chain triglycerides (e.g., MCT oil) can act as an appetite suppressant increasing the sensation of feeling full and reducing food intake.[22] Compared with long-chain triglycrides, medium-chain triglycerides decreased body weight, waist circumference, and total body fat without adversely affecting lipid profiles.[23] A starting dose is typically 20–30 gm/day in three divided doses with a maximum daily dose of 50–100 gm/day.[24]

Vitamin D deficiency is common in obesity. Supplementation is indicated to support overall health, but its role in treating obesity is unclear.

Sweeteners: Some people are unable to lose weight while consuming non-nutritive sweeteners (e.g., aspartame, saccharin, sucralose, and erythritol) and should avoid them.[25]

Paget's Disease/Osteitis Deformans

Paget's, or osteitis deformans, is a bone disease that causes one or more bones to become larger, misshaped, weaker, and more brittle. It is a disorder of bone remodeling where local areas of bone break down (resorb) followed by replacement with fibrous tissue.[1] Bone matrix that is more dense, but spongy, forms in those areas and eventually becomes somewhat harder (sclerotic). Nonetheless, these affected areas of bone are now softer and weaker than normal bone, which can lead to bone pain, deformities, and fractures. Paget's disease of bone can also cause the body to produce too many blood vessels in the affected bones, increasing the risk of serious blood loss during an operation.[2]

Paget's affects individuals older than 40 and is the second most common bone disease after osteoporosis. There may be no symptoms, or the symptoms may be very mild. Many people with Paget's disease do not know they have it. Typically, Paget's affects the pelvis, femur, skull, spine, or tibia. Pain often exists in the local area of bone involvement. Bone pain usually increases with rest, on weight bearing, when the limbs are warmed, and at night.[3] If it involves the skull, the head increases in size and there is pressure on cranial nerves. The spine can be curved, and thighs and lower legs can bow abnormally. Any bone changes that take place are irreversible.

The risk of acquiring Paget's disease increases with age. Complications can include fractures (especially of long bones), osteoarthritis, bone deformities, hearing loss, hypercalcemia, heart failure, and rarely malignant degeneration leading to bone cancer (osteosarcoma).[4]

CLINICAL CHOICES

Bisphosphonate: The current mainstay of medical treatment is with a potent bisphosphonate (pamidronate, alendronate, risedronate, or zoledronic acid) as indicated in patients with Paget's disease who have symptoms likely to respond to reduced bone turnover.

Calcium and Vitamin D: As a result of bisphosphates, because these medications have potent anti-osteoclast actions, calcium and vitamin D repletion are mandatory to avoid hypocalcemia.[5]

Vitamin D is a vital component that is also needed to optimize absorption of calcium in the intestinal tract. This calcium is then used to help strengthen the remodeled bones.[6] Women who are 50 and older and men who are 70 and older should get 1,200–1,500 mg of calcium and at least 600 IU (International Units) of vitamin D every day to maintain a healthy skeleton. Individuals who are 70 and older should increase their vitamin D intake from 400 IU to 800 IU/day.[7,8]

Exercise is important because it helps preserve skeletal health, prevent weight gain, and maintain joint mobility. Patients should discuss any new exercise program with their doctor before beginning, to avoid any undue stress on affected bones.[7]

Ipriflavone (IP) is a supplement and a derivative from the soy plant. It is used for preventing and treating weak bones and bone pain in Paget's disease.[9,10]

In one study, 16 patients (nine males and seven females) with active Paget's disease were randomly allocated to two different crossed-over dose regimens of treatment with IP (600 mg/day vs. 1,200 mg/day). Each treatment course lasted 30 days. At the end of the 1,200/600 mg/day treatment sequence, biochemical parameters for disease activity were reduced and a significant decrease in bone pain was observed. Results indicate that short-term treatment with IP can reduce biochemical parameters of disease activity and bone pain in patients with active Paget's disease.[11]

Ascorbic Acid: Sixteen patients with painful Paget's disease were treated with high doses of ascorbic acid. Of these patients, eight experienced lessening of pain within a period of five to seven days after commencing the ascorbic acid therapy. In three of these patients, pain ceased completely.[12]

Pain—Acute

Acute pain is experienced by people of all ages due to a variety of different conditions. This type of pain is a highly unpleasant experience and is classified as actual or potential tissue damage (nociceptive), or damage to the nervous system (neuropathic).

Common causes of acute pain include injuries, infections, burns, tooth pain, kidney stones, cramps, giving birth, etc. Most cases of acute back pain will resolve relatively quickly and do not have a serious underlying pathology.[1]

PALLIATIVE TREATMENTS

Topical NSAIDs, or nonsteroidal anti-inflammatory drugs (e.g., Salonpas Pain Relief Patch LARGE), with or without menthol gel, should be the first-line treatment for acute pain from musculoskeletal injuries, according to a new guideline from the American College of Physicians and the American Academy of Family Physicians.[2]

Over-the-Counter Products: Oral NSAIDs such as ibuprofen (Advil, Nuprin, Motrin IB, and others), naproxen sodium (Aleve, Naprosyn), or aspirin taken as directed can offer some relief.[3] NSAIDs relieve fever and pain and also reduce swelling from arthritis or a muscle sprain or strain. Acetaminophen (Tylenol) is no longer recommended for acute or subacute back pain.[4]

Molybdenum: Fourteen volunteers received 500 mcg/day of the trace mineral molybdenum during two separate four-week periods. Molybdenum was significantly more effective than the placebo in relieving aches and pains and improving general health.[3]

Diclofenac and B Vitamins: The prescription drug diclofenac, used to treat low-back pain, works better when vitamins B1, B6, and B12 are also taken twice a day.[5]

Methylcobalamin (MeCbl) is an activated form of vitamin B12. It exerts its neuronal protection by promoting regeneration of injured nerves and antagonizing glutamate-induced neurotoxicity.[6] Methylcobalamin has demonstrated significant positive effects on both neck and back pain.[7,8]

Magnesium: Although magnesium is not a primary analgesic in itself, it enhances the analgesic actions of more established analgesics as an adjuvant agent.[9] Magnesium 3.7–5.5 grams, in addition to pain medication, has been utilized within 24 hours after surgery to decrease pain levels.[10] Another study reported that magnesium sulfate reduced propofol, atracurium, and postoperative morphine consumption in gynecologic surgical patients.[11]

A specific magnesium lozenge (Magnesium-Diasporal) containing 610 mg of magnesium citrate salt, taken 30 minutes before surgery, has also been used with some success.[10]

Vitamin C appears to help sustain the long-term effectiveness of anti-pain therapies that patients may be using.[12]

Alternatives: Omega-3 fatty acids, vitamin E, and pycnogenol are natural alternatives to analgesics.[13]

Back or Neck Pain: The majority of patients with back pain do not need surgical treatment. Those who are symptomatic can usually be successfully treated with electrotherapy and back muscle strengthening exercises, cutaneous stimulation, behavioral modification, and spinal manipulative therapy.[14]

In their 2007 guidelines, the American College of Physicians and the American Pain Society included spinal manipulation as a treatment option for practitioners to consider when low-back pain does not improve with self-care. More recently, a 2010 Agency for Healthcare Research and Quality (AHRQ) report noted that spinal manipulation offers additional options to conventional drug treatments, which often have limited benefit in managing back and neck pain.[15]

Spinal manipulation and osteopathic manipulation have been used for over 100 years to provide relief from neck and back pain. In a blinded review study and a randomized controlled trial, spinal manipulation was the most effective treatment for neck pain vs. physiotherapy (PT) or standard medical care from a general practitioner.[16,17]

Spinal manipulation is one of only three treatments whose effectiveness for low-back pain is substantiated by rigorous research.[18] Manipulation is both safe and effective for patients.[18] A large multi-site pragmatic comparative effectiveness study found that adding chiropractic care to usual medical care resulted in better participant outcomes.[19]

Disk Herniation/Sciatica: There is little evidence to suggest that drug treatments are effective in treating herniated discs.[20] A small number of patients with sciatica may require surgical intervention in instances where nonsurgical therapies have failed to provide adequate pain relief, and if there is pathology present that is compressing the nerves.[21]

Spinal manipulation was found to be effective at relieving local or radiating pain in people with acute back pain and sciatica with disc protrusion.[20] In a recent study, researchers concluded that spinal manipulation was just as effective as microdiscectomy for patients struggling with sciatica secondary to lumbar disk herniation.[22]

Nonsurgical Disk Decompression: Thirty patients with discogenic low-back pain or disk herniation underwent decompression therapy for six weeks in a cohort study that compared disk heights using computerized tomography. Decompression therapy significantly increased disk height and decreased pain.[23] Nonsurgical spinal decompression represents a technological advance in lumbar disk treatment.[24]

Cancer: To lessen pain caused by nerve damage associated with cancer, single doses of 0.5–1 gm of magnesium sulfate have been given as 1 mL or 2 mL of a 50% magnesium sulfate injection over 5–10 minutes.[10]

Wisdom Teeth: Taking bromelain by mouth during the perioperative period for surgical removal of wisdom teeth reduced complications after third molar extraction, including pain, swelling, and limited mouth opening.[25,26,27] Patients were given oral bromelain enteric-coated capsules (30,000 units) on the day of the surgery, three times/day and continued for three days. Clove oil contains eugenol which acts as an anesthetic and antibacterial agent. Applied by cotton swab or cotton ball over the gums, clove oil may be as effective as benzocaine, the numbing ingredient in over-the-counter toothache gels.[28]

Other Conditions: For migraines, sciatica, neuropathies, neuralgias, etc., see those individual sections.

Pain—Chronic

***See also* Pain—Acute, Peripheral Neuralgia, and other specific conditions**

Ongoing or recurrent pain that lasts longer than three to six months is referred to as chronic pain. It is reported that over 30% of patients experience pain lasting longer than six months.[1] Common problems associated with chronic pain are spine problems, migraines and other headaches, arthritis, nerve damage (e.g., neuropathy), MS, infections, fibromyalgia, etc.

Chronic back pain is the leading cause of disability in the U.S. Treatment for back pain represents the most expensive medical problem in the country.[1] As many as 48% of patients with acute low-back pain may transition to chronic low-back pain. Patients with leg pain, obesity, or who are smokers are more likely to transition to chronic back pain.[2] Despite numerous treatment options and greatly increased medical care resources devoted to this problem, the functional status of persons with back pain in the U.S. has deteriorated.[3]

PALLIATIVE CARE

Nonpharmacologic Treatments: For treatment of chronic low-back pain, nonpharmacologic treatments (e.g., spinal manipulation, exercise, multidisciplinary rehabilitation, acupuncture, mindfulness-based stress reduction, tai chi, yoga, motor control exercise, progressive relaxation, electromyography biofeedback, low-level laser therapy, operant therapy, or cognitive behavioral therapy) should be employed before pharmacologic treatments.[4]

OTC Remedies: In addition to standard medical care such as opioids, tramadol (Ultram), trigger point injections, nerve blocks, etc., many patients use over-the-counter pain pills such as acetaminophen, naproxen, ibuprofen, or aspirin, in an attempt to gain additional amounts of relief.

Additional Measures: Lidocaine patches and analgesic gels, creams, and lotions are available.

Vitamin K: Researchers in Sarajevo reported on the effects of vitamin K injection on pain. They determined that vitamin K was more effective than morphine in its "thermoanalgesic" properties (relief of pain from burns) in animal testing.

Researchers also gave vitamin K injections to 115 individuals with chronic pain (due to terminal cancer) thought to be controllable only with morphine. 95 of the 115 were able to eliminate morphine and rely on the vitamin K injections alone for pain relief.[5]

Palmitoylethanolamide (PEA) (e.g., 300–1,200 mg/day), an endogenous fatty acid amide available as supplement, has become more mainstream as adjunctive medical care in the treatment of chronic pain and as a stand-alone therapy. A researcher on PEA recommends selecting a formulation containing micro-PEA, such as one containing micronized (PEA-m), ultra-micronized (PEA-um), or optimized PEA (PEA-opt).[6]

Magnesium: In one study, a two-week intravenous magnesium sulphate infusion (1g in 250 ml saline 0.9%) followed by four weeks of oral magnesium supplementation (magnesium oxide 400 mg plus magnesium gluconate 100 mg bid) reduced pain intensity and improved lumbar spine mobility during a six-month period in patients with refractory chronic low-back pain with a neuropathic component.[7]

Pancreatic Exocrine Insufficiency (PEI)

Pancreatic exocrine insufficiency is an important cause of maldigestion. Exocrine pancreatic insufficiency is caused by a generalized reduction in pancreatic exocrine (digestive) enzyme production and delivery, leading to severe impairment in fat and fat-soluble vitamin absorption.[1] Acute and chronic pancreatitis can cause such an insufficiency as can celiac and Crohn's disease, cystic fibrosis, Shwachman-Diamond syndrome, and previous pancreatic surgery. Patients with EPI manifest lethargy, weakness, abdominal pain, bloating, diarrhea, and steatorrhea. PEI is one of the major complications in chronic pancreatitis and should be considered in all chronic pancreatitis patients.

PRESCRIPTION CARE

Pancreatic Digestive Enzymes: Chymotrypsin, trypsin, and pancreatin/pancrelipase (with mixtures of amylase, lipase, and protease), either individually or in combination are key components of most pancreatic supplements.[2] Taking these enzymes with meals leads to a better quality of life even though, in most patients, steatorrhea, or fatty stool, is not completely abolished.[1] Since steatorrhea does not typically occur until >90% of pancreatic lipase activity is lost, 10% enzyme activity is the initial goal for therapy. One caveat: pancreatic enzymes may cause folic acid deficiency.[1]

NUTRITIONAL SUPPORT

Bromelain can be used as a supplement in cases of pepsin and/or trypsin deficiencies and has been used in combination with pancreatic enzymes to facilitate digestion in cases of exocrine pancreatic insufficiency. Bromealin, has been used in doses ranging from 200–2,000 mg/day in four divided doses.[3]

Deficiencies: Consequences of exocrine pancreatic insufficiency include deficiencies of fat-soluble vitamins which should be replaced:[4]

Deficiency	Outcome
Vitamin A	Night blindness
Vitamin D	Osteomalacia, hypocalcemia
Vitamin E	Neuropathy, hemolytic anemia
Vitamin K	Coagulopathy
Fat malabsorption	Weight loss
Hypoproteinemia	Edema
Carbohydrate malabsorption	Bloating, diarrhea

Lifestyle: Smoking and alcohol cessation are strongly recommended.[5]

EPI-Friendly Diet: Small frequent meals are usually better tolerated than large, high-caloric meals.[5] Avoid high-fiber meals and limit fat.[6]

Pancreatitis—Acute

Acute pancreatitis (AP) is inflammation of the pancreas that may lead to organ failure and death in severe cases. Gallstone disease and alcohol are the two leading causes of acute pancreatitis. Other causes include hypertriglyceridemia (typically >1,000 mg/dL), hypercalcemia, familial (hereditary) pancreatitis, and viral infections.[1] Different medications can also precipitate an attack of acute pancreatitis. Damage to the pancreas is the result of digestive enzymes being trapped within the pancreas and then digesting the gland itself.

Severe upper abdominal pain is the most common presenting symptom. Pain often radiates to the back, accompanied by symptoms of nausea, vomiting, and fever. The pain may be made worse by eating, drinking, or lying supine.[1] Acute pancreatitis can cause both hypocalcemia and hypomagnesemia.[2] A serious complication of acute pancreatitis is necrotizing pancreatitis where parts of the pancreas die and the dead tissue can get infected. Necrotizing pancreatitis is life-threatening. Most cases of acute pancreatitis will improve within three to seven days, but those with severe pancreatitis may have a progressively downhill course to respiratory failure, sepsis, and death (less than 10%).[3]

Treatment of pancreatitis is primarily supportive and consists of prevention of complications.[1] Pancreatic exocrine insufficiency will develop in up to 35% of all patients.[1]

THERAPY STRATEGIES

Treatment of acute pancreatitis requires early and adequate fluid resuscitation, oral feeding as tolerated, adequate pain management, and acid blocking agents.[4]

Nutritional support is necessary to counter the catabolic state that pancreatitis creates and to decrease the rate of infectious complications. Feeding by mouth was discouraged because it was thought that the inflamed pancreas would be stimulated to secrete, thereby exacerbating the disease. However, this concern has not been validated and evidence overwhelmingly supports oral nutrition with a low-fat soft or solid diet when bowel sounds have returned and pain has resolved.[1]

Calcium Caveat: Hypocalcemia correction should be done with extreme caution in patients with acute pancreatitis because calcium plays a central role in the pathogenesis of acinar injury and cell death.[5] There is no evidence to support calcium correction by parenteral calcium infusion in patients with mild to moderate hypocalcemia.[5]

Magnesium: In animal studies, magnesium administration reduced pancreatic enzyme activities, edema, tissue necrosis, and inflammation. Magnesium supplementation also significantly reduced premature protease activation and the severity of pancreatitis.[6]

Patients with acute pancreatitis and hypocalcemia commonly have magnesium deficiency despite normal serum magnesium concentrations. Magnesium deficiency may also play a significant role in the pathogenesis of hypocalcemia in patients with acute pancreatitis.[7] Magnesium supplementation should be considered in pancreatitis with hypocalcemia.

Magnesium sulphate (4,930 mg magnesium sulphate [= 20 mmol] 60 min before and six hours after ERCP) was found to be effective in preventing post-ERCP pancreatitis.

Beyond its preventive usage, magnesium may be considered a novel analgesic alternative to treat pain in acute pancreatitis.[4,8] Although magnesium is not a primary analgesic in itself, it enhances the analgesic actions of more established analgesics as an adjuvant agent.[9]

CoQ10: Administration of Coenzyme Q10 demonstrated protective effects, reducing the severity of AP and its associated pulmonary complications in animal studies.[10]

Pancreatitis—Chronic

Chronic pancreatitis is characterized by permanent and progressive structural or functional damage of the pancreas with scarring (fibrosis). This results in exocrine and endocrine insufficiency and, often, chronic disabling pain. The symptoms are identical to acute pancreatitis. Most patients with chronic pancreatitis are alcoholics. Symptoms of chronic pancreatitis can include abdominal pain, malabsorption, bleeding due to anemia, liver problems leading to jaundice, weight loss, nutritional deficiencies, and an inability to produce insulin, resulting in diabetes.[1]

METHODS OF CARE

Alcohol abstinence is of urgent necessity.[1]

Stopping tobacco use is also vital because smoking, while not a cause of pancreatitis, can accelerate the progression of the disease.[1]

Additional therapy for chronic pancreatitis includes pain management, nutrition, acid blockers, and diabetes control.[2]

Diet: Patients with chronic pancreatitis are advised to consume six to eight small low-fat meals each day.[1] A pancreas-friendly diet is high in protein from lean meats and low in animal fats and simple sugars. Add 1–2 tablespoons of medium-chain triglycerides to your daily diet. This can be continued even if one has moderately severe or severe chronic pancreatitis. Patients with mild pancreatitis can benefit from diet and lifestyle changes alone.[3]

Supplementation of vitamins A, D, E, K, B12, zinc, and folic acid is mandatory because their absorption is impaired.[3,4]

Magnesium deficiency is a common clinical condition in chronic pancreatitis that may exist despite a normal serum magnesium concentration. Appropriate supplementation could lead to symptomatic improvement in patients with severe chronic pancreatitis.[5]

Pancreatic enzyme supplementation is warranted.[6] Enteric-coated pancreatic enzymes are utilized for replacement of pancreatic function. Because of its higher enzyme content, pancrelipase formulations are favored over pancreatin preparations.[7]

Parkinson's Disease

Parkinson's disease (PD) is the most common movement disorder and the second most common neurodegenerative disorder after Alzheimer's. Parkinson's is a progressive disease that affects movement and results in three cardinal features: slowness of voluntary movement, rigidity, and a unilateral resting tremor in the hand. Later in the course of the disease, patients typically develop a stooped posture, an inability to maintain equilibrium resulting in a shuffling gait, imbalance, and falls, and the loss of automatic movements such as swinging arms during ambulation, facial expressions with decreased blinking, and difficulty swallowing. There are often negative changes in speech and writing as well.

Parkinson's is associated with the loss of dopamine-producing neurons in the substantia nigra and the presence of Lewy bodies. A common primary complaint is an overwhelming fatigue that makes it feel nearly impossible to move. Falls are a frequent complication and major detriment with almost half of individuals with PD experiencing a fall in any 90-day period.[1] Dementia occurs in 50%–80% of PD patients and affects problem-solving, the speed at which thoughts occur, memory, and mood, alongside other important cognitive functions.[2]

The exact cause of Parkinson's disease is not known. Genetics, aging, repeated head injuries, and exposure to pesticides or heavy metals are thought to increase the risk of this disorder. A Finnish study found that exposure to certain antibiotics was associated with an elevated risk of Parkinson's disease after a lag period.[3,4] Oral macrolides and lincosamides had the strongest association. Antifungal medications, sulfonamides, and trimethoprim had a 1–5 year lag period while tetracyclines and antianaerobics had a 10–15 year lag.[3,4]

Diagnosis is primarily based on the history and physical examination. For those afflicted with PD the quality of life is often poor. Parkinson's leads to disability for most patients within ten years.[5] Currently, no pharmacologic therapies prevent PD or stop its progression.

RESEARCH ANALYSIS

Diet: The sufferer should follow a diet that is high in fiber and calcium, with adequate fluid intake, to limit complications caused by constipation and osteoporosis.[6] Milk and dairy consumption should be minimized.[7]

L-dopa (Levodopa) is a direct precursor to dopamine, an amino acid, and is the cornerstone of medical treatment for motor symptoms such as tremor. However, higher oral doses can come with a number of troublesome side effects, the worst of which are hypotension and a variety of abnormal involuntary movements. The real problem is that L-dopa can stop being effective after only a few years.

Ascorbic Acid and Vitamin E: Seventy-five patients with early Parkinson's disease received supplements of vitamin C and vitamin E, 3,000 mg/day and 3,200 IU/day respectively. The time until L-dopa therapy became necessary was prolonged by an average of 2.5 years. This study suggests that vitamins C and E can slow the progression of Parkinson's disease, possibly by preventing oxidation damage to the substantia nigra.[8] In addition, a Swedish study found higher dietary vitamin E and C intake to be associated with lower risk of PD.[9]

Folic Acid: Previous research in patients with Parkinson's disease has shown that they often have low levels of folic acid in their blood. The latest research shows that animals on a low-folic-acid diet are much more likely to get Parkinson's disease than those on a normal diet.[10]

Researchers were able to finger homocysteine as the likely culprit behind the loss of brain cells in Parkinson's. When homocysteine was injected directly into the brains, the Parkinson's symptoms were much worse than in animals injected with a placebo. Folic acid decreases homocysteine levels.[10] More research is needed to see the effects of folic acid in the treatment of Parkinson's.

L-Methionine: Previous studies indicate that taking L-methionine by mouth for two weeks up to six months improves symptoms of Parkinson's disease, such as tremor, inability to control movements, and rigidity.[11] Eleven patients with previously untreated Parkinson's disease were treated with L-methionine for periods from two weeks to six months. The treatment was well-supported and good improvement in clinical signs, particularly akinesia and rigidity, appeared within approximately three weeks, the effect on tremor being less marked.[12,13]

N-Acetylcysteine (NAC): Combining clinical evaluations of a patient's mental and physical abilities with brain imaging studies that tracked the levels of dopamine showed that patients receiving NAC improved on both measures. Patients received NAC 50 mg/kg intravenously once per week and 600 mg orally twice per day on the non-IV days.[14,15]

Gamma-Amino Butyric Acid (GABA): Generally, patients with early PD have non-motor symptoms such as a decreased sense of smell, depression, and various gastrointestinal and other systemic features which have been shown to predate the classical motor features of PD[16,17] and which are undoubtedly related to a deficiency of GABA.[16] Additional research in this area is required.

L-Dopa and 5-HT: The Parkinson's disease process is known to be associated with depletion of serotonin, tyrosine hydroxylase, norepinephrine, and dopamine. L-dopa is known to deplete serotonin, serotonin precursors, tyrosine, and the sulfur amino acids. When 5-HTP and L-dopa were administered in proper balance along with L-tyrosine, L-cysteine, and cofactors, the long list of problems that can interfere with optimum administration of L-dopa became controllable and manageable or did not occur at all.[18]

In a case study, one patient within four months of initiating treatment with 5-HTP and L-dopa administered in a proper balance experienced dramatic improvement in the tremor in both the upper and lower extremities. He regained coordination in his left hand and was once again able to use the computer keyboard. He resumed his hobby of guitar playing and was able to perform proficiently. His gait and balance were restored. The depression improved significantly. Anxiety was significantly relieved. The patient had lost his fear of going out in public.[19]

In this case the doses were started at 240 mg/day L-dopa, 300 mg/day 5-HTP, 3 gm/day L-tyrosine with L-dopa doses increased to 360 mg/day after seven days. In addition, the following cofactors were administered daily: (1) vitamin C 1,000 mg; (2) calcium citrate 220 mg; (3) vitamin B6 75 mg; (4) folate 400 mcg; (5) L-lysine 500 mg; (6) L-cysteine 4,500 mg; (7) selenium 400 mcg.[19] The doses were modified for a period of two years.

Lifestyle: Walking, gardening, swimming, calisthenics, and other general physical activity improve emotional well-being.[20]

Caffeine: Caffeine intake and physical activity can slow the progression of the disease, thus representing viable options for primary prevention and disease modifying strategies in PD.[7]

Protective Factors: According to review studies, the following appear to confer a protective factor against developing Parkinson's disease: coffee and tea intake, vitamin E, vitamin B6 supplementation, gout, smoking, ibuprofen, and β2-adrenoreceptor agonists.[7,21]

Black tea, caffeine, coffee, green tea, and vitamin E are all recognized as possibly being effective for tremors in Parkinson's disease.[22]

Citicoline: In a study involving Parkinson's disease patients already taking L-dopa, it was found that injection with 500 mg citicoline daily led to improvement in symptoms, especially slow movements and rigidity. The results may be due to the impact of CDP-choline on dopamine levels.[23]

Vitamin E: Long-term, high-dose vitamin E dietary supplementation or parenteral vitamin E succinate administration has been proposed as a beneficial therapeutic strategy for the prevention or treatment of PD.[24]

Pellagra

The lack of vitamin B3, or niacin, in the body causes a disease known as pellagra. The term *pellagra* means "rough skin." Like all B vitamins, niacin plays a role in converting carbohydrates into glucose, metabolizing fats and proteins, and keeping the nervous system working properly.[1] Pellagra is a chronic wasting disease rarely found in developed countries. It can occur when the intake of both niacin and tryptophan are low. Pellagra is known as the four D disease: diarrhea, dermatitis, dementia, and eventually, if untreated, death.

REPLENISHING NIACIN STORES

Oral nicotinic acid in doses of 50 mg by mouth three times a day has been noted to improve symptoms in two to three days.[2,3] As little as 20 mg/day of niacin can prevent pellagra.[1]

Niacinamide 200 mg/day avoids the gastrointestinal and vasodilator effects of niacin.[4]

Thiamine, riboflavin, and pyridoxine should be administered at the same time as vitamin B3.[4]

Diet and B Vitamins: Because patients are often malnourished and have other vitamin deficiencies, provisions for a high-protein diet (1 gm/kg/day) and the administration of B-complex vitamins are needed for complete recovery.[4,5]

Pemphigus Vulgaris

Pemphigus is a group of rare autoimmune disorders that causes thin walled, flaccid, easily-ruptured blisters and sores on the top layer of skin and mucous membranes, such as in the mouth, throat, nose, and genitals. It is an autoimmune disorder and is not contagious. The disease occurs almost exclusively in middle-aged or older people and tends to be a long-lasting chronic condition. The type of pemphigus diagnosed depends on where the blisters form. Pemphigus vulgaris with blisters on the skin and in the mouth is the most common type of pemphigus. Wherever the blisters form, they tend to break open quickly, leaving painful sores. The disorder can sometimes be cause by certain medications such as ACE inhibitors, penicillamine, cephalosporin, pyrazolones, NSAIDs, and rifampin.[1] The goals of treatment are to promote and maintain remission, as well as to avoid complications, such as infections.[1]

CARE OPTIONS

Use a soft toothbrush and avoid spicy, crispy, or acidic foods if there are blisters in the mouth.[2]

Use anesthetic mouthwashes to relieve mouth pain, particularly before eating or brushing the teeth.[2]

DHEA level was markedly lower in pemphigoid/pemphigus. DHEA supplementation may help.[3]

Tocopherol: Good results treating skin lesions were reported using oral vitamin E (300–1,600 IU/day).[4]

Periodic Paralysis—Hyperkalemic/Hypokalemic

Primary periodic paralysis (PPP) is a group of rare inherited diseases characterized by interference with the electrochemical communications between nerve cells and skeletal muscles. In this case, muscles become unable to properly respond to nerve signals, resulting in temporary weakness, pain, or stiffness. These episodes can occur periodically or daily and can last from a few minutes to a few days, depending on the type of PPP.[1] The two major recognized forms are (A) hyperkalemic, or high-potassium form, and (B) hypokalemic, or low-potassium form. Attacks usually begin in later childhood before the age of 20, but can start later. There is no cure for patients with PPP.

(A) HYPERKALEMIC PERIODIC PARALYSIS

Hyperkalemic periodic paralysis is a condition that causes episodes of extreme muscle weakness or paralysis, usually beginning in infancy or early childhood. Attacks are usually brief, lasting a few minutes to an hour or two, but tend to occur frequently. Most often, these episodes involve a temporary inability to move muscles in the arms and legs. Some people with hyperkalemic periodic paralysis have elevated serum levels of potassium (hyperkalemia) during attacks. Hyperkalemia results when the weak or paralyzed muscles release potassium ions into the bloodstream. In most patients, potassium levels do not actually rise above normal. "Hyperkalemic" refers more to the fact that attacks may be triggered by eating potassium-rich foods or by giving the patient potassium.

The goal of treatment is to relieve symptoms and prevent further attacks.[2] The goals of pharmacotherapy are to reduce serum potassium levels and morbidity and to prevent complications.

Diet: For those with hyperkalemic periodic paralysis, ingestion of potassium-rich foods, rest after exercise, or emotional stress may provoke an attack, whereas eating carbohydrates (which results in a shift of extracellular K+ into muscle) may abort an attack.[3] While most attacks of hyperkalemic periodic paralysis are brief and do not require emergency intervention, occasionally the serum potassium level will be high enough to cause cardiac distress, or muscle stiffness may interfere with respiration.[4]

Calcium chloride contains about three times more elemental calcium than an equal volume of calcium gluconate: 1 gm of calcium chloride has 270 mg (13.5 mEq) of elemental calcium, whereas 1 gm of calcium gluconate has 90 mg (4.5 mEq). Calcium has no effect on the serum level of potassium but protects the myocardium from the deleterious effects of hyperkalemia.[5] Therefore, when hyperkalemia is accompanied by hemodynamic compromise, calcium chloride is preferred to calcium gluconate.[6]

Calcium gluconate is a primary treatment option. Calcium alleviates symptoms in hyperkalemic periodic paralysis, most likely by reducing the abnormal sodium influx.[4] It is used in part for rapid response to treatment because calcium gluconate does not require hepatic metabolization before it is active. A tablespoonful of calcium gluconate syrup stirred into a glass of Coca-Cola or other sweet beverage can stop a mild episode in the early stages and help protect the heart cells.[6] Calcium guconate syrup is a mineral supplement available over the counter and is found in most pharmacies.[6]

A cold environment and emotional stress can provoke or worsen attacks.[7]

Calcium and magnesium supplements are also recommended to prevent attacks.[8]

Sugar: Attacks can often be stopped by drinking a can of soda or other sweet drink.[9]
(B) Hypokalemic periodic paralysis

Hypokalemic periodic paralysis is the most common form of periodic paralysis. It affects males more often than females. Attacks can be periodic or occur daily and can last from hours to days. The low level of potassium in the blood during episodes of weakness results from potassium moving from the blood into muscle cells in an abnormal way.

Diet: Eating a low-carbohydrate diet may help decrease the frequency of attacks.[10]

Potassium: For those with hypokalemic periodic paralysis, the risk of attack and episodes of weakness may be prevented or shortened by ingesting potassium chloride (KCl) supplements.[3,8] A dose of 0.5–1.0 mEq/kg in aqueous form can be taken 15–30 minutes prior to exercise or before bed to prevent attacks. The same dose can also be ingested at the beginning of an attack.[11]

Exercise: Some attacks may be aborted with mild exercise.[3,8]

Periodontal Disease

Periodontal disease, or gum disease, is characterized by unhealthy gums and teeth and often reflects serious health risks. In its early stage, it is known as gingivitis. Periodontitis is a chronic infection caused predominantly by gram-negative bacteria, especially *A. actinomycetemcomitans* and *P. gingivalis* and often leads to tooth loss. Symptoms include red, swollen, and tender gums, bleeding or receding gums, loose or shifting teeth, and persistent bad breath.

MANAGEMENT APPROACHES

Good Oral Hygiene: Regular brushing and flossing on a daily basis is important to maximize oral health.

Vitamin C has long been a candidate for modulating periodontal diseases, although the exact role of vitamin C deficiency in periodontitis is not known. Periodontitis is associated with a low concentration of vitamin C in plasma. Therefore, periodontitis may well be associated with subacute vitamin C deficiency.[1,2]

Also, the negative association between plasma vitamin C levels and periodontal attachment loss suggests that vitamin C deficiency may contribute to the severity of periodontal breakdown.[3]

Avoiding tobacco is critical in helping to avoid periodontitis. Smoking makes it harder for gum tissue to repair itself.

Peripheral Neuropathy

Peripheral neuropathy refers to compressed, damaged, or diseased nerves outside the brain and spinal cord that are malfunctioning. Often, it results in numbness, tingling, burning, or stinging pain, especially in the hands or feet. Peripheral neuropathy is tied to significant morbidity and decreases in quality of life.

Although there are multiple causes of neuropathy, diabetes and alcohol are the two most common causes. Up to one-half of people with diabetes have peripheral neuropathy. Disorders of peripheral nerves are also the most common neurological complications of systemic amyloidosis. Nutritional disorders such as thiamine deficiency, also known as "dry" beriberi, may cause peripheral neuropathy. Vitamin B12 (cyanocobalamin) deficiency causes neurologic disease, most commonly a combination of spinal cord disease and peripheral nerve disease (myeloneuropathy). Vitamin B6 (pyridoxine) deficiency from severe malabsorption or as a consequence of therapy with isoniazid, cycloserine, hydralazine, or penicillamine can cause peripheral neuropathy.[1] Vasculitic neuropathy can also damage nerves. Other factors may further contribute to nerve damage such as injury, high blood pressure, high cholesterol, some drugs, metabolic problems, and smoking.[2] Despite the different etiologies leading to neuropathic pain, increased neuronal excitability is thought to be the underlying mechanism for all forms of painful neuropathies.

Neuropathic pain is challenging to manage because many patients experience pain that is refractory to existing treatments. The goals of treatment are to slow progression of the disease, relieve pain, manage complications, and restore function.[3] Although pharmacologic therapy can slow the progression of neuropathy, chronic residual symptoms typically persist for most patients.[4]

RESEARCH RESULTS

Oral analgesics (e.g., acetaminophen or NSAIDs and adjuvant analgesics) are the most commonly used treatment for neuropathic pain.[5]

Alpha-Lipoic Acid: Treatment with alpha-lipoic acid increases reduced glutathione, an important endogenous antioxidant. In clinical trials, alpha-lipoic acid (e.g., 600 mg) taken daily for five weeks improved neuropathic symptoms and deficits in patients with distal symmetric neuropathy.[6,7]

Vitamins B12 and Folate: Older adults with or without diabetes, particularly those who follow a vegetarian or vegan diet, have an increased risk of vitamin B12 deficiency. Because vitamin deficiencies, particularly of vitamin B12 and folate, can cause peripheral neuropathy, it is important to supplement both as a safety net to maximize treatment results.[8,9] Vitamin B12 deficiency causes a typical pattern of degeneration of the white matter in the central nervous system that can be manifested clinically as encephalopathy, myelopathy, peripheral neuropathy, and optic neuropathy.[10]

Multiple B Vitamins: Whether polyneuropathy results from thiamine deficiency or the lack of other vitamins (e.g., pyridoxine, pantothenic acid, or folate) is unclear. Treating this disorder with multiple B vitamins is appropriate when the etiology is obscure.[11]

Acetyl-l-carnitine (1–2 gm/day) may be effective in treating peripheral neuropathies.[12] In a study involving 294 patients with peripheral neuropathy, acetyl-l-carnitine 1,000 mg/day was injected IM followed by an oral dose of 2,000 mg/day for 355 days. The authors concluded that carnitine was effective and well-tolerated in improving neurophysiological parameters and in reducing pain over a one-year period. LAC is, therefore, a promising treatment option in patients with diabetic neuropathy.[13]

Vitamin E deficiency is often associated with symptoms of a peripheral neuropathy. The low tocopherol content of the nerves was present in three vitamin E-deficient patients, suggesting the nerve injury resulted from low nerve tocopherol content.[14] Thus, vitamin E deficiency may cause some of the symptoms of peripheral neuropathy and supplementation should be directed at any deficiencies.

Capsaicin cream depletes tissue of substance P and reduces chemically-induced pain. Several controlled studies combined in meta-analyses provide evidence of efficacy in diabetic neuropathic pain. It may be best to reserve topical capsaicin creams, lotions, ointments, gels, sticks, films, or ointments for patients with localized discomfort rather than those with widespread generalized neuropathic pain.[15]

Palmitoylethanolamide (PEA): Many patients suffering from neuropathic conditions have pain that is refractory to existing treatments. In this context, palmitoylethanolamide (PEA), an endogenous fatty acid amide, is emerging as a novel agent in the treatment of pain and inflammation.[16] Palmitoylethanolamide is available as a supplement (PeaPure and PeaPlex) and as a cream (PEA cream).

A number of patients not responding well to conventional therapy were started on PEA 600 mg sublingually twice daily for quick absorption and to avoid first-pass effects. After 10 days, they were switched to tablets of 600 mg PEA twice daily, and if pain was sufficiently reduced, the dose was thereafter reduced to 300 mg twice daily. In case studies of patients suffering with metastatic prostate cancer pain, failed low-back surgery, diabetic neuropathy, polyneuropathy, and a female with partial vulvectomy from vulvar intraepithelial neoplasia II all responded to the previous regimen. Most results were seen between weeks one and three of treatment, but some cases improved only after five weeks of treatment.[16]

Thiamine: Peripheral neurologic changes from thiamine (vitamin B1) deficiency, also known as dry beriberi, affect the lower legs symmetrically. The condition is characterized by burning of the feet, paresthesias of the toes, calf muscle cramps, and pains in the legs.[17] In mild polyneuropathies, treatment is 10–20 mg/day in divided doses. For moderate to advanced neuropathy, 20–30 mg/day is given.[18]

Vitamin B6: Peripheral neuropathy from pyridoxine deficiency is treated with supplementation 10–30 mg/day.[17,19] Pyridoxine hydrochloride is also given to patients at risk (e.g., alcoholics) or during long-term therapy with isoniazid to prevent peripheral neuropathy.[20]

Peyronie's Disease

This is a disorder in which the development of flat fibrous scar tissue, or plaque, inside the penis causes curved, painful erections. Peyronie's disease begins with inflammation, or swelling, which later becomes a hard scar. Specifically, scar tissue forms in the tunica albuginea, the thick sheath of tissue surrounding the corpora cavernosa, causing pain, abnormal curvature, erectile dysfunction, indentation, loss of girth, and shortening. Peyronie's disease is benign and not contagious or caused by any known transmittable disease. In approximately 10% of cases, there can be spontaneous remission.[1] The goal of treatment is to reduce pain and to restore and maintain the ability to have intercourse.

MEDICAL MANAGEMENT OPTIONS

Vitamin E: Studies as far back as 1948 show that taking vitamin E may make plaques smaller and help straighten the penis.[1,2] Tocopherol remains the most common nonsurgical therapy because of its safety, availability, and low cost.

Acetyl-L-carnitine is also used in the treatment of this disorder.[2]

Biagiotti and Cavallini performed a double-blind, randomized study in 2001 that compared acetyl-L-carnitine with tamoxifen, and demonstrated that acetyl-L-carnitine was more effective in reducing pain and disease progression.[3]

Cavallini et al. compared the efficacy of oral propionyl-L-carnitine or tamoxifen combined with intralesional verapamil injections. They demonstrated that the combination of propionyl-L-carnitine and verapamil improved sexual performance, halted the progression of the disease, and possibly prevented surgery in patients and, therefore, suggested it as the treatment of choice for advanced PD.[4]

Potassium para-aminobenzoate (PABA), aka potaba, is FDA-approved for use in this skin condition.[2,5] Zarafonetis and Horrax first reported on the use of potassium para-aminobenzoate (potaba) to treat PD. PABA not only significantly slowed the progression of the disease, but all 21 men in the study reported a reduction in pain, 82% noted an improvement in penile curvature, and 76% experienced a decrease in plaque size.[6]

Another trial enrolled 103 men with Peyronie's disease and followed them for one year. The results showed that use of PABA at a dose of 3 gm four times daily for three to six months significantly slowed the progression of Peyronie's disease.[7] Other studies also suggest the use of PABA for Peyronie's disease.[8,9]

PABA, or potaba, is currently a first-line therapy for PD because of its tolerability and availability.

Pick's Disease/Frontotemporal Dementia/Lobar Atrophy

Pick's is a rare disease, also known as frontotemporal dementia (FTD), where the anterior portions of the frontal and temporal lobes of the brain degenerate with loss of brain tissue. This causes progressive and irreversible dementia. There is a strong genetic component to FTD. Prominent changes in personality and behavior along with loss of language skills (e.g., difficulty communicating or understanding speech) are typically the first symptoms to appear. The disease invariably results in death usually within 2 to 10 years after the diagnosis is made.[1] Pick's disease affects more men than women and is typically diagnosed between the ages of 40 and 75. There is no known treatment to cure or stop the progression of the disease.

MANAGEMENT OPTIONS

Thiamine and multiple B complex supplementation may help to slow progressive neurodegeneration.[2]

Folic Acid: Diminished serum folate levels may mimic this disorder.[2] Supplementation would appear to be safe, cheap, and worthwhile to eliminate any complications from possible deficiency.

Pityriasis Lichenoides Chronica

Pityriasis lichenoides chronica (PLC) is a chronic infectious skin disease of unknown etiology. PLC causes the development of small, scaling, raised spots (papules) on the skin. They first appear pink and scaly, and gradually flatten and become brown in color over a period of weeks or months.[1] An individual with PLC tends to have multiple episodes of papules on the skin, meaning they experience the development of new papules after old papules have faded. The disease can last for months or a few years.

NUTRITIONAL TREATMENT METHOD

Bromelain: Oral bromelain 40 mg tid for one month, 40 mg bid for one month, and 40 mg/day for one additional month reportedly caused complete resolution of this condition.[2]

Pityriasis Versicolor/Tinea Versicolor

Pityriasis versicolor is a common fungal disorder presenting as hypopigmented scaly small flat spots (macules) on the trunk. It is a common condition in the tropics and may affect up to 40% of the population. Azole antifungals like itraconazole and ketoconazole, both in topical and systemic formulations, form the mainstay of medical treatment.[1]

TREATMENT PROTOCOLS

Selenium Sulfide 1%: Selsun Blue shampoo should be applied to the entire trunk, then allowed to dry and remain in place overnight before showering. Repeat application one week later.[2]

Zinc pyrithione 1% (Head & Shoulders, Selsun Blue Itchy Dry Scalp, Neutrogena T/Gel Daily Control, or Pyrithione Zinc Bar) is a proven treatment modality for pityriasis versicolor owing to its anti-inflammatory action and direct cytotoxic action on *Pityrosporum ovale.*[1]

Topical zinc sulphate has also been used for the management of pityriasis versicolor. A complete clinical and mycological cure after three weeks' treatment was observed with once daily application of 15% topical zinc sulphate.[1]

Pneumonia

Pneumonia is an acute inflammation of the lung parenchyma (alveoli, alveolar ducts, and bronchioles) that can cause mild to severe illness in people of all ages. Most often an infection inflames lung tissue and the small air sacs, or alveoli, inside the lungs which fill up with fluid and/or purulent material (pus) reducing oxygen intake. Pneumonia is a major public health problem in the elderly in general and especially in nursing home (NH) residents. It is also the leading infectious cause of death in children less than five years old.[1] Symptoms, which can vary from mild to serious, can include productive cough, fever, chills, chest pain, hemoptysis, and difficulty breathing. Complications include lung abscesses, ARDS, pleural effusions, empyema, and pleurisy. Overwhelming sepsis is potentially a lethal complication.

ADJUNCTIVE THERAPY

Over-the-counter medications can help manage the symptoms of pneumonia, such as reducing fever and reducing aches and pains. Cough suppressants should be avoided because suppression may interfere with airway clearance.[2]

It is crucial to rest and drink plenty of fluids. Staying hydrated helps to thin out thick phlegm and mucus, making it easier to cough up.[2]

Bromelain: Combined bromelain and antibiotic therapy was shown to be more effective than antibiotics alone in treating pneumonia.[1,3,4] It is thought that the best results occur at a dose of 750–1,000 mg/day.[5]

Zinc: A recent observational study in addition to other studies indicate that inadequate stores of zinc might be a risk factor for pneumonia in the elderly.[6,7,8] The researchers concluded that a dose of 30 mg of elemental zinc per day might be adequate to improve immune function and to reduce the risk of infections.[8] Typical daily doses range widely from 12–150 mg/day as free zinc or up to 220 mg as zinc sulfate.[9]

A WHO report states that several studies have indicated that zinc supplementation can reduce the frequency and severity of respiratory infections in children.[10] Treating young children with zinc (20 mg/day) in addition to standard antibiotics greatly reduces the duration of severe pneumonia, according to a study by researchers from the Johns Hopkins Bloomberg School of Public Health.[11] Zinc supplementation lowered the incidence pneumonia by 41%, according to an analysis of studies on children in developing countries.[12]

Vitamin C: Therapeutic vitamin C supplementation may be reasonable for pneumonia patients who have low vitamin C plasma levels because its cost and risks are low.[13] The use of proton pump inhibitors is associated with increased risk of vitamin C deficiency.[14]

Vitamin D: Vitamin D deficiency in pneumonia patients is associated with increased mortality. Adult patients admitted to the hospital with pneumonia are more likely to die if they have vitamin D deficiency.[15]

Poison Ivy/Oak/Sumac

Poison ivy, oak, and sumac are common poisonous plants on the North American continent. When these plants are touched, they deposit an oily sap called urushiol onto the skin. The sap is noted for its ability to create a localized type of allergic contact dermatitis with an uncomfortable, red, itchy, blistery rash. Poison ivy, oak, and sumac rashes are not contagious and cannot spread from one person to another even if there are open sores, because blister fluid does not contain urushiol. Only if another person touches the urushiol that is still on the affected person or his or her clothing can the rash be acquired.

Poison Ivy

Poison ivy causes characteristic thin, red, raised lines in a whip-like appearance on the skin. The rash typically takes a few days to develop in full. Poison ivy treatments are usually limited to self-care methods since the rash typically goes away on its own in two to three weeks.

Poison Oak/Sumac

In poison oak and sumac there is itching initially, followed by a rash. Painfully itchy bumps may form and eventually turn into blisters that ooze liquid. The rash usually peaks in severity about a week after exposure and lasts 5 to 12 days. In some cases, it can last a month or more.

MANAGEMENT METHODS

Wipe the affected area with rubbing alcohol or with alcohol wipes as soon as possible. This helps dissolve urushiol and should be followed up with a thorough wash of the skin with regular soap (e.g., Dial) and water within two hours of exposure.[1,2] Poison ivy soaps (e.g., Zanfel, Tecnu) claim to more effectively remove the oily urushiol and to allow it to wash away. It would be best to have rubbing alcohol, alcohol wipes, or special soaps available before contracting poison ivy and to treat the area as soon as possible after contact with the plant.[3]

Wash Clothing and the Clothes Washer: Wash affected clothing in hot water on a heavy-duty load and on the longest cycle setting. After that, run the washer with an empty load on hot with a cup of bleach to help prevent recontamination.

TOPICAL TREATMENTS

Calamine lotion, oatmeal paste, or baths (in lukewarm water), **baking soda baths and paste** may be applied to relieve itching. Adding a cup of baking soda to the tub is recommended by the American Academy of Dermatology for relief from poison ivy rash.[4] Once out of the bath, a three to one ratio of baking soda to water can be used to make a paste to be applied to the affected area.

Zinc: The FDA advises the use of products containing zinc acetate, zinc carbonate, and zinc oxide to treat the oozing and weeping sores caused by poison ivy.[4]

Vitamin C can be applied locally as a paste. Vitamin C powder can be mixed gradually with hot water until a paste is formed. This paste should be applied three times a day until symptoms subside.[5]

Alternative topical treatments for poison ivy rash can be highly effective but must be started immediately. These include:

- **Fresh aloe juice** taken straight from the leaves provides relief at the site of the rash. There is no need to rinse it.[5]
- **Cool compresses** with water or milk are also effective against poison ivy rash.[5]
- **Menthol cream** can be applied directly to the affected area. The same goes for **pantothenic acid or vitamin B5 cream.**[5]
- **Solutions** containing Tecnu, Zanfel, aluminum acetate (Domeboro solution),[6] or an over-the-counter corticosteroid cream can be used for the first few days.[7]
- **Witch hazel** is an astringent that relieves the itch of poison ivy. A cotton ball can be soaked in witch hazel and applied over the rash for relief.[8]
- **Burrow's solution** in the form of a wet dressing/compress can be applied to affected skin for 15–30 min, then reapplied as needed.
- **Bentonite Clay:** A paste of bentonite clay and water or a lotion containing 5% quaternium-18 bentonite can effectively reduce or prevent the allergic contact dermatitis caused by poison ivy and poison oak.[9]
- **Aluminum Acetate:** The American Academy of Dermatology advises the use of aluminum acetate solution (e.g., Domeboro Astringent Solution Powder Packets, Pedi-Boro Soak Paks, and Gordon's Boro-Packs) to help temporarily relieve skin irritation caused by poison ivy/oak/sumac, insect bites, athlete's foot, and contact dermatitis.[10]

ORAL TREATMENT

Ascorbic acid can be an important factor in curing a poison ivy rash. It should be taken orally at a dose of 500 mg four times a day and can also be applied locally as a paste.[5]

126 patients with moderate to severe poison oak received treatment with injectable ascorbic acid (100 mg IM every four to six hours). This was supplemented with oral ascorbic acid 1,200 mg/day in divided doses. The average period of treatment was five days. The earlier treatment was initiated, the quicker and more favorable the recovery.[11]

Ascorbic acid has also been used prophylactically against poison oak. Patients who took an oral dose of ascorbic (300 mg/day one day prior to exposure, on the day of exposure and one to two days thereafter) did not contract the condition when exposed.[11]

Antihistamines such as diphenhydramine (Benadryl) can help reduce itching and rash.

Polycystic Ovarian Syndrome (PCOS)

Women with PCOS may have excess male hormone (androgen) levels (*see* Testosterone), acne, profuse facial or body hair, anovulation, infrequent or prolonged menstrual periods, and excessive body weight. Polycystic ovary syndrome is one of the most common endocrine disorders, affecting approximately 6% of women of reproductive age. In polycystic ovary syndrome, multiple cysts in each ovary can be seen with medical imaging. These cysts are small, immature ovarian follicles.

Normally, ovarian follicles contain egg cells, which are released during ovulation. In polycystic ovary syndrome, abnormal hormone levels prevent follicles from growing and maturing to release the egg cells. Instead, these immature follicles, or collections of fluid, accumulate in the ovaries.[1]

Complications include increased risk for developing insulin resistance and prediabetes/diabetes, abnormal cholesterol, and triglyceride levels, heart disease, stroke, endometrial cancer (cancer of the inner lining of the uterus), obesity, and sleep apnea.[2] Women with polycystic ovary syndrome are also at increased risk for having mood disorders and developing metabolic syndrome (insulin resistance syndrome).[1] Spontaneous resumption of menses, along with improved pregnancy rates, has occurred.[3]

CLINICAL CARE

Weight Loss: Obesity associated with PCOS can worsen complications of the disorder. Therefore, weight loss via a low-calorie diet combined with moderate exercise activities is a goal of treatment.[4]

Myo-Inositol: Therapy that combined myo-inositol (MI) and D-chiro-inositol (DCI) was tested in young overweight women affected by polycystic ovary syndrome (PCOS).[5] Twenty-one women received MI plus DCI combined treatment at the ratio of 40:1 (the physiologic ratio of the two isomers in the body) in soft gel capsule containing 550 mg of MI, 13.8 mg of DCI, and 200 μg of folic acid twice a day.[5]

The combined therapy of MI plus DCI was effective in improving endocrine and metabolic parameters in young obese PCOS affected women.[5]

Berberine: Research shows that berberine (1.5 gm daily for 3–6 months) lowered blood sugar, improved cholesterol and triglyceride levels, reduced testosterone levels, and lowered waist-to-hip ratio in women with PCOS.[6] Berberine was as effective as metformin.

Electrolysis may be necessary for excessive hair growth.

Polyneuritis/Guillain-Barre Syndrome

Polyneuritis, also known as acute idiopathic polyneuritis or Guillain-Barre syndrome, is widespread inflammation of the peripheral nerves. The syndrome is characterized by progressive inflammation of multiple nerve trunks and results in symmetrical motor neuropathy (paralysis and loss of reflexes). Weakness and paralysis often begin in the feet and ascend to the other muscles. Symptoms can mimic fibromyalgia and include pain and paresthesias, difficulty using arms, hands, legs and feet, muscle weakness, and frequent falls. The autonomic nervous system can also be affected. The main causes are classified as infectious, nutritional, metabolic, and unknown.

TREATMENT MEASURES

B1 and B Complex: Treatment with B complex and thiamine hydrochloride (B1) (5 mg q.i.d.) is suggested.[1]

The following format is one example: intravenous 40% glucose 5% solution of thiamine chloride, 1 ml cyanocobalamin (vitamin B12) 200 mcg intramuscularly daily, oral nicotinic acid 0.03–0.05 g, ascorbic acid (vitamin C) 0.3 gm three times a day, and pangamat calcium (vitamin B15) tablets 0.05 gm three times a day.[2]

Thiamine: In a five-year study, 520 cases of polyneuritis patients were treated with thiamine chloride orally or parenterally in doses of 3–10 mg/day. An improvement usually occurred after three weeks and by nine weeks reached its peak.[3]

In another study, researchers treated 31 patients, 15 suffering from polyneuritis and 16 from other nervous complaints, with oral doses of vitamin B1 up to 3,000 units daily or subcutaneous doses up to 1,000 units daily. Good results were obtained in 19 cases, of which 12 were affected with polyneuritis of diabetic, alcoholic, or diphtheritic origin.[4]

Postherpetic Neuralgia (Pain Following Shingles)

Postherpetic neuralgia is a neuropathic pain and is the most common complication of shingles, which is a reactivation of the chickenpox, or varicella, virus. The virus causes a painful rash and blistered skin lesions that typically follow along the course of a peripheral nerve, and is characteristic of shingles (herpes zoster). Most times when the shingles or blisters fade away, so does the pain. In some cases, however, constant, or sharp, burning recurring pain lasts long after the rash and blisters clear up.[1] This is known as postherpetic neuralgia and is defined as pain that persists one to three months following the disappearance of the herpes zoster rash. About 20% of people who get shingles, particularly in patients over 60, go on to develop postherpetic neuralgia.

Although opioids and prescription or nonprescription analgesics may be medically necessary, no single treatment relieves postherpetic neuralgia in all people. In many cases, it takes a combination of treatments to reduce the pain.[1]

METHODS TO DECREASE PAIN

Ascorbic Acid: Chen et al. found ascorbic acid, or vitamin C, plasma concentrations were lower in 38 patients with postherpetic neuralgia compared with 39 healthy volunteers. In this study, restoration of vitamin C concentrations decreased spontaneous pain, but not brush-evoked pain. The authors concluded that vitamin C status is a component in postherpetic neuralgia and is a component involved in spontaneous pain relief.[2]

A case report by Byun et al. showed that in the case of postherpetic neuralgia which did not respond to conventional therapy such as analgesics and nerve blocks, an intravenous infusion of vitamin C resulted in an immediate reduction in pain.[3]

In two case series referred to by Kauffman, success was achieved in 14 of 14 cases in one series, and 7 of 8 cases in the other.[4] Vitamin C (3 gm) was given by injection every 12 hours with an additional 1 gm orally every two hours while awake. Following the work of Kauffman, Jane M Orient, MD, treated two patients using the same method with substantial positive results.[5]

Tocopherol: The neuralgia has also been reported to be responsive to vitamin E 1,200–1,600 IU/day especially when coupled with vitamin E at a concentration of 30 IU/gram applied to the skin.[6,7] Several months of continuous vitamin E use may be needed in order to see improvement.

Vitamins B1 and B12: Eighty herpetic neuralgia patients were injected with thiamine (vitamin B1) and cobalamin (vitamin B12). After seven days, thiamine yielded a significant itch relief, cobalamin yielded a significant pain relief, and their combination significantly relieved both pain and itch.[8]

Vitamin B12 is effective in treating neuralgias.[9] To help regenerate damaged nerve tissue in patients with postherpetic neuralgia, some doctors use alternative treatments such as vitamins B6 (50–100 mg/day) and B12 (500–5,000 mcg/day), folic acid (400 mcg/day), and alpha-lipoic acid (300 mg bid).[10]

Topical Capsaicin: Pain control was improved by application of capsaicin (0.025% applied four to five times a day).[11] In a double-blind study, 32 elderly patients with chronic postherpetic neuralgia were treated with either capsaicin cream or its vehicle for a six-week period. Significantly greater relief in the capsaicin-treated group compared with vehicle was observed for all efficacy variables. After six weeks almost 80% of capsaicin-treated patients experienced some relief from their pain.[12]

Peppermint Oil: Two to three drops of peppermint oil can be applied to the affected area three or four times per day for pain relief.[13]

Lidocaine ointment or a 5% lidocaine patch over the affected area can be helpful.[14]

Preeclampsia

Preeclampsia is a complication of pregnancy characterized by hypertension and signs of kidney damage (edema, proteinuria) and liver damage (elevated liver enzymes). Preeclampsia and eclampsia are the most common causes of maternal death. Therefore, prevention as well as early diagnosis and management are imperative.[1] Preeclampsia usually begins after 20 weeks of pregnancy and increases the risk of poor outcomes for both the mother and the baby. In severe preeclampsia, hypertension may be accompanied by hemolysis, elevated liver enzymes, and low platelets (HELLP). Complications of preeclampsia include seizures, fetal growth retardation, low birth weight, premature or stillbirth, and, for the mother, liver or renal compromise. Women who develop seizures are diagnosed as having eclampsia.[1]

REDUCING OR PREVENTING HYPERTENSION AND RISKS

Diet: In an observational study, pregnant women who adhered to a Mediterranean diet, characterized primarily by high intake of vegetables, fruits, and unsaturated fats, had a lower risk of preeclampsia.[2]

Calcium Supplementation: A meta-analysis has shown that calcium supplementation during pregnancy reduced all gestational hypertensive-related disorders.[1]

In one study, supplementation with calcium (500–2,000 mg/day) during pregnancy led to an important reduction in systolic and diastolic blood pressure and preeclampsia.[3] This was confirmed by a meta-analysis that concluded that calcium supplementation led to a 70% decrease in the proportion of women with new onset of hypertension and a 60% decrease in preeclampsia during pregnancy.[4]

Additionally, a Cochrane review of 12 randomized controlled trials involving 15,206 women has shown that women who received calcium supplementation were half as likely to develop PE compared with a placebo. Therefore, calcium supplementation appears to be beneficial for women at high risk of developing hypertension in pregnancy.[5]

Magnesium sulfate was shown to be superior to phenytoin for the prevention of eclampsia (seizures) in hypertensive pregnant women.[6] In another study, women who were given magnesium sulfate had a 58% lower risk of developing eclampsia than the placebo group. Maternal mortality was also lower in the treatment group.[7] Magnesium sulfate has also been found to be cost effective in preventing eclampsia with the benefit increasing with the severity of the disease.[8]

Vitamin D: While low serum levels of vitamin D have been associated with the development of preeclampsia, there are conflicting data as to whether vitamin D supplementation provides protection from the disorder. For women with vitamin D deficiency, the American College of Obstetricians and Gynecologists recommends supplementation with 1,000–2,000 IU/day but states that there is insufficient evidence at this time to recommend supplementation for the purpose of preventing preeclampsia.[9]

L-Arginine: One study showed that eating food bars containing the amino acid L-arginine and antioxidant vitamins lowered the risk of preeclampsia in high-risk women. Far fewer of the women in the L-arginine plus vitamin group developed preeclampsia (12.7%) than women in the vitamin-alone (22.5%) group and in the no-supplement (30.2%) group.[10]

Riboflavin: In women who are four months pregnant, taking riboflavin (15 mg/day) by mouth reduced the risk of preeclampsia during pregnancy.[11]

Low-Dose Aspirin: Aspirin (e.g., 50–150 mg/day) after 12 weeks gestation has been shown to be a moderately effective preventable tool for preeclampsia without significant effect on the risk of death of the fetus or baby, having a small for gestational age infant, or bleeding events for either the women or their babies.[12] A Cochrane systematic review of 59 trials including 37,560 women revealed a reduction in the risk of pulmonary embolism with the use of antiplatelet drugs, mainly low-dose aspirin.[13] As a result, it is recommended that women with a high risk of developing PE should start low-dose aspirin (75 mg) from 12 weeks until the birth of the baby.[14]

Antioxidants: In a study involving 283 women, supplementation with vitamin E (400 IU/day) and vitamin C (1,000 mg/day) at 16–22 weeks of gestation indicated that these antioxidants may be beneficial in the prevention of preeclampsia in women with increased risk of the disease.[15]

TREATING PREECLAMPSIA

Delivery: The most effective treatment for preeclampsia is delivery.[16]

Magnesium sulfate, an anticonvulsant medication, is typically given IV to treat active seizures and prevent future seizures.[10] It is also administered to stop premature labor.[17,18]

Premature Labor/Preterm Birth

A pregnancy is considered to be full term at 39 weeks, although the due date is typically set at 40 weeks. After reaching full term, uncomplicated labor and delivery can occur in a matter of days or even hours. Research shows that babies do best when they are born during weeks 39 and 40.[1] That is why preventing preterm labor and birth is important for the health of the baby.

Also known as preterm labor, premature labor is labor that begins more than three weeks before the full term 40-week due date and occurs in about 12% of all pregnancies.[1] Premature babies tend to have more health problems and longer stays in the hospital than babies born full term. In 2015, preterm birth and low birth weight accounted for about 17% of infant deaths. Babies who survive may have:

- Breathing problems
- Feeding difficulties
- Cerebral palsy
- Developmental delays
- Vision problems
- Hearing problems[2]

Premature infants are especially susceptible to nutritional rickets and may require supplemental vitamin D (400 units/day).[3] Premature babies are also predisposed to copper deficiency since copper stores are built up late in pregnancy.[4]

AVOIDING PREMATURE LABOR

Oral Magnesium Citrate: 530 women with non-risk pregnancies were recruited randomly. Half the women received 15 mmol of magnesium citrate daily. The rate of hospitalization due to risk of preterm labor was significantly lower in the magnesium group. The authors concluded that the incidence of hospitalization due to risk of preterm labor may be reduced by oral magnesium supplementation.[5]

Avoidance of smoking.[6]

Avoidance of alcohol and street drugs.[6]

Contractions: Pregnant women should call their doctor or midwife if they continue to have contractions every 10 minutes or more often, or if there is heavy spotting.[6]

Pain: If there is pain or other symptoms of labor, individuals should get off their feet and lie down.[6]

Beta-carotene (42 mg/week) by mouth before, during, and after pregnancy reduced the incidence of maternal diarrhea and fever post-childbirth.[7]

Nutritional Interventions: In a review, it was determined that fish oil and vitamins E and C were promising for preventing preeclampsia and preterm delivery. Further testing is needed. Supplementation would be cost effective and likely worthwhile for those at risk.[8]

MEDICAL TREATMENT

Magnesium sulfate is a medication that may be given intravenously if the pregnancy is less than 32 weeks, the patient is in preterm labor, and/or there is a risk of delivery within the next 24 hours.[9,10] Best evidence shows that pregnant women who received magnesium sulfate before preterm births had a reduced risk of infants with cerebral palsy.[11]

Premenstrual Syndrome/Premenstrual Dysphoric Disorder

Premenstrual syndrome is a common cyclic disorder of young and middle-aged women. It refers to physical and emotional symptoms that occur between ovulation and the onset of menstruation (luteal phase) when estrogen and progesterone levels begin to fall dramatically. A wide variety of signs and symptoms can exist, including mood swings, tender breasts, bloating, headaches, food cravings, fatigue, acne, irritability, and depression. Most women get some premenstrual symptoms. Premenstrual syndrome is a diagnosis of exclusion. When there is a pattern of symptoms without a known medical explanation that occur month after month, and affect a woman's normal life, it is known as premenstrual dysphoric disorder.

RESEARCH ANALYSIS

Vitamin B6: Vitamin B6 may help with PMS symptoms, including moodiness, irritability, forgetfulness, bloating, and anxiety.[1]

Magnesium: Magnesium may help relieve some PMS symptoms, including migraines.[1] For premenstrual syndrome, 333 mg of magnesium oxide taken daily for two menstrual cycles has been effective. A higher dose of 360 mg elemental magnesium three times daily has had positive effects when used from the 15th day of the menstrual cycle until menstrual period begins. 360 mg of elemental magnesium taken three times daily for two months helps manage PMS symptoms. A combination of 200 mg of magnesium daily plus 50 mg of vitamin B6 daily can also been used to minimize unwanted symptoms.[2]

Facchinetti and co-workers used magnesium supplementation, on the basis of a supposed magnesium deficiency both in migraine and in premenstrual syndrome sufferers. Interestingly, a positive correlation was found between clinical improvement and magnesium content in polymorphonuclear cells.[3,4]

Evening primrose oil benefits clinical mastalgia.[5]

Vitamin E: One double-blind study that compared the administration of 400 IU/day of vitamin E to a placebo in 46 women suffering from PMS showed statistically significant amelioration of PMS symptoms in the treated group and no side effects.[6]

L-Tryptophan: Taking 6 gm of L-tryptophan per day helps to decrease mood swings, tension, and irritability in women with PMDD.[7]

Vitex agnus-castus (chaste tree berry, monk's pepper). One study has shown effectiveness for vitex agnus-castus in the treatment of premenstrual symptoms.[8]

Ginger and St. John's Wort: PMS symptoms are reported by some patients to be decreased with the use of herbs, such as ginger and St. John's wort.[8]

Manganese: Previous clinical studies demonstrate that taking manganese along with calcium helps improve symptoms of PMS, including pain, crying, loneliness, anxiety, restlessness, irritability, mood swings, depression, and tension.[9]

Ginkgo Biloba: Taking ginkgo leaf extract by mouth reduced breast tenderness and other symptoms associated with PMS when started during the sixteenth day of the menstrual cycle and continued until the fifth day of the following cycle.[10]

Calcium: Studies show that calcium can help reduce some PMS symptoms, such as fatigue, cravings, and depression.[11,12]

Turmeric: In one study, taking turmeric's extract (curcumin 100 mg bid) for seven days before the menstrual period and continuing for three days after the period ends improved pain, mood, and behavior in women with PMS. PMS symptoms were significantly less in the curcumin group.[13]

Prostatic Hypertrophy/Benign Prostatic Hypertrophy (BPH)

The prostate is a walnut-shaped gland located between the bladder and the penis. An enlarged prostate, which can cause problems with urination, is termed prostatic hypertrophy or benign prostatic hypertrophy. BPH is the most common prostate problem in men older than age 50 while prostatitis is the most common prostate problem in men younger than age 50.

The prostate goes through two main growth periods as a man ages. The first occurs early in puberty, when the prostate doubles in size. In the second phase, increased numbers of epithelial and stromal cells (hyperplasia) cause a gradual noncancerous enlargement of the prostate. This begins around age 25 and continues throughout most of a man's life. Thus, an enlarged prostate is a common condition associated with aging. However, an enlarged prostate can also put pressure on the urethra. This can block the flow of urine out of the bladder and cause a weak stream, incomplete bladder emptying, nocturia, dribbling, difficulty starting a stream, urinary tract infections, hematuria, hydronephrosis, or bladder calculi. About half of all men over 50 develop symptoms of BPH but only about 10% will need medical help or surgery. BPH is not associated with cancer.

MANAGEMENT CHOICES

Diet: Avoid caffeine, spicy/acidic foods, and alcohol.

Medicines: Over-the-counter cold and sinus medicines that contain decongestants or antihistamines should also be avoided because these drugs can increase BPH symptoms.[1]

Nonpharmacologic Care: Decrease fluid intake in the evening. Exercise and weight loss can help lessen symptoms. Use bladder empying techniques such as Valsalva voiding, manual bladder compression, and double voiding.[2]

Saw palmetto inhibits the production of testosterone and reduces the size of the inner lining of the prostate. A clinical controlled study suggested that saw palmetto berries are more effective than Proscara for BPH symptoms. As many as 89% of men taking saw palmetto berries extract improved after one month of treatment.[3] Unlike Proscar, saw palmetto berries do not cause impotence; on the contrary, this herbal remedy has some reputation for being an aphrodisiac. The dosage used in most studies was 360 mg/day of a standardized extract. Saw palmetto is approved in Germany and France for the treatment of BPH.

Saw Palmetto and Lycopene: A single randomized controlled trial showed combination therapy of saw palmetto plus lycopene, selenium, and tamsulosin was more effective than single therapies alone.[4]

Vitamin F or linoleic acid (LA) and alpha-linoleic acid (LNA) are reported to improve urinary symptoms and reduce the size of the enlarged prostate.[5]

Zinc supplements have been shown to produce a similar effect.[6,7,8] Chronic zinc deficiency potentially increases the likelihood of developing BPH. Taking zinc supplements or increasing dietary intake of zinc may help reduce urinary symptoms associated with an enlarged prostate.[9]

Pumpkin seed oil (320 mg/day) improved symptoms of BPH for all patients receiving treatment with it over 12 months in comparison with a placebo. One reason may be that pumpkin seed oil is high in zinc, which is critical to normal prostate function.[10]

Beta-sitosterol (e.g., Super Beta Prostate), a phytosterol, 60–130 mg/day in a systematic review decreased symptoms of BPH and increased urinary output, but did not shrink enlarged prostates.[9,11] Because pumpkin seeds contain beta-sitosterol some studies recommend taking 10 gm of pumpkin seed extract daily for BPH symptoms.[12]

Rye Grass Pollen Extract: One systematic review involving 163 men compared rye grass pollen extract (Cernilton) versus a placebo. It found that pollen extract, typically two tablets taken tid, significantly increased self-rated improvement and significantly reduced nocturia compared with a placebo.[13]

Stinging Nettles (*Urtica dioica*): There is some limited evidence that *Urtica dioica* (600 mg bid) may improve some symptoms of BPH, including lower urinary tract symptoms. There is also evidence that *Urtica dioica* and saw palmetto (*Serenoa repens*) as in PRO 160/120 may be efficacious for lower urinary tract symptoms associated with BPH. In one RCT, researchers gave individuals either stinging nettles or a placebo for eight weeks. They found a significant reduction in symptoms for people taking stinging nettles, but not those taking the placebo.[14] In three other clinical trials on BPH patients, *Urtica dioica*, or nettle, had a better impact in reducing patients' clinical symptoms than a placebo. The results of another study showed that simultaneous consumption of higher doses of *U. dioica*, up to 7 gm/day, plus the medication prazosin (Minipress), compared with the consumption of prazosin alone, resulted in significant improvements in the clinical symptoms of BPH.[15,16,17]

Pygeum: Taking pygeum (100–200 mg/day) by mouth reduced symptoms of BPH such as low urine flow.[18]

African plum tree bark extract may help men deal with the discomfort of BPH.[19]

Proton Pump Inhibitors (PPIs)

PPIs, including omeprazole (Prilosec), lansoprazole (Prevacid), and esomeprazole (Nexium), are the most commonly prescribed agents for problems that can be corrected, or at least improved, by reducing stomach acid levels. PPI's are also available over the counter, but are not always the better medication under all circumstances. For instance, the occasional incident of mild heartburn does not need to be treated with a PPI. An antacid or H2 blocker may work just as well and sooner than a PPI.[1] Unfortunately, PPIs have been associated with an increased risk of impaired vitamin and mineral absorption.

REPLENISHING VITAMIN AND MINERAL STORES

Supplements containing vitamin B12, vitamin C, calcium, iron, and magnesium may be required.[2] Calcium deficiencies lead to increased risks of hip and vertebral fractures.[3] For this reason, calcium supplementation should be in the form of calcium citrate which does not require an acidic environment to be absorbed. Because of deficient magnesium absorption, it is considered to be reasonable practice to screen patients with a history of cardiac arrhythmias or those on antiarrhythmic agents for low serum magnesium if they are on chronic PPI therapy.[2] Magnesium citrate is the most absorbable form of supplementation.[4]

Pseudotumor Cerebri/ Idiopathic Intracranial Hypertension (IIH)

IIH causes chronic disabling headaches, visual disturbances, and, in a minority of patients, permanent visual loss. When intracranial pressure rises without a pathological explanation (i.e., space-occupying lesion), it is known as pseudotumor cerebri or idiopathic intracranial hypertension. The condition is strongly associated with obesity and its incidence is rising corresponding to population increases in body mass index (BMI).[1] The condition predominantly affects women of childbearing age.[2] The name pseudotumor means "false brain tumor" because the symptoms and signs are similar to a brain tumor. Nearly all patients have headaches, often daily, and are worse upon wakening or with eye movement. Vomiting, blurred or dimmed vision, and papilledema may be present. Pseudotumor cerebri is a difficult diagnosis to establish. The main goals of treatment are to preserve vision and to reduce the severity of headaches.

Studies have suggested associations of IIH with obesity, growth hormone treatment, Turner syndrome, hypervitaminosis A, certain medications, and deficiencies in vitamins A, D, and B12.[3,4,5] Treating the underlying cause, if known, is always the best treatment.

CONSERVATIVE CARE

Weight Loss/Diet: The definitive management for IIH is weight loss, but a minority of patients require surgery to preserve vision.[6] Most patients improve after losing 5–10% of their total body weight. Indications are that in addition to weight reduction, sodium restriction is also a useful adjunct.[7]

Vitamin B12: In the absence of a definitive cause, vitamin B12 (parenteral 100 mg/day for two weeks) has been used with success.[8]

Vitamin D deficiency can present as IIH especially in pediatric patients. A five-month-old female with vitamin D deficiency had rickets and pseudotumor cerebri. Treatment of the deficiency resulted in a complete cessation of symptoms within three days.[9]

Vitamin A: Pseudotumor cerebri in children can be associated with vitamin A deficiency, even when other manifestations of xerophthalmia do not exist. Early recognition of this condition and appropriate therapy can prevent blindness.[10]

Pseudoxanthoma Elasticum

Pseudoxanthoma elasticum (PXE), also known as Grönblad-Strandberg syndrome, causes yellow papules, or bumps, to develop on the neck, underarms, and other areas of skin friction. It is a progressive genetic disease in which calcium deposits and other minerals accumulate in elastic fibers. Mineralization of elastic fibers primarily affects the skin, the retina, and blood vessels. On occasion, the digestive tract can be also be involved. Complications include eye abnormalities which can involve bleeding and scarring of the retina, leading to vision loss. Atherosclerosis and claudication are other frequent complications.

THERAPIES

Vitamins A, C, and E and zinc supplements may reduce the risk of retinal hemorrhages.[1,2]

Smoking avoidance can help.[2]

Diet: A low calcium diet is always recommended for improvement in the number of abnormal calcified elastic fibers in the dermis.[2,3]

Exercise: Moderate physical exercise may slow the progression of the disease.[4,5,6]

Supplements: Supplemental vitamin K (90 mcg/day for adult females and 120 mcg/day for adult males) and magnesium oxide (1,000 mg bid depending on tolerability) have been used to reduce calcium deposits in the skin.[4,5,6]

Aluminum Hydroxide: Administration of aluminum hydroxide tablets or liquid in six patients produced marked improvement of skin lesions in three of those patients.[7]

Sports: To reduce the occurrence of facial trauma and the subsequent development of angioid streaks or retinal hemorrhages, playing sports that use balls of any kind and engaging in combat are contraindicated.[5]

Oral vitamin E (300–1,600) IU/day) can yield good results for skin lesions.[8] Antioxidant therapy with daily doses of tocopherol acetate and ascorbic acid were followed in one patient.[9] The skin lesions regressed at 12 months but had started to progress again at 18 months.

Psoriasis

Psoriasis is a chronic inflammatory skin disease that causes raised red patches of thick, itchy skin with silvery-white scales, most commonly on the knees, elbows, trunk, lower back, and scalp.[1] Nails, eyebrows, and other areas may also be affected. There are several types of psoriasis. Generally, psoriasis causes cells to build up rapidly on the surface of the skin and results in the raised red patches and scales. The condition tends to run in families and usually appears in early adulthood.

There is no cure for psoriasis. Patients with severe psoriasis may have an increased risk of psoriatic arthritis, obesity, uveitis, inflammatory bowel disease, diabetes, metabolic disease, high cholesterol, hypertension, depression, and cardiovascular morbidity.

The primary goals of treatment are to minimize plaques and scales, to alleviate pruritis (itching), and to lessen the frequency of flare-ups.[2] Topical medicinal treatments, including steroids or systemic medications, are the mainstay of medical treatments.

NONPHARMACOLOGIC MEASURES

Lifestyle Changes: As a general rule, more alcohol intake leads to more body surface area being affected by psoriasis. Therefore, alcohol intake should be reduced or eliminated.[3] Smoking abstinence, appropriate exercise (e.g., low impact), physical therapy, and massage therapy are all recommended. Weight loss lowered pain scores and reduced cardiovascular risk factors.[4,5,6]

UV Light Therapy: Sunlight may help to clear psoriasis. For many patients psoriasis improves significantly during summer months or on sunny holidays.[7]

Sunscreens (preferably sun protection factor [SPF] 30 or higher) should be used when outdoors.

TOPICAL MEDICATIONS

Moisturizers including emollient creams, ointments, petrolatum, lanolin, paraffin, and even hydrogenated vegetable (cooking) oils reduce scaling and are most effective when applied twice daily and immediately after bathing.[8]

Vitamin A and D topical analogs are routinely used to treat psoriasis.[4,7,9,10]

Salicylic (.5–10%) **or lactic acid** in medicated shampoos and scalp solutions are a benefit.[9,10]

Urea (5–40%) **or propylene glycol** 20% in aqueous creams[4] help reduce the thickness of the scales.

Anthralin in ointment, cream, and paste forms can also be effective. However, anthralin may be irritating and it also stains. Irritation and staining may be avoided by washing off the anthralin 20–30 minutes after application.[4,7,10,11,12]

Nicotinamide: Current treatment strategies of psoriasis are not completely satisfactory. By inhibiting inflammatory cytokines, nicotinamide may enhance the effects of current topical treatments. Preliminary studies have shown that nicotinamide, which is a vitamin B derivative, is effective in the treatment of psoriasis.[11]

Nicotinamide has an enormous moisture barrier boost, so it turns a moisturizer into a super moisturizer. Treatment with topical nicotinamide 4% in combination or calcipotriol 0.005% twice daily for 12 weeks was evaluated. The authors concluded that nicotinamide can enhance the efficacy of calcipotriol when used in combination for topical psoriasis treatment, and it may be a good adjuvant to the current treatment regimens of psoriasis.[13,14]

Coal tar (.5–33%) may be applied as a solution, lotion, cream, ointment, or gel. It has an unpleasant odor and can stain clothing and bedding. Coal tar is typically applied at night and should be allowed to dry on the skin for 10–15 minutes before getting into bed (to minimize staining of bedding and nightclothes) and is showered off in the morning. Alternatively, coal tar can be applied in the morning and showered off after 10–15 minutes.[15,16] Tar-containing shampoos are effective in the treatment of psoriasis of the scalp.[15,16]

Zinc Pyrithione: Sadeghian et al. found topical 0.25% zinc pyrithione cream, applied twice daily, to be effective for localized plaque psoriasis in a randomized double-blind controlled trial.[17]

Salicylic acid and coal tar soaps, gels, lotions, creams, and ointments are approved by the FDA for psoriasis.[18] Salicylic acid helps reduce the thickness of the scales.

Aloe vera cream may reduce redness, scaling, itching, and inflammation. Applying a cream containing 0.5% aloe extract for four weeks can reduce skin plaques. In one study, applying a cream containing aloe gel decreased the severity of psoriasis better than the corticosteroid triamcinolone.[1,19]

ORAL MEDICATIONS

Fish oil (3 gm/day) may reduce inflammation associated with psoriasis.[9]

Vitamin D can be useful in the treatment of psoriasis. Vitamin D deficiency is strongly linked to increased risk for a multitude of diseases, including psoriasis, which have historically been shown to improve dramatically with either adequate UVB exposure to the skin or to oral or topical supplementation with vitamin D.[20] Many patients report improvement in symptoms within months of taking a vitamin D supplement or using a topical lotion containing vitamin D oil.[21,22,23] Typical dosing ranges for vitamin D3 are from 5,000–50,000 IU/day.[24]

Vitamin E: At least one study has linked topical vitamin E to a reduction in psoriasis symptoms. The study also showed that there were no serious side effects.[25]

Psoriatic Arthritis (PsA)

Psoriatic arthritis is a type of joint inflammation, or arthritis, that occurs in combination with psoriasis. Up to 30% of people with psoriasis also develop psoriatic arthritis, which causes pain, stiffness, and swelling in and around the joints. Typically, large joints in the lower extremities, distal joints in the fingers and toes, and the low-back and sacroiliac joints can be affected. There can also be swelling of entire fingers and toes, giving the digits a sausage-like appearance. Other symptoms can include skin rashes, nail changes, fatigue, and eye problems.

Psoriatic symptoms tend to develop before joint symptoms. Psoriatic arthritis usually appears in individuals between the ages of 30–50, but can begin as early as childhood. For most patients, joint problems begin about 10 years after psoriasis begins.[1] Early diagnosis is essential since joint damage can occur in almost half of patients within two years of arthritis onset.[1] Children with psoriatic arthritis are at increased risk to develop uveitis (inflammation of the middle layer of the eye).

The differential diagnosis of psoriatic arthritis should include rheumatoid arthritis, systemic lupus erythematosus, osteoarthritis, and gout. Many psoriatic arthritis patients also have additional disorders (comorbidities) including obesity, metabolic syndrome, diabetes, hypertension, cardiovascular disease, inflammatory bowel disease, liver and ophthalmic diseases, and depression or anxiety. Compared with the general population, patients with PsA are at increased risk of death from cardiovascular diseases.[1] The primary purposes of psoriasis and PsA treatment are to halt organ damage as well as lessen inflammation and pain.

PHARMACOLOGIC CARE

NSAIDs: The use of nonsteroidal anti-inflammatory drugs (NSAIDs) are recommended for firstline treatment of mild symptoms. Consideration should be given for all patients using NSAIDs regarding cardiovascular, renal, and gastrointestinal risks.[2]

LIFESTYLE CHANGES

Abstaining from both alcohol and smoking is recommended.[1]

NUTRITIONAL THERAPY

Oral zinc sulphate was found to be effective for psoriatic arthritis in a double-blind crossover trial versus a placebo in 24 patients of psoriatic arthritis. However, oral zinc sulphate did not produce clinically significant improvement as a treatment modality for plaque psoriasis.[3] Zinc sulfate 220 mg tid daily for four to six weeks was effective for relief of stiffness, joint pain, and swelling, and also reduced the use of analgesics.[4,5]

NONPHARMACOLOGIC CARE

Nondrug treatments for spondyloarthritis include exercise, physical therapy, good posture practices, and other options such as applying heat/cold.[6]

Pulmonary Embolism

Pulmonary embolism (PE) is a blockage in one of the pulmonary arteries in the lungs and is the third most common cause of preventable death in hospitalized patients with at least 650,000 cases occurring annually.[1] The word "embolism" comes from the Greek *émbolos*, meaning "stopper" or "plug." In a PE, an embolus fractures off a deep vein thrombosis (DVT) or clot. Then it circulates through the blood into the inferior vena cava and ultimately to the lungs.[2] The clot eventually becomes wedged in an arterial blood vessel that is too small to allow it to continue further, and blocks the blood flow.[3]

Massive or multiple clots can lead to lung damage, low blood oxygen (because clots prevent blood from interacting with oxygen), and death, primarily due to acute right-sided heart failure. Symptoms of a PE may include shortness of breath, sharp stabbing chest pain particularly upon inspiration, dizziness, and coughing up blood. Risk factors for developing a PE include age over 60, sedentary lifestyle, obesity, recent major surgery, fractures of the leg or hip, cancer, or a history of a heart attack or stroke or hypercoagulable blood. The history and physical examination are neither sensitive nor specific for PE and the results of V/Q scanning are frequently equivocal. Therefore, documentation of DVT in a patient with suspected PE establishes the need for treatment and may preclude further testing.[4]

PREVENTION

The best treatment is the prevention of a pulmonary embolism. That means preventing and treating DVTs. (*See* Deep Vein Thrombosis.)

Raynaud's Phenomenon

Raynaud's phenomenon is a disease of the blood vessels that temporarily decreases blood flow to the fingers and toes. Cold temperatures or anxiety cause the blood vessels to overreact and they narrow more than necessary. When this happens, a sufficient amount of blood cannot get to the surface of the skin and the affected areas can turn pale or blue. During an episode, affected individuals often experience pain or a pins and needles sensation in the fingers or toes.[1] When the blood flow returns, the arteries again overreact, allowing the skin to turn red and throb or tingle.

Women are nine times more likely to have Raynaud's than men. It usually occurs between the ages of 20–40 in women and later in life in men. When Raynaud's occurs by itself, it's called primary Raynaud's. When it occurs in association with other conditions, such as scleroderma, lupus, and rheumatoid arthritis, it is known as secondary Raynaud's.[2] Secondary Raynaud's can severely restrict the blood supply, so it carries a higher risk of complications, such as ulceration of the digits, scarring, and even tissue death (gangrene) in the most serious cases. Fortunately, severe complications are rare.[3] Treatment goals are to reduce the severity of attacks, prevent or lessen ischemic tissue damage, and improve quality of life.

LESSENING BLOOD VESSEL OVERREACTION

Avoidance of cold weather/temperatures, caffeine, alcohol, and smoking is advised. Those who are affected should get regular exercise and wear gloves in cooler temperatures.[2]

Omega-3 fatty acids, found in fish oil, may reduce symptoms in individuals with primary Raynaud's, according to one study. Fish oil did not reduce symptoms in people who had secondary Raynaud's. Patients should consult their doctor before taking fish oil, especially if they already take blood thinners, such as warfarin (Coumadin), clopidogrel (Plavix), or aspirin.[2]

Evening Primrose Oil (EPO): EPO contains a different type of fatty acid that stops the body from making chemicals that narrow blood vessels. In one study, people with Raynaud's who took EPO had fewer and less severe attacks compared to those who took a placebo. More research is needed, however. Individuals who have a history of seizures should not take EPO. EPO can increase the risk of bleeding, especially if taken in combination with blood thinners.[2]

Inositol hexaniacinate, a form of vitamin B3 or niacin, 1 gm q.i.d. for several months, may reduce the frequency of Raynaud's attacks. This should be monitored by a physician since liver toxicity is a possibility.[2]

Magnesium opens up blood vessels. Some doctors suggest taking a magnesium supplement, although there are no scientific studies to show that it works. Magnesium should be taken with meals and the dosage reduced if diarrhea occurs.[2]

Ginkgo: Ginkgo biloba can open up blood vessels and increase circulation in the fingers. One preliminary study found that people with Raynaud's who took 160 mg of ginkgo per day had less pain. Patients should talk to their doctor before taking ginkgo and should not take it if they have a history of seizures. Ginkgo can interact with several herbs and medications, and can increase the risk of bleeding, especially when taken in combination with blood thinners.[2]

Respiratory Tract Infections

Respiratory infections happen in the lungs, chest, sinuses, nose, and throat. Recurrent respiratory infections are a major cause of hospitalizations. Examples of chronic respiratory infections include the common cold, pneumonia, rhinosinusitis, acute and chronic bronchitis, croup, streptococcal pharyngitis (strep throat), and influenza (flu). The symptoms of chronic respiratory infections can include shortness of breath, fatigue, mucus production, fever, sore throat, postnasal drip or nasal discharge, bad breath, and cough.

Infections affecting the respiratory tract are divided into upper (above and in the voice box) and lower respiratory tract (in the lungs and below the voice box) infections.

A. Most upper respiratory infections (URIs), such as the common cold or pharyngitis, are of viral etiology. Epiglottitis and laryngotracheitis (croup) are exceptions, with severe cases likely caused by *Hemophilus influenzae* type b. Bacterial pharyngitis is often caused by *Streptococcus pyogenes*.[1]

B. Lower respiratory tract infections, such as pneumonia, lung abscess, acute bronchitis, and bronchiolitis, can be more serious.[1]

The goals in treating respiratory tract infections are to achieve better treatment response and to prevent the affected individual from acquiring repeated infections.

ADJUVANT PROCEDURES

General Measures: The management of most viral respiratory infections consists of rest, adequate caloric and fluid intake, and management of fever and malaise.[2]

Avoidance of Smoking: Every patient should stop smoking or at least drastically curtail the habit. Adults should not smoke around children with frequent or chronic respiratory infections.

Vitamin D: A relationship between low vitamin D levels and the development or outcomes of respiratory diseases has been identified. Studies on the role of vitamin D in respiratory diseases have consistently indicated that low vitamin D levels may be associated with a higher incidence, greater severity, or poorer treatment responses in various respiratory diseases, including respiratory tract infections (e.g., community-acquired pneumonia).[3,4,5,6,7] Research shows that taking vitamin D reduces the chance of a respiratory infection in children and adults. Also, children with low blood levels of vitamin D tend to experience more upper respiratory tract infections than those with higher levels of vitamin D.[8] Perhaps most importantly, patients with vitamin D deficiency are at high risk of hospitalization and developing severe disease with quadruple the death rate for Covid-19. This is likely due to the loss in the protective action of vitamin D on the immune system and against the SARS-CoV-2–induced cytokine storm.[9] Taking oral vitamin D3 (60,000 IU/day for seven days) after Covid infection, accelerated viral clearance for a more rapid and complete recovery.[10] More studies are needed to assess the merit of vitamin D supplementation in preventing and treating respiratory tract infections. Considering the safety and low cost of treatment, supplementation of vitamin D3 (5,000–50,000 IU/day for adults)[11] would seem warranted to improve treatment response.

Zinc helps to ensure the proper action of various leukocytes such as neutrophils, monocytes, macrophages, and B and T lymphocytes. A U.S. Airforce study compared URI incidence between supplemented (zinc gluconate 15 mg/day capsules) and non-supplemented groups. This study was a seven-month, randomized, double-blind, placebo-controlled trial involving 40 cadets to evaluate zinc's effectiveness in reducing the risk of upper respiratory infections (URIs). Self-reported symptoms as recorded by a weekly website survey revealed that supplemented participants experienced significantly more symptom-free episodes than those in the placebo group.[12]

Zinc reduced the incidence of acute lower respiratory tract infections by approximately 15% in one study and had a 6% effect on reducing overall child mortality. The effect was much more substantial (18% reduction in deaths) among zinc-supplemented children who were older than 12 months of age.[13]

According to current research, adequate zinc status can bring down the likelihood of infectious respiratory diseases, pneumonia, and its complications. There are also indirect indications that zinc supplementation may be effective in the fight against coronavirus disease (e.g., COVID-19), but there is insufficient data for recommendations.[14]

Honey: In one study, children with upper respiratory tract infections (age two and over) were given up to 2 teaspoons (10 milliliters) of honey at bedtime. The honey seemed to reduce nighttime coughing and improve sleep. Honey appeared to be as effective as a common cough suppressant ingredient, dextromethorphan, in typical over-the-counter doses.[15] Children under the age of one should not be given honey.

Colchicine: Although more studies are needed, it appears that the prescription drug colchicine (0.5 mg/day) could improve the treatment of people with severe COVID-19 and reduce the COVID mortality rate by as much as 50%. Four controlled studies comprised of approximately 6,000 coronavirus patients have been published on the positive effects of colchicine.[16]

Quercetin, a flavonoid, taken at a dose of 1,000 mg/day, along with exercise, reduced the incidence of upper respiratory tract infections during winter.[17] Quercetin (500–1,000 mg/day) has also been proven to potentialize the effects of routine drugs against coronavirus.[18]

Restless Legs

Restless legs syndrome (RLS) is a neurological disorder in the nervous system that causes unpleasant and uncomfortable sensations in the legs and an irresistible urge to move them. Moving the legs or walking eases the urge and discomfort temporarily. Most patients also experience involuntary periodic limb movements. Since symptoms increase in severity during the night, these urges and movements seriously interfere with sleep. That is why some doctors consider RLS to be a sleep disorder. In most cases, doctors do not know the cause of this disorder.

RLS is twice as common among female patients, with increased severity of symptoms after menopause. Considerable evidence suggests that RLS is related to dysfunction in the basal ganglia of the brain that uses the chemical dopamine to control movement. Perhaps not coincidentally, individuals with Parkinson's have in increased risk of developing RLS.[1]

ADJUVANT TREATMENT OPTIONS

General Approach: A trial of brief walking, hot baths, or leg massage before bedtime may be beneficial.[2]

Iron Deficiency: In patients with iron deficiency and RLS, treatment with iron is curative.[3] Sometimes, treating any underlying condition greatly relieves the symptoms of RLS.[4,5]

Folic acid can be a significant benefit.[6,7] One physician identified 45 individuals from five families in whom folic-acid therapy relieved restless legs. The amount of folic acid needed to prevent their symptoms from recurring was 5–30 mg/day.[6] Most other patients respond to 5–10 mg/day.[8]

L-Tryptophan: In another study, 2 gm/day of L-tryptophan ameliorated symptoms.[9]

Inositol Hexaniacinate (IHN): IHN 1,500–4,000 mg/day in two or three divided doses has provided relief for restless legs syndrome.[10,11]

Selenium: Sixty patients with primary RLS were enrolled in a clinical trial. It was based on three periods of drug prescription with a one month wash-out period. As a placebo, 50 and 200 μg of selenium were administered in each separated month. Improvement was significantly higher in the selenium (50 and 200 μg) group than in the placebo group. The authors concluded that selenium prescription in a daily recommended dose of 50 μg instead of a dopamine agonist would be an alternative treatment for improvement of RLS symptoms.[12]

Biotin: In one study, three patients with severe symptoms were given high doses of biotin (10 mg IM daily for six weeks, then 10 mg IM three times per week for six weeks, and then 5 mg/day orally). Within four to eight weeks after the biotin administration, there was disappearance of restless leg syndrome in all patients.[13]

Retinopathy (Diabetic)

Retinopathy is any damage to the retina of the eyes (e.g., microaneurysms, retinal infarcts, or hemorrhages) with or without macular edema and proliferative retinopathy that may cause vision impairment. The two most typical causes of retinopathy are high blood pressure and diabetes (type 1 or type 2). In diabetic patients, retinopathy occurs after 10–20 years. It is the most common cause of blindness in middle-aged and elderly patients.[1]

In diabetes, pathologic angiogenesis often occurs where new blood vessels form, but do not develop as they should underneath the retina. Instead, they grow into the retina itself resulting in retinal damage in the elderly or even blindness in infants.[2]

Patients with diabetes are at risk for not only diabetic retinopathy, but also cataracts and glaucoma. The prevalence of diabetic retinopathy increases with the duration of diabetes mellitus, poor glycemic control, and the presence of comorbid vascular risk factors (e.g., hypertension, poor control of lipids, etc.). In some patients with diabetic retinopathy, blood vessels may close off or swell or leak fluid, making the retina swell. Swelling of the retina's central macula is the most common reason why patients with diabetes lose their vision.[2]

Three major types of diabetic retinopathy (DR):

1. Nonproliferative diabetic retinopathy (NPDR) occurs when retinal microaneurysms form due to a lack of perfusion. In this early stage of diabetic retinopathy, the walls of the blood vessels in the retina weaken. Tiny bulges, or microaneurysms, protrude from the vessel walls, sometimes leaking or oozing fluid and blood into the retina.
2. Proliferative diabetic retinopathy (PDR) occurs when abnormal new blood vessels grow on the surface of the retina due to ischemia from capillary closure. In PDR, new fragile blood vessels which are easily damaged can hemorrhage into the retinal area of the eye. Diabetic vitreous hemorrhage secondary to PDR is a cause of severe vision loss in many diabetic patients.[3] Patients with severe vision loss (e.g., of 5/200 or less) due to diabetic vitreous hemorrhage that does not clear spontaneously after one year typically require surgery.[3]
3. Diabetic macular edema (DME). Diabetic retinopathy usually affects both eyes and is the leading cause of blindness in developed countries.

Goals of treatment are to control blood pressure, diabetes, including A1c level, and to preserve vision.

APPROACHES TO LOWER RISK

Magnesium: Diabetics are often deficient in magnesium, and the deficiency is most severe in those with retinopathy.[4] Although there is no evidence that supplementing with magnesium will prevent retinal damage, magnesium deficiency should not go untreated.[5]

Vitamin B12: In one study, 15 type 1 (juvenile onset) diabetics with retinopathy (retinal damage due to diabetes) received 100 mcg/day of vitamin B12 mixed with their daily insulin injection. After one year, all signs of retinopathy had disappeared in 7 of 15 cases and an additional 3 had partial improvement.[6] Vitamin B12 was not helpful for adult diabetics with pre-existing eye damage.[6] Similar results were reported by others.[7]

Vitamin C: Clinical trials have suggested that doses of vitamin C (1,000–2,500 mg/day) reduce the microvascular complications of DM2 such as retinopathy, nephropathy, and diabetic foot pain. Apart from this, there is evidence that vitamin C in higher doses reduces A1c levels and low-density lipoproteins.[8]

Vitamin C and E: Diabetes is associated with various microvascular and macrovascular complications. Supplementation with vitamins C and E reduced neovascularization and prevented the inhibition of retinal glutathione reductase, glutathione peroxidase, and superoxide dismutase activities. Vitamin C and E prevent oxidative stress-induced retinopathy.[9,10,11,12]

APPROACHES TO PREVENT HEMORRHAGES

The ideal prevention is good control of the underlying diabetic disease process and intensive control of hypertension along with procedures to minimize bleeding.

Rutin: Rutin treatment significantly arrested the biochemical disturbances of diabetic retinopathy in animal studies.[13]

Resveratrol: Resveratrol treatment effectively blocks blood vessel leakage and loss of pericytes which, in turn, helps in the prevention of diabetic retinopathy.[14] Significant beneficial antidiabetic observations in an animal study were reported by researchers who concluded that resveratrol may be considered as a therapeutic supplement to prevent diabetic retinopathy.[15] A typical daily dose of resveratrol for a 150-pound person is 450 mg.

Bilberry: Bilberry extract (360–600 mg/day of an extract standardized for 25% anthocyanosides) has been shown to strengthen blood vessels in the eye and to improve vision in people with diabetic retinopathy.[16]

Retinopathy (Hypertensive)

Hypertensive retinopathy is a condition that damages the retina of the eye due to high blood pressure. Chronically elevated blood pressure causes retinal vascular damage such as arteriolar vasoconstriction, arteriovenous nicking, and arteriosclerosis. More severe hypertension can cause hemorrhages, retinal ischemia (cotton wool spots), and/or swelling of the optic nerve which requires emergency medical treatment. The primary goal in treatment is to lower the risk and progression of retinopathy through control of high blood pressure with medications, achieving and maintaining weight loss, and exercise. (*See* Hypertension.)

MANAGEMENT TECHNIQUES

Nicotine Avoidance: Smoking further worsens the adverse effects of hypertensive retinopathy.[1]

Bilberry: Bilberry extract (360–600 mg/day of an extract standardized for 25% anthocyanosides) has been shown to strengthen blood vessels in the eye and to improve vision in people with diabetic and hypertensive retinopathy.[2]

Dark Chocolate: A meta-analysis of 13 randomized controlled trials that compared dark chocolate with a placebo confirmed a significant reduction of systolic blood pressure in hypertensive and prehypertensive subgroups. It is believed that dark chocolate can help lower BP via improved vascular endothelial function and increased formation of nitric oxide.[3]

Nonpharmacologic Measures: Lowering salt (sodium chloride intake) is recommended to help lower blood pressure. Dietary or supplemental potassium, calcium, and magnesium consumption helps to lower BP.[3]

Rheumatoid Arthritis

Rheumatoid arthritis (RA) is a systemic inflammatory arthritic disease that can deform and destroy joints and cause damage throughout the body. It is characterized by symmetric (e.g., both hands, wrists, knees) chronic hypertrophic synovitis (inflammation of the joint linings) causing cartilage destruction and bone erosion. RA can also cause complications outside the affected joints which can adversely affect the eyes skin, lungs, heart, and blood vessels. As an example, patients with RA are more susceptible to atherosclerosis and have a 60% higher risk of heart attack just one year after the diagnosis.[1]

Currently, no official clinical diagnostic criteria exist for RA.[2] Prolonged morning stiffness of finger joints, autoantibody positivity, and pain and swelling in the metacarpophalangeal and metatarsophalangeal joints may indicate the diagnosis.[2] RA typically results in painful, warm, swollen, and deformed joints that are limited in movement. Individuals with RA often find pain to be their most serious problem. RA is one of the most disabling types of arthritis and can reduce life expectancy by three to seven years.

Generally, a good outcome for a disease is considered total recovery or clinical remission. Since total recovery from RA is not possible, clinical remission is considered a good outcome or target goal. Additional goals are to control inflammation, relieve pain, prevent or limit joint damage, optimize quality of life, avoid complications of therapy, and improve or preserve function.

RESEARCH RESULTS

Smoking Cessation: It is essential to draw attention to the expected beneficial effect of smoking cessation. Smoking influences the course of RA in a negative way, although its extent differs in the various studies.[3]

Acetaminophen: Acetaminophen should be tried as the initial therapy in patients with mild to moderate pain for reasons of safety and cost.[4]

NSAIDs: Nonprescription and prescription NSAIDs are frequently used as first-line agents for symptomatic relief of pain, swelling, and stiffness.[4]

Diet: Inflammation can be modulated by diet. It is best to consume higher amounts of fruits, vegetables, and whole grains, and to limit lean red meats, processed foods, and gluten. Those with celiac disease experience many of the same symptoms as those with RA, and many RA patients report decreased inflammation by following a gluten-free diet.[5]

Weight reduction is important if obese.

Deficiencies: The most commonly observed vitamin and mineral deficiencies in patients with RA are folic acid, vitamin C, vitamin D, vitamin B6, vitamin B12, vitamin E, folic acid, calcium, magnesium, zinc, and selenium.Methotrexate which is used to treat RA can also cause folic acid and other vitamin and mineral deficiencies.[6]

Calcium: Because RA patients are at risk for vitamin D and calcium deficiencies, they are at greater risk for developing osteoporosis. Supplementation of calcium and vitamin D is recommended to decrease the risk of osteoporosis that results from interference with calcium absorption due to menopause and from concurrent steroid therapy.[6]

Vitamins A and E: Rheumatoid arthritis and lupus seem to be associated with low levels of vitamins A and E. Researchers tested vitamin levels and then tracked the donors to see who eventually developed the diseases. Those who developed rheumatoid arthritis were especially deficient in beta-carotene.[7]

EPA/DHA: A meta-analysis reviewed research on fish oil and RA. Controlled trials indicate a reduction in tender joint counts and decreased use of non-steroidal anti-inflammatory drugs with fish oil supplementation. The researchers concluded that when collateral benefits of fish oil are included within efficacy, the argument for its adjunctive use in RA is strong.[8]

One recent study found that patients who received 5.5 gm daily of fish oils in combination with an anti-rheumatic drug treatment (methotrexate, sulphasalazine, and hydroxychloroquine) were more likely to achieve remission. These findings suggest that medication and fish oil supplements may be a powerful combination in helping people with RA.[9]

Folic Acid: Common rheumatoid arthritis drugs like methotrexate and sulfasalazine interfere with how the body uses folic acid, so it is very important to supplement folic acid (400–600 mcg/day).[10]

Vitamin D: Historically, rheumatoid arthritis has been shown to improve dramatically with either adequate UVB exposure to the skin, or to oral or topical supplementation with vitamin D.[11] RA tends to be worse in people who are low in vitamin D. Also, corticosteroids taken to control inflammation with RA interfere with the absorption of calcium needed for normal bones. Therefore, vitamin D3 (5,000–50,000 IU/day for adults) supplements are very important along with calcium (1,200 mg/day or higher).[10]

Vitamin D deficiency is highly prevalent in patients with RA, and low vitamin D levels are associated with increased disease severity, inflammatory cytokines, and bone loss.[12,13,14,15] The Vitamin D Council recommends supplementing with between 5,000–10,000 IU/day and maintaining a vitamin D level of between 40–80 ng/ml (100–200 nmol/l).[16] However, vitamin D supplementation at far higher doses than suggested above may sometimes be necessary. Another study recommends a safe weekly bolus of oral vitamin D3 100,000 IU/wk for one to four weeks (depending on the base levels measured) plus 800–2,000 IU/day.[17]

Turmeric: In a study posted to *Arthritis and Rheumatology*, researchers found that turmeric extract depleted of essential oils profoundly inhibited joint inflammation and periarticular joint destruction in a dose-dependent manner. Patients who are also taking Warfarin should avoid turmeric.[18,19]

Vitamin E taken along with standard treatment is better than standard treatment alone for reducing pain in people with RA.[19] Vitamin E (1,632 IU/day) and diclofenac (a prescription NSAID) treatments were compared over three weeks in hospitalized chronic polyarthritis patients. Physicians and patients rated therapy as more successful in vitamin E patients as compared to diclofenac patients.[20,21]

Borage: There is some evidence that borage seed oil (1,300 mg/day) in combination with conventional painkilling or anti-inflammatory medications might help decrease symptoms of RA after six weeks of treatment. The improvement appears to last for up to 24 weeks. Improvement is measured as a decrease in the number and severity of tender and swollen joints.[22]

Lactobacillus: Research indicates that taking lactobacillus for eight weeks reduces tender and swollen joints in women with RA.[23] Probiotic supplementation may be an appropriate adjunct therapy for RA patients and may help alleviate symptoms and improve inflammatory cytokines.[24]

Ringworm/Dermatophytosis/Tinea Infections

Ringworm, also known as dermatophytosis, is not a worm but a fungal (tinea) infection of the skin. The fungi live on the dead tissues of the skin, hair, and nails. Tinea infections are commonly referred to as ringworm due to the characteristic circular lesions. These infections are named for the affected body part, such as tinea pedis (feet), tinea capitis (scalp), and tinea corporis (body). Typically, it results in a circular red, itchy, scaly rash. Ringworm occurs in people of all ages, but it is particularly common in children. It occurs most often in warm, moist climates. Ringworm is a contagious disease and can be passed from person to person by contact with infected skin areas or by sharing combs and brushes, other personal care items, or clothing.[1]

CARE CONSIDERATIONS

Topical antifungal creams, liquids, or sprays such as clotrimazole (Lotrimin Ultra), econazole (Spectrazole), and terbinafine (Lamisil) are commonly recommended treatments for tinea corporis, tinea cruris, and tinea pedis. Ketoconazole should not be used to treat tinea infections.[2]

Oral Antifungals: Tinea capitis (ringworm of the scalp) must be treated with oral antifungals (e.g., terbinafine sold under the brand name Lamisil or fluconazole sold as Diflucan)[2] because topical agents are unable to penetrate the hair shaft.[1]

Selenium Sulfide: Treatment with 1% or 2.5% selenium sulfide (Selsun) shampoo or 2% ketoconazole shampoo should be used for the first two weeks because it may reduce disease transmission.[2]

Zinc: Topical 20% zinc-undecylenate powder (e.g., Fungi-Nail, Myco Nail A, Tineacide) applied twice daily for four weeks is an effective treatment for tinea pedis (athlete's foot).[3]

Rosacea/Acne Rosacea

Rosacea is a chronic inflammatory skin condition that causes redness and visible blood vessels on the cheeks, nose, chin, and forehead. It is more common among fair-skinned people and its cause is unknown. Small facial arteries under the skin tend to stay dilated, causing a tendency to blush or flush easily. Near the nose, cheeks, and eyes, over time, inflammatory papulopustular eruptions with red bumps and facial pustules (acne-like eruptions) develop. Skin becomes more coarse and thin thread-like red lines (telangiectasis) can develop. Rosacea is distinct from acne, but can be mistaken for acne or eczema.

There are four subtypes of rosacea which affect primarily middle-aged people and tend to worsen with age. It has been suggested that loss of integrity of upper dermal connective tissue may permit vascular dilatation and that this may have an important role in the pathogenesis of the disease.[1] There is no cure for rosacea, but control is possible.

COSMETIC CONSIDERATIONS

Avoid common triggers that can worsen symptoms such as irritating cosmetics, heat (weather, hot baths, saunas), wind, and sunlight. Photoprotection is universally recommended.[2] Therefore, broad-spectrum sunblock (UV-A and UV-B) with an SPF 15 or higher should be used daily.[3]

Diet: Once the diagnosis is established, it is wise to avoid alcohol, spicy foods, caffeine, and hot liquids.[4]

Zinc Sulphate: Oral zinc sulphate was found useful in the management of rosacea by Sharquie et al. They used zinc sulphate 100 mg three times daily in 25 patients of rosacea in a double-blind randomized control trial and observed a statistically significant decrease in disease activity after three months of therapy without any serious adverse effects.[5]

The anti-inflammatory and antioxidant actions of zinc have also been utilized for the management of other follicular occlusion disorders like hidradenitis suppurativa, acne conglobata, and folliculitis decalvans. Brocard et al. observed clinical response without significant side effects in all 22 patients of hidradenitis suppurativa when treated with zinc gluconate 90 mg/day.[6] Similarly, Kobayashi et al. reported complete cure of acne conglobata and dissecting cellulitis with oral zinc sulphate.[7] However, the overall benefit of zinc in these disorders remains understudied.[8]

Ox bile salts (one tablet three times per day) and **vitamin B2 (riboflavin)** 10 mg bid have been used to treat acne rosacea.[9]

Chromium Picolinate: Chromium (150–500 mcg/day) appears to have value as an acne treatment.[10]

Mild cleansing and moisturizing regimens can be beneficial. Cleansers should be fragrance and abrasive-free with a mildly acidic to neutral pH. Recommended skin cleansers include lipid-free, nonalkaline cleansers (e.g., Cetaphil) and sensitive skin synthetic detergent bars (e.g., Dove Sensitive Skin Bar).[2]

Sarcoidosis

Sarcoidosis is a rare chronic, progressive disease of unknown cause that induces inflammatory cells (CD+4 T cells) to gather into small lumps, or granulomas, and grow in different tissues and organs in the body. Granulomas can affect the organ's structure and function and possibly lead to permanent scarring or thickening of the organ tissue.[1] African Americans are three times more likely to be diagnosed with sarcoidosis than Caucasians and tend to have more severe disease.

The lungs are the primary target of the disease (88% of patients) where symptoms such as dry cough, wheezing, and shortness of breath dominate. Skin lesions (35%–50%) with raised patches or open sores are common. Lymph glands (27%), eye (27%) disease especially uveitis, and the liver (20%) can be affected while kidney involvement is relatively rare (1%). Bone sarcoidosis occurs in 3%–4% of patients. It most frequently affects the hands and feet, and is associated with soft tissue swelling, joint stiffness, and pain.[2] Diagnosis is difficult because sarcoidosis is a great imitator of other diseases. Most young and middle-aged adult patients are not disabled by the illness. For a small number of people, sarcoidosis is a chronic condition that may result in the deterioration of the affected organ. Rarely, sarcoidosis can be fatal and is usually the result of complications with the lungs, heart, or brain.[3]

About half of all patients with sarcoidosis get better without treatment. Therefore, the decision to provide treatment must be weighed against the risks of using corticosteroids, the most common therapy. A general rule is to consider instituting corticosteroid treatment when organ function is threatened.[4] The relapse rate after corticosteroid therapy is withdrawn may be as high as 70%.[5] Goals in the treatment of sarcoidosis are to control symptoms, prevent complications, and improve outcomes in patients with persistent sarcoidosis.

NUTRITIONAL MANAGEMENT TECHNIQUES

Melatonin: In one study, treatment with 20 mg/day of melatonin was followed by gradual disappearance of nodules in the lungs.[6]

Various NSAIDs: Nonsteroidal anti-inflammatory drugs, such as ibuprofen (Advil, Nuprin, Motrin IB), naproxen sodium (Aleve, Naprosyn), aspirin, or others, may help reduce acute joint inflammation and relieve pain and fever.[7]

Avoidance of High-Dose Vitamin D: Sarcoidosis is considered a contraindication for high-dose vitamin D supplements. In one study, administration of vitamin D3 to patients with sarcoidosis increased the circulating concentration of 1,25-dihydroxy vitamin D3. This resulted in hypercalcemia, thus accounting for their hypersensitivity to vitamin D and sunlight.[8]

Calcium and Vitamin D: Current corticosteroid dose, low dietary calcium, and low vitamin D3 levels are associated with bone fragility. In sarcoidosis, calcium and vitamin D supplementation may be warranted, but desirable D3 serum levels might be lower than those advised for the general population.[9]

Cessation of Smoking: Giving up cigarette smoking can help alleviate lung symptoms. Sarcoidosis can be a lasting disease, so improving general health with regular exercise and a healthy diet is important.[10]

Schizophrenia

Schizophrenia, formerly known as dementia praecox, is a chronic severe mental disorder characterized by significant alterations in perception, thoughts, mood, and behavior. The disorder affects how a person feels, thinks, and perceives reality (e.g., delusions, false beliefs, hallucinations, impaired cognitive ability, unclear or confused thinking, or hearing voices that do not exist). As a result, schizophrenia is characterized by behavioral problems, flat affect, trouble focusing or learning, and difficulty relating to others. Individuals with schizophrenia seem to have lost touch with reality. There is no cure for schizophrenia. Managing symptoms is the best way of managing the illness.

DESIGNS FOR BETTER MANAGEMENT

Medications are the cornerstone of schizophrenia treatment, and antipsychotic medications are the most commonly prescribed drugs. They are thought to control symptoms by affecting the brain neurotransmitter dopamine.[1]

B Vitamins: A meta-analysis has found that add-on treatment with high-dose B-vitamins, including B6, B8, and B12, can significantly reduce symptoms of schizophrenia, more than standard treatments alone.[2]

Vitamin Supplementation: Another study found that vitamin supplementation, particularly with folic acid, vitamin B12, and vitamin D, may play an important role in the treatment of schizophrenia within certain subgroups. In those patients who are vitamin D deficient (darker skin, living at latitudes with less sunlight), supplementation with vitamin D may be protective among those vulnerable to psychosis. Among those patients with specific genetic variants in the folate metabolic pathway, supplementation with both folate and vitamin B12 can be beneficial, especially in improving negative symptoms.[3]

Ascorbic Acid: Very few studies have examined the effect of vitamin C with typical antipsychotics in the treatment of schizophrenia. In one study, it was observed that vitamin C level was significantly lower in the plasma and urine of schizophrenics as compared to normal controls. Oral supplementation of vitamin C with antipsychotic medications reversed low ascorbic acid levels, reduced oxidative stress, and improved the BPRS score, hence both drugs in combination can be used in the treatment of schizophrenia. The findings of another study suggest that antioxidant supplement therapy as an adjuvant therapy is useful in patients with stress-induced psychiatric disorders.[4]

Glycine: Taking glycine by mouth along with conventional medicines reduces negative symptoms of schizophrenia in some patients who do not respond to treatment with conventional medicines alone.[5,6] High doses (30 gm/day) of glycine have been shown to reduce more subtle symptoms of schizophrenia, such as social withdrawal, emotional flatness, and apathy, which do not respond to most of the existing medications.[7]

Sciatica

Sciatica is pain that radiates along the course of the longest and widest nerve in the body, the sciatic nerve. Sciatica is a symptom, not a diagnosis. There are several medical causes of sciatica, but it is most commonly a result of a bulging or herniated lumbar disk directly pressing on or inflaming a sciatic nerve root. Pain can extend from the low back into the buttock and down the side or back of the leg and, in severe cases, into the foot and toes. Tingling, numbness, or weakness may accompany the pain. Sciatica typically affects only one side of the body. There may or may not be associated neurological deficits on examination.

It is estimated that 10%–15% of sciatic patients submit to surgical procedures to relieve the pain.[1] Recently updated clinical guidelines in Denmark, the U.S., and the U.K. highlight the role of conservative treatment for sciatica.[2] NSAIDs and painkillers are the foundation for symptomatic medical treatment.

CONSERVATIVE NONSURGICAL CARE

Thiamine: Sciatica is reported only by a few people who take thiamine HCl. Thiamine 20–50 mg/day for moderate to advanced neuropathy and continued for several weeks after symptoms disappear is recommended and should eliminate any deficiency as a co-cause.[3,4] For mild polyneuropathy, 10–20 mg by mouth once/day for two weeks is suggested.[4]

Vitamin B12 has also been reported to help and cure sciatica.[5] Oral tablets or injections of this vitamin can help to prevent nerve damage, especially for those lacking sufficient levels of dietary B12 required for healthy nerve function.[6] B12 helps reduce and treat the complications of painful peripheral neuropathy.[7]

Gamma linolenic acid is a fatty substance that may help to restore healthy nerve function by reducing the pain, numbness, tingling, and burning sensations associated with nerve damage.[6]

Magnesium: This mineral may help relieve nerve pain by blocking certain pain receptors and acting as an anti-inflammatory in order to regulate pain.[6]

Palmitoylethanolamide (PEA) (orally) has proved to be effective and safe in various clinical trials for nerve compression syndromes. PEA is an endogenous fatty acid amide and is available as a supplement (PeaPure and PeaPlex). In a pivotal randomized, double-blind, placebo-controlled clinical trial of 636 patients with sciatic pain, a significant and clinically relevant analgesic effect was documented for 300 mg and 600 mg PEA.[8] Similar results were obtained in a randomized clinical trial with 85 chronic sciatic patients. Quality of life and functionality related to the back improved significantly in favor of the PEA groups in both studies.[9,10]

Spinal Manipulation: Apart from surgery and epidural injections, manipulative treatment offers a more conservative and noninvasive approach.[11] The American College of Physicians recommends spinal manipulation as a first line treatment for back pain with or without sciatic (radicular) pain.[11]

Scleroderma

Scleroderma refers to a range of disorders causing hardening and tightening of the skin and connective tissues (blood vessels, muscles, and internal organs). Scleroderma results from an overproduction and accumulation of collagen in body tissues. It affects women four times more often than men and most commonly occurs between the ages of 30 and 50.

Scleroderma is a chronic autoimmune disease with two main types. (1) Localized scleroderma has two subtypes and only affects the skin. It often appears as thick, hard waxy patches (morphea type) or streaks (linear type) on the skin.Symptoms tend to come and go with flare-ups and periods of relatively stability. It is not uncommon for the condition to go away or to stop progressing without treatment.[1] Tightening of the skin can cause fingers to curl and lose their mobility. (2) Systemic scleroderma has three subtypes and can result in changes in the skin and muscles, circulation of blood, and extend to internal organs, especially the kidneys, lungs, heart, or digestive tract.

Symptoms may include generalized hardening, thickening, and tightening of the skin. or localized thickening over the skin on the face and fingers with telangiectasis, stiffness, feeling tired, poor blood flow to the fingers or toes with cold exposure (Raynaud's phenomenon), difficulty swallowing (esophageal dysmotility), and GERD. The most common early symptoms are Raynaud's and swelling of the distal extremities with thickening of the skin on the fingers of both hands. About 90% of systemic scleroderma patients will develop GI tract involvement during the course of the disease with the most common GI manifestation being gastroesophageal reflux disease (GERD). Interstitial lung disease and renal crisis are the major complications.[2] There is no cure for scleroderma and treatment is aimed at improving skin appearance and reducing tightness while limiting organ damage.

SKIN CARE MEASURES

Potassium Para-Aminobenzoate (PABA): It has been known for years that, in scleroderma, excess collagen is being produced in the skin and other organs. Several drugs are used that have in vitro (in the tissue culture) ability to reduce collagen production or to destabilize tissue collagen. The older medications in this category include colchicine and para-aminobenzoic acid (PABA).[3] Para-aminobenzoic acid has anti-fibrosis effects due to an ability to increase oxygen consumption by tissues which thereby decreases the progression of skin fibrosis and improves survival.[4]

PABA is an effective treatment for limited scleroderma.[5] In patients who received this treatment, the skin gradually became softer and progression of fibrosis decreased with subsequent increased range of motion. A retrospective study done to assess 390 scleroderma patients' response to PABA therapy showed a significant slowing in the progression of limited pulmonary function and vital capacity. Also, it showed a significant improvement in the 5-year and 10-year survival rate in patients who received adequate treatment.[6,7,8] PABA is FDA-approved for scleroderma.[9] A typical therapeutic dosage is 300–400 mg/day. Side effects have been noted in doses above 8,000 mg/day.[10]

Inositol Hexaniacinate (IHN): One patient with sclerodermal skin lesions was reported to have improved significantly on 1,200 mg IHN daily.[11]

Scorpion Stings

Scorpion stings present with immediate pain, numbness, and burning around the area of the injection site. Localized redness and edema occur shortly thereafter. Children are particularly sensitive to scorpion stings. Fortunately for healthy adults, most scorpion stings don't need medical treatment. If a child is stung, however, immediate medical care is necessary. The FDA has approved Anascorp as the first treatment specifically for young children and adults with a severe reaction to the sting of the *Centruroides* scorpion, the most common type in the U.S.

FIRST AID TREATMENT

- **Clean the wound** with mild soap and water.
- **Elevation of the affected limb** to the same level as the heart
- **Application of a cool compress** to the affected area for 10 minutes, followed by removal for 10 minutes, then reapplication for 10 minutes. This helps reduce pain and slow the venom's spread. This is most effective in the first two hours after a sting occurs.
- **Restriction of Diet:** The patient should not consume food or liquids if they are having difficulty swallowing.
- **Over-the-Counter Pain Relievers:** NSAIDs such as ibuprofen (Advil, Nuprin, Motrin IB, Children's Motrin), naproxen sodium (Aleve, Naprosyn), aspirin, or others, given as directed, can help ease discomfort.[1] NSAIDs relieve fever and pain and also reduce swelling.
- **Ascorbic Acid:** One physician reported a potent therapeutic action of ascorbic acid when given in larger repeated doses, 500–1,000 mg every four hours, preferably intravenously or intramuscularly. The effect in acute infectious processes is favorably comparable to that of the sulfonamide or the mycelial antibiotics. He used a single IV injection of vitamin C (1 gm) and obtained rapid recovery in a patient with a scorpion sting.[2]

Scurvy

Scurvy is a disease resulting from a lack of vitamin C. Humans cannot synthesize vitamin C which is necessary for making collagen, an important component in connective tissues including blood vessels. Vitamin C is also needed for synthesizing dopamine, norepinephrine, epinephrine, and carnitine, needed for energy production.[1]

Inadequate production of collagen can lead to anemia (due to vascular fragility and subsequent subcutaneous hemorrhages), weakness, exhaustion, swelling and pain in the limbs (especially the legs), slow healing, perifollicular hyperkeratotic papules (reddish/bluish bruise-like spots surrounding hair follicles) on the shins, ulceration of the gums with loose and lost teeth, and possibly even death.[1] In infants there can be malformation of bones and teeth. Modern cases of scurvy are relatively rare, but can still affect individuals who do not consume enough vitamin C.[2]

RESTORING VITAMIN C AVAILABILITY

Ascorbic Acid: Adult treatment involves administering vitamin C supplements by mouth or by injection at the following recommended doses:

- 1–2 gm/day for two to three days
- 500 mg/day for the next seven days
- 100 mg/day for one to three months[1]

Infants should be treated with 50 mg of ascorbic acid up to four times per day.[3]

Within 24 hours, patients can expect to see an improvement in fatigue, lethargy, pain, anorexia, and confusion. Bruising, bleeding, and weakness start to resolve within one to two weeks.

Seborrhea/Seborrheic Dermatitis/Dandruff

Seborrheic dermatitis (SD), or dandruff, is a chronic noncontagious inflammatory skin disorder that affects millions of Americans of all ages. The condition causes a red, flaking skin rash that can have a swollen and greasy appearance especially in the folds of the skin. It chiefly affects areas of body where sebaceous glands are most prominent such as the scalp, face, sides of the nose, eyebrows, behind the ears, or on the eyelids. The ear canals and chest or armpits can also be involved. On top of that rash, white to yellowish crusty scales accumulate on the surface and flake off.[1] Most individuals with seborrhea complain of itchy skin and dandruff where white flakes of dead skin fall off the scalp and onto the shoulders. It is a lifelong condition that comes and goes. Severe medical illnesses such as AIDS, Parkinson's disease, head injury, and stroke are associated with seborrheic dermatitis.[1] When a baby gets seborrhea, it is called "cradle cap."

COSMETIC SKIN CARE

Cleansing: Frequent cleansing with soap removes oils from affected areas and improves seborrhea.[2]

Shampoos: Standard medical treatment involves the frequent use of dandruff shampoos containing selenium sulfide (Selsun Blue) or zinc pyrithione (Head & Shoulders, Zincon, Dandrex) or ketoconazole (Nizoral A-D) and topical steroids if necessary.[3,4] Apply the shampoo to the scalp at the first part of the bathing/showering routine and then wait until the end to rinse it off. This technique maximizes the shampoo's contact time on the skin. For severe disease, keratolytics such as salicylic acid (Neutrogena T/Sal) or coal tar (Neutrogena T/Gel, DHS Tar) preparations may be used to suppress and remove dense scale.[4]

Hydrocortisone: For SD behind the ears, in the nasolabial folds, eyelid margins, and bridge of the nose, 1% hydrocortisone cream should be rubbed in two or three times daily, decreasing to once/day when SD is controlled.[5]

Vitamin B12: A group of patients with seborrheic dermatitis received vitamin B12 injections every one to three weeks. The results were that 43.5% were cured or greatly improved and an additional 43.5% showed moderate improvement.[6,7]

Riboflavin: Riboflavin deficiency is a cause of seborrheic dermatitis. Riboflavin 5–10 mg po once/day can be given until recovery. Other water-soluble vitamins should also be given because riboflavin deficiency occurs with other B vitamin deficiencies.[8] The diagnosis can be confirmed by a successful therapeutic trial.

B6, Biotin, or Zinc Deficiency: Seborrheic dermatitis can be a symptom of vitamin B6, biotin, and zinc deficiency.[9] B6 (pyridoxine) deficiency can cause itchy scaly SD rashes.[10] The medical rationale for using biotin to treat seborrheic dermatitis is that the vitamin intercepts the main metabolic pathways underlying the pathogenesis of the disease.[11] One symptom of zinc deficiency is dry scaly skin.[12] Deficiencies need to be corrected via supplementation.

Pyridoxine Cream: A topical cream containing vitamin B6 (50 milligrams per gram) was used by a group of patients. The seborrheic dermatitis cleared up in a large majority of the cases. In some cases, the seborrhea became abruptly worse for a day or two before improving.[13]

The following treatments have helped some individuals manage their seborrheic dermatitis:[14]

- **Tea tree oil** (Melaleuca oil), an essential oil from a shrub native to Australia, can be used either alone or in a shampoo that is applied to the affected area. Tea tree oil appears to be effective and well-tolerated when used daily as a 5% shampoo.[8] Tea tree oil has long been studied as a treatment for many skin conditions. It has antibacterial, antifungal, and anti-inflammatory qualities. Topical use of tea tree oil is safe, but it should be diluted with a carrier oil such as coconut or olive oil. 3–5 drops of tea tree oil can be mixed in one ounce of carrier oil before applying. This can help reduce itching and promote healing of scaly skin patches.[14,15]
- **Fish oil** (omega-3 fatty acids) is known for its anti-inflammatory qualities. Studies have shown that taking fish oil supplements (up to 3 gm/day) causes a reduction in the symptoms of various inflammatory skin conditions.[15,16]
- **Aloe Vera Gel:** Applying aloe gel may help manage redness and itching during SD flare-ups.[15,16]
- **Aloe vera supplements** have anti-inflammatory properties and research has shown that it is effective in treating SD. Aloe vera supplements (50–300 mg bid is a standard dose)[17] help suppress flare-ups and lessen their severity.[16]

- **Raw Honey:** Honey has long been recognized for antimicrobial and wound-healing properties. Raw honey, without any of the wax filtered out, improves its effectiveness in various skin conditions. Honey's ability to resolve seborrheic dermatitis was demonstrated in a small study where 20 patients applied 90% honey diluted in warm water and gently rubbed it onto their lesions every other day. The mix was left on for 2–3 hours. Itching and scaling disappeared in all patients after four weeks.[18]
- **Zinc Pyrithione Cream:** In addition to zinc pyrithione containing shampoos, a cream (DermaHarmony) has the same ingredient to treat symptoms and can be left on the skin.

CRADLE CAP

Cradle cap is harmless and usually goes away on its own within a few months.[2]

Shampoo: In infants, baby shampoo should be used daily and a 1% hydrocortisone cream rubbed in twice daily until the thick scale is gone.[19] For extra thick lesions on the scalp of a young child, 2% salicylic acid in olive oil or a corticosteroid gel (e.g., Alevicyn) can be applied at bedtime to affected areas and rubbed in with a toothbrush.

Biotin: Studies indicate that a deficiency of biotin can cause cradle cap.[17,20] Earlier studies recommended biotin (oral or parenteral doses of 10–30 mcg/day for two to three weeks) as a treatment for seborrheic dermatitis (cradle cap) in infants.[21,22,23]

Sepsis/Septic Shock

Sepsis is a life-threatening medical emergency. It is often the consequence of bacteria in the bloodstream (bacteremia). The body's overwhelming and detrimental response to a blood infection can lead to tissue damage, organ failure, and death. For example, in attempting to fight the infection, the body sends inflammatory cytokines and nitric oxide into the blood stream which can lead to vasodilation (from smooth muscle relaxation), blood clots, and leaky blood vessels (vascular permeability). As a result, blood flow is impaired and organs are deprived of nutrients and oxygen, leading to organ damage.[1] Sepsis occupies a continuum that ranges from mild to severe sepsis to septic shock and multiple organ dysfunction syndrome (MODS).[2]

Patients typically present with confusion or disorientation, in addition to fever or hypothermia, tachycardia, and low blood pressure, which is often refractory despite adequate fluid resuscitation.[3] Circulatory, cellular, and metabolic abnormalities are associated with a greater risk of mortality than with sepsis alone.[4] In critically ill patients, severe sepsis and septic shock are known as prime causes of mortality.[4]

NUTRITIONAL SUPPORT

Ascorbic Acid: In one study, 14 patients with septic shock who required a vasopressor drug to maintain mean arterial pressure >65 mm Hg were assigned to receive either 25 mg/kg intravenous ascorbic acid every six hours or a matching placebofor 72 hours.[4]

Administration of high-dose ascorbic acid significantly decreased the requirement for vasopressor's dose and duration in surgical critically ill patients with septic shock. Several mechanisms including anti-oxidant, anti-inflammatory, nitric oxide (NO) synthase inhibitory, reversing vascular hyporesponsiveness to vasopressors, increasing catecholamines and cortisol synthesis in adrenal medulla, and improving vascular endothelium integrity properties may justify the role of ascorbic acid in septic shock. In addition, no adverse event was detected in critically ill patients with burn injury who received ascorbic acid with a dose of 66 mg/kg/hour for 24 hours.[4]

High-dose ascorbic acid may be considered as an effective and safe adjuvant therapy in surgical critically ill patients with septic shock.[4]

In another study, 24 septic patients were randomized in a 1:1:1 ratio to receive high-dose ascorbic acid (200 mg/kg), low-dose ascorbic acid (50 mg/kg), or a placebo. Patients who received ascorbic acid had more rapid reduction in measures of organ injury, inflammation, and procalcitonin. There also appeared to be a dose-response relationship, with patients who received higher doses of ascorbic acid having more rapid clinical improvement.[5]

In a more recent study, 28 patients with vasopressor-dependent septic shock were randomized to 25 mg/kg of ascorbic acid every six hours or a placebo. Those in the ascorbic acid group required lower vasopressor doses and had lower mortality.[4]

Selenium: Two recent meta-analyses of randomized controlled trials found that intravenous selenium supplementation (as sodium selenite) in critically ill patients with systemic inflammatory response syndrome, sepsis, or septic shock resulted in significantly reducing the risk of mortality by 17% to 27%.[6,7]

Bromelain, Trypsin, and Rutin: A combination of bromelain, trypsin, and rutin has been administered as an adjuvant therapy in combination with antibiotics for children with sepsis.[8] Compared to antibiotics and a placebo, combining bromelain, trypsin, and rutin resulted in earlier improvement on the Glasgow Coma Scale, suggesting a benefit for children with sepsis.

Magnesium: Hypomagnesemia is a common development in critically ill sepsis patients and indicates a poor prognosis. Magnesium can be administered parenterally as a sulfate salt.[9]

Glutamine: A decrease in plasma concentration of glutamine is a prognostic factor for a poor outcome in sepsis. Supplementation (e.g., 20–25 gm/24 h) in critical situations such as trauma, burns, and sepsis has been shown to improve gut function, decrease septic complications, improve insulin sensitivity, and benefit survivability.[10,11]

REDUCTION AND/OR PREVENTION OF ENDOTOXIN-INDUCED INJURY AND MORTALITY

Choline Chloride: Apparently, choline diminishes endotoxin shock by preventing macrophage activation.[12] One method of treatment is with choline chloride 1.5–20 gm administered daily.[13] In animal studies, choline supplementation increased survival in a dose-dependent manner and prevented mortality completely after 2.5 or 5 mg/kg LPS. Choline also improved the microscopic appearance of the lungs and blunted increases in serum aspartate aminotransferase levels.

Glycine and Choline Chloride: Another method of treatment involves a mixture of glycine and choline. Glycine (2–60 gm/day) and choline (1.5–20 gm/day) can be combined in a ratio of choline/glycine at 1:5 or 1:20.[13]

Sickle Cell Anemia/Hemoglobin SS Disease

Sickle cell disease (SCD) is an inherited type of anemia affecting mostly people of African ancestry. An abnormal oxygen-carrying protein (hemoglobin S) found in red blood cells causes cells to deform into rigid, sickle-like shapes under circumstances (e.g., low oxygenation such as being at high altitudes, dehydration, illness, or going from a warm to a cold environment). These irregularly shaped cells do not flow well and can get stuck in small blood vessels, slowing or blocking blood flow and oxygen to parts of the body.

Early signs and symptoms of sickle cell disease include swelling of the hands and feet; symptoms of anemia, including fatigue, or extreme tiredness; and jaundice. Over time, sickle cell disease can lead to complications such as infections, delayed growth, and episodes of pain, called pain crises.[1] Neurologic complications are also common in sickle cell disease and include ischemic and hemorrhagic stroke, seizures, CNS infection, hearing loss, cognitive impairment, and, rarely, spinal cord infarction.[2] SCD can cause lifelong disabilities and reduces average life expectancy to about 40 years in the U.S.

CLINICAL APPROACHES

Smoking/Alcohol: SCD patients should avoid smoking and excessive alcohol intake.

Low oxygen levels (e.g., flying, climbing mountains, or visiting cities at a high altitude) tend to trigger painful episodes and should be avoided.

Iron Supplements: Taking iron supplements could harm a person with sickle cell disease and is to be avoided because the extra iron builds up in the body (hemosiderosis) and can cause damage to the organs.[1]

Vitamin E: The administration of 450 units of vitamin E per day for six to 36 weeks to patients with sickle cell anemia has been found to produce a significant reduction in the number of irreversibly sickled erythrocytes. Adult patients with sickle cell anemia have been reported to have significantly lower serum tocopherol values than do normal control subjects. In children with sickle cell anemia, those with vitamin E deficiency were found to have significantly more irreversibly sickled cells than did children without vitamin E deficiency.[3,4]

Vitamin D: Vitamin D deficiency is associated with acute pain in SCD.[5]

Zinc: Zinc supplements appear to decrease the risk for complications and infections related to sickle cell disease. Oral zinc helps reduce symptoms of sickle cell disease in patients who also have zinc deficiency.[6]

Sinusitis (Acute)

Inflammation or infection of any of the sinuses surrounding the nose is sinusitis, or rhinosinusitis. Inflammation causes nasal passages to become swollen with nasal obstruction due to a mucus buildup. There are acute and chronic types of sinusitis. Most cases will resolve without treatment.[1]

MEASURES FOR CARE

Symptom Relief: Topically or orally administered decongestants, proteolytic enzymes, nasal irrigation with salt water, mucolytic agents, and antihistamines have all been used for symptom relief in acute bacterial sinusitis.[2]

Amoxicillin of No Effect: Some 214 patients with acute maxillary sinusitis were randomly assigned to receive amoxicillin (750 mg three times a day for seven days) or a placebo, in a double-blind trial. Amoxicillin had no effect on the clinical course of the sinusitis. The incidence of side effects was significantly greater in the antibiotic group than in the placebo group (28% vs. 9%).[3]

Glutathione: A small study performed in the Netherlands found that people suffering with sinusitis have low amounts of glutathione, an antioxidant compound that can be found in fruits and vegetables such as watermelon, grapefruit, oranges, asparagus, potatoes, and broccoli. The glutathione contained in these foods may help the cells that line the respiratory tract keep free radicals in check.[4]

Bromelain: In a double-blind trial, 48 patients with moderately severe to severe sinusitis received bromelain or a placebo for six days. All patients were placed on standard therapy for sinusitis, which included antihistamines, analgesics, and antibiotics. Upon completion of the study, inflammation was reduced in 83% of those taking bromelain compared to 52% of the placebo group.[5]

Gentian: Research studies show that taking gentian as part of a combination herbal product (containing 12 mg of gentian root and 36 mg each of European elder flower, verbena, sorrel, and cowslip flower) three times daily improves symptoms from sinus infections. Taking gentian as part of a combination herbal product along with a prescription steroid nasal spray (Nasonex) seems to reduce the symptoms of a sinus infection better than taking the steroid nasal spray alone.[6]

Ancillary treatments, such as humidifiers, vaporizers, and saline nasal sprays or drops used to moisturize the nasal canal and impair crusting of secretions, benefit many patients.

Smell Perception/Anosmia/Parosmia

Anosmia is the complete loss of smell. Nasal congestion is a common cause of temporary anosmia. Loss of smell from nasal polyps, sinusitis, upper respiratory tract infection, or fractures is due to intranasal swelling or other obstruction that prevents odors from gaining access to the olfactory area. Neurologic causes include head trauma and viral infections, as well as aging or Alzheimer's. A number of other conditions can cause anosmia as well. Parosmia, or dysosmia, describes a distortion or perversion of the sense of smell. What typically happens is that natural and pleasant odors are perceived as offensive and disgusting. Additional causes can include Alzheimer's, Huntington's, or Parkinson's, and olfactory damage from head injury, bacterial or viral infection, toxic chemicals, radiation, or chemotherapy, etc. Neurologists have used sodium valproate, gabapentin, and pregabalin to treat parosmia for decades with good results.[1]

THERAPEUTIC MEASURES

Medications and compounds such as alcohol, nicotine, and organic solvents, or the direct application of zinc salts may alter normal smell sensitivity. Offending medications or substances should be avoided. Neurologists have used sodium valproate (to be avoided in women with childbearing potential), gabapentin, and pregabalin to treat parosmia for decades with good results.[1]

Zinc Sulfate (ZnSO4): In addition to correcting any underlying known causes, zinc sulphate has been utilized with success in the management of anosmia. In a prospective study with 95 patients suffering from post-traumatic olfactory disorders, significant improvement of self-assessed olfactory performance was reported in two of four patients receiving zinc sulfate (300 mg/day) for longer than one month.[2]

Vitamin A: The epithelial degeneration associated with vitamin A deficiency can cause anosmia.[3] Vitamin A has been reported to normalize olfactory performance in malabsorption conditions or A-β-lipoproteinemia. One study reported a significant improvement in a patient with vitamin A deficiency due to alcoholic liver cirrhosis undergoing a 4-week therapy with oral vitamin A (10 mg/day).[4]

B12: Olfactory losses also occur in vitamin B12 deficiency.[3]

Salt Water Rinse: Rinsing the inside of the nose with a salt water solution may help if the sense of smell is affected by an infection or allergy.[5]

Smoking (Cessation)

Cigarette smoking is the leading preventable cause of death in the U.S. Smokers are far more likely to develop coronary heart disease, stroke, lung cancer, and COPD. Smoking increases the chances of acquiring type 2 diabetes, rheumatoid arthritis, bladder cancer, leukemia, and many other types of cancer.[1] Smoking is a practice wherein tobacco smoke is breathed in and absorbed into the bloodstream. Nicotine in cigarette smoke is an appetite suppressant that speeds up the heart and elevates blood pressure, as well as increasing the calories that the body burns. It is also a highly addictive drug. To quit smoking is a very difficult endeavor for most. Cessation counseling may be necessary for some patients.

QUITTING STRATEGIES

Nicotine Replacement: The most popular method to quit smoking is nicotine replacement. Many products are available without prescription in patches, gum, inhalers, and lozenges.

L-Tryptophan (5-HTP): Tryptophan (50 mg/kg/day) relaxes and eases nicotine cravings. It helps people quit smoking when used with conventional treatment.[2,3,4,5] 5-HTP reduces some nicotine withdrawal symptoms such as teeth chattering and shakes by increasing brain serotonin, which improves mood.

High CHO Diet: A low-protein, high-carbohydrate diet increases the synthesis of brain serotonin and thus helps with mood.[6]

Vitamin C: Women who are unable to quit smoking during their pregnancy may reduce the harm smoking does to their baby's lungs by taking vitamin C (500 mg/day), according to a new randomized controlled trial.[7] Vitamin C can also largely stop the serious depletion of vitamin E that occurs in smokers.[8]

Vitamin E (Gamma Tocopherol): A total of 30 smokers in their twenties who had smoked at least half a pack per day for a year participated in a study. All participants stopped smoking and 16 received 500 milligrams daily of gamma tocopherol while 14 received a placebo.[9] After seven days of not smoking, participants who took gamma tocopherol saw an increase in their vascular function by an average of 4.3%. This translates to a 55.9 % drop in the risk of developing heart disease later in life.

E-Cigarettes: Individuals attempting to quit smoking should try FDA-approved smoking cessation products before e-cigarettes because of the lack of evidence that e-cigarettes aid in smoking cessation.[10] Multiple studies have not supported the efficacy of using e-cigarettes for cigarette cessation.[11,12]

Solar Urticaria/Sun Allergy

Solar urticaria, also known as sun allergy, is a rare allergy to sunlight that causes a red rash to form on skin that is exposed to the sun. Itchy, reddish spots or welts usually appear within minutes of sun exposure.[1] The reaction may subside in a few minutes or last an hour or more. If large areas of the body are affected, the loss of fluid into the skin may result in light-headedness, headache, nausea, and vomiting. The mean age of onset is 35 years, but it has occurred in infants and individuals up through the age of 70.[1]

CLINICAL CARE

Avoidance of Sun Exposure: Prevention is the most important treatment, so sun exposure should be avoided and, if that is not possible, then exposure should be minimized by wearing a broad spectrum sunscreen with SPF >30.

Vitamin D: Chronic spontaneous urticaria (CSU) is associated with low D3 concentrations and a higher prevalence of vitamin D deficiency. If the serum level of vitamin D was less than 30 ng/ml, subjects in one study were treated with a vitamin D2 supplement at a dose of 20,000 IU/day.[2] After six weeks, these patients showed significant improvements compared with the non-vitamin D supplement group. This study revealed a significant association of lower serum vitamin D concentrations with CSU. Vitamin D supplements might improve symptoms and quality of life in CSU patients.[2]

Beta-Carotene: It has recently been reported that, in one case, oral beta-carotene was a useful therapeutic agent for solar urticaria.[3,4]

Antihistamines: Whether prescription or over-the-counter, antihistamines are a treatment mainstay to block wheal response and to minimize pruritus.[5] However, antihistamines are generally inadequate because most patients have an extremely low UV threshold.[6]

Steatorrhea

Steatorrhea is the presence of excess fat in the feces with symptoms of foul-smelling, foamy, frothy, or mucous-filled stools, bloating, and diarrhea. Steatorrhea can happen simply from eating a meal high in fat and fiber or potassium oxalate.[1] Severe or long-term symptoms of steatorrhea may be a sign of a medical condition, such as a malabsorption disorder, enzyme deficiency, or gastrointestinal disease.[2] Since steatorrhea is caused by decreased absorption of fat by the intestine, there are also typically significant losses of calcium, magnesium, and fat-soluble vitamins. Many different medical conditions can cause steatorrhea. For that reason, the best treatment is contingent upon the underlying diagnosed condition causing the fatty stools.

GENERAL MEASURES

Smoking should be stopped or reduced.

Diet: Maintaining an adequate diet that is rich in fresh fruits and vegetables, with a reduced fat intake, is recommended to prevent steatorrhea (fatty stool). Alcohol intake should be reduced or even completely eliminated. Foods high in potassium oxalate should also be limited.[3]

- Dietary intake of fat-soluble vitamins by taking supplemental fat-soluble vitamins A, D, E, and K should be increased.
- Dietary intake of vitamin B12, folic acid, iron, magnesium, and calcium should also be increased.

Over-the-counter antidiarrheal medications, including loperamide (Imodium) and bismuth subsalicylate (Kaopectate, Pepto-Bismol), can be helpful.

Over-the-counter antacids, anti-bloating, and gas medications can also be helpful.[2]

Supplements like pancreatic enzymes (e.g., lipase, protease, and amylase) can be helpful and are good for those who are suffering from pancreatic enzyme deficiency.[4]

Magnesium and calcium levels should be monitored and supplementation given accordingly.

Bile salt therapy was effective in a case study where a patient underwent a colectomy, partial ileectomy, and ileostomy for Crohn's disease. There was concern that bile salt therapy would cause or exacerbate severe diarrhea, but this did not happen.[3] Oral bile acid supplementation reduced fat excretion markedly, but did not aggravate diarrhea in this case and in another study.[5,6]

Stroke

A stroke is the sudden death or damage of brain cells (neurological deficit) caused by a lack of oxygen and nutrients due to a disruption of blood supply. Stroke is the fifth leading cause of death in the U.S. and is a major cause of serious disability for adults.[1] When the blood supply to a specific region of the brain is blocked (88% of cases), or ruptures out (12% of cases), those affected areas begin to die within minutes. Therefore, a stroke is a medical emergency. The advent of a stroke is sudden with potentially long-lasting and far-reaching negative consequences.

Ideally, a stroke patient should receive treatment at a hospital within three hours of their symptoms first appearing.[1] Initial symptoms can include weakness or numbness in the face, arm, or leg; loss of speech or difficulty communicating; unstable walking or loss of balance; and a sudden, severe headache, or loss of vision. Stroke is both preventable and treatable.

Major risk factors associated with stroke include old age, hypertension, smoking, diabetes mellitus, hyperlipidemia, atrial fibrillation, myocardial infarction, congestive heart failure, and acute alcohol abuse. African Americans have about twice the risk of a first-time stroke and a significantly higher risk of death from stroke.

RESEARCH RESULTS FOR STROKE PREVENTION

Minimize Risk Factors: As part of preventing stroke, risk factors must be reduced or eliminated. These include:

- High blood pressure
- Cigarette smoking or exposure to secondhand smoke
- High cholesterol
- Diabetes

- Obesity
- Obstructive sleep apnea
- Cardiovascular disease, including heart failure, heart defects, heart infection, or abnormal heart rhythm
- Illicit drug use (e.g., cocaine, heroin, PCP, amphetamines, etc.)

Folic Acid: There is a benefit of taking folic acid for stroke prevention. Folate supplementation (0.5–15 mg/day) reduced the risk for stroke by 18%, a significant benefit compared with a placebo.[1] The largest improvements in stroke risk were seen in people who took folic acid supplements for more than three years (29% lower risk).[1]

In two of seven RCTs, folic acid reduced the risk for stroke (RR, 0.80; 95% CI, 0.69–0.93; $P = .003$), with no heterogeneity and moderate-quality evidence. A meta-analysis of seven studies also showed a similar benefit for folic acid driven by the China Stroke Primary Prevention Trial (CSPPT).[2]

Magnesium: Stroke patients have been shown to have a deficiency of magnesium, both in the blood stream and in the cerebrospinal fluid (the fluid that surrounds the brain).

Magnesium deficiency increases the risk that the carotid arteries (in the neck) or the arteries in the brain will go into spasm and choke off the blood supply to the brain. This impairment of cerebral blood flow could lead to a transient ischemic attack (TIA aka pre-stroke) or a stroke.[3,4]

B Vitamins: High doses of B vitamins may also help prevent stroke in high-risk people. People who took the B vitamins were 25% less likely to suffer a stroke.[5] For decades, physicians have known that a rare, inherited form of severe hyperhomocysteinemia causes premature heart attacks and strokes. Most researchers believe that the evidence supports a causal relationship between hyperhomocysteinemia and coronary heart disease. B vitamin deficiencies are reported to be the prime determinant of elevated hyperhomocysteine levels in the blood.[6] One study looked at 1,160 adults aged 67–96 years and found that 29.3% had homocysteine levels greater than 14 umol/L.[7] Low levels of B vitamins played a role in 67% of these cases. People can safely reduce their homocysteine level with B vitamin supplements.[8]

Riboflavin: Taking riboflavin by mouth for 12 weeks decreased levels of homocysteine by up to 40% in some people. Also, taking riboflavin along with folic acid and pyridoxine lowers homocysteine levels by 26% in people with high homocysteine levels caused by drugs that are used to prevent seizures.[9]

Ascorbic Acid: A new study found a link between vitamin C depletion and increased risk for intracerebral hemorrhage (ICH). In a case-control study, researchers found vitamin C depletion was more common among ICH cases than matched controls. This original study suggested that a low plasma vitamin C concentration is a risk for spontaneous intracerebral hemorrhages. This link is probably associated with the role of vitamin C in blood pressure regulation and collagen biosynthesis.[10]

Aspirin is an antiplatelet agent approved by the Food and Drug Administration for secondary stroke prevention. Studies reflect that daily low-dose aspirin demonstrated a statistically significant reduction in nonfatal strokes.[11,12] One study involved more than 14,000 Japanese patients over 60 years old and found that the positive benefits of aspirin therapy outweighed the risks for those 50–59 years of age who have a 10-year cardiovascular risk of < 10%.[12,13]

Reducing LDL helps to lower the risk of recurrent stroke. In a French study, reducing LDL to a mean of 66 mg/dL was associated with a 26% risk reduction for the composite endpoint of ischemic stroke, MI, new symptoms requiring urgent coronary or carotid revascularization, and vascular death.[14]

Post-Stroke Management (Brain Hypoxia/Ischemic Damage)

Brain function is characterized by high expenditure of energy and low energy reserve. Therefore, the brain is extremely sensitive to hypoxia, particularly in specific brain regions, such as the cortex and hippocampus. The goals during and after ischemia and hypoxia from a stroke are to reduce ongoing neurologic injury, prevent stroke recurrence, and lessen the risk for mortality.

MINIMIZING SECONDARY BRAIN DAMAGE

Ginkgo biloba protects the brain during hypoxia/ischemia (stroke) and seizure. There is substantial experimental evidence to support the view that ginkgo biloba extracts have neuroprotective properties under conditions such as hypoxia/ischemia, seizure activity, and peripheral nerve damage.[1]

Glycine is used as therapy for ischemic stroke.[2,3] Sublingual application of glycine (1.0–2.0 gm/day) started within six hours after the onset of acute ischemic stroke in the carotid artery territory (and continued for five days) helped limit brain damage, was safe, and can exert favorable clinical effects.[3]

Vitamin E is well known to have neuroprotective effects. Studies have demonstrated brain protection in animals with induced hypoxia who were given vitamin E.[4,5,6]

Vitamin D: Several lines of evidence show that vitamin D has neuroprotective effects following ischemic brain injury. Results show a direct protective effect of vitamin D3 against ischemic injury in vitro in cerebral endothelial cells.[7,8]

Docosahexaenoic Acid (DHA): DHA, a component of fish oil, is a powerful therapeutic agent that can protect brain tissue and promote recovery per an experimental model of acute ischemic stroke, even when treatment is delayed by up to five hours.[9]

Citicoline: In treatment of patients with acute ischemic cerebrovascular disease (stroke), citicoline accelerated recovery of consciousness and motor deficit, achieved a better final outcome, and facilitated rehabilitation of these patients.[10] Stroke patients who took citicoline (e.g., 500–2,000 mg/day) by mouth within 24 hours of having an ischemic stroke were more likely than other ischemic stroke patients to have a complete recovery within three months.[11]

PREVENTING RECURRENCE OF ISCHEMIC STROKE

Aspirin (50–350 mg/day): The early use of early aspirin (e.g., 48 hours after ischemic stroke) to reduce long-term death and disability is supported by two large, randomized clinical trials. In the International Stroke Trial (IST), aspirin 300 mg/day significantly reduced stroke recurrence within the first two weeks resulting in a significant decrease in death and dependency at six months. Aspirin should not be taken within 24 hours of the administration of tPA.[12]

Lifestyle Factors: In addition to minimizing risk factors (*see* Stroke), healthy, low-salt, and Mediterranean diets, along with regular physical activity are are recommended for preventing a second ischemic stroke.[13]

LESSENING MORTALITY

Exercise: The results of a large Canadian study demonstrated that 10 hours of exercise per week (measured in metabolic equivalents) reduced the risk of death by over 50%. There was a 79% reduction in mortality risk in those under 75.[14]

Subacute Combined Degeneration of the Spinal Cord

Subacute combined degeneration of the spinal cord refers to the progressive degeneration of the posterior and lateral columns of the spinal cord as a result of vitamin B12 deficiency (most common), vitamin E deficiency,[1] copper or folic acid deficiency, or recreational use of nitrous oxide inhalation.[2]

The disorder is characterized by progressive symptoms of paresthesias (sensation of pins and needles) in both hands and feet along with spastic paralysis. These sensations tend to be constant and gradually worsen. Affected individuals may not be able to feel vibrations and may lose the sense of where their limbs are (position sense). The limbs can feel stiff, movements become clumsy, and walking may become difficult. Reflexes may be decreased, increased, or absent.[3] Subacute combined degeneration can further be characterized by mild distal weakness in the lower limbs, bilateral Babinski responses, unsteady gait, and positive Romberg sign. Paraplegia, incontinence, dementia, and visual loss can result from continued degeneration.

THERAPEUTIC OPTIONS

Vitamin B12 is necessary for the formation and maintenance of myelin (fatty sheath) surrounding nerve cells and speeding transmission of nerve signals.[4] Atrophy of the gastric mucosa is followed after several months, in some cases by subacute combined degeneration of the spinal cord because the body cannot absorb vitamin B12.[5] Older adults, particularly those who follow a vegetarian or vegan diet, have an increased risk of vitamin B12 deficiency. Certain drugs (metformin, proton pump inhibitors, and histamine [H-2] receptor antagonists) may also lead to a B12 deficiency.[6] Treatment is with vitamin B12 (100 mcg cyanocobalamin) intramuscularly daily for one week, then weekly for one month, and then monthly for the remainder of the patient's life.[7] Large doses of vitamin B12 taken by mouth can be used if vitamin B12 deficiency is mild and symptoms of nerve damage have not developed.[3] When the cause is vitamin B12 deficiency, treatment with cyanocobalamin will fully or partially reverse the disorder.

Vitamin E supplementation is needed if deficiency is the underlying cause.

Copper: There is growing clinical evidence supporting a connection between copper deficiency and subacute combined degeneration.[8] Copper deficiency must be corrected as this may partially reverse the clinical findings.[9]

Subcorneal Pustular Dermatosis (SPD)

SPD is a rare skin disease in which discreet pus-filled pimples or blisters (pustules) or grouped vesicles form in crops under the top (subcorneal) layer of the skin, predominantly on the flexor surfaces. They usually appear on the trunk, particularly in the skin folds such as the armpits and groin. They may appear on otherwise normal skin, but often are present within a red patch. The pustules resolve over a few days and are replaced by fine scale before there is another relapse and new pustules form again.[1] This condition is more common in middle-aged adults, especially women, but has also been reported in children.[2]

DERMATOLOGICAL CARE

Vitamin E: Good results have been reported using oral vitamin E (300–1,600 IU/day). Owing to the safety and good results from this therapy, it should be added onto any ongoing medical treatment.[3,4]

Sunburn

Excessive exposure of the skin to the rays of the sun or other UV light burns the skin. The result is red, tender, or painful skin that feels hot to the touch. Blisters may develop later. The burn is usually evident about 2–6 hours after exposure. Sunburns are graded as pink, red, and blistering. Severe cases can be complicated by extensive burning, blistering, dehydration, electrolyte imbalance, and possible infection. One or more blistering sunburns in childhood or adolescence more than doubles a person's chances of developing melanoma later in life, according to the Skin Cancer Foundation.[1]

PREVENTION

Sunscreen or Sunblock: Para-aminobenzoic acid (PABA) 5% or its esters in ethyl alcohol or in a cream or gel are quite effective in helping to prevent sunburn from ultraviolet B rays. Sunscreens with SPF rating at 15 or higher are recommended. Fair-skinned people need an SPF rating of 30 or more. For protection against ultraviolet A rays, it is recommended to use a sunscreen that contains at least one of the following: ecamsule, avobenzone, oxybenzone, titanium dioxide, sulisobenzone, or zinc oxide.[2]

Ascorbic Acid: Taking vitamin C by mouth along with vitamin E might prevent sunburn. But taking vitamin C alone does not prevent sunburn.[3] Vitamin C can also be applied topically to the skin for extra protection.

Selenium (plus copper) and a vitamin complex (with tocopherol and retinal) were examined for their ability to prevent sun burn cell formation in human skin. After three weeks of oral supplementation, there was relative protection (versus a placebo) against ultraviolet-induced cell damage. Supplementation was ineffective in preventing light-induced skin redness (erythema).[4]

Vitamin A: In one study, 1,668 adult vacationers with sunburn received tablets containing 35,000 IU of vitamin A combined with 120 mg of calcium carbonate.[3] The usual dosage was two tablets per day starting two days before sun exposure. Two-thirds of the people who took vitamin A rated their sunburn as less severe than usual. Of the 630 individuals who had a history of severe or moderately severe sunburn, 90.6% reported improvement, with 51% experiencing complete freedom from the symptoms of sunburn. Individuals with blonde hair seemed to benefit the most, whereas those with auburn hair benefited the least.[5]

TREATMENT

Vitamins E and C: Taking high doses of vitamin E by mouth together with vitamin C protects against skin inflammation after exposure to UV radiation.[6]

Over-the-counter pain relievers can help.

Cool compresses with equal parts of milk and water, or cold tap water compresses, or cold compresses with a Burow's solution from any pharmacy can soothe burned skin.

Aloe vera gel or lotion applied to the burn area can be beneficial.

Witch hazel has soothing anti-inflammatory properties. Apply witch hazel directly to sunburn using a cloth or cotton ball. It may be especially soothing to combine witch hazel with aloe vera.[7]

Tardive Dyskinesia (TD)

Tardive dyskinesia (TD) is an involuntary repetitive movement disorder mostly affecting the face, lips, jaws, and tongue. TD causes frequent grimacing, tongue protrusion, lip smacking, puckering and pursing, or rapid eye blinking. Repetitive, stiff, jerky body movements of the upper extremities, lower extremities, and trunk can also occur.

TD is the result of treatment with neuroleptic medications that function as dopamine blockers in the treatment of psychiatric disorders and can induce extrapyramidal symptoms. Not everyone who takes neuroleptics will acquire the disorder. Some drugs that treat nausea (e.g., Compazine, Reglan) can also cause TD if they are taken for more than three months.[1]

TD can be associated with significant and often irreversible functional impairment, reducing the quality of life and increasing social withdrawal. Major risk factors for TD include older individual and cumulative exposure to dopamine receptor blocking agents. There are two FDA-approved prescription treatments for TD: valbenazine and deutetrabenazine.

SUPPLEMENTAL MANAGEMENT OPTIONS

Pyridoxine, or vitamin B6, starting at 100 mg/day and increasing over four weeks to 400 mg/day with doses of 1,200 gm/day, in one study demonstrated significant benefit for tardive dyskinesia.[2] Higher doses up to 1,400 mg/day may have even greater benefits.[3]

Tocopherol: Taking vitamin E (600–1,600 IU/day) by mouth is reported to improve symptoms associated with the movement disorder.[4,5] At least 12 studies on the use of vitamin E in treating tardive dyskinesia were performed before 1996. Nine of the 12 studies reported some improvement with vitamin E in at least a portion of the study subjects. The dosages of vitamin E used were from 1,200–1,600 IU/day for periods of four weeks to a few months.[6,7]

Manganese and Vitamin B3 (Nicotinic Acid): Manganese is found in high concentration in the extrapyramidal system (corpus striatum/putamen). One researcher demonstrated dramatic results in treating TD with manganese (15–60 mg/day) and vitamin B3 (100–500 mg/day).[8]

Ginkgo biloba may also be effective in diminishing symptoms from tardive dyskinesia.[9] Research shows that taking a specific ginkgo extract (EGb 761) for 12 weeks can reduce the severity of tardive dyskinesia symptoms in people with schizophrenia who are taking antipsychotic drugs.[10]

Choline Chloride: When choline chloride (150–200 mg/kg/day, orally) was given to patients with tardive dyskinesia, several patients improved.[11]

Taste Disorders

Taste disorders have three broad descriptions. Hypogeusia is a reduced ability to taste things while dysgeusia is a distortion in taste sensation. A complete lack of taste is referred to as ageusia. The complaint of "loss of taste" is more often related to a loss of smell than to true impairment of taste. (*See also* Smell Perception.)[1] Causes of hypogeusia can include nutritional deficiencies; upper respiratory tract and middle ear infections; radiation therapy (head and neck cancers); exposure to some chemicals; head injury; surgery to the ear, nose, and throat; poor oral hygiene; dental problems; and certain antibiotics and antihistamines.[2] Illnesses such as chronic renal failure or stroke, idiopathic causes, and medicines such as phenytoin may also be responsible.[3,4]

IMPROVING SENSORY FUNCTION

General Measures: Offending chemicals and medications should be avoided if possible and any underlying causes addressed.

Nutritional Deficiencies: Distortion or decrease in taste sensation associated with zinc or magnesium deficiency is well documented.[5] There are other nutritional causes of hypogeusia including decreased copper and nickel levels.[6]

Vitamin B: Nutritional deficiencies including a lack of vitamin B can affect taste and may be caused by anorexia, malabsorption, and/or increased urinary losses. Restoring normal vitamin B levels can help achieve normal taste sensation.[3,4]

Nicotine: Patients who quit smoking typically have improved olfactory function and flavor sensation over time.[4]

ALA, Ginkgo Biloba, Pilocarpine: Various treatment methods have been used to improve taste sensation. These include the use of pilocarpine, alpha lipoic acid, and ginkgo biloba.[7]

Zinc Sulphate: Taking zinc supplements (zinc sulphate 220 mg tid) may be beneficial in treating taste disorders.[7,8]

Testosterone

Testosterone is a steroid hormone that stimulates development of male secondary sexual characteristics. Testosterone is a male sex hormone, but females also produce small amounts of it. It is produced mainly in the testes, but also in ovaries and the adrenal cortex.[1] Falling testosterone levels are a normal part of aging in males, but certain medical conditions can hasten the decline. Unfortunately, testosterone can fuel the growth of prostate cancer so supplements should not be taken in certain medical situations without consulting a physician.[2] For females, high testosterone levels can lead to symptoms of such as acne, deep voice, excess hair on the face and body, thinning hair, irregular periods, etc.

ELEVATING FREE TESTOSTERONE LEVELS

Oral DHEA supplementation (50 mg/day) increased circulating DHEA-S and free testosterone levels well above baseline in a middle-aged group, with no significant effect on total testosterone levels. A younger group of men in the same study had no significant changes in testosterone levels. These results demonstrate that oral DHEA supplementation can elevate free testosterone levels in middle-aged men.[3]

Fish oil as a source of omega-3 fatty acids for three months has been found to be associated, in a dose response manner, with a higher free testosterone to luteinizing hormone ratio in young men.[4]

LOWERING TESTOSTERONE LEVELS

Stinging nettle appears to interfere with the synthesis of dihydrotestosterone. Research suggests that taking nettle leaf extract (e.g., 770 mg bid) for about four months was as effective as standard therapy for improving menstrual cycle conditions and for decreasing facial hair, oily skin, or acne in women with high testosterone levels.[5]

Saw palmetto (e.g., 160 mg twice a day) has estrogenic activity and reduces plasma testosterone concentration.[6]

Thrombophlebitis/Superficial Vein Thrombosis

Thrombophlebitis is an inflammation of a superficial vein wall causing a clot, or thrombus formation. Most cases of superficial vein thrombosis occur in the legs (e.g., long or short saphenous veins) in association with varicosities. In the upper extremity, the condition can develop after use of an IV line or other trauma to the vein wall. Pain, warmth, swelling, and tenderness are often present over the clot site. Superficial thrombophlebitis is generally a benign and short-term condition. Symptoms typically resolve in one to two weeks.[1] Most times, treatment of superficial thrombophlebitis is directed to managing pain and inflammation.[2]

MANAGEMENT METHODS

NSAIDs: Using over-the-counter anti-inflammatory medications and warm compresses may be helpful for treating pain.[3]

Bromelain: Bromelain is a complex mix of proteolytic enzymes. Combined bromelain and antibiotic therapy was shown to be more effective than antibiotics alone in the treatment of thrombophlebitis.[4,5] In a study involving 73 patients, bromelain decreased symptoms of inflammation including skin temperature, tenderness, edema, pain, and disability.[5,6] It is thought that the best results occur at a dose of 750–1,000 mg/day.[7]

Heat application with rest and elevation of the legs is a standard treatment method if there is an elevated risk of a DVT.[3]

Compression stockings can also be used to lower risks of developing a DVT.[3]

Tick Bites

Ticks get onto the skin, tend to move to a warm moist location, and then bite onto the skin to attach themselves. Next, they burrow into the skin and feed on blood. Ticks are most often found on the head, scalp, or neck. Most tick bites are painless and cause minor redness and swelling. However, some ticks can cause illness or infection such as Lyme disease, anaplasmosis/ehrlichiosis, spotted fever rickettsiosis, babesiosis, tularemia, and Powassan virus. A tick should be removed as soon as it is found to help prevent disease. Symptoms of weakness, paralysis, fever, lethargy, numbness, headache, or rash (especially an expanding rash) are reasons to seek medical care. According to the CDC, tick-borne diseases are increasing nationally.[1]

TREATMENT STRATEGIES

Removal: The tick can be grasped with clean, fine-tipped forceps or tweezers. The tick should be pulled out smoothly and gently without twisting. After the tick is removed, the bite area should be cleaned with rubbing alcohol or soap and water. For tick paralysis, tick removal is curative.[2]

Medical Assistance: If there is difficulty removing the tick, medical assistance may be required.

Kill the Tick: If the tick cannot be removed, another option is to kill it. The Australasian Society of Clinical Immunology and Allergy (ASCIA) recommends using aerosol "freezing" sprays normally associated with wart treatments (e.g., Wart-Off Freeze). Avoid spraying on the face, groin, and armpit areas. Once killed, the tick can then be left to fall out naturally.[3]

Tinnitus

Tinnitus, or ringing in the ears, is a perceived sound that is unrelated to an external noise source. The sensation is often described as a high-pitched ringing, roaring, buzzing, hissing, screeching, whistling, whooshing, or other sounds. Tinnitus can be temporary, or chronic and persistent. Symptoms are often worse when background noise is minimal, so the individual is often most aware of it at night when trying to fall asleep.

Tinnitus affects about 50 million Americans and usually occurs after the age of 50. Causes include chronic hearing loss, diseases of the ear or head, neck trauma, and acoustic trauma (exposure to loud noises). It can lead to problems getting to sleep and getting back to sleep, difficulty with concentration, poor work or school performance, frustration, anxiety, and depression. Medications such as aspirin, methotrexate or cisplatin, bumetanide, ethacrynic acid or furosemide (Lasix), and certain antidepressants can cause or worsen tinnitus.[1]

REDUCING TINNITUS SYMPTOMS

Medications: Large aspirin doses (e.g., 12 or more 325 mg tablets per day) typically cause or worsen tinnitus.[1] For many patients, tinnitus can improve by eliminating ototoxic medications as listed above.

Ginkgo Biloba: Many patients have taken ginkgo biloba or minerals such as magnesium with varying results.[2]

Zinc Supplementation: In one study, taking 50 mg of zinc daily for two months reduced tinnitus symptoms in 46% of subjects.[3]

Glutamic acid functions as the primary and secondary afferent cochlear transmitter or at least an agonist of the main transmitter. Supplementation at 1,000–2,000 mg/day can be quite beneficial.[3]

Niacin has been used as a therapy for tinnitus for years with variable success. Niacin is thought to provide smooth muscle relaxation and increase blood flow to the tiny blood vessels that supply the inner ear. Patients often sustain a blush when taking niacin in effective doses. About half of all patients with tinnitus report successful treatment with niacin.[4] Nicotinic acid improves microcirculation to the inner ear and thus increases oxygenation to cochlear structures. Niacin up to 2,000 mg/day is helpful when tinnitus is associated with diminished circulation.[5]

Vitamin A: Individuals with dietary deficiencies of vitamin A acquired both improvement in their hearing and reduction of tinnitus with vitamin A therapy. However, those with more normal diets did not benefit from increased intake of vitamin A.[6]

Alcohol: Curiously, some tinnitus sufferers apparently find that small amounts of alcohol assist in tinnitus control.[7] Of theoretical and practical interest is the nature of the assistance. It is possible that the primary contribution of alcohol is to foster general relaxation and improve coping ability.[6]

B vitamins may also be an effective treatment.[8]

Removing ear wax can lessen tinnitus symptoms.[9]

Tooth Loss

See also Periodontal Disease

Tooth loss is a process in which one or more teeth come loose and fall out. Periodontal disease is the leading reason for tooth loss.

PREVENTION

Calcium (500 mg/day) and vitamin D3 (700 IU/day) by mouth for three years appear to help prevent tooth loss in elderly people.[1,2]

Traumatic Brain Injury

Traumatic brain injury (TBI) is a disruption in the normal function of the brain and is a major cause of death and disability in the U.S. TBI results from a violent bump, blow, jolt, or other head injury that damages the brain. TBI has a broad spectrum of different symptoms and types of disabilities. Symptoms may not appear until days or weeks following the injury. Initial treatment is to stabilize the patient following brain injury. Acute treatment is aimed at minimizing secondary brain injury. Rehabilitative care helps prepare the patient for participation in daily life.[1] The following modes of care are in the sphere of acute treatment.

IMPROVING RECOVERY

Creatine is an amino acid-like compound that is produced in the liver, kidney, and pancreas, and is ingested from dietary sources.

Neuroprotective effects of creatine in an oral suspension of 0.4 gm/kg given within the first four hours after the time of injury and then once a day for six months were examined in TBI patients between the ages of one and eighteen.[2] Patients who received creatine displayed greater improvements in cognitive functioning, self-care, sociability, and communication skills. The number of children with headaches, dizziness, and fatigue during a six-month observation period was significantly lower in the creatine-supplemented group.[3]

Studies performed found that levels of brain creatine are inversely proportional to the severity of a depressive episode following brain trauma.[4,5] Support for the potential usefulness of creatine in the treatment of depression comes from open-label studies demonstrating that creatine given orally 3–5 gm/day elevated mood in depressed patients who were resistant to antidepressant drugs and in patients with comorbid post-traumatic stress disorder.[6,7,8]

Choline/Citicoline: A systematic review of clinical data from TBI suggested that citicoline could hasten the resorption of cerebral edema and improve the recovery of consciousness and neurologic disorders in severe TBI cases (classified by Glasgow Coma Scale [GCS] scores of ≤8). Citicoline also appeared to limit memory deficits and the duration and severity of other post-traumatic symptoms (e.g., headache, dizziness, attention disorder) in TBI patients with mild-to-moderate injuries (GCS scores, 9–15).[9,10]

Citicoline is currently included in the TBI therapeutic regimen in 59 countries.[11]

Panaz Ginseng: Ginseng total saponins can decrease post-TBI brain edema, which is partly responsible for the focal neurological deficits seen in TBI. It also decreases the pro-inflammatory cytokines IL-6 and IL-1β, and increases IL-10, which is anti-inflammatory.[12] It has also been shown to alleviate oxidative stress post-TBI. Randomized controlled studies are still needed to assess clinical results, however.

Transient Ischemic Attack (TIA)

A TIA is a ministroke, or warning stroke, as a result of a temporary disruption of blood flow to the brain. The disruption results in a brief lack of oxygen to the brain. Therefore, it does not cause permanent damage. Symptoms of a TIA are characteristic stroke symptoms that typically have a duration of only a few minutes, but by definition last less than 24 hours, so no lasting damage is done.[1] TIAs are highly predictive of a subsequent disabling ischemic stroke within hours or days. Because a stroke can have serious long-lasting negative effects and be life-threatening, a TIA is a major warning and should not be ignored.[2] Immediate help is needed and must be sought. The goal of treatment following after a TIA is to correct the abnormality that caused the TIA and prevent a stroke.

PREVENTION OF AN ADDITIONAL TIA OR STROKE

General Measures: Following a TIA, an individual should, within 24 hours, be on an antiplatelet medication to prevent ischemic stroke. That person needs to also stop smoking and make sure blood pressure, diabetes, and serum lipids are well-controlled.[3]

Taking a daily low-dose aspirin (81 mg/day) is an easy and well-known way to reduce the chances of having a heart attack or stroke. However, it was found in one study that too many patients did not have adequate antiplatelet activity. It turned out that 325 mg/day was more effective for most people.[4] The FDA approved dose for aspirin is 81–325 mg/day.[4]

Vitamin E potentiates the antiplatelet effect of acetylsalicylic acid in vitro.[5] Vitamin E has antiatherosclerotic and antiplatelet effects that may reduce the rate of ischemic stroke.[6]

The combination of vitamin E with aspirin is becoming an attractive therapeutic approach to prevent thrombotic vascular accidents. The role of vitamin E in reducing platelet adhesion to collagen was studied.[7] The findings provide a clear rationale for combining aspirin and vitamin E to prevent thrombotic complications in atherosclerotic patients.[5]

Fish Oil: In a month-long study, the addition of 1 gm of omega-3 fatty acids to dual antiplatelet therapy with aspirin and clopidogrel significantly potentiated the platelet response to clopidogrel.[8]

Tremors

Essential tremor (ET) is the most common adult-onset movement disorder. It involves an unintentional, rhythmic muscle movement with to-and-fro movements (oscillations) of one or more parts of the body. Ninety percent of patients have arm and hand tremor. Most patients never seek medical attention, because the tremor remains mild.[1]

The disorder generally affects men and women equally and is more common in people aged 40 and older. Essential tremors include postural or intention (action) types. There are many different causes of tremors including neurological disorders, certain drugs (e.g., corticosteroids, or amphetamines or antipsychotics), alcohol withdrawal, mercury poisoning, hyperthyroidism, and liver failure.[2] Reducing the tremor is the goal of treatment.

THERAPY CHOICES

Magnesium: Tremors are an indication that magnesium supplementation is needed.[3,4]

Black tea, caffeine, coffee, green tea, and vitamin E are all recognized as possibly being effective for Parkinson's disease with tremors.[5]

Riboflavin: According to one study, riboflavin in high doses will likely improve essential tremor without any adverse effects. Results on the analysis on 16 patients showed that riboflavin reduced tremor severity in eight patients with hand tremor and two patients with head tremor. Moreover, 50% of the patients reported moderate improvement while 20% reported slight improvement.[6,7]

Limb Weighting: In some patients, tremors can be reduced by weighting the limb, usually by applying wrist weights.[8]

Supplements such as vitamin C, iron, protein, zinc, and magnesium may also be necessary to reduce tremors.[9,10]

Vitamin B12: Vitamin B12 deficiency has been implicated as a cause of involuntary tremor.[11]

Trigeminal Neuralgia

Trigeminal neuralgia (TN), also known as tic douloureux, is a chronic condition that affects the fifth cranial nerve. It is a form of neuropathic pain and typically affects people over the age of 50. Episodic but extreme burning, stabbing, or shock-like facial pain is transmitted along the trigeminal nerve. It is sometimes described as the most excruciating pain known to humanity and is considered to be one of the most painful conditions. Episodes last a few seconds for up to two minutes or can occur in quick succession, or volleys, lasting as long as two hours.[1] Horrific painful jolts seem to come spontaneously out of nowhere or they can be triggered by mild stimulation such as washing the face, shaving, brushing the teeth, or putting on makeup. Just talking, smiling, or being in a light breeze may set off an electric jolt.

Attacks typically continue for weeks or months, tending to get more frequent with time, usually followed by a pain-free period for months or even years. The exact cause of tic douloureux is not known although some patients report that it started after a vehicular accident, a blow to the face, or dental surgery.

RESEARCH RESULTS

Vitamin B12: Researchers explored vitamin B12 injections and pills as a TN treatment as early as the 1940s and 1950s. In three separate studies between 1952 and 1954, more than three-quarters of the 49 patient participants got complete or marked relief from vitamin B12 (1,000 micrograms IM) given daily for 10 days.[2,3] The daily doses ranged up to 1,000 micrograms.[2] In one of the studies, 17 patients with trigeminal neuralgia were treated with cyanocobalamin (vitamin B12) 1,000 micrograms IM daily for 10 days to maintain a more consistent therapeutic level. There was remarkable relief of pain in all the cases with complete remission in nine patients.[3]

Niacin: Eight patients with trigeminal neuralgia were treated with daily intravenous injections of niacin.[4] Treatment resulted in four complete cures and three partial cures. When an injection was given during an attack, pain relief was immediate.[5]

Fortunately, orally-administered niacin is also helpful for some individuals with trigeminal neuralgia, providing varying degrees of relief.

Alternate Treatments: Some patients have found improvement with treatments, such as chiropractic, acupuncture, and vitamin or nutritional therapy.[6]

Avoidance of Coffee: Evidence suggests that caffeine may be one of the triggers of this painful condition.[7]

Triglycerides/Hypertriglyceridemia

Triglycerides are a type of lipid, or fat, found in the blood. The body converts extra calories into triglycerides and stores them in fat cells. Untreated or uncontrolled high blood triglyceride levels increase the risk of serious complications such as coronary heart disease, cardiovascular events, and stroke. Very high blood triglycerides can also increase the risk of acute pancreatitis, which is inflammation of the pancreas that causes severe pain in the abdomen.[1] High triglycerides can be a sign of other comorbid conditions that increase the risk of heart disease and stroke, such as obesity and metabolic syndrome (also known as insulin resistance syndrome) which is a cluster of conditions that includes too much fat around the waist, high blood pressure, high triglycerides, high blood sugar, and abnormally low high-density lipoprotein (HDL) cholesterol levels).[2]

Causes of elevated blood levels of triglycerides include obesity, high-carbohydrate diet, type 2 diabetes, excess alcohol intake, liver disease, and chronic renal failure. High triglycerides can also be a side effect of taking certain medications, such as diuretics, estrogen and progestin, retinoids, steroids, beta blockers, some immunosuppressants, and certain HIV medications.[2] The goal of treating high triglycerides is a blood level of less than 150 mg/dL.

CLINICAL RESEARCH OUTCOMES

Lifestyle modifications (e.g., smoking cessation, higher fiber and low saturated fat diet, exercise, and caloric restriction leading to weight reduction) are first-line treatment measures usually initiated before any pharmacologic therapy to reduce triglyceride levels.[3]

Nicotinic Acid (Vitamin B3): Niacin is a first-line pharmacologic agent for treating hypertriglyceridemia.[1] Niacin blocks the release of free fatty acid from adipose tissue and reduces the rate of secretion of very-low-density lipoprotein particles.[4] Clinically, niacin reduces triglycerides by 30%–50%, raises HDL cholesterol by 20%–30%, and lowers LDL cholesterol levels by 5%–25%.[1] Niacin is not as potent as fibrates for lowering triglyceride levels but is more effective at raising HDL cholesterol levels.[1] Patients on nicotinic acid are usually started on low daily doses and gradually increased to an average daily dose of 1.5–3 gm/day to avoid hepatotoxicity.[2] Flushing from nicotinic acid can be decreased by taking the extended-release form and by taking niacin during or after meals, or by the use of an aspirin 30 minutes before niacin ingestion.[5] Patients should be made aware that niacin can interact with other medications and cause side effects. Low-dose niacin combined with a statin has been associated with a significant decrease in cardiovascular events.[6]

EPA/DHA: Fish oil with DHA and EPA is another primary pharmacologic agent for treating hypertriglyceridemia.[1] Omega-3 fatty acids are being used as an adjunct to statins or other drugs in patients with moderately elevated triglyceride levels. Omega-3 ethyl esters inhibit the secretion of triglycerides from the liver and reduce blood TG levels. They also activate lipoprotein lipase to stimulate clearance of TG from plasma.[4]

Fish oil with 2–4 gm of total EPA/DHA daily can lower triglyceride levels by 30%–50%. Studies indicate that even a modest fish oil consumption (approximately 250 mg/day of EPA/DHA) may reduce the risk of CHD death and sudden cardiac death.[3] Fish oil can also help reduce atherogenicity.[4] A dose of 2–4 gm of total EPA/DHA per day is recommended.[1,4,7]

Psyllium as a source of fiber is a great cholesterol-buster and part of a healthy diet. Fiber also helps to lower triglycerides and total cholesterol, especially for people with type 2 diabetes.[5]

Ground flaxseed may help lower triglycerides.[8]

Dehydroepiandrosterone (DHEA) enhanced tissue insulin sensitivity and lowered serum triglycerides in one study.[9]

Biotin: A double-blind, placebo-controlled study showed that biotin (15 mg/day) lowered plasma triglyceride concentrations in both diabetic (type 2) and nondiabetic patients with hypertriglyceridemia. Supplying extra biotin reduced the triglyceride concentration in the blood by 35%.[10]

Tropical Sprue

Tropical sprue is a malabsorption disease commonly found in tropical regions. The name sprue derives from a Dutch word describing inflammation of the mouth, wherein a sore tongue (glossitis) is a frequent symptom. In tropical sprue, the small intestine's ability to absorb nutrients is impaired due to abnormal flattening of the villi and inflammation of the lining. The proximal small bowel is involved in absorption and maintenance of an adequate supply of folic acid, whereas the distal portion is essential for absorption of vitamin B12. Therefore, nutritional deficiencies, especially of folate and vitamin B12, eventually develop after several months to years. This condition is characterized by abdominal cramps, abundant nonbloody diarrhea that is pale and foul-smelling, glossitis, anorexia, weight loss, bloating, abdominal cramps, fatigue, and megaloblastic anemia resulting in general weakness.[1]

TREATMENT APPROACHES

Folic acid has been utilized to treat tropical sprue. In one study, 18 patients with chronic diarrhea resulting from tropical sprue had marked improvements after receiving 5–10 mg/day of folic acid.[2] Krupp & Chaton recommend 10–20 mg of folic acid daily by mouth to correct diarrhea, anorexia, weight loss, glossitis, and anemia.[3] Combined therapy with folic acid and tetracycline for three to six months seems to rapidly reduce the severity of the symptoms and also heal unhealthy tissue in the small intestine.[4]

Vitamin B12 should be given 1 mg intramuscularly weekly for several weeks.[5]

Other Nutrients: Additional nutrients (e.g., iron) should be given as needed.[5]

Tuberculosis (TB)

Tuberculosis is an infectious disease caused by *Mycobacterium tuberculosis* bacteria. It is characterized by the growth of nodules (tubercles) in tissues, especially the lungs. Worldwide, TB is the second most common cause of death from infection, after HIV/AIDS. The emergence of resistant strains of tuberculosis and an increase in immunosuppressed patients are significant clinical concerns. The inability to control this infection stems from the fact that the vaccines and drugs that were once effective against TB are no longer as efficacious. This has led to a search for new antituberculous agents and adjuvant therapy.[1]

The disease is spread from one person to another through tiny droplets released into the air. Not everyone infected with TB bacteria becomes sick.[2] As a result, two TB-related conditions exist: latent TB infection (LTBI) and TB disease. Only patients with active TB disease are contagious.

The bacteria usually attack the lungs, but can attack other parts of the body, such as the kidney, spine, and brain. Classic signs and symptoms of TB disease include fever, night sweats, cough, hemoptysis, weight loss, and malaise. Complications of TB can include back pain and stiffness, arthritis, meningitis, and liver or kidney problems. If not treated properly, TB disease can be fatal.

CARE CONSIDERATIONS

Ascorbic Acid: Bioavailability of the antibiotic rifampicin (RIF) from fixed dose combination (FDC) products remains problematic for effective control of tuberculosis (TB). This is due to rifampin's degradation in the presence of isoniazid (INH) in the stomach acid environment. Ascorbic acid added to the dissolution medium as well as the plasma sample as an anti-oxidant helps prevent degradation of resistance-inducing factor (RIF), and daily intake of ascorbic acid is recommended to control TB infection.[2] One study demonstrates that co-administration of ascorbic acid with INH can protect RIF from degradation in the acid environment and improve its bioavailability with effective control of TB.[3]

Another study has noted that drug resistant *Mycobacterium tuberculosis* bacteria is highly sensitive to being destroyed by vitamin C.[4] This is due to a large iron content in the bacterium which is reduced from Fe^{3+} to Fe^{2+} and causes pro-oxidative effects after reacting with oxygen.[5]

Vitamin B6: It is well known that isoniazid used to treat TB inactivates vitamin B6, which may result in pyridoxine deficiency and peripheral neuropathy. A dose of 50–100 mg of pyridoxine daily should prevent peripheral neuropathy.[6]

Vitamin A: People with low levels of vitamin A were at least 10 times more likely to develop TB after exposure to the disease. Vitamin A supplementation among individuals at high risk of tuberculosis may provide an effective means of preventing the disease.[7] Low levels of vitamin A are common in people with tuberculosis. However, taking vitamin A once the disease is acquired does not appear to improve symptoms or to decrease the risk of death in people with tuberculosis.[8]

Vitamin D: Vitamin D has been shown to possess antimycobacterial properties.[9] In a placebo controlled clinical study, high-dose vitamin D supplementation (600,000 IU intramuscularly x2) accelerated clinical and radiographic recovery from TB.[10] Vitamin D deficiency is strongly linked to increased risk for a multitude of diseases including tuberculosis.[11] Studies on the role of vitamin D in respiratory diseases have consistently indicated that low vitamin D levels may be associated with a higher incidence, greater severity, or poorer treatment responses in various respiratory diseases, including pulmonary TB. Oral vitamin D3 dosing typically ranges from 5,000–50,000 IU/day for adults.[11]

Tyrosinemia

Tyrosinemia is a genetic disorder that affects infants. The disorder is characterized by disruptions in the multistep process that breaks down the amino acid tyrosine. If untreated, tyrosine and its byproducts build up in tissues and organs, which can lead to serious health problems. There are three types of tyrosinemia, each distinguished by their symptoms and genetic cause. The presentation includes herpetiform corneal ulcers and hyperkeratotic (skin thickening) lesions of the digits, palms, and soles, as well as intellectual disability. About 10% of newborns have temporarily elevated levels of tyrosine (transient tyrosinemia). In these cases, the cause is not genetic. The most likely causes are vitamin C deficiency or immature liver enzymes due to premature birth.[1]

ALTERNATIVE TREATMENT

Vitamin C: Taking vitamin C by mouth or as an injection improves the genetic disorder in newborns whose blood levels of the amino acid tyrosine are too high.[2]

Ulcerative Colitis

Ulcerative colitis (UC) is a chronic inflammatory disease that affects the large intestine (cecum and colon) and rectum, while sparing the anus. It is the most common form of inflammatory bowel disease (IBD) and causes long-term inflammation and ulceration in continuous areas of the large intestine's inner lining (primarily the mucosa and submucosa).

The disease is characterized by crampy abdominal pain, rectal bleeding leading to intermittent bloody diarrhea, and pus and mucus in the stool. Additional symptoms may include nausea and anorexia (loss of appetite) resulting in weight loss, as well as fever, fatigue, and anemia.

This disorder can occur in people of any age but begins most frequently between the ages of 15 and 30 or after age 60. Ulcerative colitis is more likely to develop in individuals who have a family member with IBD or are of Jewish descent. Relatively minor local complications that occur in the majority of patients include hemorrhoids, anal fissures, and perirectal abscesses. Toxic megacolon and colorectal cancer are well-known major complications of long-standing chronic ulcerative colitis. Screening for colorectal cancer via colonoscopy should be accomplished eight years after the diagnosis is established and then every one to two years thereafter.[1] There is no cure for ulcerative colitis so symptom management is the primary goal of treatment.

ADJUVANT THERAPIES

Diet: Decrease dietary fiber during increased disease activity. A low-residue diet may decrease the frequency of BMs.[2]

Nutritional Support: Proper nutritional support via oral supplementation is an important aspect in the management of patients with IBD, not because specific diets are useful in treatment, but because patients with moderate to severe disease are often malnourished. This is because the inflammatory process results in significant malabsorption or maldigestion, or because of the catabolic effects of the disease process.[3] Administration of vitamin B12, folic acid, fat-soluble vitamins, and iron may be needed to prevent or treat deficiencies.[4]

Strawberries: Recent research suggests that eating about 3.5 ounces of strawberries per day can reduce inflammation and improve IBD symptoms.[5]

EPA/DHA: Previous studies have accordingly proposed a protective role from supplementary dietary intake of (n-3) PUFAs (EPA and DHA) in inflammatory bowel disease (IBD) such as UC, potentially comparable to the effects of mesalazine, which has clear efficacy in the treatment of acute ulcerative colitis and in the maintenance of its remission.[6]

In one study, 18 patients with ulcerative colitis were given 3.2 gm of EPA and 2.16 gm of DHA daily for four months. The treatment group showed a 61% reduction in leukotriene B4 compared to a 2% reduction in the placebo group. Seven patients who received concurrent treatment with prednisone were able to reduce their medication by 50%.[7]

In another study, 11 patients with ulcerative colitis received 2.7 gm of EPA or 1.8 gm EPA or a placebo for eight months. Mean disease activity decreased 56% in the treatment group and only 4% in the control group.[8]

Butyrate, a short-chain fatty acid formed in the colon by bacterial fermentation, is a key nutrient for the cells that line the colon. Just as some cells in the body use glucose for fuel, colonic cells require butyrate. Individuals with ulcerative colitis have decreased levels of butyrate in their stool.[9]

In a recent study, 10 patients with distal (near the rectum) ulcerative colitis received butyrate enemas each night for six weeks.[9] Six of the patients improved and in four of those individuals there was a complete response (i.e., all symptoms disappeared and there was no longer evidence of colonic inflammation on sigmoidoscope examination).

Bromelain: Previous studies indicate that bromelain (e.g., 400–500 mg with each meal) helped alleviate ulcerative colitis symptoms.[10] Bromelain also improved some symptoms of ulcerative colitis in patients who had persistent disease despite ongoing standard therapy.[11] Two patients who were not responding to conventional medical care took bromelain in addition to their usual drug regimen. This resulted in rapid improvement of symptoms, which was confirmed by endoscopy.[12]

Thiamine: Fatigue in inflammatory bowel diseases can be treated with large doses of thiamine.[13]

Probiotics: Lactobacillus probiotics increase remissions in patients with ulcerative colitis. The best evidence of benefit is for a multi-species probiotic containing lactobacillus, bifidobacterium, and streptococcus. Taking this product can increase remission rates almost two-fold when used with standard ulcerative colitis treatment. Taking a single strain of lactobacillus can improve symptoms, but lactobacillus alone does not seem to prevent ulcerative colitis relapse.[14]

Turmeric/Curcumin: Turmeric's extract curcumin taken by mouth (2 gm/day for six months)[15] or as an enema[16] improves symptoms and increases the number of people who go into remission. Patients in the curcumin group had significantly lower disease activity index and endoscopic index scores at six months than patients in the placebo group. No serious side effects were reported.

For people already in remission, curcumin (2 gm/day) increased the likelihood of staying in remission when added to sulfasalazine or mesalamine, and significantly reduced clinical and endoscopic activity indices at six months in patients with UC in remission.[17]

Vitamin D supplementation may lead to significant improvements in ulcerative colitis patients, based on a placebo-controlled trial involving 60 patients with active disease.[18]

A study found that patients utilizing vitamin D supplementation demonstrated a lower risk of relapse in Crohn's disease. Another study showed that injectable vitamin D could reduce inflammation as documented in lower erythrocyte sedimentation rate (ESR) and C-reactive protein (CRP) levels.[18]

Wheatgrass Juice: A randomized controlled trial of wheatgrass juice in the management of ulcerative colitis has demonstrated some efficacy. Sigmoidoscopic evaluation failed to demonstrate a statistically significant difference between the treatment and control group, but it was demonstrated that there was a significant difference in symptomatic indicators of disease activity, such as rectal bleeding.[19]

Aloe Vera Gel: A randomized, double-blind, placebo-controlled trial of aloe vera gel (100 mL bid for four weeks) in patients with mild to moderate ulcerative colitis demonstrated clinical remission, histological remission, and sigmoidoscope remission.[19]

Smoking: As odd as it seems, smoking is somewhat protective against ulcerative colitis, reducing the risk of acquiring it by about 40%. Smoking also helped prevent flare-ups.[20]

Calcium: Patients with IBS are at higher risk for kidney stones, especially oxalate stones. Calcium carbonate and calcium acetate (e.g., 365–500 mg with each meal) can be used to restrict oxalate absorption and minimize the risk of kidney stones.[21]

Ulcers—Leg/Foot

Open sores or lesions on the legs or feet that do not heal over a long period of time or return are ulcers. The three most common types of leg and foot ulcers are venous stasis ulcers which occur below the knee; neurotrophic (diabetic) ulcers on the bottom of the feet; and arterial (ischemic ulcers) ulcers that occur most often on the heels, tips of toes, and between the toes. Venous ulcers are the most common cause of lower-extremity ulceration. Weakened (venous insufficiency) or blocked vein valves increase venous pressure and, when combined with blood back-up, make it difficult for oxygen and nutrients to get to the affected tissue. When this happens, cell death and tissue damage occur, causing wounds to develop.[1] Causes of ischemic ulcers include trauma, atherosclerosis, and peripheral vascular diseases.[2]

THERAPY CONSIDERATIONS

Compression is the gold standard treatment for venous ulcer disease.[3]

Leg elevation to minimize edema in patients with venous insufficiency is recommended as adjunctive therapy for venous ulcers. The recommended regimen is 30 minutes, three or four times per day.[4]

Aspirin (300 mg/day) is effective when used with compression therapy for venous ulcers.[4]

Smoking must be stopped.

Deficiencies: Identified deficiencies implicated in slow or incomplete healing of diabetic foot wounds include deficiencies of magnesium, calcium, zinc, riboflavin, folate, and vitamin A.[5]

Vitamin D: Vitamin D plays a significant role in wound healing, participating in cell growth and differentiation, reversal of corticosteroid-induced epidermal atrophy, and the inhibition of hyperplastic epidermal tissue formation. Vitamin D deficiency has been shown to have increased incidence in patients with venous ulcers.[6] Vitamin D supplementation results in increased rates of wound healing and increased wound tensile strength.[5]

Zinc Oxide: Topical preparations containing zinc oxide have been used in the management of arterial and venous leg ulcers, pressure ulcers, and diabetic foot ulcers. The reported response rate was 83% in a study on efficacy of topical zinc oxide paste in both arterial and venous ulcers.[7]

Zinc Sulphate: In a double-blind study, 104 patients with leg ulcers received an oral dose of zinc sulphate (50 mg) three times a day or a placebo for 16 weeks. The ulcers in the zinc-treated group healed more than twice as fast as did those in the placebo group (on average, 32.3 vs. 77.2 days).[8] Henzel et al. have reported on the therapeutic use of oral zinc (220 mg tid for one month) to completely heal leg ulcers.[9]

Folic Acid: Large doses of folic acid (e.g., 15 mg tid) promoted the healing of chronic leg ulcers caused by venous stasis and atherosclerosis. Four patients (two with large varicose ulcers and two with ischemic ulcers) received an additional 20 mg dose of folic acid twice weekly, intravenously. In nine of the 10 cases, complete healing was achieved in 6 to 12 weeks. In the tenth case there was definite improvement but not complete healing of a toe ulcer.[10] High-dose folic acid also appears to prevent the progression of atherosclerosis.[11]

Calendula: Previous clinical studies demonstrate that applying a calendula ointment (7.5%) to the skin speeds up the healing of leg ulcers caused by poor blood circulation.[12] Patients with leg ulcers treated with *Calendula officinalis* extract had a significant four-fold increase in percentage healing velocity per week.[13] Research also indicates that using a calendula spray in addition to standard care and hygiene might prevent infection and decrease odor in people with long-term foot ulcer from diabetes.[13]

Ulcers—Peptic/Gastroduodenal

Peptic ulcer disease is a chronic disorder affecting up to 10% of the world's population. Peptic ulcers include both gastric and duodenal ulcers. The only difference between gastric and duodenal ulcers is the location of the lesion. The same goals apply to treating duodenal ulcers as for gastric ulcers. The risk of complications with peptic ulcer is increased four times in NSAID users.[1]

If stomach acid burns through the protective mucus layer in the stomach, this causes the erosions or sores in the lining of the stomach and upper small intestine known as peptic ulcers. Peptic ulcers include gastric and duodenal ulcers. Peptic ulcers can be present even if there are no symptoms or if symptoms are mild, but can cause significant problems if left untreated. A dull, biting, gnawing, or burning pain in the upper abdomen is the most common symptom of a peptic ulcer. Additional symptoms may be bloating, gas, indigestion, and nausea. Abdominal pain is often worse at night or in between meals when the stomach is empty. The pain can often be briefly ameliorated by eating or taking antacids. Peptic ulcers can lead to internal bleeding. The most common causes of peptic ulcers are *Helicobacter pylori* (*H. pylori*) infection, excess stomach acid, and long-term use of aspirin and other nonsteroidal anti-inflammatory drugs (NSAIDs, e.g., Motrin, Advil, Aleve, etc.). The goals of therapy are to: (1) resolve symptoms; (2) reduce acid secretion; (3) promote epithelial healing; (4) prevent ulcer-related complications; and (5) prevent ulcer recurrence.

TREATMENT COURSES

Medical treatment typically includes eliminating or reducing NSAIDs, if possible, and helping the ulcer heal with medications that lower stomach acid levels, as well as killing *H. pylori* bacterium if it is present.[2]

Antacids are rarely used as primary therapy for PUD but antacids neutralize existing stomach acid and can provide rapid pain relief.[3] Over-the-counter products that neutralize stomach acid include aluminum hydroxide (Amphojel, AlternaGEL), magnesium hydroxide (Phillips' Milk of Magnesia), aluminum hydroxide and magnesium hydroxide (Maalox, Mylanta), calcium carbonate (Rolaids, Titralac, Tums), and sodium bicarbonate (Alka-Seltzer).[4]

Acid blockers, also called histamine (H-2) blockers, reduce the amount of acid released into the digestive tract, relieving gastritis pain and encouraging healing. Available by prescription or over-the-counter, acid blockers include ranitidine (Zantac), famotidine (Pepcid), cimetidine (Tagamet HB), and nizatidine (Axid AR).[2] Recently, the FDA alerted the public that the drug ranitidine (Zantac) can contain a cancer-causing impurity called N-nitrosodimethylamine (NDMA). No recall of the drug has been issued.

Proton pump inhibitors (PPIs) reduce acid by blocking the action of the parts of cells that produce acid. These drugs include the prescription and over-the-counter medications omeprazole (Prilosec), lansoprazole (Prevacid), and esomeprazole (Nexium).[2] PPIs are usually preferred to treat NSAID-induced ulcers because they provide more rapid ulcer healing than acid blockers (H2RAs) or sucralfate.[5] Research shows that taking L-tryptophan in combination with the ulcer medication omeprazole improves ulcer healing rates compared to taking omeprazole alone.[6]

Diet: Spicy foods, excessive alcohol, coffee and caffeinated drinks, fatty, and fried foods should be avoided.[4] Individuals should be encouraged to eat balanced meals at regular intervals. There is no scientific justification for bland or restrictive diets.

NSAIDs: If NSAIDs must be continued in a patient despite ulceration, consideration should be given to reducing the NSAID dose and taking it with food and/or antacids. If possible, alternative agents such as acetaminophen or nonacetylated salicylate/aspirin (e.g., salsalate) should be used for relief of pain.[7] Patients should NOT stop any prescribed medication without first talking to their doctor.

Deglycyrrhizinated Licorice (DGL): Carbenoxolone is a derivative of the licorice compound glycyrrhizinic acid and has been found to promote healing of both gastric and duodenal ulcers. Deglycyrrhizinated licorice (DGL) has shown promise in the treatment of peptic ulcers.[8] The standard dose is two to four 380 mg DGL tablets taken before meals and at bedtime.

In another study, 100 patients with gastric ulcers received either DGL (760 mg three times a day between meals) or Tagamet (200 mg, three times a day and 400 mg at bedtime). Ulcers healed after 6 weeks and 12 weeks were similar in both groups. DGL (760 mg, two times a day) was been found to work as well as cimetidine (Tagamet) for both short-term treatment and maintenance therapy.[9]

A preliminary study suggests that DGL might help prevent ulcers caused by aspirin and related medication such as ibuprofen.[10]

In one study, 33 patients with gastric ulcers received either deglycyrrhizinated licorice (DGL) 760 mg, three times a day initially, or a placebo for one month. There was a significant reduction in ulcer size in the DGL group (78%). Complete healing occurred in 44% of those receiving DGL.[11] In another study, DGL was at least as effective as antacids, and possibly even more beneficial.[12]

DGL's anti-ulcer properties seem to be related to its ability to protect the cells that line the stomach and duodenum against damage. Animal studies have shown that DGL increases the number of cells that produce protective mucus. In human volunteers, aspirin-induced gastrointestinal blooding was also reduced by 20% with DGL.[10]

DGL is effective in treating duodenal ulcers. This is perhaps best illustrated by one study of patients with severe duodenal ulcers. In the study, 40 patients with chronic duodenal ulcers of 4 to 12 years duration and with more than six relapses during the previous year were treated with DGL.[13] All of the patients had been referred for surgery because of relentless pain, sometimes with frequent vomiting, despite treatment with bed rest, antacids, and powerful drugs. Half of the patients received 3 gm of DGL daily for eight weeks; the other half received 4.5 gm/day for 16 weeks. All 40 patients showed substantial improvement, usually within five to seven days, and none required surgery by the one-year follow-up. Although both dosages were effective, the higher dose was significantly more effective than the lower dose.

In another more recent study, the therapeutic effect of DGL was compared to that of antacids, or cimetidine, in 874 patients with confirmed chronic duodenal ulcers.[14] 91% of all ulcers healed within 12 weeks and there was no significant difference in healing rate in the groups. However, there were fewer relapses in the DGL group (8.2%) than in the group that received cimetidine (12.9%), or antacids (16.4%). These results, coupled with DGL's protective effects, suggest that DGL is a superior treatment for duodenal ulcers.

Zinc: In another study, 15 individuals with gastric (stomach) ulcers were given either zinc or a placebo for three weeks. The reduction in ulcer size was about three times as great in the zinc group as in the placebo group and zinc therapy resulted in rapid relief of pain.[15]

Ascorbic Acid: In one study, administration of vitamin C (500 mg/day intravenously) along with iron accelerated gastric ulcer healing in patients.[16]

In 1955, Weiss et al. evaluated the use of vitamin C in treating bleeding ulcers. The author graded the response of patients to vitamin C, based on recurrence of symptoms and scheduled guaiac tests, as "good" in 12 of 14 subjects with duodenal ulcers and in two patients with gastric ulcer.[17]

More recently, McAlindon et al. evaluated vitamin C for the prevention of aspirin-induced gastroduodenal injury and noted a statistically significant reduction in duodenal injury and bleeding in the vitamin C group as assessed by the Lanza score.[18]

Ascorbic acid supplementation has been associated with a decreased incidence of bleeding from peptic ulcer disease and with a reduction in NSAID-associated gastric mucosal damage. Pharmacologic doses of ascorbic acid may also improve the effectiveness of *H. pylori* eradication therapy.[19]

Bismuth therapy (Pepto-Bismol) has shown efficacy against peptic ulcer disease. In peptic ulcer disease, it is as effective as the H2-receptor antagonists, costs considerably less, and offers a lower rate of relapse.[20]

Taurine: Previous clinical studies indicate that taking 500 mg of taurine twice daily together with conventional treatments for six weeks reduces *H. pylori* infection and improves ulcer healing.[21]

Spinal Manipulation: Preliminary evidence suggests that spinal manipulation may benefit a number of patients with uncomplicated gastric or duodenal ulcers. In one clinical study, researchers compared the effectiveness of medication to spinal manipulation in patients with gastric and duodenal ulcers over a period of up to 22 days. Those who received spinal manipulation had significant pain relief after an average of four days, and were completely free of symptoms on average ten days earlier than those who took medication.[22] Osteopathic treatment, as an adjunctive therapy to medication, has been proven to reduce the pain and to shorten the healing time in patients with peptic ulcers.[23]

S-Methylmethionine (SMM): Also known as vitamin U, SMM was initially evaluated for the treatment of peptic ulcers in older American studies.[24] Vitamin U was administered as raw cabbage juice (one quart daily in four or five divided doses) to 100 patients with peptic ulcers. The result was rapid pain relief and significantly decreased crater healing time.[24,25] More recently, SMM has been studied in France, Germany, Italy, and Japan and its therapeutic effect has been deemed to be clinically proven.[26]

Zinc ascorbate, magnesium ascorbate and vitamin A have a direct role in helping to heal the intestinal membranes.[27]

Cigarette smoking doubles the risk of peptic ulcer development, delays healing, and promotes recurrence; therefore, cessation of cigarette smoking should be encouraged.[28]

Ulcers—Pressure Ulcers/Decubitus Ulcers/Bedsores

A decubitus ulcer, also known as a pressure ulcer, pressure sore, or bedsore, is an open wound on the skin. *Decubitus* in Latin means "lying down." These ulcers are usually the result of lying in one position for too long so that the circulation in the skin is compromised or cut off by the weight of the body against the mattress or chair.[1] This leads to a breakdown of the skin. A bedsore initially presents as persistently red, broken, blistered, or necrotic skin. As it further develops, the ulceration can extend into underlying structures including bone, ligaments, and muscle. It is particularly common over bony prominences like on the sacrum, ankles, hips, or heels.

Pressure ulcers often become chronic wounds that are difficult to treat and that tend to recur after healing.[2] Two major groups of pressure ulcer patients are those with spinal cord injuries and the elderly. Pressure ulcers are usually graded on a scale of 1 to 4, with a higher grade indicating greater ulcer severity.[3] Potential complications from grade 3 or grade 4 pressure ulcers include infections, sepsis, tissue loss, scarring, deformity, squamous cell cancer, and death.[4]

Prevention has been a primary goal of pressure ulcer research. Ulcer wounds should not be cleaned with skin cleansers or antiseptic agents (e.g., Betadine, hydrogen peroxide, or acetic acid) because they destroy granulation tissue that is needed to repair the wound.[5]

GENERAL MEASURES AND NUTRITIONAL SUPPORT

General Measures: Follow a repositioning schedule. Keep the head of the bed at lowest safe position to prevent shear. Assess nutrition and provide the supplementation needed to reverse catabolic nutritional status.[6,7]

Zinc: Monitoring for nutritional deficiencies, including zinc, is essential for optimal patient outcomes. Zinc supplementation in older patients improved outcomes, decreased healing time, and mitigated comorbidities.[8] In another study, supplementation with zinc appeared to promote healing of decubitus ulcers in six elderly patients.[9]

Vitamin C: In one study, 20 surgical patients received ascorbic acid supplementation for one month. The result was a mean reduction in pressure-sore area of 84% after one month compared with 42.7% in the placebo group.[10]

Arginine: With supplementation containing 3–9 gm of arginine, 10 out of 11 studies showed a beneficial effect of the arginine-enriched oral nutritional supplementation on the healing of pressure ulcers.[11]

Oral Nutrition Supplementation: In a review of six clinical studies aimed at examining the effect of oral nutritional supplementation enriched with arginine, vitamin C, and zinc in pressure ulcer care, ONS was found to have positive effects on pressure injury healing and potentially to reduce the risk of developing these injuries.[12,13]

Calendula: A study found that cleaning venous ulcers, burns, and skin lesions with a 10% calendula solution followed by daily application of 2% calendula gel resulted in a greater number of healed wounds, as well as a reduction in the median time to heal when compared to using calendula solution alone.[14]

Vitamin D deficiency has been shown to have an increased incidence in patients with pressure ulcers.[15]

ADJUNCTIVE THERAPIES

Additional therapies for nonhealing ulcers include electrical stimulation, radiant heat, negative pressure therapy, and surgical intervention.[16]

Uremia/Uremic Syndrome

Uremia is defined as elevated concentrations of urea, creatinine, and other nitrogenous end products of metabolism in the blood that are normally excreted by the kidneys into the urine. It is a serious condition and when left untreated can lead to death. Uremia occurs after the kidneys are damaged (chronic kidney disease) and cannot filter the blood normally. Symptoms include itchy skin, nausea, loss of appetite, weight loss, leg cramps, and fatigue. Common causes of chronic kidney disease are hypertension, polycystic kidney disease, diabetes (DM1 and DM2), glomerulitis, some cancers, and recurrent kidney stones or infections. Complications of untreated uremia can be seizures, coma, bleeding, cardiac arrest, and death.

CLINICAL CARE

Zinc depletion associated with uremia has been shown to be reversible via zinc supplementation (25 mg t.i.d for six months). Zinc also lowered high plasma ammonia levels in uremic patients as well as lowering elevated prolactin levels in male patients with uremia.[1]

Folic Acid: High plasma homocysteine levels are a common finding in uremia; indeed, they are almost the rule. Administration of 5 mg/day of folic acid to uremic patients can decrease the blood homocysteine level.[2]

Urethritis

Urethritis is inflammation and swelling of the urethra, the structure that transports urine from the bladder to the outside of the body. Pain or burning with urination is the main symptom of urethritis along with increased urinary frequency and/or urgency. The urethral opening is typically red due to inflammation. Urethritis can be caused by bacterial infections (e.g., *Staphylococcus aureus* or *E. coli*) and STDs (*Neisseria gonorrhoeae*, non-gonococcal urethritis, *Chlamydia trachomatis*, or *Mycoplasma genitalium*) and also by trauma or irritating chemicals (e.g., antiseptics or spermicides). In females, pelvic inflammatory disease and tubo-ovarian abscess are well-known complications. In males, complications such as epididymitis and prostatitis can occur.

REMEDIAL TREATMENT

Ascorbic Acid: One study reported that 3 gm of ascorbic acid daily by mouth for four days completely relieved all symptoms of urethritis. The author asserted that the urethral irritation and pain were caused by phosphatic crystals formed in the urine because of insufficient acidity and that ascorbic acid acidified the urine enough to force the crystals back into solution.[1]

Urinary Tract Infection (UTI)

An infection anywhere in the kidneys, ureters, bladder, or urethra is a urinary tract infection. This is divided into infections of the upper tract (i.e., kidneys and/or ureters) or lower tract (i.e., bladder, also known as cystitis, and/or urethra). Women are at greater risk of developing a UTI and it is most common in young sexually active women and women over 65 years. Typical UTI symptoms include dysuria, urinary urgency and frequency, dark or cloudy or bloody urine, strong-smelling urine, and fever or chills.

UTIs are one of the most common infections in seniors especially those who have a catheter or reside in a hospital or care facility. Asymptomatic bacteriuria and pyuria are also common in older adults. Serious UTI complications include kidney infections and sepsis. Antibiotics are the primary treatment for UTIs. However, overutilization of antibiotics can lead to negative consequences, including development of multidrug resistant organisms and unwanted side effects (e.g., *Clostridium difficile* infection).

TREATMENT OPTIONS

Bromelain: Bromelain is a complex mixture of proteolytic enzymes. Bromelain has been documented to increase blood and urine levels of certain antibiotics in humans. In one double-blind study, 28 patients with a urinary-tract infection received, in addition to antibiotics, either bromelain or a placebo. Signs of infection cleared up in 100% of the patients receiving bromelain, compared to only 46% of those given the placebo.[1,2]

MANAGEMENT OF RECURRENT UTIs

Cranberry extracts do not help treat existing UTIs but may help prevent their development. This is because cranberries contain a compound called proanthocyanidin (PAC) that helps prevent *E. coli* from sticking to the walls of the digestive and urinary tracts.[3]

One study demonstrated that among women living in nursing homes and assisted living facilities, 10 ounces (300 ml) of cranberry juice cocktail (36 mg of PAC as a supplement, e.g., Ellura, TheraCran One) reduced bacteriuria plus pyuria at six months of follow-up.[4,5]

In a large meta-analysis, researchers found that women with recurrent UTIs who took cranberry extract over 12 months had a 35% reduction in infections.[3]

Another large clinical trial found that 500 mg of cranberry extract taken daily for six months reduced the rate of UTI to the same extent as 100 mg of trimethoprim, an antibiotic, without posing a risk of antimicrobial resistance or super-infection in women with recurrent UTIs.[3]

Cranberry extract tablets appear to be twice as effective as cranberry juice for preventing UTIs, which may be due in part to the sugar content of cranberry juice. Cranberry extracts also contain anthocyanins and salicylic acid. This may have a pain-killing and anti-inflammatory effect that can further help alleviate UTI symptoms.[3]

In one study, taking proanthocyanidin-A for 12 weeks reduced bacterial adhesion, bacterial MRHA negativity, urine pH reduction, and prevented recurrent-UTI (dysuria, bacteriuria, and pyuria).[6] The Society of Obstetricians and Gynecologists of Canada recommends cranberry products to prevent recurrent UTIs, but not for active UTIs.

Probiotics, in particular *Bifidobacterium longum*, has shown an ability to prevent undesirable bacteria sticking to the walls of the intestinal tract, in addition to enhancing production of natural antibacterial chemicals and organic acids, thereby reducing the likelihood of UTI.[3,7]

Lactobacillus: Recurrent urinary tract infections are a common problem among women. Frequent use of antibiotics can disrupt normal intestinal bacteria or allow resistant bacterial strains to grow. In one study, 42 women with an acute UTI were given either lactobacillus intravaginal suppositories (500 mg) or a placebo beginning on the last day of antibiotic treatment to be used twice per week for two weeks. This was followed by suppository use once a month for two months. UTIs recurred more than twice as often (47% vs. 21%) in women taking the placebo compared to those using the lactobacillus suppositories.[8]

Methionine: Methionine makes urine more acidic and can be used effectively to prevent urinary tract infections (UTIs). This is because *E. coli*, which is usually responsible for cystitis, cannot survive in an acidic environment. A 2002 study showed that taking methionine supplements (500 mg tid) markedly reduced the tendency for urinary tract infections.[9]

Because methionine discourages bacteria from sticking to the wall of the bladder, it has been useful in the treatment of recurrent bladder infections. However, the evidence that it works is limited to one small trial without a placebo control.[10]

D-Mannose: The sugar D-mannose was studied in 308 women with acute UTI and a history of recurrent UTI. Of the women who received D-mannose (2 gm/day for six months) only 15% had another UTI in six months compared to 60% in women with no prophylaxis.[11]

Urticaria/Hives

Urticaria, also known as hives, are swollen, pale red elevated bumps, patches, or welts on the skin that appear suddenly because of allergies. The pink-to-red raised patches can show up anywhere on the body, including the face, lips, tongue, throat, and ears. These raised areas, or wheals, usually itch but they may also burn or sting. They range in size from a pencil eraser to the size of a dinner plate and may join together to form larger areas known as plaques.

There are two types of urticaria. An acute bout typically lasts less than 24 hours, but certainly less than six weeks, and chronic or recurrent urticaria lasts longer than six weeks.

In the majority of cases, a cause cannot be found. Known causes include certain foods (nuts, shellfish, eggs, milk, chocolate, cheese, tomatoes, and fresh berries), increased body temperature, sun exposure, insect bites or stings, and some medications (e.g., penicillin, sulfa, aspirin, ibuprofen, codeine, ACE inhibitors, etc.).[1,2]

PREVENTION

Known Triggers such as medications, foods, insect bites, or sun exposure should be avoided if possible.

ACUTE URTICARIA

Oral antihistamines (e.g., diphenhydramine 50–100 mg q four hours) are a standard form of medical care.

Vitamin B12: In one study, 100 patients with urticaria improved after treatment with vitamin B12 injections, even though blood levels of the vitamin were normal before treatment.[3,4]

CHRONIC URTICARIA

Diet: Aspirin, alcohol, coffee, and tobacco should be avoided because they can aggravate symptoms.

Pyridoxine: In chronic urticaria, pyridoxine dependency may exist. Taking 50–100 mg of pyridoxine (vitamin B6) orally per day can alleviate the problem.[5,6]

Uveitis

Uveitis is eye inflammation and swelling that can destroy eye tissues. The most common form of uveitis is anterior uveitis. Signs and symptoms include eye redness and pain, severe photosensitivity, and blurred vision with floating dark spots in the field of vision. Uveitis can lead to poor vision or blindness. The swelling most often affects the part of the eye called the uvea (the iris, the ciliary body, and the choroid) between the white part of the eye, or sclera, and the inner layers of the eye.[1] Symptoms and signs tend to come on suddenly and get worse quickly.

Many times, a cause of uveitis cannot be identified but causes can include an autoimmune disease (sarcoidosis, ankylosing spondylitis), inflammatory disorder (Crohn's disease or ulcerative colitis), infection (herpes zoster, TB, Lyme disease, West Nile virus, etc.), or eye injury. Uveitis can lead to permanent vision loss. A painful red eye with sensitivity to light signals the need to see an ophthalmologist as soon as possible.

CONSERVATIVE CARE APPROACHES

Vitamin E: Numerous studies recommend the use of oral vitamin E in uveitis.[2]

Vitamins C and E: Taking vitamin E with vitamin C by mouth improves vision but does not, for reasons that are unknown, reduce the swelling in uveitis.[3] In one study, 145 patients with acute uveitis took vitamin C (500 mg bid) and vitamin E (100 IU bid) and this had a significant positive effect (i.e., better visual acuity) after eight weeks. The results appear to indicate that vitamins C and E exert a protective effect in patients with acute anterior uveitis.[4]

Vitamin D: Supportive evidence exists for a potential causal role of vitamin D deficiency in anterior uveitis. The data adds to the increasing body of literature showing that vitamin D may play a role in autoimmune disease.[5]

A daily multivitamin that contains antioxidant vitamins A, C, and E, the B vitamins, and trace minerals such as magnesium, calcium, zinc, and selenium, can be helpful. These vitamins and minerals are good for eye health and for overall health.[6]

EPA/DHA: Omega-3 fatty acids, such as fish oil, may help lower inflammation and boost the immune system. Patients taking blood-thinning medications, such as aspirin, warfarin (Coumadin), or clopidogrel (Plavix), should consult their doctor before taking omega-3 fatty acid supplements.[6]

Lutein is an antioxidant that is important for eye health.[6]

Deficiencies: Kandi et al. have shown that the levels of vitamins E, C, B1, B2, and flavin mononucleotide were significantly lower in affected patients compared to the control group.[2,7]

Benfotiamine: Recently, beneficial effects of a vitamin B1 analogue, benfotiamine, have been demonstrated on uveitis in animal studies.[8]

Vaginal or Vulvovaginal Atrophy/Atrophic Vaginitis/ Genitourinary Syndrome of Menopause (GSM)

Vaginal symptoms associated with menopause are common, affecting 40%–60% of postmenopausal women.[1] Vulvovaginal atrophy, or atrophic vaginitis, is thinning and inflammation of the vaginal walls leading to a loss of elasticity. This leads to symptoms of uncomfortable or painful intercourse (dyspareunia), localized dryness, burning, pruritus, dysuria, and urinary incontinence. Loss of libido is also possible.

Atrophic vaginitis is commonly due to the body having less estrogen after menopause.[2] Unfortunately, symptoms are expected to persist or worsen over time without treatment.

MANAGEMENT CHOICES

Nicotine: Smoking should be avoided because it impairs blood circulation, depriving the vagina and other tissues of oxygen. Tissue thinning occurs especially where blood flow is decreased or restricted. Smokers are also less responsive to estrogen therapy in pill form.[3]

Vitamin E oil can be used as a lubricant.[3]

Over-the-counter moisturizers (Me Again, Replens, Silk-E, etc.) or water-based, glycerine-free lubricants (Astroglide, K-Y, and others) help treat the dryness.[3]

DHEA: In a prospective, randomized, double-blind, and placebo-controlled clinical trial, dehydroepiandrosterone (DHEA) was applied intravaginally for 12 weeks. All three doses (0.25%, 0.5%, and 1.0%) of DHEA (Prasterone) ovules induced highly significant beneficial changes in the pH as well as in dyspareunia and vaginal dryness at two weeks.[4,5]

The researchers concluded that DHEA causes a rapid and efficient reversal of all the symptoms and signs of vaginal atrophy with no or minimal changes in serum steroids, which remain well within the normal postmenopausal range.[4,5]

According to a published report from Genazzani and colleagues in Italy, 25 mg of oral DHEA per day worked very well in the treatment of vaginal atrophy. A daily dose of a 10 mg DHEA pill worked as well as two different types of standard hormone therapy in improving sexual function and frequency of intercourse.[6,7]

Vitamin D vaginal suppositories (1,000 IU) used daily for eight weeks had protective effects that decreased the mean pain during intercourse, vaginal pH, dryness and paleness, and helped increase the vaginal maturation value compared to the placebo suppositories.[8]

Oral Vitamin D: In one study, the vitamin D group received oral vitamin D2 at 40,000 IU/week for 12 weeks. The vitamin D group at six weeks showed significant improvement in VVA symptoms, pH, and VMI.[9] Another evaluation was undertaken in a cross-sectional study of 60 women, half of whom had taken vitamin D3 orally for at least one year and half of whom had not. The prevalence of vaginal atrophy was significantly higher in the group who did not use vitamin D.[10]

Calendula: Previous clinical studies demonstrate that applying a gel (Estromineral Gel) containing calendula, *Lactobacillus sporogenes*, isoflavones, and lactic acid to the vagina for four weeks reduces symptoms of vaginal atrophy such as vaginal itching, burning, dryness, and pain during intercourse.[11]

Oral Sea Buckthorn (SB) Oil: Ninety-eight women with symptoms of vaginal atrophy took 3 gm of sea buckthorn oil daily for three months. Compared to a placebo, there was a significantly higher rate of improvement in the integrity of vaginal epithelium in the SB group. SB oil showed beneficial effects on vaginal health, indicating that it is a potential alternative for mucosal integrity for those women not able to use estrogen treatment for vaginal atrophy.[12]

Vaginitis (Candida/Yeast Infection)

Candida vaginitis is inflammation of the vagina due to a yeast infection. Symptoms of vaginitis can include vaginal pain, itching, discharge, and odor, along with pain on urination or during sexual intercourse. Vaginitis is probably the most common manifestation of candidiasis and represents infection by a microorganism that normally resides on the vaginal mucosal surface. Trichomonas is also a common cause of vaginitis, as is physical or chemical irritation.

RESEARCH RESULTS

OTC agents to treat candida vaginitis include Clotrimazole, Miconazole, Tioconazole, Butoconazole, Tercoconazole, and Flucoconazole.[1]

Probiotics: Fifty-five women diagnosed with vulvovaginal candidiasis associated with at least one symptom (itching and burning vaginal feeling, dyspareunia, and dysuria) were treated with single dose of fluconazole (150 mg) supplemented every morning for the following four weeks with two placebo or two probiotic capsules (containing *Lactobacillus rhamnosus* GR-1 and *Lactobacillus reuteri* RC-14). At four weeks, the probiotic-treated group showed significantly less vaginal discharge associated with any of the above mentioned symptoms and lower presence of yeast detected by culture. The authors report that this study has shown that probiotic lactobacilli can increase the effectiveness of an anti-fungal pharmaceutical agent in curing disease.[2]

A significant decrease in infections also occurred when patients consumed yogurt containing lactobacillus. The authors concluded that daily ingestion of 8 oz. of yogurt with *L. acidophilus* decreased both candida colonization and infections.[3]

Boric Acid: Intravaginal boric acid has been employed for over a 100 years to treat vaginal infections. Boric acid is inexpensive, accessible, and has shown to be an effective treatment for infections including vaginal candidiasis.[4]

Varicose Veins/Venous Insufficiency

Varicose veins cause bulging, swollen, twisted, bluish or dark purple cords just beneath the surface of the skin. Veins carry blood back to the heart, and valves in the veins allow blood to flow from superficial veins into deeper veins to return to the heart. When veins have difficulty in efficiently returning blood from the limbs back to the heart, it is known as venous insufficiency. In venous insufficiency, blood pools in the leg veins and the ankles swell. If veins cannot effectively move blood towards the heart or stop the backflow of blood, varicose veins can develop. In the majority of cases, there is no pain, but if symptoms occur, they can include aching legs, swollen ankles, and spider veins.

Potential complications associated with varicose veins are ulcers (due to venous stasis), localized bleeding, skin color changes, and deep vein thrombosis (blood clots). Most individuals who have varicose veins will not develop complications and tend to view varicose veins as primarily a cosmetic issue. The goals of treatment are to relieve symptoms, improve appearance, and prevent complications.[1]

REDUCING SWELLING

Compression Treatment: Whether with stockings or bandages, compression is the primary treatment for varicose veins.[2]

Weight loss, exercise, and elevation of the legs can also be a benefit along with avoiding prolonged sitting or standing.[2]

Flavonoids (diosman, troxerutin, and horse chestnut extract) are widely used for the treatment of chronic venous insufficiency (CVI).[3] Research has revealed flavonoids to be a supportive treatment, suitable to reduce varicose vein pathophysiology and to regularize venous tone.[4]

Horse chestnut seed extract (HCSE) (e.g., 300 mg bid, or escin, the active ingredient of the extract, 100–150 mg/day) alone has been shown to reduce swelling in the legs due to venous insufficiency. In one study, HCSE was found to be as effective as compression treatment, as determined by the reduction in swelling in the legs.[5] In a Cochrane review, HCSE was considered efficacious and safe for the short-term therapy for chronic venous insufficiency.[6] Studies have shown both an improvement in pain, as well as swelling, in patients with chronic venous insufficiency. Oral tinctures and topical gels containing 2% escin are available.

Additional therapies that may be effective include:[6,7]

- Butcher's broom
- Grape leaves, sap, seed, and fruit
- Sweet clover

Methylsulfonylmethane (MSM) and EDTA: Research shows that applying MSM and EDTA (ethylenediaminetetraacetic acid) to the skin can reduce swelling in the calf, ankle, and foot in people with chronic venous insufficiency. However, applying MSM alone seems to increase swelling.[8]

Omega-3 oils (1,000 mg/day) by mouth helps restore elasticity to blood vessels.[9]

Coenzyme Q10 (100 mg/day) improves circulation and tissue oxygenation.[9]

Bilberry Extract: Research shows that taking bilberry extract with 173 mg of anthocyanins (173 mg/day for 30 days) can improve symptoms of swelling, pain, bruising, and burning due to chronic venous insufficiency.[10]

Pycnogenol: French maritime pine bark extract, better known as pycnogenol, (100 mg tid for 60 days) induced a significant reduction in subcutaneous edema, as well as heaviness and pain in the legs. Approximately 60% of patients treated with pycnogenol experienced a complete disappearance of edema and pain at the end of the treatment.[11] A study was undertaken to assess various products to treat chronic venous insufficiency (CVI). The best improvement in CVI symptoms score were obtained with pycnogenol (100 mg tid for 60 days) along with compression.[12]

Vertigo—Cervical Vertigo/Cervicogenic Dizziness

Cervical vertigo, or cervicogenic dizziness, is not a true vertigo, but a sensation in which a person feels dizzy, lightheaded, unsteady, or unbalanced in a way that is related to the neck. Certain head or neck movements tend to make the dizziness worse.

Position receptors located in the facets of the cervical spine are important physiologically in the coordination of head and eye movements. Cervical proprioceptive dysfunction is a common cause of vertigo triggered by neck movements.[1] When abnormal sensory input from neck proprioceptors does not match inner ear and visual information in the central nervous system, a sensation of unsteadiness, dizziness, or imbalance can occur.[2]

TREATMENT METHODS

Manual Techniques: Several studies have reported that approximately 75% of patients improve with conservative treatment of the neck, such as gentle spinal mobilization, exercise, and instruction in proper posture and use of the neck.[2,3,4]

Pain Medications: Reducing neck pain with acetaminophen or NSAIDs is sometimes effective for cervical vertigo.[5]

Vitamin E Deficiency

A deficiency of vitamin E is uncommon. The classic abnormalities in vitamin E deficiency may produce a disorder somewhat similar to Friedreich's ataxia. It can progress from muscle weakness, hyporeflexia, ataxia (difficulty with coordination), limitations in upward gaze and strabismus to long-tract defects, profound muscle weakness, and visual field constriction.

Lack of vitamin E can also cause mild hemolytic anemia and infertility.[1] Patients with severe, prolonged deficiency may develop complete blindness, dementia, and cardiac arrhythmias. Vitamin E deficiency often runs in families. Medical causes include celiac disease, cholestatic liver disease, chronic pancreatitis, and cystic fibrosis.[2]

Deficiency is also common in newborns and low birth weight infants.[2] Treatment must be tailored to the underlying cause of the vitamin E deficiency.[3]

REPLENISHING VITAMIN E STORES

Vitamin E: 60–75 units orally once daily to correct deficiency or 30 units orally once daily to prevent deficiency.[4]

Vitiligo

Vitiligo is a cosmetic problem caused by the loss of cells (melanocytes) that produce skin color (melanin) resulting in white blotches on the skin. Often the patches begin on areas of skin that are exposed to the sun and effect both sides of the body. Vitiligo tends to expand over time, causing larger areas of skin to lose pigment. It may begin at any age, but the average age of onset is in the mid-twenties.[1] Vitiligo is more common in people with autoimmune diseases. There is no cure for vitiligo, but available treatments may stop its progression and induce varying degrees of re-pigmentation. A combination of therapies is usually more effective than any single therapy.[1]

COSMETIC CARE

Nonpharmacologic Care: Individuals with vitiligo should strive for good general health and a balanced nutritious diet enriched with adequate proteins, vitamin B complex, vitamin E, and minerals such as copper, zinc, and iron.[2]

Zinc: As vitiligo patients have been found to have significant lower serum zinc levels than normal controls, zinc was postulated to play a role in the management of vitiligo. Definitive results, however, have not been forthcoming.[3]

Alpha Lipoic Acid (ALA) and Vitamins C and E: Taking a product containing alpha-lipoic acid, vitamins C and E, and polyunsaturated fatty acids along with light therapy daily for eight months improved skin discoloration in people with patchy white skin due to vitiligo.[4]

Folic Acid: Taking folic acid by mouth improves vitiligo.[5]

Phenylalanine: Taking L-phenylalanine by mouth in combination with UVA exposure or applying L-phenylalanine to the skin in combination with UVA exposure is effective for treating vitiligo in adults and in children.[6]

Picrorhiza: Taking picrorhiza rhizome powder (200 mg twice a day) by mouth for up to one year, in combination with a drug called methoxsalen that is taken by mouth and applied to the skin, helps to treat vitiligo in adults and children.[7]

Antioxidant Vitamins and Minerals: Antioxidant supplementation with vitamins A, C, and E, along with zinc, selenium, and polyphenol, is significantly beneficial in contributing superior clinical efficacy to improve vitiligo.[8]

Ginkgo Biloba: Limited studies show that ginkgo biloba may return skin color in people with vitiligo.[9]

Vitamins B12 and C: Small studies have shown that vitamin C and vitamin B12 plus phototherapy may restore skin color for some people.[9]

Warts

Warts are rough, raised, grainy bumps on the skin that occur most often on the fingers or hands and are caused by the human papillomavirus (HPV). Wart viruses are contagious. Common warts often feature a pattern of tiny black dots, which are small, clotted blood vessels. There are many different types of warts that respond variably to a variety of treatment measures. Warts may recur even after successful treatment.

TREATMENT MEASURES

Salicylic acid preparations (e.g., Compound W, Duofilm, Occlusal-HP, and Mediplast are offered as a solution, gel, cream, or pad in concentrations from 10% to 60%)[1] are available over the counter as a treatment.

Cryotherapy: Freeze sprays (e.g., Compound W Nitrofreeze, Dr. Scholl's Freeze Away, Wart-Off Freeze) are available over the counter to help remove warts.

Topical Zinc: 5%–10% zinc sulphate lotion, 20% zinc oxide paste, and 2% intralesional zinc sulphate injection were all effective in the treatment of plane warts.[2,3]

Oral zinc sulphate 10 mg/kg/day for two months was an effective treatment modality for recalcitrant warts.[2]

Pumice Stone/Callus File: Repeated application, with pumice stone or callus file use, results in cure rates of 60% to 80%, but takes several weeks to work.[1]

Wernicke-Korsakoff Syndrome

Wernicke-Korsakoff syndrome is a neurodegenerative disorder named for two conditions that often happen together: Wernicke's encephalopathy (WE) and Korsakoff syndrome (KS).

A deficiency of thiamine causes WE. In most cases, heavy, long-term alcohol use causes a deficiency of vitamin B1, or thiamine, which helps the brain turn glucose (sugar) into energy.[1] Brain cells are particularly sensitive to low levels of thiamine, so symptoms are neurological.[2] Wernicke's encephalopathy typically comes on suddenly after repeated vomiting or diarrhea.[3] It begins with a global confusional state, evolving over days or weeks, with inattentiveness, indifference, decreased spontaneous speech, impaired memory, lethargy, loss of balance, and trouble with vision. Initially, the eyes can be looking in different directions from each other, which helps to account for complaints of double vision.[1] Undiagnosed and/or undertreated Wernicke's encephalopathy can result in permanent brain damage, long-term institutionalization, and death.

Symptoms of Korsakoff syndrome usually begin as the signs of Wernicke encephalopathy start to go away. The telltale sign is the severe loss of short-term memory (amnesia). Memory loss, confabulation, and problems managing day-to-day tasks are key features of KS.

Wernicke's encephalopathy can often be reversed, but Korsakoff syndrome typically cannot.

CLINICAL OPTIONS

Thiamine and Multivitamins: Treatment includes oral thiamine, 50–100 mg/day, plus multivitamins.[4] Effective management also involves intravenous thiamine daily for several months, abstaining from alcohol, and eating a balanced sensible diet.[5] For patients with suspected WE, thiamine 500 mg/day for three to five days has also been advised. If there is clinical improvement at that dosage, the supplementation is continued for a total of two weeks.[6] The European Federation of Neurologic Societies recommends thiamine 200 mg three times a day until improvement stops.[7]

Caveat: Thiamine should be administered prior to any carbohydrate to avoid iatrogenic Wernicke's encephalopathy precipitation.[7]

B Complex and Vitamin C: Due to chronic malnutrition and the gastric malabsorption that follows chronic alcohol abuse, many clinicians advise multivitamin supplements (B1, B2, B6, nicotinamide, vitamin C) in parenteral form for the initial three to five days.[6]

Whooping Cough/Pertussis

Whooping cough is a highly contagious respiratory tract infection which is more common in children than adults. It is caused by the bacterium *Bordetella pertussis*. In its early stages, pertussis appears to be nothing more than the common cold. After one to two weeks, more severe symptoms start to appear. In many people, whooping cough is marked by severe uncontrollable coughing fits followed by a high-pitched intake of breath that sounds like "whoop." The coughing fit may be so severe as to obstruct breathing, cause vomiting, or even crack ribs.[1] Despite vaccinations, worrisome outbreaks of whooping cough have been seen in the past decade.[2]

NUTRITIONAL MANAGEMENT TECHNIQUE

Ascorbic acid definitely shortened the paroxysmal stage of the disease, particularly in doses of 500 mg/day for seven days and then reduced to 250 mg/day.[3,4]

Vitamin C therapy was tried in 81 cases of whooping cough. In 34 cases, a clear improvement of the symptoms or perfect healing was obtained; in 32 cases improvement of the symptoms was achieved; and in 15 cases the effects were indeterminate.

In light cases of pertussis, "Roche" (L-ascorbic acid sodium) in injectable solution, 0.1 gm per ampule, was administered at 50–100 mg; in moderately severe cases 100–150 mg; and in severe cases over 200 mg once daily (sometimes twice). Injections started daily at first; after improvement of the symptoms, injections continued every other day with a total of 5 to 12 injections.[5]

As a result, the vitamin C therapy can be viewed as an effective specific therapy. This treatment exhibited no side effects compared to other treatments and had the advantage that it could be applied to pertussis in infancy. Success with specific vaccine injections has been achieved with difficulty so far because of insufficient production of immune bodies.[5]

The clinical success of the vitamin C therapy can be explained by the fact that, among the different pathogenic bacteria, the growth of *B. pertussis* is suppressed specifically by vitamin C and is finally killed. In addition, vitamin C detoxified the pertussis bacterial toxin.[5]

Wilson's Disease

Wilson's disease, also known as hepatolenticular degeneration, is an inherited disease that prevents the body from removing extra copper. This causes copper to build up in the liver, brain (basal ganglia), eyes (corneas), and kidneys.[1]

Common signs of associated liver disease include a yellow discoloration (jaundice) of the skin, mucous membranes, and the membranes (sclera) that line the eye, swelling (edema) of the legs and abdomen (ascites) due to abnormal retention of fluid, presence of abnormally enlarged or swollen veins (varices) in the esophagus that may bleed, a tendency for bruising and prolonged bleeding, and excessive tiredness (fatigue). Wilson's disease presents clinically in the teenage years or early twenties. Hepatic copper accumulation leads to chronic liver disease, which can further lead to cirrhosis. Without medical chelation treatment, which is a lifetime process, high copper levels can cause life-threatening organ damage, central nervous system dysfunction, and death.[2]

ADJUVANT THERAPY

Diet: Patients should generally avoid eating foods with a high copper content, such as liver, chocolate, nuts, mushrooms, legumes, and shellfish (especially lobster). Drinking water from atypical sources (e.g., well water) should be analyzed for copper content and replaced with purified water if the copper content is greater than 0.2 parts per million.[3]

Lipoic Acid: There is some evidence that children afflicted with inborn errors of pyruvate metabolism may derive some benefit from lipoic acid treatment. Therefore, those with Wilson's disease may be helped by lipoic acid as well.[4,5]

Zinc Acetate (Galzin): Zinc acts by blocking the absorption of copper in the intestinal tract. This action both depletes accumulated copper and prevents its reaccumulation.[6,7] Zinc interferes with the uptake of copper from the gastrointestinal tract. The effectiveness of zinc has been shown by more than 30 years of considerable experience overseas. A major advantage of zinc therapy is its lack of side effects.[6]

Zinc salts, 50 mg tid, are indicated in patients with chronic hepatitis and cirrhosis in the absence of hepatic failure. Other than gastric irritation, zinc has an excellent safety profile.[8]

Antioxidants, mainly vitamin E, may have a role as adjunctive treatment. Serum and hepatic vitamin E levels have been found to be low in WD.[9,10,11,12,13] Symptomatic improvement when vitamin E was added to the treatment regimen has been reported, but no rigorous studies have been conducted.[14,15]

Vitamin D: There is some question of whether more frequent bone disease is present in patients with Wilson's disease because their chronic liver disease may have impaired vitamin D metabolism, and so osteoporosis and osteopenia may develop.[16] Therefore, vitamin D supplements are recommended.

Pyridoxine: Patients also will need to take vitamin B6 (25–50 mg/day) and follow a low-copper diet, which means avoiding mushrooms, nuts, chocolate, dried fruit, liver, and shellfish.[17,18]

Iron and/or Calcium: Supplementation of iron or calcium during penicillamine or trientine therapy is to be avoided.[19]

Wound Care (Chronic)/Delayed Healing

Chronic wounds are those that do not progress through a normal, orderly, and timely sequence of repair. Common lower extremity wounds include arterial, diabetic, pressure, and venous ulcers.[1] The rate of open wound healing is dependent on the location, size, and depth of the wound as well as nutritional status.[2]

Healing is normally achieved through four precise and highly-programmed phases: hemostasis (clotting to stop the bleeding), inflammation (wound area becomes fluid-filled due to increased vascular permeability so neutrophils and macrophages can be delivered to remove bacteria), proliferation (fibroblasts proliferate and angiogenesis and epithelialization occur with collagen crosslinking and the resulting wound contraction), and remodeling (collagen maturation and stabilization occur). The remodeling phase starts approximately two weeks after injury and can last up to two years.[3] For a wound to heal successfully, all four phases must occur in the proper sequence and time frame. Nutrition deficiencies interfere with the normal processes that allow progression through the stages of wound healing.[4]

If there is no significant healing after about four weeks, a wound is becoming chronic. Leg ulcers are the most common type of chronic wound infections and are responsible for considerable illness and degradation of health. *Staphylococcus aureus* and *Pseudomonas aeruginosa* are the most common bacteria associated with chronic wound infections.

Examples of wound healing issues include poor nutrition (i.e., low protein levels), diminished oxygenation, decreased circulation, diabetes, smoking, obesity, low hemoglobin levels, and infection (e.g., hepatitis C). Inflammation is a normal part of the wound-healing process, and is important to facilitate the removal of contaminating micro-organisms.[5] The presence of bacterial biofilms in wound infections can cause persistence of chronic infections due to antibiotic tolerance.[6] Debridement (except for arterial ulcers) and infection control are the first steps in medical management.

RESEARCH RECOMMENDATIONS

Moisture balance is an essential part of wound care. Chronic wounds should never be exposed to air to "dry out," as is often recommended. Moist wounds heal more quickly and have less risk of infection.[1]

Glucocorticoids should be avoided or reduced, if possible, because they are used as anti-inflammatory agents, and are well-known to inhibit wound repair via global anti-inflammatory effects and suppression of cellular wound responses, including fibroblast proliferation and collagen synthesis.[5]

NSAIDs should be avoided or limited. Non-steroidal anti-inflammatory drugs such as ibuprofen, which have demonstrated an anti-proliferative effect on wound healing, should be avoided because they result in decreased numbers of fibroblasts, weakened breaking strength, reduced wound contraction, and delayed epithelialization.[5]

Weight loss should be encouraged. Obese individuals frequently face wound complications, including skin wound infection, dehiscence, hematoma and seroma formation, pressure ulcers, and venous ulcers.[5]

Avoidance of Alcohol: Clinical evidence and animal experiments have shown that exposure to alcohol impairs wound healing and increases the incidence of infection.[5]

Avoidance of Nicotine: The negative effects of smoking on wound-healing outcomes have been known for a long time. Postoperatively, patients who smoke show a delay in wound healing and an increase in a variety of complications such as infection, wound rupture, anastomotic leakage, wound and flap necrosis, epidermolysis, and a decrease in the tensile strength of wounds.[5]

Vitamin A: Vitamin A deficiency also leads to impaired wound healing.[5]

Micronutrients: Several micronutrients, such as zinc, magnesium, and iron, have been shown to be important for optimal repair.[5]

Ascorbic acid plays a pivotal role in collagen synthesis and, thus, wound healing. A deficiency in this vitamin has multiple negative effects on tissue repair.[5] In one study, four case reports with very positive results led to the authors' recommendation that patients suffering from poor wound healing should be supplemented with at least 500–1,000 mg of ascorbic acid twice a day until the healing process is finished. If a patient must undergo surgery while being deficient, it is suggested that the patient should start supplementation with ascorbic acid post-surgery, during a normoxic state, to prevent possible damage caused by its pro-oxidant effects, although evidence for its harmful effects seems largely hypothetical. Invasive procedures, especially if accompanied by severe infections or sepsis, could lead to a detrimental depletion of ascorbic acid storage.[7]

The clinical cases presented above demonstrate that treating deficient patients with ascorbic acid leads to more rapid improvement of the wound-healing process post-surgery, thereby reducing the costs of elaborate wound treatment and extensive hospital stays.[7]

Glutamine: Oral glutamine supplementation has been shown to improve wound-breaking strength and to increase levels of mature collagen.[8]

Arginine: Arginine supplementation has been shown to be an effective adjuvant therapy in wound healing.[9]

Topical Honey: In clinical practice, Manuka honey produced by Australian honey bees (*Apis mellifera*) is used topically for its antibacterial and antiseptic effects in the management of superficial wound infections.[10]

Acetic Acid (1%): Acetic acid is known for its antimicrobial effect on bacteria. Acetic acid is present in vinegar in a 3%–5% concentration and has been used in medicine for thousands of years. In vitro and in vivo testing of acetic acid against bacterial biofilms has been shown to be effective against planktonic and biofilm bacteria.[11] The recurrence of soft tissue deterioration despite antibiotic treatment and/or surgical debridement would be an indication for treatment with acetic acid. Another indication is chronic *P. aeruginosa* soft tissue infection.[11] Application of 1% acetic acid solution in isotonic saline was applied for an average of nine days. Treatment completely eradicated *P. aeruginosa* biofilms (i.e., no viable counts on plates) and completely eradicated of *S. aureus.*[11]

Zinc deficiency affects all phases of wound healing. Zinc supplementation (40–220 mg bid for 14 days) is recommended. A review by Lansdown et al. looked at enteral vs. topical zinc in wound healing and found that topical zinc applied to surgical wounds consistently augmented wound healing, regardless of serum or plasma zinc levels.[12]

General Advice: Increase protein intake to 1.5 g per kg body weight and supplement vitamins A and C along with zinc.[1]

Wrinkles

Wrinkles, also known as a rhytides, are folds, lines, or creases that form in the skin. Wrinkles are shallow (fine surface lines) or deep, forming crevices or furrows. Skin wrinkles typically appear as a result of the aging processes especially around the eyes, mouth, and neck. Treatment for fine surface lines is typically more effective than for deeper wrinkles.

MINIMIZING PHOTO-AGING

Alpha hydroxy acid in a lotion, cream, or solution can decrease wrinkles and other signs of sun-damaged skin.[1]

Moisturizers are a time-tested remedy for wrinkles. Moist skin looks younger and better. Aging causes oil producing glands to become less active and thus skin becomes drier. A wide variety of moisturizers with different ingredients are available. A medical professional should be consulted to obtain the best product and result for your age, skin type, and any underlying conditions.[2]

Retinol: The only FDA-approved topical treatment for wrinkles is tretinoin, known commercially as Retin-A and available by prescription. Retinol is a natural form of vitamin A and in high concentrations may be as effective as Retin-A without the side effects.[3]

Ascorbic Acid: Vitamin C (ascorbic acid) is one of the four most important ingredients in skin care products. It is proven to increase collagen production when applied topically to improve the appearance of wrinkled skin.[4,5]

In a clinical study, a stabilized 10% solution of vitamin C was applied directly to the skin of individuals with wrinkles and sun-induced spotting with good results.[6] In a 2015 study of 60 healthy female subjects, Crisan et al. used high-frequency ultrasound to determine that the use of a topical vitamin C formulation yielded significant increases in collagen synthesis, revealing the solution to be an effective rejuvenation therapy.[7] The L-ascorbic acid form of vitamin C appears to be the most effective for wrinkle relief.

Alpha-Lipoic Acid (ALA): Thirty-three women with a mean age of 54.4 years were included in a controlled study. After randomization, half the face of each woman was treated twice daily for 12 weeks with alpha-lipoic acid cream 5% and the other half with the control cream. The following methods of assessment were used: self-evaluation by the test subjects, clinical evaluation, photographic evaluation and laser profilometry. All four methods of assessment showed a statistically significant improvement on the alpha-lipoic acid-treated half of the face. Twelve weeks of treatment with a cream containing 5% alpha-lipoic acid improved clinical characteristics related to facial skin photo-aging.[8,9]

Vitamin B3, niacinamide, reduced the appearance of aging on the face.[10]

Copper-Zinc Malonate: Mahoney et al. evaluated the effects of a bi-metal, 0.1% copper-zinc malonate-containing cream on elastin biosynthesis and elastic tissue accumulation in 21 female patients with photo-aged facial skin. After eight weeks of therapy, significant elastic fiber regeneration was seen in the papillary dermis leading to effacement of wrinkles.[11]

Cross-sectional studies have reported that higher dietary intakes of EFAs are associated with more youthful skin appearance and photoprotection.[12]

Para-Aminobenzoic Acid (PABA): PABA taken by mouth can make skin look younger.[13,14] A typical therapeutic dose of PABA is 300–400 mg/day.[15]

Idebenone: In one study, just six weeks of applying a 1.0% idebenone cream topically twice a day resulted in a 29% decrease in lines and wrinkles, a 37% increase in hydration, and a 26% reduction in skin dryness and roughness.[16]

Xanthelasma

Xanthelasma is a localized deposit of fat and cholesterol near the inner canthus of the eyelid. Xanthelasmas appear as a yellowish, raised plaque, more often on the upper lid than on the lower lid. Some xanthelasmas can be indicative of hyperlipidemia that can be associated with increased risk of coronary heart disease or occasionally with pancreatitis (due to hypertriglyceridemia). About half the people with xanthelasma have high cholesterol. These patches will not go away on their own and may grow in size. Removal, although not without some unwanted side effects, may be the best option, but the growths can come back.

COSMETIC IMPROVEMENT

B12 Injections: Twenty-five patients with xanthelasma received vitamin B12 injections (500–1,000 mcg) once a week for 6 to 20 weeks. The skin lesions became smaller in 92% of the patients, with marked improvement occurring in 20% of cases.[1,2]

DIETARY MEASURES TO TREAT HYPERLIPIDEMIA AND HYPERTRIGLYCERIDEMIA

- Prepare most meals from vegetables, salads, cereals, and fish.
- Minimize saturated fats (found in meat, butter, other dairy produce, coconut oil, and palm oil).
- Minimize intake of simple, refined sugars found in fizzy drinks, sweets, biscuits, and cakes.
- If obese or overweight, the aim is to slowly reduce weight by reducing caloric intake and increasing exercise.[3]

Xeroderma Pigmentosum

Xeroderma pigmentosum, commonly known as XP, is an inherited condition characterized by an extreme sensitivity to ultraviolet (UV) rays from sunlight. In this genetic disorder, there is a decreased ability to repair DNA damage caused by ultraviolet light. This condition mostly affects the eyes and areas of skin exposed to the sun. The signs of xeroderma pigmentosum usually appear in infancy or early childhood. Patients with xeroderma pigmentosum have a greatly increased risk of developing skin cancer.[1] About 30% of people with xeroderma pigmentosum develop progressive neurological abnormalities in addition to problems involving the skin and eyes.[1]

THERAPY FOR SKIN LESIONS

Topical Zinc: A 20% topical zinc sulphate solution was applied to 19 patients with xeroderma pigmentosa. Improvement in all types of skin lesions, including softening and lightening of the skin color, and clearance of solar keratosis and small malignancies was observed in 15 patients who continued the study during monthly follow-ups for two years. There was no exacerbation of old lesions and no development of new malignancy.[2,3]

NOTES

Acetaminophen (Tylenol) Poisoning

1 https://emedicine.medscape.com/article/820200-overview. Accessed Dec. 16, 2018.

2 https://wwwrxlist.com/methionine/supplements.htm. Accessed Nov. 17, 2018.

3 M.J. Ellenhorn and D.G. Barceloux, *Medical Toxicology: Diagnosis and Treatment of Human Poisoning* (New York, NY: Elsevier Science Publishing Co., Inc., 1988), 80.

4 https://pubmed.ncbi.nlm.nih.gov/26250417/. Accessed Feb. 19, 2021.

5 https://www.webmd.com/vitamins/ai/ingredientmono-1018/n-acetyl-cysteine-nac. Accessed Feb. 19, 2021.

6 https://www.webmd.com/vitamins/ai/ingredientmono-42/methionine. Accessed Nov. 17, 2018. Please note that a free, one-time registration is required in order to view the full linked article and all other content on the Medscape/WebMD sites.

7 National Center for Biotechnology Information, PubChem Compound Database. CID=84815. https://ncbi.nlm.gov/compound/84815. Accessed Nov. 14, 2018.

8 https://pubmed.ncbi.nlm.nih.gov/26250417/.

Acne Vulgaris

1 M. Gupta et al., "Zinc Therapy in Dermatology: A Review," *Dermatol Res Pract* 2014 (2014): 709152. Published online July 10, 2014. DOI: 10.1155/2014/709152.

2 E.T. Bope and R.D. Kellerman, *Conn's Current Therapy*, 14th ed. (Philadelphia: Elsevier/ Saunders), 237.

3 L.K. Oge, A. Broussard, and M.D. Marshall, "Acne Vulgaris: Diagnosis and Treatment," *Am Fam Physician* 100 (2019): 475-484.

4 M.A. Chisolm-Burns et al., *Pharmacotherapy Principles & Practice* (McGraw-Hill Medical, 2008), 962.

5 T. Arif, "Salicylic Acid as a Peeling Agent: A Comprehensive Review," *Clin Cosmet Investig Dermatol* 8 (2015): 455-461.

6 https://www.webmd.com/vitamins/ai/ingredientmono-977/alpha-hydroxy-acids. Accessed Jan. 21, 2018.

7 https://www.mayoclinic.org/diseases-conditions/acne/in-depth/acne-products/art-20045814. Accessed Jan. 21, 2018.

8 https://pubmed.ncbi.nlm.nih.gov/27416309/. Accessed May 19, 2021.

9 https://www.hindawi.com/journals/drp/2014/709152/. Accessed Feb. 1, 2021.

10 https://www.researchgate.net/publication/314425582_High_dose_niacin_in_the_treatment_of_acne_vulgaris_a_pilot_study. Accessed Nov. 14, 2018.

11 Z. Shahmoradi et al., "Comparison of Topical 5% Nicotinamide Gel versus 2% Clindamycin Gel in the Treatment of the Mild-Moderate Acne Vulgaris: A Double-Blinded Randomized Clinical Trial," *J Res Med Sci* 18, no. 2 (Feb. 2013): 115-117.

12 A.R. Shalita et al., "Topical Nicotinamide Compared with Clindamycin Gel in the Treatment of Inflammatory Acne Vulgaris," *Int J Dermatol.* 34 (1995): 434-437.

13 https://www.mdedge.com/dermatology/article/215102/acne/ketogenic-diet-and-dermatology-primer-current-literature. Accessed Jan. 30, 2020.

14 https://www.ncbi.nlm.nih.gov/pmc/articles/PMC7847434/. Accessed Jan. 6, 2022.

15 D.A. Fomin, DO, and K. Handfield, MD, "The Ketogenic Diet: A Primer on Current Literature," *Cuti* 105, no. 1 (Jan. 2020): 40-43.

16 J.J. Russell, MD, "Topical Therapy for Acne," *Am Fam Physician.* 61, no. 2 (Jan. 15, 2000): 357-365.

17 https://www.medicalnewstoday.com/articles/71702#risk_factors. Accessed May 14, 2020.

18 https://www.mayoclinic.org/diseases-conditions/seobrrheic-dernatitis/diagnosis-treatment/drc-20352714. Accessed Jan. 2, 2019.

19 https://www.medicalnewstoday.com/articles/319113.php. Accessed Jan. 2, 2019.

20 https://www.ncbi.nlm.nih.gov/pmc/articles/PMC7847434/. Accessed Jan. 6, 2022.

Acrodermatitis Enteropathica

1 M. Gupta et al., "Zinc Therapy in Dermatology: A Review," *Dermatol Res Pract* 2014 (2014): 709152. Published online July 10, 2014. DOI: 10.1155/2014/709152.

2 https://www.webmd.com/drugs/2/drug-4086/zinc-sulfate-oral/details. Accessed Sept. 4, 2018.

3 K. Weismann and H. Hoyer, "Zinc Deficiency Dermatoses: Etiology, Clinical Aspects and Treatment," *Hautarzt* 33, no. 8 (Aug. 1982): 405-410. [article in German]

Actinic Keratosis

1 https://www.ncbi.nlm.nih.gov/pmc/articles/PMC3339136/. Accessed Jan. 4, 2019.

2 P. Star, "Oral Nicotinamide Prevents Common Skin Cancers in High-Risk Patients, Reduces Costs," *Am Health Drug Benefits* 8, spec. issue (Aug. 2015): 13-14.

3 https://pubmed.ncbi.nlm.nih.gov/21921960/.

4 https://pubmed.ncbi.nlm.nih.gov/11359487/.

Adult-Onset Spinocerebellar Syndrome

1 https://onlinelibrary.wiley.com/doi/abs/10.1002/ana.410220119. Accessed Dec. 16, 2018.

2 http://practicalneurology.com/2013/04/overview-of-adult-onset-cerebellar-ataxia. Accessed Mar. 23, 2019.

3 T. Yokota et al., "Adult-Onset Spinocerebellar Syndrome with Idiopathic Vitamin E Deficiency," *Ann Neurol* 22, no. 1 (1987): 84.

4 A. Costantini et al., "Thiamine and Spinocerebellar Ataxia Type 2," *BMJ Case Reports.* Published online Jan. 10, 2013.

5 https://www.sciencedirect.com/science/article/pii/0022510X81901623. Accessed Jan. 6, 2019.

6 H. Sarva and V.L. Shanker, "Treatment Options in Degenerative Cerebellar Ataxia: A Systematic Review," *Movement Disorders Clinical Practice* 1, no. 4 (2014). DOI: 10.1002/mdc3.12057.

Alcohol Withdrawal Syndrome

1 M.G. Griswold et al., "Alcohol Use and Burden for 195 Countries and Territories, 1990-2016: A Systematic Analysis for the Global Burden of Disease Study 2016," *The Lancet* 392 (2018): 1015-1035. DOI: 10.1016/S0140-6736(18)31310-2.

2 https://www.emedicinehealth.com/alcoholism/article_em.htm#what_is_the_treatment_for_alcoholism. Accessed Dec. 21, 2018.

3 https://www.ncbi.nlm.nih.gov/pmc/articles/PMC4085800/. Accessed Dec. 21, 2018.

4 https://www.webmd.com/vitamins/ai/ingredientmono-834/acetyl-l-carnitine. Accessed Sept. 4, 2018.

5 https://wwwrxlist.com.acetyl-l-carnitine/supplements.htm. Accessed May 31, 2019.

6 J.F. Sullivan et al., "Magnesium Metabolism in Alcoholism," *Am J Clin Nutr* 13 (1963): 297-303.

7 J.C.M. Brust, *Current Diagnosis and Treatment Neurology*, 2nd ed. (McGraw-Hill, 2012), 518.

8 https://www.medscape.com/answers/819502-80779/which-medications-in-the-drug-class-vitamins-are-used-in-the-treatment-of-withdrawal-syndromes. Accessed Dec. 21, 2018.

9 https://medlineplus.gov/ency/article/002149.htm. Accessed Dec. 21, 2018.

10 K. Doheny, "Chinese Herb Kudzu May Help Drinkers Cut Down." https://www.webmd.com/mental-health/addiction/news/20120517/chinese-herb-kudzu-may-help-drinkers-cut-down#1. Accessed Sept. 2, 2019.

11 H.E. Sartori, "Lithium Orotate in the Treatment of Alcoholism and Related Conditions," *Alcohol* 3, no. 2 (1986) 97-100. 3718672.

Alertness

1 A.B. Clemetson, *Vitamin C, Vol. III* (Boca Raton, FL: CRC Press, 1989), 93.

2 https://www.webmd.com/vitamins/condition-1380/mental+alertness.aspx. Accessed Nov. 19, 2018.

3 G. Vorberg, "Ginkgo Biloba Extract (GBE): A Long-Term Study of Chronic Cerebral Insufficiency in Geriatric Patients," *Clin Trials J* 22 (1985): 149-157.

4 J. Taillandier et al., "Ginkgo Biloba Extract in the Treatment of Cerebral Disorders Due to Aging," *Presse Med* 15 (1986): 1583-1587.

5 https://www.independent.co.uk/news/science/herbal-cocktail-gives-an-instant-boost-to-memory-and-alertness-280552.html. Accessed Nov. 19, 2018.

6 https://www.webmd.com/vitamins/ai/ingredientmono-1024/taurine. Accessed Nov. 28, 2018.

7 https://www.webmd.com/vitamins/ai/ingredientmono-1037/tyrosine. Accessed Nov. 28, 2018.

8 https://www.rxlist.com/tyrosine/supplements.htm. Accessed Nov. 28, 2018.

9 http://www.medicaldaily.com/dark-chocolate-found-lengthen-attention-span-and-improve-brain-alertness-332720. Accessed Jan. 9, 2019.

10 https://www.medicaldaily.com/brain-boosters-foods-can-help-improve-your-intelligence-alertness-focus-and-memory-289182. Accessed Jan. 9, 2019.

Allergies

1 R.R. Widmann and J.D. Keye, "Epinephrine Precursors in Control of Allergy," *Northwest Med* 51 (1952): 588-590.

2 https://www.medicalnewstoday.com/articles/323276.php. Accessed Mar. 2, 2019.

3 https://www.webmd.com/allergies/news/20050822/butterbur-may-be-effective-hay-fever-remedy#1. Accessed Mar. 2, 2019.

Alopecia Areata/Hair Loss

1 https://www.mdedge.com/familymedicine/quiz/9968/obesity/obesity-test-your-skills-these-5-questions?ecd=wnl_fam_210121_mdedge_4am. Accessed Jan. 21, 2021.

2 K.E. Sharquie, A.A. Noaimi, and E.R. Shwail, "Oral Zinc Sulphate in Treatment of Alopecia Areata," *Journal of Clinical and Experimental Dermatology Research* 3 (2012): 150.

3 https://pubmed.ncbi.nlm.nih.gov/22741940/. Accessed Jan. 21, 2021.

4 https://www.medicalnewstoday.com/articles/321673.php. Accessed Dec. 20, 2018.

5 https://www.ncbi.nlm.nih.gov/pubmed/23428658. Accessed Dec. 20, 2018.

6 S. Famenini and C. Goh, "Evidence for Supplemental Treatments in Androgenetic Alopecia," *J Drugs Dermatol* 13, no. 7 (2014): 809-812.

7 https://lpi.oregonstate.edu/mic/vitamins/biotin#reference46. Accessed Jan. 5, 2019.

8 https://www.medicalnewstoday.com/articles/318724.php. Accessed Jan. 5, 2019.

9 https://www.rxlist.com/biotin/supplements.htm. Accessed Jan. 5, 2019.

10 https://www.emedicinehealth.com/para-aminobenzoic_acid_paba/vitamins-supplements.htm. Accessed Dec. 26, 2018.

11 https://pubmed.ncbi.nlm.nih.gov/33313047/. Accessed June 18, 2021.

Altitude Sickness

1 https://med.stanford.edu/news/all-news/2012/03/ibuprofen-decreases-likelihood-of-altitude-sickness-researchers-find.html. Accessed Nov. 19, 2018.

Alzheimer's Disease (AD)

1 J.P.T. Higgins and L. Flicker, "Lecithin for Dementia and Cognitive Impairment," *Cochrane Database Syst Rev* 3 (2003): CD001015.

2 https://www.mayoclinic.org/diseases-conditions/vascular-dementia/symptoms-causes/syc-20378793.

3 https://lpi.oregonstate.edu/mic/other-nutrients/choline#reference59. Accessed Nov. 23, 2018.

4 N. Tabet, "Acetylcholinesterase Inhibitors for Alzheimer's Disease: An Anti-Inflammatories in Acetylcholine Clothing," *Age and Aging* 35, no. 4 (July 2006): 336-338.

5 https://www.mayoclinic.org/diseases-conditions/alzheimers-disease/diagnosis-treatment/drc-20350453. Accessed Nov. 23, 2018.

6 V. Parisi et al., "Cytidine-5'-diphosphocholine (Citicoline): A Pilot Study in Patients with Non-Arteritic Ischemic Optic Neuropathy," *Eur J Neurol* 15, no. 5 (2008): 465-474.

7 https://pubmed.ncbi.nlm.nih.gov/8709678/. Accessed Mar. 7, 2021.

8 L. Ottobelli et al., "Citicoline Oral Solution in Glaucoma: Is There a Role in Slowing Disease Progression?," *Ophthalmologica* 229, no. 4 (2013): 219-226.

9 G. Douaud et al., "Preventing Alzheimer's Disease-Related Gray Matter Atrophy by B-Vitamin Treatment," *Proc Natl Acad Sci* 110, no. 23 (2013): 9523-9528.

10 A.D. Smith et al., "Homocysteine-Lowering by B Vitamins Slows the Rate of Accelerated Brain Atrophy in Mild Cognitive Impairment," *Public Library of Science One*. DOI: 10.1371/journal.pone0012244.

11 J.M. Kim et al., "Changes in Folate, Vitamin B12 and Homocysteine Associated with Incident Dementia," *J Neurol Neurosurg Psychiatry* 79, no. 8 (Aug. 2008): 864-868. DOI: 10.1136/jnnp.2007.131482. Epub Feb. 5, 2008.

12 M.A. Chisolm-Burns et al., *Pharmacotherapy Principles & Practice* (McGraw-Hill Medical, 2008), 519, 521.

13 M. Sano et al., "A Controlled Trial of Selegiline, Alpha-Tocopherol, or Both as Treatment for Alzheimer's Disease," *N Engl J Med* 336 (1997): 1216-1222.

14 M.W. Dysken et al., "Effect of Vitamin E and Memantine on Functional Decline in Alzheimer Disease: The TEAM-AD VA Cooperative Randomized Trial," *JAMA* 311, no. 1 (2014): 33-44.

15 https://www.webmd.com/alzheimers/news/20020114/vitamin-c-may-improve-alzheimers-treatments. Accessed Mar. 18, 2021.

16 https://www.ncbi.nlm.nih.gov/pmc/articles/PMC3783921/. Accessed Sept. 6, 2018.

17 https://www.webmd.com/vitamins/ai/ingredientmono-333/ginkgo. Accessed Nov. 26, 2018.

18 https://alzheimersnewstoday.com/resveratrol/. Accessed Jan. 9, 2019.

19 https://www.ncbi.nlm.nih.gov/pubmed/12804452. Accessed May 31, 2019.

20 A. Spagnoli et al., "Long-Term Acetyl-L-Carnitine Treatment in Alzheimer's Disease," *Neurology* 41, no. 11 (Nov. 1991): 1726. DOI: 10.1212/WNL.41.11.1726.

21 https://www.webmd.com/vitamins/ai/ingredientmono-834/acetyl-l-carnitine. Accessed May 31, 2019.

22 https://www.rxlist.com/acetyl-l-carnitine/supplements.htm. Accessed May 31, 2019.

23 https://www.ncbi.nlm.nih.gov/pmc/articles/PMC3930088/. Accessed May 31, 2019.

24 M.G. Sullivan, "Seaweed Floats to the Top of Alzheimer's News," *MDEdge Neurology* (Nov. 15, 2019). Accessed Dec. 2, 2019.

25 https://www.ncbi.nlm.nih.gov/pmc/articles/PMC2600464/. Accessed Mar. 6, 2020.

26 https://www.mdedge.com/neurology/article/99259/alzheimers-cognition/moderate-adherence-mind-diet-may-protect-against. Accessed Mar. 15, 2021.

27 https://www.mdedge.com/clinicalneurologynews/article/216430/alzheimers-cognition/dietary-flavonol-intake-linked-reduced. Accessed Mar. 11, 2020.

28 https://www.mdedge.com/neurology/article/118918/alzheimers-cognition/how-does-physical-activity-differ-mild-alzheimers. Accessed Mar. 15, 2021.

29 J. Kingsland, "Could Viagra Reduce Alzheimer's Risk," *Medical News Today* (Dec. 7, 2021). https://www.medicalnewstoday.com/articles/could-viagra-reduce-alzheimers-risk. Accessed Dec. 7, 2021.

Amblyopia (Nutritional)

1 "Nutritional Amblyopia and B Complex Vitamin Deficiencies," *Handbook of Nutrition and Ophthalmology* (Nutrition and Health, Humana Press, 2007), 281-354.

2 D.L. Knox et al., "Nutritional Amblyopia: Folic Acid, Vitamin B12, and Other Vitamins," *Retina* 2, no. 2 (1982): 288-293.

Amyotrophic Lateral Sclerosis

1 https://www.intechopen.com/books/current-advances-in-amyotrophic-lateral-sclerosis/pathophysiology-of-amyotrophic-lateral-sclerosis. Accessed May 5, 2021.

2 https://www.ninds.nih.gov/Disorders/Patient-Caregiver-Education/Fact-Sheets/Amyotrophic-Lateral-Sclerosis-ALS-Fact-Sheet. Accessed Mar. 12, 2019.

3 E.J. O'Reilly et al., "Long-Term Vitamin E Intake Linked to Reduced ALS Risk," *American Journal of Epidemiology* 173 (2011): 595-602.

4 https://www.medscape.com/viewarticle/739860. Accessed Sept. 5, 2018.

5 See also https://www.ncbi.nlm.nih.gov/pmc/articles/PMC2631353/. Accessed Sept. 5, 2018.

6 E. Beghi et al., "Randomized Double-Blind Placebo-Controlled Trial of Acetyl-L-Carnitine for ALS," *Amyotroph Lateral Scler Frontotemporal Degener* 14 (2013): 397-405.

7 Y. Kira et al., *Brain Res* 1070, no. 1 (2006): 206-214.

8 https://pubchem.ncbi.nlm.nih.gov/compound/L-carnitine#section=Therapeutic-Uses. Accessed Jan. 6, 2019.

9 R. Mancuso et al., "Resveratrol Improves Motoneuron Function and Extends Survival in SOD1 (G93A) ALS Mice," *Neurotherapeutics* 11 (2014): 419-432.

10 L. Song et al., "Resveratrol Ameliorates Motor Neuron Degeneration and Improves Survival in SOD1 (G93A) Mouse Model of Amyotrophic Lateral Sclerosis," *Biomed Res Int* 2014 (2014): 483501.

11 R. Mancuso et al., "Lack of Synergistic Effect of Resveratrol and Sigma-1 Receptor Agonist (PRE-084) in SOD1 G93A ALS Mice: Overlapping Effects or Limited Therapeutic Opportunity?," *Orphanet J Rare Dis* 9 (2014): 7.

12 C. Karam et al., "Vitamin D Deficiency and Its Supplementation in Patients with Amyotrophic Lateral Sclerosis," *J Clin Neurosci* 20, no. 11 (2013): 1550-1553.

13 J.W. Nieves et al., "Association Between Dietary Intake and Function in Amyotrophic Lateral Sclerosis," *JAMA Neurology*. Published online ahead of print Oct. 24, 2016. Accessed Nov. 22, 2016.

Anal Fissures

1 https://www.medicinenet.com/anal_fissure/article.htm. Accessed Nov. 21, 2018.

2 S.M. Ebinger et al., "Operative and Medical Treatment of Chronic Anal Fissures—A Review and Network Meta-Analysis of Randomized Controlled Trials," *J Gastroenterol* 52, no. 6 (2017): 663-676.

3 https://www.webmd.com/drugs/2/drug-159295/nitroglycerin-rectal/details. Accessed Nov. 21, 2018.

4 *The Merck Manual of Diagnosis and Therapy*, 19th ed., 247.

5 https://www.webmd.com/vitamins/ai/ingredientmono-235/calendula. Accessed Nov. 21, 2018.

6 S. Naseer and S. Lorenzo-Rivero, "Role of Calendula Extract in Treatment of Anal Fissures," *Am Surg* 78, no. 8 (2012): E377-E378. PMID: 22856483.

Anemia

1 D.C. Heimburger and J.D. Ard, *Clinical Nutrition*, 4th ed. (Mosby Elsevier, 2006), 523.

Anemia (Chronic Kidney Disease)

1 https://www.webmd.com/vitamins/ai/ingredientmono-954/vitamin-e. Accessed Sept. 5, 2018.

2 https://www.webmd.com/vitamins/ai/ingredientmono-1017/folic-acid. Accessed Feb. 11, 2019.

3 https://www.ncbi.nlm.nih.gov/pmc/articles/PMC3884187/. Accessed June 18, 2020.

4 https://www.ncbi.nlm.nih.gov/pmc/articles/PMC3155231/. Last accessed Jan. 6, 2019.

5 https://academic.oup.com/ndt/article/19/9/2319/1836244. Accessed Nov. 6, 2020.

6 W.H. Hörl, "Is There a Role for Adjuvant Therapy in Patients Being Treated with Epoetin?," *Nephrol Dial Transplant* 14, suppl. 2 (1999): 50-60.

Anemia (Copper Deficiency)

1 https://www.ncbi.nlm.nih.gov/pubmed/22080848. Accessed Mar. 2, 2019.

2 "Anemia Due to Other Nutritional Deficiencies," *Williams Hematology* (2011): ch. 29.

3 https://www.ncbi.nlm.nih.gov/pmc/articles/PMC2872358/. Accessed Feb. 7, 2019.

4 D.N. Fiske, H.E. McCoy III, and C.S. Kitchens, "Zinc-Induced Sideroblastic Anemia: Report of a Case, Review of the Literature, and Description of the Hematologic Syndrome," *Am J Hematol* 46 (1994): 147-150.

5 https://www.sciencedirect.com/science/article/pii/0016508588904453. Accessed Mar. 2, 2019.

6 http://www.bloodjournal.org/content/106/11/1681?sso-checked=true. Accessed Feb. 7, 2019.

Anemia (Hemolytic)

1 https://ghr.nlm.nih.gov/condition/glucose-6-phosphate-dehydrogenase-deficiency. Accessed Mar. 3, 2019.

2 https://emedicine.medscape.com/article/201066-treatment. Accessed Nov. 16, 2018.

3 J.H. Ritchie et al., "Edema and Hemolytic Anemia in Premature Infants: A Vitamin E Deficiency Syndrome," *N Engl J Med* 279, no. 22 (Nov. 28, 1968): 1185-1190.

4 *The Merck Manual of Diagnosis and Therapy*, 12th ed. (1973), 1047.

5 A. Cheema et al., "Hemolytic Anemia an Unusual Presentation of Vitamin B12 Deficiency," *J Hematol Thrombo Dis* 6, no. 1 (2018).

Anemia (Macrocytic)

1 https://www.sciencedirect.com/topics/medicine-and-dentistry/macrocytic-anemia. Accessed Apr. 12, 2020.

2 https://www.merckmanuals.com/professional/hematology-and-oncology/anemias-caused-by-deficient-erythropoiesis/megaloblastic-macrocytic-anemias. Accessed Apr. 12, 2020.

3 https://www.msdmanuals.com/professional/nutritional-disorders/vitamin-deficiency,-dependency,-and-toxicity/vitamin-b12-deficiency. Accessed Apr. 12, 2020.

4 "Vitamin Deficiency and Excess," *Harrison's Principles of Internal Medicine*, 13th ed., 475.

Anemia (Microcytic)

1 https://www.rightdiagnosis.com/m/microcytic_anemia/symptoms.htm#symptom_list. Accessed Mar. 24, 2019.

2 J.T. DiPiro et al., *Pharmacotherapy: A Pathophysiologic Approach*, 6th ed. (McGraw-Hill, 2005), 1814-1815.

3 https://www.medscape.org/viewarticle/551577. Accessed Nov. 29, 2018.

4 https://www.emedicinehealth.com/vitamin_c_ascorbic_acid/vitamins-supplements.htm. Accessed Nov. 28, 2018.

5 https://www.webmd.com/vitamins/ai/ingredientmono-1024/taurine. Accessed Nov. 28, 2018.

Anemia (Normochromic and Normocytic)

1 http://www.medicalhealthtests.com/diseases-and-tests/anemia/normocytic-anemia.html. Accessed Mar. 24, 2019.

2 "Vitamin Deficiency and Excess," *Harrison's Principles of Internal Medicine*, 13th ed., 475.

Aneurysms

1 https://onlinelibrary.wiley.com/doi/abs/10.1111/j.1651-2227.1998.tb01381.x. Accessed Dec. 9, 2018.

Angina Pectoris

1 https://www.medscape.com/answers/150215-69337/what-is-the-role-of-aspirin-in-the-treatment-of-angina-pectoris. Accessed Dec.28, 2020.

2 https://www.webmd.com/vitamins/ai/ingredientmono-998/magnesium. Accessed Sept. 5, 2018.

3 T. Kamikawa et al., "Effects of L-Carnitine on Exercise Tolerance in Patients with Stable Angina Pectoris," *Jpn Heart J* 25 (1984): 587597.

4 A. Cherchi et al., "Effects of L-Carnitine on Exercise Tolerance in Chronic Stable Angina: A Multicenter, Double-Blind, Randomized, Placebo-Controlled Crossover Study," *Int J Clin Pharm Ther Toxicol* 23 (1985): 569-572.

5 P. Davini et al., "Controlled Study on L-Carnitine Therapeutic Efficacy in Post-Infarction," *Drugs Exp Clin Res* 18, no. 8 (1992): 355-365.

6 L. Cacciatore et al., "The Therapeutic Effect of L-Carnitine in Patients with Exercise-Induced Stable Angina: A Controlled Study," *Drugs Exp Clin Res* 17, no. 4 (1991): 225-235.

7 A. Salachas et al., "Effects of a Low-Dose Fish Oil Concentrate on Angina, Exercise Tolerance Time, Serum Triglycerides, and Platelet Function," *Angiology* 45 (1994): 1023-1031.

8 A.R. Gaby, "Research Review," *Nutrition and Healing* 2, no. 1 (1995).

9 K.A. Oster, "The Treatment of Bovine Xanthine Oxidase Initiated Atherosclerosis by Folic Acid," *Clin Res* 24 (1976).

10 https://www.ncbi.nlm.nih.gov/pmc/articles/PMC509066/. Accessed Apr. 12, 2020.

11 https://today.oregonstate.edu/archives/1998/jun/vitamin-c-may-reduce-angina-heart-attack-risks. Accessed Mar. 18, 2019.

12 https://www.webmd.com/vitamins/ai/ingredientmono-1018/n-acetyl-cysteine. Accessed Nov. 17, 2018.

13 A. Blum et al., "Clinical and Inflammatory Effects of Dietary L-Arginine in Patients with Intractable Angina Pectoris," *Am J Cardiol* 83, no. 10 (1999): 1488-1490.

14 https://www.drugs.com/npp/l-arginine.html. Accessed Nov. 28, 2018.

15 M.T. Tran et al., "Role of Coenzyme Q10 in Chronic Heart Failure, Angina, and Hypertension," *Pharmacotherapy* 21, no. 7 (2001): 797-806.

16 H.A. Nieper, "Effects of Bromelain on Coronary Heart Disease and Angina Pectoris," *Acta Med Empirica* 5 (1978): 274-278.

17 S.J. Taussig and H.A. Nieper, "Bromelain: Its Use in Prevention and Treatment of Cardiovascular Disease, Present Status," *JIAPM* 6 (1979): 139-156.

18 http://www.altmedrev.com/archive/publications/15/4/361.pdf. Accessed Oct. 14, 2019.

Anorexia Nervosa

1 C.L. Birmingham et al., "Controlled Trial of Zinc Supplementation in Anorexia Nervosa," *Int J Eating Disorders* 15 (1994): 251-255.

2 D. Bryce-Smith and R.I. Simpson, "Case of Anorexia Responding to Zinc Sulphate," *Lancet* 2 (1984): 350.

3 D. Paige, *Manual of Clinical Nutrition* (1983): 26.

4 https://www.webmd.com/vitamins/ai/ingredientmono-982/zinc. Accessed Jan. 29, 2019.

5 https://pubmed.ncbi.nlm.nih.gov/11054793/. Accessed June 20, 2021.

6 K.D. Tripathi, *Essentials of Medical Pharmacology*, 7th ed. (2013), 914.

Antacids

1 A. Travalto, D.N. Nuhlicik, and J.E. Midtling, "Drug-Nutrient Interactions," *Am Fam Phys* 44, no. 5 (Nov. 1991): 1651-1658.

Anticonvulsants

1 https://www.ncbi.nlm.nih.gov/pubmed/789046. Accessed Mar. 12, 2019.

2 H.A. Schneider, ed., *Nutritional Support of Medical Practice* (Harper and Row, 1983).

Anxiety

1 H. Mohler et al., "Nicotinamide Is a Brain Constituent with Benzodiazepine-Like Actions," *Nature* 278 (1979): 563-565.

2 *PDR for Nonprescription Drugs* (Oradell, NJ: Medical Economics Co., Inc., 1988), 542.

3 https://www.ncbi.nlm.nih.gov/pmc/articles/PMC2486454/. Accessed Sept. 6, 2018.

4 www.ncbi.nlm.nih.gov/pubmed/11386498. Accessed Sept. 6, 2018.

5 https://www.webmd.com/vitamins/condition-1001/anxiety.aspx. Accessed Sept. 6, 2018.

6 A. Palatnik et al., "Double-Blind, Controlled, Crossover Trial of Inositol Versus Fluvoxamine for the Treatment of Panic Disorder," *J Clin Psychopharmacol* 21, no. 3 (June 2001): 335-339.

7 https://www.webmd.com/vitamins/ai/ingredientmono-333/ginkgo. Accessed Nov. 26, 2018.

8 M. Smriga et al., "Oral Treatment with L-Lysine and L-Arginine Reduces Anxiety and Basal Cortisol Levels in Healthy Humans," *Biomed Res* 28, no. 2 (2007): 85-90.

9 https://hospitalnews.com/nutritional-treatments-to-combat-anxiety-disorders/. Accessed Jan. 7, 2019.

10 https://www.webmd.com/diet/health-benefits-gaba#1. Accessed Jan. 20, 2021.

11 V.P. Arcangelo and A.M. Peterson, *Pharmacotherapeutics for Advanced Practice: A Practical Approach*, 3rd ed. (Wolters Kluwer/Lippincott Williams & Wilkins, 2013), 124.

12 Ibid., 125.

Aortic Aneurysm

1 https://www.sciencedirect.com/topics/biochemistry-genetics-and-molecular-biology/copper-deficiency. Accessed Sept. 26, 2020.

2 C.E. Hunt and W.W. Carlton, "Cardiovascular Lesions Associated with Experimental Copper Deficiency in the Rabbit," *J Nutr* 87 (1965): 385.

3 A.R. Gaby, "The Essentials of Copper: A Maligned but Important Mineral," *Nutrition and Healing* 2, no. 3 (1995).

4 https://www.cbsnews.com/news/fruit-heavy-diet-may-prevent-against-dangerous-aneurysm/. Accessed Dec. 9, 2018.

Arsenic Toxicity

1 https://www.ncbi.nlm.nih.gov/pmc/articles/PMC1297497/. Accessed Feb. 7, 2019.

2 https://www.medicalnewstoday.com/articles/241860.php. Accessed Feb. 7, 2019.

3 https://link.springer.com/article/10.1007%2Fs12011-019-01691-w.

4 https://www.ncbi.nlm.nih.gov/pmc/articles/PMC3783921/. Accessed Sept. 8, 2018.

Asthma/Bronchial Asthma

1 *The Washington Manual of Medical Therapeutics*, 34th ed., 424.

2 http://jaoa.org/article.aspx?articleid=2099473. Accessed Nov. 15, 2018.

3 https://www.pulmonologyadvisor.com/home/decision-support-in-medicine/pulmonary-medicine/asthma-clinical-manifestations-and-management/. Accessed Oct. 23, 2019.

4 W-J Song and Y-S Chang. "Magnesium Sulfate for Acute Asthma in Adults: A Systematic Literature Review," *Asia Pac Allergy* 2, no. 1 (2012): 76-85.

5 B.H. Rowe et al., "Intravenous Magnesium Sulfate Treatment for Acute Asthma in the Emergency Department: A Systematic Review of the Literature," *Ann Emerg Med* 36 (2000): 181-190.

6 https://www.aafp.org/afp/2009/0715/p157.html. Accessed Mar. 25, 2021.

7 J. Britton et al., "Dietary Magnesium, Lung Function, Wheezing, and Airway Hyperreactivity in a Random Adult Population Sample," *Lancet* 344, no. 8919 (Aug. 6, 1994): 357-362.

8 B. Anibarro et al., "Asthma with Sulfite Intolerance in Children: A Blocking Study with Cyanocobalamin," *J Allergy Clin Immunol* 90 (1992): 103-109.

9 A.R. Gaby, "Nutrient of the Month: Vitamin B12, Part 11," *Nutrition and Healing* 5, no. 7 (Aug. 1995): 4.

10 J.A. Crocket, "Cyanocobalamin in Asthma," *Acta Allergologica* 11 (1952): 261-268.

11 M. Caruselli, "Therapy of Asthma with Vitamin B12," *JAMA* 150 (1952): 1731.

12 F.T. Antonions and G.A. MacGregor, "Deleterious Effects of Salt Intake Other Than Effects on Blood Pressure," *Clin Exp Pharmacol Physiol* 22 (1995): 180-184.

13 A.R. Gaby, "Research Review," *Nutrition and Healing* 2, no. 10 (1995): 7.

14 J. Britton et al., "The Effects of Dietary Antioxidants on Lung Function in the General Population," *Am Rev Respir Dis* 146 (1993): 369.

15 H. Hemila, "Vitamin C May Alleviate Exercise-Induced Bronchoconstriction: A Meta-Analysis," *BMJ Open* 3, no. 6 (2013).

16 https://www.ncbi.nlm.nih.gov/pubmed/12391710. Accessed Feb. 27, 2019.

17 F.A. Paul and B.R. Buser, "Osteopathic Manipulative Treatment Applications for the Emergency Department Patient," *J Am Osteopath Assoc* 96 (1996): 403-409.

18 J. Alcantara, J.D. Alcantara, and J. Alcantara, "Chiropractic Treatment for Asthma? You Bet!" *J Asthma* 47, no. 5 (June 2010): 597-598. The authors revisit a previous study: J. Balon et al., "A Comparison of Active and Simulated Chiropractic Manipulation as Adjunctive Treatment for Childhood Asthma," *N Engl J Med* 339, no. 15 (Oct. 8, 1998): 1013-1020.

19 P.A. Guiney, DO, et al., "Effects of Osteopathic Manipulative Treatment on Pediatric Patients with Asthma: A Randomized Controlled Trial," *The Journal of the American Osteopathic Association* 105 (Jan. 2005): 7-12.

20 https://www.webmd.com/vitamins/ai/ingredientmono-436/choline. Accessed Nov. 23, 2018.

21 https://www.webmd.com/vitamins/ai/ingredientmono-999/beta-carotene. Accessed Nov. 27, 2018.

22 B.W. Jhun, MD, et al., "Vitamin D Status in South Korean Military Personnel with Acute Eosinophilic Pneumonia: A Pilot Study," *Tuberc Respir Dis (Seoul)* 78, no. 3 (July 2015): 232-238. Published online June 30, 2015. DOI: 10.4046/trd.2015.78.3.232.

23 J.M. Brehm et al., "Serum Vitamin D Levels and Severe Asthma Exacerbations in the Childhood Asthma Management Program Study," *J Allergy Clin Immunol* 126 (2010): 52-58.

24 J. Jaura, G. Kelsberg, and S. Safranek, "Does Vitamin D Reduce Asthma Exacerbations?," *J Fam Pract* 69, no. 4 (May 2020): E4-E6. Accessed May 13, 2020.

25 A. Okpap, A.J. Friend, and S.W. Turner, "Acute Asthma and other Recurrent Wheezing Disorders in Children," *Am Fam Physician* 88, no. 2 (July 15, 2013): 130v131. https://www.aafp.org/afp/2013/0715/p130.html. Accessed Oct. 23, 2019.

Ataxia

1 http://www.ajnr.org/content/29/7/1420. Accessed Mar. 24, 2019.

2 J.C.M. Brust, *Current Diagnosis and Treatment Neurology,* 2nd ed. (McGraw-Hill, 2012): 233.

3 https://my.clevelandclinic.org/health/diseases/17748-ataxia. Accessed May 2, 2021.

4 https://www.hopkinsmedicine.org/neurology_neurosurgery/centers_clinics/ataxia/conditions/ataxia_treatment.html.

5 https://www.webmd.com/vitamins/ai/ingredientmono-954/vitamin-e. Accessed Oct. 11, 2018.

6 *The Merck Manual of Diagnosis and Therapy,* 16th ed. (1992), 1435.

7 https://www.sciencedirect.com/science/article/pii/0022510X81901623. Accessed Jan. 6, 2019.

8 https://www.webmd.com/vitamins/ai/ingredientmono-436/choline. Accessed Nov. 23, 2018.

9 https://www.medicalnewstoday.com/articles/162368#symptoms. Accessed May 20, 2020.

Atherosclerosis

1 https://www.nhlbi.nih.gov/health-topics/atherosclerosis. Accessed May 2, 2021.

2 https://www.ncbi.nlm.nih.gov/pmc/articles/PMC3755365/. Accessed Mar. 14, 2019.

3 T.L. Kopjas, "Folic Acid for the Treatment of Chronic Leg Ulcers in Elderly Patients," *Am Soc* 16 (1968): 338-342.

4 K.A. Oster, "The Treatment of Bovine Xanthine Oxidase Initiated Atherosclerosis by Folic Acid," *Clin Res* 24 (1976): 512A.

5 M. Suzukawa et al., "Effect of In Vivo Supplementation with Low-Dose Vitamin E on Susceptibility of Low-Density Lipoprotein and High-Density Lipoprotein to Oxidative Modification," *J Am Coll Nutr* 14, no. 1 (Feb. 1995): 46-52.

6 https://www.webmd.com/vitamins/ai/ingredientmono-137/policosanol. Accessed Nov. 16, 2018.

7 https://www.ncbi.nlm.nih.gov/pubmed/12126462. Accessed Jan. 6, 2019.

8 R. Más et al., "Effects of Policosanol on Lipid Profile and Cardiac Events in Older Hypercholesterolemic Patients with Coronary Disease," *Clinical Drug Investigation* 21, no. 7 (2001): 485-497.

9 N. Gokce et al., "Long-Term Ascorbic Acid Administration Reverses Endothelial Vasomotor Dysfunction in Patients with Coronary Artery Disease," *Circulation* 99, no. 25 (1999): 3234-3240.

10 D. Versari et al., "Endothelium-Dependent Contractions and Endothelial Dysfunction in Human Hypertension," *Br J Pharmacol* 157, no. 4 (2009): 527-536.

11 H. Frikke-Schmidt and J. Lykkesfeldt, "Role of Marginal Vitamin C Deficiency in Atherogenesis: In Vivo Models and Clinical Studies," *Basic Clin Pharmacol Toxicol* 104, no. 6 (2009): 419-433.

12 K.F. Gey et al., "Increased Risk of Cardiovascular Disease at Suboptimal Plasma Concentrations of Essential Antioxidants: An Epidemiological Update with Special Attention to Carotene and Vitamin C," *Am J Clin Nutr* 57, suppl. (1993): 787S-797S.

13 J.E. Digby, Neil Ruparelia, and Robin P. Choudhury, "Niacin in Cardiovascular Disease: Recent Preclinical and Clinical Development," *Arterioscler Thromb Vasc Biol* 32, no. 3 (Mar. 2012): 582-588.

14 "Clofibrate and Niacin in Coronary Heart Disease," *JAMA* 231 (1975): 360-381.

15 P.L. Canner et al., "Fifteen Year Mortality in Coronary Drug Project Patients: Long-Term Benefit with Niacin," *J Am Coll Cardiol* 8 (1986): 1245-1255.

16 https://www.medscape.com/viewarticle/504813. Accessed Nov. 19, 2018.

17 https://www.mdedge.com/familymedicine/article/221972/cardiology/hypertriglyceridemia-strategic-approach. Accessed May 14, 2020.

18 C. von Schacky et al., "The Effect of Dietary Omega-3 Fatty Acids on Coronary Atherosclerosis. A Randomized, Double-Blind, Placebo-Controlled Trial," *Ann Intern Med* 130 (1999): 554-562.

19 *The Merck Manual of Diagnosis and Therapy*, 19th ed., 2239.

Autism

1 https://www.nimh.nih.gov/health/topics/autism-spectrum-disorders-asd/index.shtml. Accessed Mar. 24, 2019.

2 B. Rimland, "The Use of Megavitamin B6 and Magnesium in the Treatment of Autistic Children and Adults," in *Neurobiological Issues in Autism*, ed. E. Schopler and G. Mesibov (New York: Plenum Press, 1987), 389-405.

3 C. Barthélémy et al., "Behavioral and Biological Effects of Oral Magnesium, Vitamin B6, and Combined Magnesium-B6 Administration in Autistic Children," *Magnes Bull* (1981): 3: 150-153.

4 J. Martineau et al., "Comparative Effects of Oral B6, B6-Mg, and Mg Administration on Evoked Potentials Conditioning in Autistic Children," in *Proceedings, Symposium on Event-Related Potentials in Children*, ed. A. Rothenberger (Amsterdam: Elsevier, 1982), 411-416.

5 J. Martineau et al., "Vitamin B6, Magnesium and Combined B6-Mg: Therapeutic Effects in Childhood Autism," *Biol Psychiatry* 20 (1985): 467-468.

6 G. Lelord et al., "Clinical and Biological Effects of Vitamin B6 and Magnesium in Autistic Subjects," in *Vitamin B6 Responsive Disorders in Humans*, ed. J. Leklem and R. Reynolds (New York: Liss, 1988), 219-230.

7 https://www.webmd.com/vitamins/ai/ingredientmono-294/quercetin. Accessed Mar. 2, 2019.

8 https://www.drugs.com/npp/quercetin.html. Accessed Mar. 24, 2019.

Basal Cell Carcinoma (BCC)/Squamous Cell Carcinoma (SCC)

1 https://www.cancer.org/content/dam/CRC/PDF/Public/8821.00.pdf. Accessed May 2, 2021.

2 K.E. Sharquie, A.A. Al-Nuaimy, and F.A. Al-Shimary, "New Intralesional Therapy for Basal Cell Carcinoma by 2% Zinc Sulphate Solution," *Saudi Medical Journal* 26, no. 2 (2005): 359-361.

3 https://www.mdedge.com/dermatology/article/215102/acne/ketogenic-diet-and-dermatology-primer-current-literature/page/0/1. Accessed Jan. 30, 2020.

4 P. Star, "Oral Nicotinamide Prevents Common Skin Cancers in High-Risk Patients, Reduces Costs," *Am Health Drug Benefits* 8 (Spec Issue) (Aug. 2015): 13-14.

5 https://www.ncbi.nlm.nih.gov/pmc/articles/PMC4314970/. Accessed May 23, 2019.

6 T.E. Moon et al., "Effect of Retinol in Preventing Squamous Cell Skin Cancer in Moderate-Risk Subjects: A Randomized, Double-Blind, Controlled Trial," *Cancer Epidemiol Biomarkers Prev* 6 (1997): 949-956.

7 https://www.consumerlab.com/rdas/. Accessed July 25, 2021.

8 J. Kim et al., "Association with Vitamin A Intake with Cutaneous Squamous Cell Carcinoma Risk in the United States," *JAMA Dermatol.* Published online July 31, 2019. DOI: 10.1001/jamadermatol.2019.1937.

Becker's Muscular Dystrophy

1 J. Seiler and E.T. Bope, "The Muscular Dystrophies," *Am Fam Phys* 34, no. 1 (1986): 128-130.

2 https://medlineplus.gov/ency/article/000705.htm. Accessed Sept. 8, 2018.

Behcet's Disease

1 A.B.M. Abdullah, *Practical Manual in Clinical Medicine* (Philadelphia: Jaypee—The Health Sciences Publisher, 2017), 825.

2 K.E. Sharquie et al., "Oral Zinc Sulfate in the Treatment of Behcet's Disease: A Double Blind Cross-Over Study," *Journal of Dermatology* 33, no. 8 (2006): 541-546.

3 http://www.behcets.com/site/c.8oIJJRPsGcISF/b.9196317/k.904C/Behcets_Disease.htm. Accessed Mar. 24, 2019.

4 https://www.dermnetnz.org/topics/potassium-iodide/. Accessed May 15, 2020.

Belching/Burping

1 *Physician's Desk Reference*, 36th ed. (1982), 1559.

Bell's Palsy

1 https://jamanetwork.com/journals/jamaotolaryngology/fullarticle/2759437?guestAccessKey=d517f277-3838-46f6-b8f9-e5cad9ce4e20&utm_content=weekly_highlights&utm_term=020120&utm_source=silverchair&utm_campaign=jama_network&cmp=1&utm_medium=email. Accessed Feb. 1, 2020.

2 https://www.uspharmacist.com/article/bells-palsy-to-treat-or-not-to-treat. Accessed Dec. 16, 2018.

3 https://www.mdedge.com/jfponline/article/60117/are-drug-therapies-effective-treating-bells-palsy. Accessed Dec. 9, 2018.

Beta Thalassemia

1 https://ghr.nlm.nih.gov/condition/beta-thalassemia. Accessed Oct. 6, 2018.

2 https://www.webmd.com/vitamins/ai/ingredientmono-954/vitamin-e. Accessed Oct. 6, 2018.

3 https://www.medicinenet.com/beta_thalassemia/article.htm#the_treatment_of_thalassemia_major. Accessed Oct. 6, 2018.

4 https://www.hopkinsmedicine.org/healthlibrary/conditions/hematology_and_blood_disorders/beta_thalassemia_cooleys_anemia_85,P00081. Accessed Oct. 6, 2018.

5 https://journals.lww.com/ebp/Abstract/2016/02000/does_folic_acid_supplementation_have_a_role_in_the.17.aspx. Accessed Feb. 3, 2021.

6 *Standards of Care Guidelines for Thalassemia.* http://www.thalassemia.com/documents/SOCGuidelines2012.pdf. Accessed Jan. 6, 2018.

7 https://www.emedicinehealth.com/l-carnitine/vitamins-supplements.htm. Accessed Nov. 26, 2018.

8 https://www.ncbi.nlm.nih.gov/pmc/articles/PMC3155231/. Accessed Jan. 6, 2019.

9 https://www.ncbi.nlm.nih.gov/pmc/articles/PMC4024502/. Accessed June 18, 2020.

Bile Acid Sequestrants

1 https://www.drugs.com/drug-class/bile-acid-sequestrants.html. Accessed Dec. 16, 2018.

2 A. Travalto, D.N. Nuhlicik, and J.E. Midtling, "Drug-Nutrient Interactions," *Am Fam Phys* 44, no. 5 (Nov. 1991): 1651-1658.

Biliary Atresia

1 https://www.ncbi.nlm.nih.gov/pmc/articles/PMC4790131/.

2 http://www.adhb.govt.nz/starshipclinicalguidelines/_Documents/Biliary%20Atresia.pdf. Accessed Nov. 7, 2018.

Bipolar Disorder

1 https://www.nimh.nih.gov/health/topics/bipolar-disorder/index.shtml. Accessed Mar. 24, 2019.

2 https://www.aafp.org/afp/2021/0215/p227.html. Accessed May 2, 2021.

3 G.M. Skutsch, "Manic Depression: A Multiple Hormone Disorder?," *Biol Psychiatry* 20, no. 6 (1985): 662-668.

4 S.E. Lakhan and Karen F. Vieira, "Nutritional Therapies for Mental Disorders," *Nutritional Journal* 7, no. 2 (Feb. 2008). DOI: 10.1186/1475-2891-7-2. [PubMed]

5 G.J. Naylor, "Vanadium and Manic Depressive Psychosis," *Nutr Health* 3 (1984): 79-85.

6 G.J. Naylor and A.H. Smith, "Vanadium: A Possible Etiological Factor in Manic Depressive Illness," *Psychol Med* 11 (1981): 249-256.

7 T. Botiglieri, "Folate, Vitamin B12, and Neuropsychiatric Disorders," *Nutr Rev* 54 (1996): 382-390.

8 C.I. Hasanah et al., "Reduced Red-Cell Folate in Mania," *J Affect Disord* 46 (1997): 95-99.

9 H.A. Nieper, "The Clinical Applications of Lithium Orotate: A Two Year Study," *Agressologie* 14, no. 6 (1973): 407-411.

10 H.E. Sartori, "Lithium Orotate in the Treatment of Alcoholism and Related Conditions," *Alcohol* 3, no. 2 (1986): 97-100.

11 https://www.drugs.com/npp/lithium-orotate.html. Accessed Dec. 24, 2020.

12 T. O'Donnell et al., "Effects of Chronic Lithium and Sodium Valproate on Concentrations of Brain Amino Acids," *Eur Neuropsychopharmacol* 13, no. 4 (2003): 220-227.

Black Hairy Tongue

1 www.nejm.org/doi/full/10.1056/NEJMicm1800351. Accessed Nov. 8, 2018.

2 https://www.webmd.com/oral-health/guide/black-hairy-tongue#2. Accessed Nov. 8, 2018.

3 G.M. Sarti et al., "Black Hairy Tongue," *Am Fam Physician* 41, no. 6 (1990): 1751-1755.

4 https://dimensionsofdentalhygiene.com/article/black-hairy-tongue/. Accessed Nov. 8, 2018.

Body Odor/Bromhidrosis

1 https://www.medicaldaily.com/natural-body-odor-remedies-4-ways-eliminate-body-odor-good-hygiene-300446. Accessed Nov. 20, 2018.

2 M. Gupta et al., "Zinc Therapy in Dermatology: A Review," *Dermatol Res Pract* 2014 (2014): 709152. Published online July 10, 2014. DOI: 10.1155/2014/709152.

3 M.D. Scribner, "Zinc Sulfate and Axillary Perspiration Odor," *Arch Dermatol* 113, no. 9 (1977): 1302.

Boils/Styes

1 P.R.N. Sutton, "Does the Daily Ingestion of a Small Amount of 'Raw' Wheat Cause Boils to Resolve?," *Med Hypothesis* 44 (1995): 194.

2 A.R. Gaby, "Research Review," *Nutrition and Healing* 2, no. 10 (1995): 7.

Bronchitis (Acute)

1 https://www.aafp.org/afp/2016/1001/p560.html.

2 https://www.medicalnewstoday.com/articles/10278. Accessed Dec. 5, 2020.

3 B.M. Killeen and A.B. Wolfon, "Antibiotics for Acute Bronchitis," *Am Fam Physician* 102, no. 9 (Nov. 1, 2020): online.

4 https://www.aafp.org/afp/2016/1001/p560.html.

5 https://www.ncbi.nlm.nih.gov/pmc/articles/PMC4998156/. Accessed Oct. 14, 2019.

6 R.A. Neubauer, "A Plant Protease for Potentiation of and Possible Replacement of Antibiotics," *Exp Med Surg* 19 (1961): 143-160.

7 https://www.aafp.org/afp/2010/1201/p1345.pdf.

Bronchitis (Chronic)

1 https://www.ncbi.nlm.nih.gov/pmc/articles/PMC4951627/.

2 A.B. Tattersall et al., "Acetylcysteine (Fabrol) in Chronic Bronchitis: a Study in General Practice," *J Int Med Res* (1983): 11.

3 B.W. Jhun, MD, et al., "Vitamin D Status in South Korean Military Personnel with Acute Eosinophilic Pneumonia: A Pilot Study," *Tuberc Respir Dis (Seoul)* 78, no. 3 (July 2015): 232-238. Published online June 30, 2015. DOI: 10.4046/trd.2015.78.3.232.

4 W. Janssens et al., "Vitamin D Beyond Bones in Chronic Obstructive Pulmonary Disease: Time to Act," *Am J Respir Crit Care Med* 179 (2009): 630-636.

5 W. Janssens et al., "Vitamin D Deficiency Is Highly Prevalent in COPD and Correlates with Variants in the Vitamin D Binding Gene," *Thorax* 65 (2010): 215-220.

6 M. Zhu et al., "The Association Between Vitamin D and COPD Risk, Severity, and Exacerbation: An Updated Systematic Review and Meta-Analysis," *Int J Chron Obstruct Pulmon Dis* 11 (2016): 2597-2607.

7 https://www.consumerlab.com/rdas/. Accessed July 25, 2021.

8 A.B. Tattersall et al., "Acetylcysteine (Fabrol) in Chronic Bronchitis a Study in General Practice," *J Int Med Res* (1983): 11.

9 M. Decramer et al., "Effects of N-Acetylcysteine on Outcomes in Chronic Obstructive Pulmonary Disease (Bronchitis Randomized on NAC Cost-Utility Study, BRONCUS): A Randomized, Placebo-Controlled Trial," *Lancet* 365 (2005): 1552-1560.

10 https://www.mayo.edu/research/clinical-trials/cls-20266947.

11 *Physician's Desk Reference*, 36th ed. (1982), 1131.

12 T.G. Saxe, "Toxicity of Medicinal Herbal Preparations," *Am Fam Phys* 35, no. 5 (May 1987): 135-142.

13 https://www.webmd.com/vitamins/ai/ingredientmono-464/gaba-gamma-aminobutyric-acid. Accessed Nov. 27, 2018.

14 https://www.aafp.org/afp/1998/0515/p2365.html. Accessed Dec. 31, 2020.

Bronchopulmonary Dysplasia (BPD)

1 https://www.nhlbi.nih.gov/health-topics/bronchopulmonary-dysplasia. Accessed Mar. 2, 2019.

2 Council on Scientific Affairs, "Vitamin Preparations as Dietary Supplements and as Therapeutic Agents," *JAMA* 257, no. 14 (Apr. 1987): 1929-1936.

3 https://www.researchgate.net/publication/353809465_An_Update_on_the_Prevention_and_Management_of_Bronchopulmonary_Dysplasia. Accessed Aug. 15, 2021.

Bulimia Nervosa

1 M. Mira and S. Abraham, "L-tryptophan as an Adjunct to Treatment of Bulimia Nervosa," *Lancet* 2 (1989): 1162-1163.

Burns

1 https://dailymed.nlm.nih.gov/dailymed/fda/fdaDrugXsl.cfm?setid=d05200cb-cf29-4bc7-bf0c-b42ab2d20958. Accessed Nov. 17, 2018.

2 B.A. Araneo et al., "Dehydroepiandrosterone Reduces Progressive Dermal Ischemia Caused by Thermal Injury," *Surg Reg* 59, no. 2 (Aug. 1995): 250-262.

3 J.C. Houck, C.M. Chang, and G. Klein, "Isolation of an Effective Debriding Agent from the Stems of Pineapple Plants," *International Journal of Tissue Reactions* 5, no. 2 (1983): 125-134.

4 https://www.ncbi.nlm.nih.gov/pmc/articles/PMC3529416/. Accessed Oct. 4, 2019.

5 https://www.webmd.com/vitamins/ai/ingredientmono-895/bromelain. Accessed Nov. 19, 2018.

6 J.G. Miller, H.R. Carruthers, and D.A.R. Burd, "An Algorithmic Approach to the Management of Cutaneous Burns," *Burns* 18, no. 3 (1992): 200-211.

7 R.L. Sheridan, R.G. Tompkins, and J.F. Burke, "Management of Burn Wounds with Prompt Excision and Immediate Closure," *Journal of Intensive Care Medicine* 237 (1994): 68-75.

8 R.E. Salisbury, "In-Thermal Burns," in *Plastic Surgery*, ed. J.C. McCarthy (1990): Vol. 1: 787-830.

9 https://www.woundsresearch.com/article/9064. Accessed Nov. 21, 2018.

10 M. Parry-Billings Dphil et al., "Does Glutamine Contribute to Immunosuppression after Major Burns?," *The Lancet* 336, no. 8714 (Sept. 1990): 523-525.

11 https://www.webmd.com/vitamins/ai/ingredientmono-878/glutamine. Accessed Nov. 28, 2018.

12 https://www.webmd.com/vitamins/ai/ingredientmono-607/aloe. Accessed Jan. 5, 2019.

13 https://www.ncbi.nlm.nih.gov/pmc/articles/PMC4158441/. Accessed May 8, 2019.

14 F.E. Brölmann et al., "Evidence-Based Decisions for Local and Systemic Wound Care," *Br J Surg* 99 (2012): 1172-1183.

15 M. Kasovic et al., "Analgesic Properties of Vitamin K," *Proc Soc Exp Biol Med* 90 (1955): 660-662.

Bursitis

1 https://www.medicalnewstoday.com/articles/175596. Accessed May 14, 2020.

2 https://www.arthritis.org/about-arthritis/types/bursitis/. Accessed Oct. 23, 2019.

3 I.S. Klemes, "Vitamin B12 in Acute Subdeltoid Bursitis," *Industrial Med Surg* 26 (1957): 290-292.

4 A.R. Gaby, "Nutrient of the Month: Vitamin B12, Part 11," *Nutrition and Healing* 5, no. 7 (Aug. 1995): 3.

5 http://pennstatehershey.adam.com/content.aspx?productId=107&pid=33&gid=000022. Accessed Nov. 20, 2018.

Cadmium Toxicity

1 https://www.ncbi.nlm.nih.gov/pmc/articles/PMC2831915/. Accessed June 11, 2020.

2 https://www.ncbi.nlm.nih.gov/pmc/articles/PMC3783921/. Accessed Nov. 20, 2018.

3 *PDR for Nutritional Supplements*, 2nd ed. (Montvale, NJ: Thomson Reuters, 2008), 25.

4 https://pubchem.ncbi.nlm.nih.gov/compound/dl-Thioctic_acid#section=Therapeutic-Uses. Accessed Nov. 20, 2018.

5 https://www.ncbi.nlm.nih.gov/pmc/articles/PMC5596182/. Accessed Jan. 19, 2022.

6 https://www.ncbi.nlm.nih.gov/pmc/articles/PMC4303853/#B58-nutrients-07-00552. Accessed Nov. 16, 2018.

7 https://www.ncbi.nlm.nih.gov/pmc/articles/PMC3686085/. Accessed Jan. 19, 2022.

Calcinosis Cutis

1 https://www.dermnetnz.org/topics/calcinosis-cutis/. Accessed Feb. 7, 2019.

2 S. Ayres Jr. and R. Mihan, "Vitamin E in Dermatology," *Cutis* 16 (1975): 1017-1021.

3 T. Nakagawa and T. Takaiwa, "Calcinosis Cutis in Juvenile Dermatomyositis Responsive to Aluminum Hydroxide Treatment," *The Journal of Dermatology* 20, no. 9 (1993): 558-560.

4 https://emedicine.medscape.com/article/1103137-treatment. Accessed Feb. 7, 2019.

Cancer (Bladder)

1 https://www.nih.gov/news-events/nih-research-matters/smoking-bladder-cancer. Accessed Mar. 24, 2019.

2 E.J. Jacobs et al., "Vitamin C and Vitamin E Supplement Use and Bladder Cancer Mortality in a Large Cohort of US Men and Women," *Am J Epidemiol* 156 (2002): 1002-1010.

3 https://www.webmd.com/vitamins/ai/ingredientmono-954/vitamin-e. Accessed Nov. 9, 2018.

4 J.W. Schlegel, *Trans of the Amer Assoc of Genito-Urinary Surgeons* 61 (1969): 85-89.

5 I. Stone, *The Healing Factor: Vitamin C Against Disease* (Grosset & Dunlap, 1972), 140.

Cancer (Breast)

1 M.A. Kosir, "Breast Cancer," *Merck Manual Professional Version.* https://www.merckmanuals.com/professional/gynecology-and-obstetrics/breast-disorders/breast-cancer. Accessed Apr. 17, 2020.

2 National Cancer Institute, "Breast Cancer Treatment (Adult) (PDQ®)—Health Professional Version." Content last updated May 7, 2020. https://www.cancer.gov/types/breast/hp/breast-treatment-pdq?cid=eb_govdel#_551_toc. Accessed June 6, 2020.

3 https://www.merckmanuals.com/professional/gynecology-and-obstetrics/breast-disorders/breast-masses-breast-lumps. Accessed Aug. 11, 2020.

4 https://pubmed.ncbi.nlm.nih.gov/25993238/. Accessed May 15, 2021.

5 https://academic.oup.com/advances/advance-article-abstract/doi/10.1093/advances/nmab015/6174025?redirectedFrom=fulltext. Accessed May 15, 2021.

6 https://pubmed.ncbi.nlm.nih.gov/25993238/. Accessed May 15, 2021.

7 A. Hoyt-Austin et al., *Obstet Gynecol* (Dec. 2020). DOI: 10.1097/AOG.0000000000004162.

8 J.L. Freudenheim, "Alcohol's Effects on Breast Cancer in Women," *Alcohol Res* 40, no. 2 (2020): 11.

9 T. Wang et al., *Cancer* (Aug. 12, 2019). DOI: 10.1002/cncr.32364. Accessed Aug. 12, 2019.

10 https://www.webmd.com/breast-cancer/news/20170501/low-dose-aspirin-may-lower-risk-for-common-breast-cancer-by-20-percent#1. Accessed Aug. 12, 2019.

11 P.D. Chandler et al., "Effect of Vitamin D3 Supplements on Development of Advanced Cancer: A Secondary Analysis of the VITAL Randomized Clinical Trial," *JAMA Netw Open* 3, no. 11 (2020): e2025850. DOI: 10.1001/jamanetworkopen.2020.25850.

12 Isabel Peraita-Costa, Paula Carrillo Garcia, and María Morales-Suárez-Varela, "Is There an Association Between β-Carotene and Breast Cancer? A Systematic Review on Breast Cancer Risk," *Nutrition and Cancer* (2020). DOI: 10.1080/01635581.2020.1865422.

13 K. Lockwood et al., "Progress on Therapy of Breast Cancer with Vitamin Q10 and the Regression of Metastases," *Biochem Biophys Res Commun* 212 (1995): 172-177.

14 K. Lockwood et al., "Partial and Complete Regression of Breast Cancer in Patients in Relation to Dosage of Coenzyme Q10," *Biochemical and Biophysical Research Communications* 199, no. 3 (1994): 1504-1508.

15 M. Holmes et al., "Aspirin Intake and Survival after Breast Cancer," *Journal of Clinical Oncology* (Mar. 20, 2010). DOI: 10.1200/JCO.2009.22.7918.

Cancer (Esophagus, Oral Cavity, Stomach, Pancreas, Cervix, Colon, Rectum, Breast, Lung, and Prostate)

1 https://www.health.harvard.edu/newsletter_article/The-10-commandments-of-cancer-prevention. Accessed Nov. 20, 2018.

2 National Cancer Institute, "Harms of Cigarette Smoking and Health Benefits of Quitting." https://www.cancer.gov/about-cancer/causes-prevention/risk/tobacco/cessation-fact-sheet. Reviewed Dec. 19, 2017. Accessed June 20, 2018.

3 American Cancer Society, "What Are the Risk Factors for Penile Cancer?." https://www.cancer.org/cancer/penile-cancer/causes-risks-prevention/risk-factors.html. Revised October 19, 2017. Accessed June 20, 2018.

4 World Health Organization, *WHO Report on the Global Tobacco Epidemic, 2011: Warning About the Dangers of Tobacco* (Geneva, Switzerland: World Health Organization, 2011).

5 E. Cameron and A. Campbell, "The Orthomolecular Treatment of Cancer. II. Clinical Trial of High-Dose Ascorbic Acid Supplements in Advanced Human Cancer," *Chem Biol Interact* 9 (1974): 285-315.

6 E. Cameron and Linus Pauling, "Supplemental Ascorbate in the Supportive Treatment of Cancer: Prolongation of Survival Times in Terminal Human Cancer," *Proc Natl Acad Sci USA* 73 (1976): 3685-3689.

7 E. Cameron and L. Pauling, "Supplemental Ascorbate in the Supportive Treatment of Cancer: Re-Evaluation of Prolongation of Survival Times in Terminal Human Cancer," *Proc Natl Acad Sci USA* 75 (1978): 4538-4542.

8 A. Murata, F. Morishige, and H. Yamaguchi, "Prolongation of Survival Times of Terminal Cancer Patients by Administration of Large Doses of Ascorbate," *Int J Vit Nutr Res* 2, no. 23 (1982): 103-113.

9 G. Block, "Vitamin C and Cancer Prevention: The Epidemiologic Evidence," *Am J Clin Nutr* 53, no. 1 (1991): 270S-282S.

10 G. Block, "Epidemiologic Evidence Regarding Vitamin C and Cancer," *Am J Clin Nutr* 54, no. 6 (1991): 1310S.

11 https://www.ncbi.nlm.nih.gov/pmc/articles/PMC3783921/. Accessed Nov. 20, 2018.

12 M.J. Larriba et al., "Vitamin D Receptor Deficiency Enhances Wnt/β-Catenin Signaling and Tumor Burden in Colon Cancer," *PLoS ONE* 6, no. 8 (2011): e23524. DOI: 10.1371/journal.pone.0023524.

13 K. Ng et al., "Effect of High-Dose vs Standard-Dose Vitamin D_3 Supplementation on Progression-Free Survival among Patients with Advanced or Metastatic Colorectal Cancer: The SUNSHINE Randomized Clinical Trial," *JAMA* 321, no. 14 (2019): 1370-1379. DOI: 10.1001/jama.2019.2402.

14 https://www.ncbi.nlm.nih.gov/pmc/articles/PMC7686489/. Accessed Dec. 15, 2020.

15 https://pubmed.ncbi.nlm.nih.gov/30611908/.

16 L.C. Clark et al., "Decreased Incidence of Prostate Cancer with Selenium Supplementation: Results of a Double-Blind Cancer Prevention Trial," *Br J Urol* 81, no. 5 (1998): 730-734.

17 https://ods.od.nih.gov/factsheets/Selenium-HealthProfessional/.

18 A.T. Kunzmann et al., "Dietary Fiber Intake and Risk of Colorectal Cancer and Incident and Recurrent Adenoma in the Prostate, Lung, Colorectal, and Ovarian Cancer Screening Trial," *Am J Clin Nutr* 102, no. 4 (Oct. 2015): 881-890. DOI: 10.3945/ajcn.115.113282. Epub Aug. 12, 2015.

19 https://www.ncbi.nlm.nih.gov/pmc/articles/PMC3070119/. Accessed Nov. 23, 2018.

20 https://www.webmd.com/vitamins/ai/ingredientmono-982/zinc. Accessed Jan. 29, 2019.

21 https://jamanetwork.com/journals/jamanetworkopen/fullarticle/2756258. Accessed Dec. 20, 2019.

22 D.K. Smith, T. Demetriou, and C. Weber, "Aspirin for Primary Prevention: USPSTF Recommendations for CVD and Colorectal Cancer," *J Fam Pract* 68, no. 3 (Apr. 2019): 146-151.

23 H. Risch et al., "Aspirin Use and Reduced Risk of Pancreatic Cancer," *Cancer Epidemiol Biomarkers Prev* 26 (2016): 68-74.

24 F. Islami et al., "A Prospective Study of Tea Drinking Temperature and Risk of Esophageal Squamous Cell Carcinoma," *Int J Cancer.* Published online Mar. 20, 2019. Accessed Mar. 21, 2019.

25 https://www.webmd.com/vitamins/ai/ingredientmono-42/methionine. Accessed June 6, 2019.

26 https://bmccomplementalternmed.biomedcentral.com/articles/10.1186/1472-6882-10-24. Accessed Aug. 8, 2019.

27 https://www.cancer.gov/about-cancer/treatment/cam/hp/coenzyme-q10-pdq. Accessed Dec. 10, 2020.

Cancer (Gastric)

1 https://www.cancer.org/cancer/stomach-cancer/causes-risks-prevention/prevention.html.

2 *J Natl Cancer Inst* 92 (2000): 1868-1869, 1881-1888.

3 https://www.webmd.com/vitamins/ai/ingredientmono-957/riboflavin. Accessed Nov. 14, 2018.

4 https://pubmed.ncbi.nlm.nih.gov/14684401/. Accessed Jan. 19, 2021.

Cancer (Ovarian, Pancreatic, Breast, Mesothelioma, and Incurable Cancer)

1 https://www.emedicinehealth.com/vitamin_c_high_dose_benefits_side_effects/article_em.htm#is_high-dose_vitamin_c_approved_by_the_fda_for_cancer_treatment. Accessed Nov. 20, 2018.

2 https://onlinelibrary.wiley.com/doi/abs/10.1002/mnfr.200700222. Accessed Aug. 8, 2019.

3 A.B. Awad, R. Roy, and C.S. Fink, "Beta-Sitosterol, a Plant Sterol, Induces Apoptosis and Activates Key Capsases in MDA-MB-231 Human Breast Cancer Cells," *Oncol Rep* 10, no. 20 (Mar.-Apr. 2003): 497-500.

4 https://www.cancer.gov/about-cancer/treatment/cam/hp/coenzyme-q10-pdq. Accessed Dec. 10, 2020.

5 B. Trabert et al., "Aspirin, Nonaspirin Nonsteroidal Anti-Inflammatory Drug, and Acetaminophen Use and Risk of Invasive Epithelial Ovarian Cancer: A Pooled Analysis in the Ovarian Cancer Association Consortium," *J Natl Cancer Inst* 106 (2014).

6 P.D. Chandler et al., "Effect of Vitamin D3 Supplements on Development of Advanced Cancer: A Secondary Analysis of the VITAL Randomized Clinical Trial," *JAMA Netw Open* 3, no. 11 (2020): e2025850. DOI: 10.1001/jamanetworkopen.2020.25850.

Cancer—Prostate (PCa)

1 Y. Al-Jebari et al., "Risk of Prostate Cancer for Men Fathering through Assisted Reproduction: Nationwide Population Based Register Study," *BMJ* 366 (2019): l5214.

2 O.P. Heinonen et al., "Prostate Cancer and Supplementation with Alpha-Tocopherol and Beta-Carotene: Incidence and Mortality in a Controlled Trial," *J Natl Cancer Inst.* 90, no. 6 (Mar. 18, 1998): 440-446. DOI: 10.1093/jnci/90.6.440.

3 https://www.cancer.gov/about-cancer/treatment/cam/hp/prostate-supplements-pdq. Accessed Nov. 1, 2018.

4 https://www.webmd.com/prostate-cancer/guide/alternative-treatments-for-prostate-cancer2#2. Accessed Nov. 1, 2018.

5 https://clinicaltrials.gov/ct2/show/NCT00524680. Accessed Nov. 1, 2018.

6 https://www.ncbi.nlm.nih.gov/pmc/articles/PMC4616444/. Accessed Nov. 2, 2019.

7 M. Etminan, B. Takkouche, and F. Caamano-Isorna, "The Role of Tomato Products and Lycopene in the Prevention of Prostate Cancer: A Meta-Analysis of Observational Studies," *Cancer Epidemiol Biomarkers Prev* 13 (2004): 340-345.

Canker Sores/Recurrent Aphthous Stomatitis (RAS)/Oral Aphthosis

1 https://www.ncbi.nlm.nih.gov/pmc/articles/PMC3227248/. Accessed Nov. 20, 2018.

2 https://www.cedars-sinai.org/blog/canker-sores.html.

3 https://www.mayoclinic.org/diseases-conditions/canker-sore/diagnosis-treatment/drc-20370620. Accessed Nov. 18, 2018.

4 A.B. Skaare, B.B. Herlofson, and P. Barkvoll, "Mouth Rinses Containing Triclosan Reduce the Incidence of Recurrent Aphthous Ulcers (RAU)," *J Clin Periodontol* 23 (1996): 778-781.

5 https://www.dermatologyadvisor.com/dermatology/aphthous-stomatitis-canker-sores-recurrent-aphthous-stomatitis-simple-aphthosis-complex-aphthosis/article/691617/. Accessed Nov. 18, 2018.

6 E.T. Bope and R.D. Kellerman, *Conn's Current Therapy*, 14th ed. (Philadelphia: Elsevier/Saunders), 270.

7 K.E. Sharquie et al., "Oral Zinc Sulfate in the Treatment of Behcet's Disease: A Double-Blind Cross-Over Study," *Journal of Dermatology* 33, no. 8 (2006): 541-546.

8 M.W Dronfield et al., "Zinc Sulfate Supplementation for Treatment of Recurring Oral Ulcers," *Gut* 18 (1977): 33-36.

9 K.E. Sharquie et al., "The Therapeutic and Prophylactic Role of Oral Zinc Sulfate in Management of Recurrent Aphthous Stomatitis (RAS) in Comparison with Dapsone," *Saudi Medical Journal* 29, no. 5 (2008): 734-738.

10 H.W. Merchant et al., "Zinc Sulfate Supplementation for Treatment of Recurring Oral Ulcers," *South Med J* 70, no. 5 (May 1977): 559-561.

11 http://www.medic8.com/healthguide/mouthulcers/treatment.html. Accessed Nov. 20, 2018.

12 B.C. Demoss, "Letters to the Editor," *Am Fam Physician* 51, no. 1 (Jan. 1995): 47.

13 https://www.webmd.com/vitamins/ai/ingredientmono-237/lysine. Accessed Nov. 27, 2018.

14 I. Volkov et al., "Effectiveness of Vitamin B12 in Treating Recurrent Aphthous Stomatitis: A Randomized, Double-Blind, Placebo-Controlled Trial," *J Am Board Fam Med* 22 (2009): 9-16.

15 L. Baccaglini et al., "Urban Legends: Recurrent Aphthous Stomatitis," *Oral Dis* 17 (2011): 755-770.

16 D. Compilato et al., "Hematological Deficiencies in Patients with Recurrent Aphthosis," *J Eur Acad Dermatol Venerol* 24 (2010): 667-673.

17 K. Yasui et al., "The Effect of Ascorbate on Minor Recurrent Aphthous Stomatitis," *Acta Paediatrica* 99, no. 3 (2010): 442-445.

18 N.R. Edgar, DO; D. Saleh, DO; and R.A. Miller, "Recurrent Aphthous Stomatitis: A Review," *J Clin Aesthet Dermatol* 10, no. 3 (2017): 26-36.

Capillary Fragility

1 https://www.omicsonline.org/open-access/treatment-of-capillary-fragility-in-subjects-with-spontaneous-hematomas-2165-7920-10001152-103433.html. Accessed Mar. 24, 2019.

2 https://www.sciencedirect.com/science/article/abs/pii/S0002870344910422. Accessed June 15, 2021.

3 https://nutrition.bmj.com/content/early/2018/12/04/bmjnph-2018-000010. Accessed Mar. 24, 2019.

4 B. Cox and W.J.H. Butterfield, "Vitamin C Supplements and Diabetic Cutaneous Capillary Fragility," *British Medical Journal* 3 (1975): 205. DOI: 10.1136/bmj.3.5977.205.

5 G. Elmer, "Vitamins: Part 4," *Nurse Pract* 7, no. 2 (Feb. 1982): 26-29.

6 K.D. Tripathi, *Essentials of Medical Pharmacology*, 7th ed. (2013), 616.

7 https://wa.kaiserpermanente.org/kbase/topic.jhtml?docId=hn-1181000. Accessed Mar. 24, 2019.

8 J.L. Blonstein, "Control of Swelling in Boxing Injuries," *Practitioner* 185 (1960): 78. And *Practitioner* 203, no. 214 (Aug. 1969): 206.

9 http://www.altmedrev.com/archive/publications/15/4/361.pdf. Accessed Oct. 14, 2019.

Carbon Monoxide Poisoning

1 https://www.webmd.com/vitamins/ai/ingredientmono-1018/n-acetyl-cysteine. Accessed Nov. 17, 2018.

2 https://www.bmj.com/rapid-response/2011/10/30/ascorbate-little-known-flash-oxidiser-carbon-monoxide. *BMJ* 311 (1995): 437. Accessed Nov. 20, 2018.

3 F. Klenner, "The Role of Ascorbic Acid in Therapeutics," *Tri-State Medical J*, letter (Nov. 1955): 34.

Cardiac Arrythmias

1 https://www.medscape.com/viewarticle/951623. Accessed May 26, 2021.

2 https://www.ncbi.nlm.nih.gov/pubmed/11105328/. Accessed May 14, 2020.

3 https://academic.oup.com/ehjcvp/article/3/2/108/2669829. Accessed May 14, 2020.

4 https://www.webmd.com/vitamins/ai/ingredientmono-998/magnesium. Accessed Oct. 10, 2018.

5 H. Holzgartner, E. Maier, and W. Vierling, "High-Dosage Oral Magnesium Therapy in Arrhythmias. Results of an Observational Study in 1,160 Patients with Arrhythmia," *Fortschritte der Medizin* 108, no. 28 (Oct. 1990): 539-542.

6 M. Zehender et al., "Antiarrhythmic Effects of Increasing the Daily Intake of Magnesium and Potassium in Patients with Frequent Ventricular Arrhythmias," *J Am Coll Cardiol* 29 (1997): 1028-1034. DOI: 10.1016/S0735-1097(97)00053-3.

7 T. Shiga et al., "Magnesium Prophylaxis for Arrhythmias after Cardiac Surgery: A Meta-Analysis of Randomized Controlled Trials," *The American Journal of Medicine* 117, no. 5 (Sept. 2004): 325-333.

8 https://www.ncbi.nlm.nih.gov/pubmed/3523053. Accessed Sept. 7, 2018.

9 https://www.medicine.net.com/magnesium/supplements-vitamins.htm. Accessed Dec. 16, 2018.

10 G. Eby and W.W. Halcomb, "Elimination of Cardiac Arrhythmias Using Oral Taurine with L-Arginine with Case Histories: Hypothesis for Nitric Oxide Stabilization of the Sinus Node," *Med Hypotheses* 67, no. 5 (2006): 1200-1204. Epub Jun 23, 2006.

11 K. Buchanan Keller, RN, PhD, and L. Lemberg, MD, "The importance of Vitamin C in the Incidence of Atrial Fibrillation," *Am J Crit Care* 17, no. 3 (May 2008): 270-272.

12 https://www.emedicinehealth.com/vitamin_c_ascorbic_acid/vitamins-supplements.htm. Accessed Sept. 7, 2018.

13 J.J. DiNicolantonio et al., "L-Carnitine in the Secondary Prevention of Cardiovascular Disease: Systematic Review and Meta-Analysis," *Mayo Clin Proc* (2013). DOI: 10.1016/j.mayocp.2013.02.007. Available at: http://www.mayoclinicproceedings.org.

Cardiogenic Shock

1 G.C. Corbucci and F. Loche, "L-Carnitine in Cardiogenic Shock Therapy: Pharmacodynamic Aspects and Clinical Data," *Int J Clin Pharm Res* 13 (1993): 87-91.

2 A.R. Gaby, "Nutrient of the Month: The Story of L-Carnitine," *Nutrition and Healing* 2, no. 4 (1995): 3.

Cardiomyopathy

1 https://www.nhlbi.nih.gov/health-topics/cardiomyopathy. Accessed Mar. 24, 2019.

2 *The Washington Manual of Medical Therapeutics*, 34th ed. (2010): 263.

3 B. Wasi, *Standard Treatment Guidelines: A Manual for Medical Therapeutics*, 1st ed. (2014): 77.

4 J.B. Levy, H.W. Jones, and A.C. Gordon, "Selenium Deficiency, Reversable Cardiomyopathy and Short-Term Intravenous Feeding," *Postgrad Med J* 70, (Oct. 1994): 764-765.

5 *Md Med J* 42, no. 7 (July 1993): 669-674.

6 S. Iliceto et al., "Effects of L-Carnitine Administration on Left Ventricular Remodeling after Acute Anterior Myocardial Infarction: The L-Carnitine Ecocardiografia Digitalizzata Infarto Miocardico (CEDIM) Trial," *J Am Coll Cardiol* 26 (1995): 380-387. DOI: 10.1016/0735-1097(95)80010-E.

7 https://www.ncbi.nlm.nih.gov/pmc/articles/PMC3875693/. Accessed Nov. 25, 2018.

8 L. Zhang et al., "Alpha-Lipoic Acid Attenuates Cardiac Hypertrophy via Downregulation of PARP-2 and Subsequent Activation of SIRT-1," *European Journal of Pharmacology* 744, no. 5 (Dec. 2014): 203-210.

9 F. Jeejeebhoy et al., "Nutritional Supplementation with MyoVive Repletes Essential Cardiac Myocyte Nutrients and Reduces Left Ventricular Size in Patients with Left Ventricular Dysfunction," *Am Heart J* 143 (2002): 1092-1100.

10 J. Azuma, A. Sawamura, and N. Awata, "Usefulness of Taurine in Chronic Congestive Heart Failure and Its Prospective Application," *Jpn Circ J* 56 (1992): 95-99.

11 D. Juilus, J.B. Militante, and J. Lombardini, "Increased Cardiac Levels of Taurine in Cardiomyopathy: The Paradoxical Benefits of Oral Taurine," *Nutrition Research* 21, no. 1 (2001): 93-102.

12 J.C.M. Brust, *Current Diagnosis and Treatment Neurology,* 2nd ed. (McGraw-Hill, 2012), 240.

13 https://openheart.bmj.com/content/5/2/e000775. Accessed Feb. 20, 2021.

14 B.G. Katzung, *Basic & Clinical Pharmacology,* 14th ed., A Lange Medical Book (2018), 1142.

Carpal Tunnel Syndrome (CTS)

1 https://www.wci360.com/cdc-releases-report-on-carpal-tunnel-statistics/.

2 https://www.ncbi.nlm.nih.gov/pmc/articles/PMC1949298/. Accessed Nov. 21, 2018.

3 A.L. Bernstein and J.S. Dinesen, "Brief Communication: Effect of Pharmacologic Doses of Vitamin B6 on Carpal Tunnel Syndrome, Electroencephalographic Results, and Pain," *J Am Coll Nutr* 12 (1993): 73-76.

4 J.M. Ellis et al., "Response of Vitamin B-6 Deficiency and the Carpal Tunnel Syndrome to Pyridoxine," *Proc Natl Acad Sci USA* 79, no. 23 (1982): 7494-7498.

5 K. Folkers et al., "Biochemical Evidence for a Deficiency of Vitamin B6 in the Carpal Tunnel Syndrome Based on a Crossover Clinical Study," *Proc Natl Acad Sci USA* 75, no. 7 (1978): 3410-3412.

6 M. Kasdan and C. Janes, "Carpal Tunnel Syndrome and Vitamin B6," *Plast Reconstr Surg* 79 (1987): 456-458.

7 G. Di Geronimo et al., *Eur Rev Med Pharmacol Sci* 13, no. 2 (2009): 133-139.

8 https://pubchem.ncbi.nlm.nih.gov/compound/dl-Thioctic_acid#section=Therapeutic-Uses. Accessed Nov. 20, 2018.

9 https://www.ncbi.nlm.nih.gov/pmc/articles/PMC4045922/. Accessed Nov. 20, 2018.

10 https://www.researchgate.net/publication/311340986_A_Topical_Gel_From_Flax_Seed_Oil_Compared_With_Hand_Splint_in_Carpal_Tunnel_Syndrome_A_Randomized_Clinical_Trial. Accessed Nov. 20, 2018.

Cataracts (Diabetic)

1 https://www.ncbi.nlm.nih.gov/pmc/articles/PMC3589218/.

2 C.J. Bates, T.D. Cowen, and P.H. Evans, "Effect of Vitamin C on Sorbitol in the Lens of Guinea Pigs Made Diabetic with Streptozotocin," *Br J Nutr* 67, no. 3 (June 1992): 445-456.

3 C. Hammond et al., "Genetic and Dietary Factors Influencing the Progression of Nuclear Cataract," *Ophthalmology* (Mar. 2016). DOI: http://dx.doi.org/10.1016/j.ophtha.2016.01.036.

4 M. Kuzniarz et al., "Use of Vitamin Supplements and Cataract: The Blue Mountains Eye Study," *Am J Ophthalmol* 132, no. 1 (2001): 19-26.

5 https://www.webmd.com/vitamins/ai/ingredientmono-964/vitamin-a. Accessed Nov. 27, 2018.

Cataracts (Prevention)

1 P.F. Jacques et al., "Long-Term Vitamin C Supplement Use and Prevalence of Early Age-Related Lens Opacities," *Am J Clin Nutr* (1997): 66.

2 K.S. Bhat, "Nutritional Status of Thiamine Riboflavin and Pyridoxine in Cataract Patients," *Nutr Rep Int* 36, no. 3 (1987): 685-692.

3 https://www.webmd.com/vitamins/ai/ingredientmono-754/lutein. Accessed Nov. 19, 2018.

4 https://www.webmd.com/vitamins/ai/ingredientmono-964/vitamin-a. Accessed Nov. 27, 2018.

Cavities/Dental Caries

1 https://www.emedicinehealth.com/vitamin_d/vitamins-supplements.htm. Accessed Dec. 28, 2018.

2 https://www.eurekalert.org/pub_releases/2012-11/uow-nra112712.php. Accessed Dec. 28, 2018.

3 https://www.webmd.com/children/news/20080528/kids-may-need-10-times-more-vitamin-d#1. Accessed Dec. 28, 2018.

Celiac Disease/Nontropical Sprue/Gluten Intolerance

1 J.C.M. Brust, *Current Diagnosis and Treatment Neurology*, 2nd ed. (McGraw-Hill, 2012): 492.

2 Ibid., 234.

3 https://www.mayoclinic.org/diseases-conditions/celiac-disease/diagnosis-treatment/drc-20352225. Accessed Nov. 29, 2018.

4 *Physician's Desk Reference*, 36th ed. (1982), 1862.

5 J. Gilroy and J.S. Meyer, *Medical Neurology*, 2nd ed. (New York: The Macmillan Co., 1969), 285.

6 C. Hallert et al., "Vitamin B Supplementation Improves the Health and Well-Being of Patients with Celiac Disease," *Aliment Pharmacol Ther* 29, no. 8 (Apr. 15, 2009): 811-816.

7 https://www.emedicinehealth.com/l-carnitine/vitamins-supplements.htm. Accessed Nov. 26, 2018.

8 https://familydoctor.org/condition/anemia/. Accessed Dec. 31, 2018.

Cerebellar Ataxia (Intermittent)

1 https://rarediseases.info.nih.gov/diseases/9851/episodic-ataxia.

2 J.C.M. Brust, *Current Diagnosis and Treatment Neurology*, 2nd ed. (McGraw-Hill, 2012): 233.

3 https://www.ncbi.nlm.nih.gov/pubmed/7436398. Accessed Apr. 18, 2020.

4 "Vitamin Deficiency and Excess," *Harrison's Principles of Internal Medicine*, 13th ed., 475.

5 H. Kinoshita and I. Nonaka, "Recurrent Muscle Weakness and Ataxia in Thiamine-Responsive Pyruvate Dehydrogenase Complex Deficiency," *J Child Neurology* 12, no. 2 (Feb. 1997): 141-144.

6 L.M. Blasco, "Cerebellar Syndrome in Chronic Cyclic Magnesium Depletion," *Cerebellum* 12 (2013): 587-588. https://doi.org/10.1007/s12311-012-0431-1.

Cerebellar Degeneration—Alcoholic

1 "Cerebellar Degeneration, Subacute," *NORD* (2007): https://rarediseases.org/rare-diseases/cerebellar-degeneration-subacute/. Accessed Dec. 12, 2018.

2 *The Merck Manual of Diagnosis and Therapy*, 16th ed. (1992), 1434.

Cerebral Palsy

1 K.B. Nelson and J.K. Grether, "Can Magnesium Sulfate Reduce the Risk of Cerebral Palsy in Very Low Birthweight Infants?," *Pediatrics* 95 (1995): 263-269.

2 A.R. Gaby, "Research Review," *Nutrition and Healing* 2, no. 10 (1995): 8.

3 https://www.rxlist.com/gaba_gamma-aminobutyric_acid/supplements.htm. Accessed Nov. 27, 2018.

4 https://www.ncbi.nlm.nih.gov/pmc/articles/PMC4339555/. Accessed Apr. 18, 2020.

Cervical Dysplasia

1 https://www.emedicinehealth.com/cervical_dysplasia/article_em.htm#when_is_surgery_necessary_to_treat_cervical_dysplasia. Accessed Oct. 13, 2019.

2 S.L. Romney et al., "Retinoids and the Prevention of Cervical Dysplasia," *Am J Obstet Gynecol* 141 (1981): 890-894.

3 S. Wassertheil-Smoller et al., "Dietary Vitamin C and Uterine Cervical Dysplasia," *Am J Epidemiol* 114, no. 5 (Nov. 1981): 714-724.

4 https://www.ncbi.nlm.nih.gov/pmc/articles/PMC3070119/. Accessed Nov. 19, 2018.

5 C.E. Butterworth Jr. et al., "Improvement in Cervical Dysplasia Associated with Folic Acid Therapy in Users of Oral Contraceptives," *Am J Clin Nutr* 35 (1982): 73-82.

6 C.E. Butterworth Jr. et al., "Oral Folic Acid Supplementation for Cervical Dysplasia. A Clinical Intervention Trial," *Am J Obstet Gynecol* 166 (1992): 803-809.

7 C.E. Butterworth Jr. et al., "Folate Deficiency and Cervical Dysplasia," *JAMA* 267, no. 4 (1992): 528-533. DOI: 10.1001/jama.1992.03480040076034.

Chediak-Higashi Syndrome

1 L.A. Boxer et al., "Correction of Leukocyte Function in Chediak-Higashi Syndrome by Ascorbate," *N Engl J Med* 295 (1976): 1041-1045.

Cheilitis/Angular Cheilitis

1 S.B. Marchbein and R. Hunt, "Angular Cheilitis (Perleche, Angular Stomatitis, Cheilosis)," *Dermatology Advisor.* https://wwwdermatologyadvisor.com/dermatology/angular-cheilitis-perleche-angular-stomatits-cheilosis/article/691377/. Accessed Feb. 8, 2019.

2 B. Barankin, "Answer: Can You Identify This Condition?," *Can Fam Physician* 53, no. 6 (June 2007): 1022-1023.

3 J.A. Rose, "Folic-Acid Deficiency as a Cause of Angular Cheilosis," *Lancet* 2, no. 7722 (1971): 453-454.

Chicken Pox/Varicella

1 https://www.cdc.gov/chickenpox/about/prevention-treatment.html. Accessed May 2, 2021.

2 https://www.mayoclinic.org/diseases-conditions/chickenpox/diagnosis-treatment/drc-20351287. Accessed May 2, 2021.

3 S. Ozsoylu et al., "Vitamin A for Varicella," *J Pediatr* 125 (1994): 1017-1018.

Chilblains/Pernio

1 https://www.dermnetnz.org/topics/chilblains/. Accessed Nov. 17, 2020.

2 https://www.medicalnewstoday.com/articles/172191.php. Accessed May 10, 2019.

3 https://chilblains.org/compare-treatments. Accessed May 10, 2019.

4 R.J. Gourlay, "Treatment of Chilblains," *Br Med J* 1, no. 5074 (1958): 831. https://www.ncbi.nlm.nih.gov/pmc/articles/PMC2027991/?page=1. Accessed May 10, 2019.

Cholera

1 https://www.cdc.gov/cholera/general/index.html. Accessed Feb. 8, 2019.

2 https://medlineplus.gov/druginfo/natural/924.html. Accessed Nov. 21, 2018.

3 T.L. Mynott et al., "Bromelain Prevents Secretion Caused by *Vibrio cholerae* and *Escherichia coli* Enterotoxins in Rabbit Ileum in Vitro," *Gastroenterology* 113 (1997): 175-184.

4 https://www.cdc.gov/cholera/treatment/zinc-treatment.html. Accessed Nov. 13, 2020.

Cholesterol/Hypercholesterolemia/Hyperlipidemia

1 B.G. Wells et al., *Pharmacotherapy Handbook*, 9th ed. (McGraw Hill Education, 2012), 66.

2 *The Washington Manual of Medical Therapeutics*, 34th ed. (Philadelphia: Lippincott Williams & Wilkins), 139-140.

3 https://www.acc.org/latest-in-cardiology/ten-points-to-remember/2019/03/07/16/00/2019-acc-aha-guideline-on-primary-prevention-gl-prevention.

4 A.J. Nordmann et al., "Effects of Low-Carbohydrate vs Low-Fat Diets on Weight Loss and Cardiovascular Risk Factors: A Meta-Analysis of Randomized Controlled Trials," *Arch Intern Med* 166, no. 3 (2006): 285-293. [Published correction appears in *Arch Intern Med* 166, no. 8 (2006): 932.]

5 https://www.aafp.org/afp/2010/0501/p1097.html#afp20100501p1097-b22. Accessed Aug. 26, 2020.

6 https://www.medicinenet.com/statins_vs_niacin/article.htm#what_drugs_interact_with_statins_and_niacin. Accessed Nov. 21, 2018.

7 W.E. Boden, M.S. Sidhu, and P.P. Toth, "The Therapeutic Role of Niacin in Dyslipidemia Management," *J Cardiovasc Pharmacol Ther* 19, no. 2 (2014): 141-158.

8 K.W. Jones, "Do Patients on Statins Also Need Niacin?," *JAAPA* 26, no. 7 (2013): 9-10.

9 https://www.medicinenet.com/script/main/art.asp?articlekey=9487. Accessed Dec. 17, 2018.

10 J.T. DiPiro et al., *Pharmacotherapy: A Pathophysiologic Approach*, 6th ed. (McGraw-Hill, 2005), 441.

11 *Physician's Desk Reference*, 54th ed. (Montvale, NJ: Medical Economics Co., 2000), 1519-1524.

12 B.G. Wells et al., *Pharmacotherapy Handbook*, 9th ed. (McGraw Hill Education), 68.

13 R.M Bakhit, B.P. Klein, and D. Essex-Sorlie, "Intake of 25g of Soybean Protein with or without Soybean Fiber Alters Plasma Lipids in Men with Elevated Cholesterol Concentrations," *J Nutr* 124 (1994): 213-222.

14 J.W. Anderson, B.M. Johnstone, and M.E. Cook-Newell, "Meta-Analysis of the Effects of Soy Protein Intake on Serum Lipids," *N Engl J Med* 333 (1995): 276-282.

15 J.A. Eden, D.C. Knight, and J.B. Howes, "A Controlled Trial of Isoflavones for Menopausal Symptoms," abstract from the Eighth International Congress on the Menopause, Nov. 3-7, 1996, Sydney, Australia.

16 M.P. McRae, "Vitamin C Supplementation Lowers Serum Low-Density Lipoprotein Cholesterol and Triglycerides: A Meta-Analysis of 13 Randomized Controlled Trials," *J Chiro Med* 7, no. 2 (2008): 48-58.

17 https://www.webmd.com/vitamins/ai/ingredientmono-998/magnesium. Accessed Nov. 20, 2018.

18 P.M. Royce and B. Steinmann, "Markedly Reduced Activity of Lysyloxidase in Skin and Aorta from a Patient with Menkes Disease Showing Unusually Severe Connective Tissue Manifestations," *Pediatr Res* 28, no. 2 (Aug. 1990): 13-41.

19 M. Janikula, "Policosanol: A New Treatment for Cardiovascular Disease?," *Altern Med Rev* 7, no. 3 (June 2002): 203-217.

20 https://www.webmd.com/vitamins/ai/ingredientmono-1061/pantethine. Accessed May 10, 2019.

21 https://www.drugs.com/npp/pantothenic-acid.html. Accessed May 10, 2019.

22 https://universityhealthnews.com/heart-health/natural-berberine-supplements-to-lower-cholesterol-more-effective-and-better-tolerated-than-prescription-ezetimibe-zetia/. Accessed May 6, 2020.

23 https://www.ncbi.nlm.nih.gov/pmc/articles/PMC3761874/#R150. Accessed Dec. 13, 2020.

24 V.P. Arcangelo and A.M. Peterson, *Pharmacotherapeutics for Advanced Practice: A Practical Approach*, 3rd ed. (Wolters Kluwer/Lippincott Williams & Wilkins, 2013): 124.

Cluster Headaches

1 J. Weaver-Agostoni, "Cluster Headache," *Am Fam Physician* 88 (2013): 122-128.

2 J. Hoffmann and A. May, "Diagnosis, Pathophysiology, and Management of Cluster Headache," *Lancet Neurol* 17 (2018): 75-83.

3 R.C. Peatfield, "Lithium in Migraine and Cluster Headache: A Review," *J R Soc Med* 74, no. 6 (1981): 432-436. 7252959.

4 B. Wasi, *Standard Treatment Guidelines: A Manual for Medical Therapeutics*, 1st ed. (2014): 112.

5 M. Leone et al., "Melatonin versus Placebo in the Prophylaxis of Cluster Headache: A Double-Blind Pilot Study with Parallel Groups," *Cephalgia* 16 (1995): 494-496.

6 A.C. Miller et al., "Intravenous Magnesium Sulfate to Treat Acute Headaches in the Emergency Department: A Systematic Review," *Headache*. DOI: 10.1111/head.13648. Published online September 30, 2019.

7 http://www.nyheadache.com/blog/emergency-treatment-of-headaches-with-intravenous-magnesium/. Accessed Jan. 3, 2020.

8 D.Y. Wei, M. Khalil, and P.J. Goadsby, "Managing Cluster Headache," *Pract Neurol*. Published online ahead of print July 5, 2019. Accessed July 15, 2019.

9 I.C. Schmidt, "The Etiology and Treatment of Headache," *Osteopathic Annals* 11, no. 12 (1983): 21-31.

10 C. Theisler, "Conservative Headache Management. Cluster Headaches: Pathologic Complexities and Conservative Management Techniques: Part II," *American Journal of Pain Management* 4, no. 1 (1994): 32-35.

11 *The Merck Manual of Diagnosis and Therapy*, 19th ed., 1884.

Cognitive Impairment (Mild)

1 P. Anderson, "Dietary Fat Tied to Better Cognition in Older Adults," *MDEdge Neurology Reviews* (Feb. 4, 2022). https://www.mdedge.com/neurology/article/251471/alzheimers-cognition/dietary-fat-tied-better-cognition-older-adults?

2 M. Fioravanti and M. Yanagi, "Cytidinediphosphocholine (CDP-Choline) for Cognitive and Behavioural Disturbances Associated with Chronic Cerebral Disorders in the Elderly," *Cochrane Database Syst Rev* 2 (2005): CD000269.

3 https://pubmed.ncbi.nlm.nih.gov/22433803/. Accessed Mar. 16, 2021.

4 S. Putignano et al., "Retrospective and Observational Study to Assess the Efficacy of Citicoline in Elderly Patients Suffering from Stupor Related to Complex Geriatric Syndrome," *Clin Interv Aging* 7 (2012): 113-118.

5 D.W. Dysken et al., "Effect of Vitamin E and Memantine on Functional Decline in Alzheimer Disease: The TEAM-AD VA Cooperative Randomized Trial," *JAMA* 311, no. 1 (2014): 33-44.

6 G. Douaud et al., "Preventing Alzheimer's Disease-Related Gray Matter Atrophy by B-Vitamin Treatment," *Proc Natl Acad Sci* 110, no. 23 (2013): 9523-9528.

7 M.I. Botez et al., "Folate-Responsive Neurological and Mental Disorders: Report of 16 Cases," *Eur Neurol* 16 (1977): 230-246.

8 https://jamanetwork.com/journals/jamanetworkopen/fullarticle/2767693?guestAccessKey=67665a32-b597-48f5-ae0a-ca646e87c062&utm_content=weekly_highlights&utm_term=070520&utm_source=silverchair&utm_campaign=jama_network&cmp=1&utm_medium=email. Accessed July 6, 2020.

9 https://www.mdedge.com/neurology/article/244147/alzheimers-cognition/flavonoids-dietary-powerhouses-cognitive-decline? Accessed Aug. 14, 2021.

10 J. Kingsland, "Could Viagra Reduce Alzheimer's Risk," *Medical News Today* (Dec. 7, 2021). https://www.medicalnewstoday.com/articles/could-viagra-reduce-alzheimers-risk. Accessed Dec. 7, 2021.

Colds/Coryza

1 R. Hawkins, "Zinc Lozenges to Treat Colds," *J Family Pract* 43 (1996): 529.

2 https://www.webmd.com/vitamins/ai/ingredientmono-1001/vitamin-c-ascorbic-acid. Accessed Nov. 14, 2018.

3 G. Eby, "Therapeutic Effectiveness of Ionic Zinc for Common Colds," *Clinical Infectious Diseases* 46, no. 3 (Feb. 2008): 483-484. https://doi.org/10.1086/527479.

4 A.S. Prasad et al., "Duration and Severity of Symptoms and Levels of Plasma Interleukin-1 Receptor Antagonist, Soluble Tumor Necrosis Factor Receptor, and Adhesion Molecules in Patients with Common Cold Treated with Zinc Acetate," *J Infect Dis* 197, no. 6 (Mar. 15, 2008): 795-802. DOI: 10.1086/528803.

5 A.R. Gaby, *Nutrition and Healing* (Feb. 1997).

6 M. Singh and R.R. Das, "Zinc for the Common Cold," *Cochrane Database Syst Rev* (Feb. 16, 2011): 2: CD001364. Accessed Dec. 31, 2018.

7 https://lpi.oregonstate.edu/mic/vitamins/vitamin-C. Accessed Nov. 14, 2018. Accessed Nov. 21, 2018.

Cold Sores/Herpes Simplex/Herpes Labialis

1 G.T. Terezhalmy, W. Bottomly, and G. Pelleu, "The Use of Water Soluble Bioflavinoid Ascorbic Acid Complex in the Treatment of Recurrent Herpes Labialis," *Oral Surg* 45, no. 1 (1978): 56-62.

2 A.R. Gaby. "Natural Remedies for Herpes Simplex," *Alternative Medical Review* 11, no. 2 (June 2006): 93-101. Pubmed.gov.

3 M.A. McCune et al., "Treatment of Recurrent Herpes Simplex Infections with L-Lysine Monohydrochloride," *Cutis* 34 (1984): 366-373.

4 R.S. Griffith et al., "Success of L-Lysine Therapy in Frequently Recurrent Herpes Simplex Infection," *Dermatologica* 175 (1987): 183-190.

5 F.A. Tomblin Jr. and K.H. Lucas, "Lysine for Management of Herpes Labialis," *American Journal of Health-System Pharmacy*. Medscape Sept. 2, 2018. https://www.medscape.com/viewarticle/406943_1.

6 https://advancedimdenver.com/hl/?/21654/Topical-Zinc. Accessed Nov. 21, 2018.

7 H.R. Godfrey et al., "A Randomized Clinical Trial on the Treatment of Oral Herpes with Topical Zinc Oxide/Glycine," *Altern Ther Health Med* 7, no. 3 (2001): 49-56.

8 W. Kneist, B. Hempel, and S. Borelli, "Clinical Double-Blind Trial of Topical Zinc Sulfate for Herpes Labialis Recidivans," *Arzneimittelforschung* 45, no. 5 (1995): 624. [German]

9 G. Eby, *Med Hypothesis* 17 (June 1985): 157-165.

10 http://www.george-eby-research.com/html/herpes.html. Accessed Nov. 21, 2018.

Complex Regional Pain Syndrome/Reflex Sympathetic Dystrophy

1 https://www.webmd.com/vitamins/ai/ingredientmono-1001/vitamin-c-ascorbic-acid. Accessed Nov. 14, 2018.

2 P.E. Zollinger et al., "Effect of Vitamin C on Frequency of Reflex Sympathetic Dystrophy in Wrist Fractures: A Randomized Trial," *Lancet* 354 (1999): 2025-2028.

3 https://www.mayoclinic.org/diseases-conditions/complex-regional-pain-syndrome/symptoms-causes/syc-20371151. Accessed Nov. 20, 2018.

4 https://www.researchgate.net/publication/316142454_The_role_of_vitamin_C_in_the_treatment_of_pain_New_insights. Accessed Apr. 12, 2020.

Conjunctivitis/Pinkeye

1 https://www.cdc.gov/conjunctivitis/about/treatment.html. Accessed Apr. 18, 2020.

2 https://www.cdc.gov/features/conjunctivitis/index.html. Accessed Dec. 23, 2018.

3 https://www.merckmanuals.com/en-ca/professional/nutritional-disorders/vitamin-deficiency,-dependency,-and-toxicity/riboflavin. Accessed Dec. 10, 2018.

4 https://jamanetwork.com/journals/jamaophthalmology/article-abstract/617578. Accessed Dec. 10, 2018.

5 H.J. Stern, "Riboflavin Treatment of Spring Catarrh," *Am J Ophth* 32, no. 11 (Nov. 1949): 1553-1556.

6 L. Castellanos, "Ariboflavinosis as a Probable Cause of Vernal Conjunctivitis," *Arch Ophth* 31 (1944): 214.

Constipation

1 B.G. Wells et al., *Pharmacotherapy Handbook*, 9th ed. (McGraw Hill Education), 195.

2 https://www.mayoclinic.org/diseases-conditions/constipation/diagnosis-treatment/drc-20354259. Accessed Nov. 15, 2018.

3 J. Yang et al., "Effect of Dietary Fiber on Constipation: A Meta-Analysis," *World J Gastroenterol* 18, no. 48 (Dec. 28, 2012): 7378-7383.

4 https://www.webmd.com/diet/supplement-guide-aloe-vera#1. Accessed Mar. 5, 2019.

5 https://www.medicalnewstoday.com/articles/318694.php. Accessed Nov. 15, 2018.

6 J.C. Cash and C.A. Glass, *Family Practice Guidelines*, 4th ed. (Springer, 2017), 260.

7 https://www.webmd.com/vitamins/ai/ingredientmono-652/senna. Accessed Nov. 4, 2019.

8 https://www.medicalnewstoday.com/articles/318694.php. Accessed Nov. 15, 2018.

9 http://www.med.umich.edu/1libr/MBCP/Magnesium.pdf. Accessed Jan. 3, 2020.

10 M. Taylor, "Alternatives in Conventional Hormone Replacement Therapy," *Compr Ther* 23, no. 8 (1997): 514-532.

11 https://www.webmd.com/vitamins/ai/ingredientmono-998/magnesium. Accessed Nov. 15, 2018.

12 B.G. Wells et al., *Pharmacotherapy Handbook*, 9th ed. (McGraw Hill Education, 2012), 197.

13 B.G. Wells et al., *Pharmacotherapy Handbook*, 9th ed. (McGraw Hill Education, 2012), 196.

14 https://www.webmd.com/vitamins/ai/ingredientmono-853/pantothenic-acid-vitamin-b5. Accessed Nov. 19, 2018.

15 https://www.webmd.com/vitamins/ai/ingredientmono-790/lactobacillus. Accessed Jan. 12, 2019.

16 R. Hari Krishnan, "A Review on Squat-Assist Devices to Aid Elderly with Lower Limb Difficulties in Toileting to Tackle Constipation," *Proc Inst Mech Eng H* 233, no. 4 (2019): 464-475. DOI: 10.1177/0954411919838644.

17 A. Wald, "Update on the Management of Constipation," *JAMA* 322, no. 22 (2019): 2239-2240. DOI: 10.1001/jama.2019.16029. Accessed Nov. 4, 2019.

18 K.D. Tripathi, *Essentials of Medical Pharmacology*, 7th ed. (2013), 914.

19 https://www.ncbi.nlm.nih.gov/pmc/articles/PMC3293077/. Accessed June 20, 2021.

Corneal Ulcer/Keratitis

1 https://www.webmd.com/eye-health/corneal-ulcer#1. Accessed Dec. 17, 2018.

2 T.A.S. Boyd and F.W. Campbell, "Ascorbic Acid and Healing of Corneal Ulcers," *Br Med J* (Nov. 18, 1950): 2(4689): 1145-1148.

3 R.R. Pfister, C.A. Paterson, and S.A. Hayes, "Topical Ascorbate Decreases the Incidence of Corneal Ulceration after Experimental Alkali Burns," *Investigative Ophthalmology & Visual Science* 17 (1978): 1019-1024.

4 https://www.ncbi.nlm.nih.gov/pmc/articles/PMC3214675/. Accessed May 31, 2019.

Coronary Heart Disease/Coronary Artery Disease (CAD)/ Ischemic Heart Disease/Coronary Atherosclerosis

1 https://www.nhlbi.nih.gov/health-topics/coronary-heart-disease. Accessed June 6, 2021.

2 *BMJ* 308 (1994): 81. *Lancet* 114 (1992): 1421.

3 N.J. Talley, B. Frankum, and D. Currow, *Essentials of Internal Medicine*, 3rd ed. (Churchill Livingstone/Elsevier, 2015), 174.

4 M. Poplawski, N.K. Nelson, and J.S. Earwood, "Rethinking Daily Aspirin for Primary Prevention," *J Fam Pract* 69, no. 9 (2020): 461-462. DOI: 10.12788/jfp.0092.

5 https://emedicine.medscape.com/article/126187-overview. Accessed Nov. 15, 2018.

6 N.G. Stephens et al., "Randomized Controlled Trial of Vitamin E in Patients with Coronary Disease: Cambridge Heart Antioxidant Study (CHAOS)," *Lancet* 347 (1996): 781-786.

7 https://pubmed.ncbi.nlm.nih.gov/15330276/. Accessed Mar. 11, 2021.

8 *Eur Heart J* 32, no. 20 (Oct. 2011): 2573-2584. DOI: 10.1093/eurheartj/ehq501. Epub Jan. 31, 2011: pubmed.ncbi.nlm.nih.gov/21285075.

9 https://www.aafp.org/afp/1998/0315/p1299.html. Accessed Mar. 11, 2021.

10 C. von Schacky et al., "The Effect of Dietary Omega-3 Fatty Acids on Coronary Atherosclerosis. A Randomized, Double-Blind, Placebo-Controlled Trial," *Ann Intern Med* 130 (1999): 554-562.

11 M.L. Burr et al., "Effects of Changes in Fat, Fish, and Fiber Intakes on Death and Myocardial Reinfarction: Diet and Reinfarction Trial (DART)," *Lancet* 334 (1989): 757-761.

12 https://www.ahajournals.org/doi/full/10.1161/CIR.0000000000000709. Accessed Mar. 5, 2020.

13 H.I. Morrison et al., "Serum Folate and Risk of Fatal Coronary Heart Disease," *JAMA* 275 (1996): 1893-1896.

14 A. Tawakol, MD, et al., "High-Dose Folic Acid Acutely Improves Coronary Vasodilator Function in Patients with Coronary Artery Disease," *J Am Coll Cardiol* 45, no. 10 (May 17, 2005): 1580-1584. Published online Apr. 26, 2005. DOI: 10.1016/j.jacc.2005.02.038.

15 B.G. Brown et al., "Simvastatin and Niacin, Antioxidant Vitamins, or the Combination for the Prevention of Coronary Disease," *N Engl J Med* 345, no. 22 (2001): 1583-1592.

16 J.E. Digby, N. Ruparelia, and R.P. Choudhury, "Niacin in Cardiovascular Disease: Recent Preclinical and Clinical Developments," *Arterioscler Thromb Vasc Biol* 32, no. 3 (Mar. 2012): 582-588.

17 "Clofibrate and Niacin in Coronary Heart Disease," *JAMA* 231 (1975): 360-381.

18 P.L. Canner et al., "Fifteen Year Mortality in Coronary Drug Project Patients: Long-Term Benefit with Niacin," *J Am Coll Cardiol* 8 (1986): 1245-1255.

19 W.E. Boden, M.S. Sidhu, and P.P. Toth, "The Therapeutic Role of Niacin in Dyslipidemia Management," *J Cardiovasc Pharmacol Ther* 19, no. 2 (2014): 141-158.

20 https://lpi.oregonstate.edu/mic/vitamins/vitamin-C. Accessed Nov. 18, 2018.

21 N. Gokce et al., "Long-Term Ascorbic Acid Administration Reverses Endothelial Vasomotor Dysfunction in Patients with Coronary Artery Disease," *Circulation* 99, no. 25 (1999): 3234-3240.

22 L.K. Kothari and P. Sharma, "Aggravation of Cholesterol Induced Hyperlipidemia by Chronic Vitamin C Deficiency: Experimental Study in Guinea Pigs," *Acta Biol Hung* 39, no. 1 (1988): 4.

23 J.L. Anderson et al., "Relation of Vitamin D Deficiency to Cardiovascular Risk Factors, Disease Status, and Incident Events in a General Healthcare Population," *Am J Cardiol* 106, no. 7 (2010): 963-968.

24 https://www.ncbi.nlm.nih.gov/pmc/articles/PMC4678494/. Accessed Nov. 6, 2021.

Cracked Skin/Tennis Shoe Dermatitis

1 https://www.medicalnewstoday.com/articles/cracked-skin#definition. Accessed Nov. 28, 2021.

2 https://www.seattlechildrens.org/conditions/a-z/cracked-or-dry-skin/. Accessed Mar. 12, 2019.

Crohn's Disease

1 B. Jansen, "Some with Mild Crohn's Disease Need No Treatment," *MDEdge Internal Medicine* (Dec. 10, 2019). Accessed Dec. 10, 2019.

2 B.G. Wells et al., *Pharmacotherapy Handbook*, 9th ed. (McGraw Hill Education), 224.

3 *The Washington Manual of Medical Therapeutics*, 34th ed., 859.

4 J.C. Cash and C.A. Glass, *Family Practice Guidelines*, 4th ed., (Springer, 2017), 264.

5 M.A. Chisolm-Burns et al., *Pharmacotherapy Principles & Practice* (McGraw-Hill Medical, 2008), 285.

6 https://www.ncbi.nlm.nih.gov/pmc/articles/PMC2984332/. Accessed Nov. 19, 2018.

7 A. Belluzzi et al., "Effect of an Enteric-Coated Fish-Oil Preparation on Relapses in Crohn's Disease," *N Engl J Med* 334 (1996): 1557-1560.

8 A. Aslan and G. Triadafilopoulos, "Fish Oil Fatty Acid Supplementation in Active Ulcerative Colitis: A Double-Blind, Placebo-Controlled, Crossover Study," *American Journal of Gastroenterology* 87, no. 4 (Apr. 1992): 432-437.

9 W.F. Stenson et al., "Dietary Supplementation with Fish Oil in Ulcerative Colitis," *Annals of Int Med* 116, no. 8 (Apr. 1992): 609-614.

10 https://www.mayoclinic.org/diseases-conditions/crohns-disease/diagnosis-treatment/drc-20353309. Accessed Nov. 19, 2018.

11 K.A. Sharkey and W K. MacNaughton, "Pharmacotherapy for Gastric Acidity, Peptic Ulcers, and Gastroesophageal Reflux Disease," in *Gilbert & Goodman's: The Pharmacological Basis of Therapeutics*, 13th ed. (2018), 951.

12 T.D. Nolan and P.A. Friedman, "Agents Affecting Mineral Ion Homeostasis and Bone Turnover," in *Gilbert & Goodman's: The Pharmacological Basis of Therapeutics*, 13th ed. (2018), 896.

13 https://familydoctor.org/condition/anemia/. Accessed Dec. 31, 2018.

14 H. Gerhardt et al., "Therapy of Active Crohn's Disease with Boswellia Serrata Extract H15," *Z Gastroenterol* 39 (2001): 11-17.

15 I. Gupta et al., "Effects of Gum Resin of Boswellia Serrata in Patients with Ulcerative Colitis," *Eur J Med Res* 2 (1997): 37-43.

16 https://www.medscape.com/viewarticle/553039_17. Accessed Dec. 17, 2018.

17 L. Yang et al., "Therapeutic Effect of Vitamin D Supplementation in a Pilot Study of Crohn's Patients," *Clin Transl Gastroenterol* 4 (2013): e33.

18 *Nutrients* 11, no. 5 (May 11, 2019). DOI: 10.3390/nu11051059.

19 https://pubmed.ncbi.nlm.nih.gov/17240130/.

20 https://www.medicalnewstoday.com/articles/322751#Strawberries-and-inflammation.

21 A. Costantini et al., "Thiamine and Spinocerebellar Ataxia Type 2," *BMJ Case Reports*. Published online Jan. 10, 2013.

22 *The Washington Manual of Medical Therapeutics*, 34th ed., 856.

Cryptosporidiosis

1 K.R. Rasmussen et al., "Effects of Dehydroepiandrosterone in Immunosuppressed Adult Mice Infected with *Cryptosporidium parvum*," *J Parasitol* 81, no. 3 (June 1995): 429-433.

Cushing's Syndrome/Hypercortisolism

1 https://www.mayoclinic.org/diseases-conditions/cushing-syndrome/symptoms-causes/syc-20351310. Accessed Jan. 3, 2019.

2 *The Merck Manual of Diagnosis and Therapy*, 19th ed., 929.

3 https://www.ncbi.nlm.nih.gov/pmc/articles/PMC5881435/. Accessed May 3, 2021.

4 https://www.rxlist.com/gaba_gamma-aminobutyric_acid/supplements.htm. Accessed Jan. 3, 2019.

Cutaneous Amyloidosis

1 M.A. Keen and I. Hassan, "Vitamin E in Dermatology," *Indian Dermatol Online J* 7, no. 4 (July-Aug. 2016): 311-315. DOI: 10.4103/2229-5178.185494.

2 http://pennstatehershey.adam.com/content.aspx?productId=107&pid=33&gid=000328. Accessed Nov. 16, 2018.

3 https://www.dermcoll.edu.au/atoz/cutaneous-amyloidosis/. Accessed Apr. 18, 2020.

Cutaneous Leishmaniasis

1 M. Gupta et al., "Zinc Therapy in Dermatology: A Review," *Dermatol Res Pract* 2014 (2014): 709152. Published online July 10, 2014. DOI: 10.1155/2014/709152.

2 K.E. Sharquie and K. Al-Azzawi, "Intralesional Therapy of Cutaneous Leishmaniasis with 2% Zinc Sulphate Solution," *J Pan Arab League Dermatol* 7 (1996): 41-46.

Cyanide Poisoning

1 C.E. Sanders and M.T Ho, *Current Emergency Diagnosis and Treatment*, 4th ed. A Lange Medical Book (1993), 739, 748.

2 https://www.emsworld.com/pressrelease/10407871/fda-approves-cyanokitr-treatment-cyanide-poisoning. Accessed Nov. 21, 2018.

Cystic Fibrosis

1 https://www.medscape.com/answers/1001602-31201/what-are-the-primary-treatment-goals-of-cystic-fibrosis-cf. Accessed May 4, 2021.

2 M.A. Chisolm-Burns et al., *Pharmacotherapy Principles & Practice* (McGraw-Hill Medical, 2008), 248.

3 V. Quick and C. Byrd-Bredbenner, "Disordered Eating and Body Image in Cystic Fibrosis," *Diet and Exercise in Cystic Fibrosis* (San Diego, CA: Academic Press, 2015), 11-12.

4 https://www.mayoclinic.org/diseases-conditions/cystic-fibrosis/symptoms-causes/syc-20353700. Accessed Nov. 28, 2018.

5 https://www.webmd.com/vitamins/ai/ingredientmono-1024/taurine. Accessed Nov. 28, 2018.

6 A.R. Gaby, "Taurine: The Cellular Buffer," *Nutrition and Healing* 4, no. 1 (Jan. 1997): 4.

7 https://www.medscape.com/answers/2038394-35996/how-does-cystic-fibrosis-cause-hypomagnesemia. Accessed Mar. 19, 2021.

8 C. Gontijo-Amaral, E.V. Guimaraes, and P. Camargos, "Oral Magnesium Supplementation in Children with Cystic Fibrosis Improves Clinical and Functional Variables: A Double-Blind, Randomized, Placebo-Controlled Crossover Trial," *Am J Clin Nutr* 96, no. 1 (July 2012): 50-56.

9 https://nutritionguide.pcrm.org/nutritionguide/view/Nutrition_Guide_for_Clinicians/1342064/all/Cystic_Fibrosis. Accessed Jan. 15, 2021.

Darier's Disease/Keratosis Follicularis

1 https://rarediseases.org/rare-diseases/keratosis-follicularis/. Accessed Nov. 11, 2020.

2 https://emedicine.medscape.com/article/1107340-treatment. Accessed Nov. 25, 2018.

3 S. Günther, "Vitamin A Acid in Darier's Disease," *Acta Derm Venereol Suppl (Stockh)* 74 (Jan. 27-29, 1975): 146-151.

4 J.R. Thomas 3rd, J.P Cooke, and R.K. Winkelmann, "High-Dose Vitamin A Therapy for Darier's Disease," *Arch Dermatol* 118, no. 11 (Nov. 1982): 891-894.

5 K.N. Mohamed, "Darier's Disease: Response to Combination of Vitamins A and E," *Singapore Medical Journal* 28, no. 1 (1987): 80-82. http://smj.sma.org.sg/2801/2801smj15.pdf.

6 K.D. Tripathi, *Essentials of Medical Pharmacology*, 7th ed. (2013), 910.

Deep Vein Thrombosis (DVT)

1 https://orthoinfo.aaos.org/en/diseases--conditions/deep-vein-thrombosis/. Accessed Apr. 8, 2020.

2 https://pubmed.ncbi.nlm.nih.gov/29656974/. Accessed Sept. 20, 2020.

3 https://www.mayoclinic.org/diseases-conditions/deep-vein-thrombosis/symptoms-causes/syc-20352557. Accessed Dec. 17, 2018.

4 R.J. Glynn et al., "Effects of Random Allocation to Vitamin E Supplementation on the Occurrence of Venous Thromboembolism: Report from the Women's Health Study," *Circulation* 116, no. 13 (Sept. 25, 2007): 1497-1503.

5 https://www.webmd.com/women/news/20070911/vitamin-e-may-lower-blood-clot-risk#2. Accessed Dec. 9, 2018.

6 J. Livesey et al., "Low Serum Iron Levels Are Associated with Elevated Plasma Levels of Coagulation Factor VIII and Pulmonary Emboli/Deep Venous Thromboses in Replicate Cohorts of Patients with Hereditary Hemorrhagic Telangiectasia," *Thorax* (Dec. 14, 2011). DOI: 10.1136/thoraxjnl-2011-201076.

7 R. Jasuja et al., "Protein Disulfide Isomerase Inhibitors Constitute a New Class of Antithrombotic Agents," *J Clin Invest* 122, no. 6 (2012): 2104-2113. DOI: 10.1172/JCI61228.

8 J.H. Choi et al., "Anti-Thrombotic Effect of Rutin Isolated from *Dendropanax morbifera* Leveille," *Journal of Bioscience and Bioengineering* 120, no. 2 (2015): 181-186.

Dementia/Cognitive Decline

1 *The Merck Manual of Diagnosis and Therapy*, 19th ed., 1840.

2 Y. Moriguchi, "Physiological Aging and Atherosclerosis: Prophylaxis of Arteriosclerosis with Vitamins," *Int J Vit Nutr Res Suppl* 26 (1984): 121-124.

3 M.A. Papadakis and S.J. McPhee, *Current Medical Diagnosis & Treatment* (2019): ch. 24, 1032.

4 *The Merck Manual of Diagnosis and Therapy,* 19th ed., 1843.

5 P. Knekt et al., *Prev Med Rep* (2020). DOI: 10.1016/j.pmedr.2020.101221.

6 J.W. Miller, D.J. Harvey, and L.A. Becket, "Vitamin D Status and Rates of Cognitive Decline in a Multiethnic Cohort of Older Adults," *JAMA Neurol* 72, no. 11 (2015): 1295-1303. DOI: 10.1001/jamaneurol.2015.2115.

7 https://www.alzheimers.net/8-27-14-vitamin-d-and-dementia/. Accessed Nov. 25, 2018.

8 http://pennstatehershey.adam.com/content.aspx?productId=117&pid=1&gid=000683.

9 K. Pham et al., "High Coffee Consumption, Brain Volume and Risk of Dementia and Stroke," *Nutritional Neuroscience* (2021). DOI: 10.1080/1028415X.2021.1945858.

10 https://www.webmd.com/alzheimers/types-dementia#2-7. Accessed Nov. 25, 2018.

11 M. Tanyel and L. Mancano, "Neurologic Findings in Vitamin E Deficiency," *Am Fam Phys* (Jan. 1997): 197.

12 https://www.webmd.com/vitamins/ai/ingredientmono-333/ginkgo. Accessed Nov. 26, 2018.

13 https://www.ncbi.nlm.nih.gov/pmc/articles/PMC1123448/. Accessed May 15, 2020.

14 M.I. Botez et al., "Folate-Responsive Neurological and Mental Disorders: Report of 16 Cases," *Eur Neurol* 16 (1977): 230-246.

15 J. Runcie, "Folate Deficiency in the Elderly," *Folic Acid in Neurology, Psychiatry and Internal Medicine*, eds. M.I. Botez and E.H. Reynolds (New York: Raven, 1979), 493-499.

16 https://pubmed.ncbi.nlm.nih.gov/29424298/. Accessed Aug. 15, 2021.

Depression

1 G.A. Eby and K.L. Eby, "Rapid Recovery from Major Depression using Magnesium Treatment," *Medical Hypotheses* 67, no. 2 (2006): 362-370.

2 V.P. Arcangelo and A.M. Peterson, *Pharmacotherapeutics for Advanced Practice: A Practical Approach,* 3rd ed. (Wolters Kluwer/Lippincott Williams & Wilkins, 2013), 125.

3 https://www.webmd.com/fibromyalgia/guide/fibromyalgia-herbs-and-supplements#2.

4 J. Keough, "Common Herbal Therapies," in *Shaum's Outlines in Pharmacology* (The McGraw-Hill Companies, Inc., 2010), 72.

5 O.M. Wolkowitz et al., "Antidepressant and Cognition-Enhancing Effects of DHEA in Major Depression," *Ann NY Acad Sci* 774 (Dec. 29, 1995): 337-339.

6 B.E. Murphy, D. Filipini, and A.M. Ghadirian, "Possible Use of Glucocorticoid Receptor Antagonists in the Treatment of Major Depression: Preliminary Results Using RU 486," *J Psychiatry Neuroscience* 18, no. 5 (Nov. 1993): 20.

7 O.M. Wolkowitz et al., "Double-Blind Treatment of Major Depression with Dehydroepiandrosterone," *Am J Psychiatry* 156, no. 4 (Apr. 1999): 646-649.

8 P.J. Schmidt, R.C. Daly, and M. Bloch, "Dehydroepiandrosterone Monotherapy in Midlife-Onset Major and Minor Depression," *Arch Gen Psychiatry* 62, no. 2 (2005): 154-162. DOI: 10.1001/archpsyc.62.2.154.

9 A.C. Logan, "Omega-3 Fatty Acids and Major Depression: A Primer for the Mental Health Professional," *Lipids Health Dis* 3 (2004): 25.

10 https://www.webmd.com/vitamins/ai/ingredientmono-662/turmeric. Accessed Nov. 14, 2018.

11 https://ods.od.nih.gov/factsheets/Folate-HealthProfessional/. Accessed Feb. 11, 2019.

12 S.N. Young, "Folate and Depression: A Neglected Problem," *J Psychiatry Neurosci* 32, no. 2 (2007): 80-82.

13 M.I. Botez et al., "Neuropsychological Correlates of Folic Acid Deficiency: Facts and Hypotheses," *Folic Acid in Neurology, Psychiatry and Internal Medicine*, eds. M.I. Botez and E.H. Reynolds (New York: Raven, 1979), 435-461.

14 https://www.psychologytoday.com/us/blog/the-integrationist/201310/depression-wont-go-away-folate-could-be-the-answer. Accessed Jan. 8, 2019.

15 D. Maes et al., "Hypozincemia in Depression," *J Affect Disord* 31, no. 2 (June 1994): 135-140.

16 http://www.if-pan.krakow.pl/pjp/pdf/2003/6_1143.pdf. Accessed Jan. 29, 2019.

17 https://www.mountsinai.org/health-library/supplement/vitamin-b1-thiamine. Accessed July 28, 2021.

18 M.A. Hollinger, *Introduction to Pharmacology*, 2nd ed. (Tayor & Francis, 2003), 845.

19 S. Alghamdi et al., *J Mol Neurosci* (Dec. 13, 2019). DOI: 10.1007/s12031-019-01461-2.

20 *Psychiatric Bulletin* 28, no. 5 (May 2004): 183. https://doi.org/10.1192/pb.28.5.183.

Diabetes Mellitus Type 1 (DM1)/Juvenile Diabetes/ Insulin Dependent Diabetes Mellitus (IDDM)

1 B.G. Wells et al., *Pharmacotherapy Handbook*, 9th ed. (McGraw Hill Education), 162.

2 P. Vague et al., "Nicotinamide May Extend Remission Phase in Insulin-Dependent Diabetes," *Lancet* 1 (1987): 619-620.

3 T. Mandrup-Poulsen et al., "Nicotinamide Treatment in the Prevention of Insulin Dependent Diabetes Mellitus," *Diabetes/Metab Rev* 9 (1993): 295-309.

4 S.M. Brichard and J.C. Henquin, "The Role of Vanadium in the Management of Diabetes," *Trends Pharmacol Sci.* 16, no. 8 (Aug. 1995): 26.

5 J.C. Coggeshall et al., "Biotin Status and Plasma Glucose in Diabetics," *Ann NY Acad Sci* 447 (1985): 389-393.

6 M. Maebashi et al., "Therapeutic Evaluation of the Effects of Biotin on Hyperglycemia in Patients with Non-Insulin Dependent Diabetes Mellitus," *J Clin Biochem Nutr* 14 (1993): 211-218.

7 A. Reddi et al., "Biotin Supplementation Improves Glucose and Insulin Tolerances in Genetically Diabetic KK Mice," *Life Sci* 42 (1988): 1323-1330.

8 J.C. Coggeshall et al., "Biotin Status and Plasma Glucose in Diabetics," *Ann NY Acad Sci* 447 (1985): 389-393.

9 F. Franconi et al., "Plasma and Platelet Taurine Are Reduced in Subjects with Insulin-Dependent Diabetes Mellitus: Effects of Taurine Supplementation," *Am J Clin Nutr* 61 (1995): 1115-1119.

10 D. Shahbah, MD, et al., "Oral Magnesium Supplementation Improves Glycemic Control and Lipid Profile in Children with Type 1 Diabetes and Hypomagnesaemia," *Medicine* 96, no. 11 (Mar. 2017): e6352. DOI: 10.1097/MD.0000000000006352.

11 http://internalmedicine.medscape.com/r11/4/2000. Accessed Nov. 17, 2018.

12 https://www.rxlist.com/consumer_vanadium/drugs-condition.htm. Accessed Nov. 5, 2021.

Diabetes Mellitus Type 2 (DM2)/Adult Onset Diabetes

1 "Expert Roundtable—Diabetes," *The Journal of Family Practice* 68, no. 9 (Nov. 2019). Accessed Feb. 15, 2020.

2 C. Celis-Morales et al. Institute of Cardiovascular and Medical Sciences, University of Glasgow, Glasgow, UK. EASD 56th Annual Meeting, 2020.

3 National Institutes of Health, *Diabetes in America*, 3rd ed. (Bethesda, MD: NIH, Pub No. 17-1468, 2017).

4 https://www.mayoclinic.org/diseasesconditions/type-2-diabetes/diagnosis-treatment/drc-20351199. Accessed Nov. 25, 2018.

5 E.T. Bope and R.D. Kellerman, *Conn's Current Therapy*, 14th ed. (Philadelphia: Elsevier/Saunders), 737.

6 https://www.mdedge.com/endocrinology/article/229158/diabetes/exercise-cuts-diabetes-death-risk-third-two-studies?ecd=wnl_evn_200928_mdedge_8pm&uac=. Accessed Sept. 29, 2020.

7 American Diabetes Association, "Nutrition Principles and Recommendations in Diabetes," *Diabetes Care* 27, suppl. 1 (Jan. 2004): s36-s36. https://doi.org/10.2337/diacare.27.2007.S36. http://care.diabetesjournals.org/content/27/suppl_1/s36. Accessed Nov. 25, 2018.

8 G.N. Dakhale, H.V. Chaudhari, and M. Shrivastava, "Supplementation of Vitamin C Reduces Blood Glucose and Improves Glycosylated Hemoglobin in Type 2 Diabetes Mellitus: A Randomized, Double-Blind Study," *Advances in Pharmacological Sciences* 2011, Article ID 195271 (2011). https://doi.org/10.1155/2011/195271.

9 M. Afkhami-Ardekani and A. Shojaoddiny-Ardekani, "Effect of Vitamin C on Blood Glucose, Serum Lipids & Serum Insulin in Type 2 Diabetes Patients," *Indian J Med Res* 126, no. 5 (Nov. 2007): 471-474.

10 J. Kositsawat and V.L. Freeman, "Vitamin C and A1 Relationship in the National Health and Nutrition Examination Survey (NHANES) 2003-2006," *J Am Coll Nutr* 30, no. 6 (2011): 477-483.

11 Y. Song et al., "Multivitamins, Individual Vitamin and Mineral Supplements, and Risk of Diabetes among Older US adults," *Diabetes Care* 34, no. 1 (2011): 108-114.

12 H.N. Santosh and C.M. David, "Role of Ascorbic Acid in Diabetes Mellitus: A Comprehensive Review," *Journal of Medicine, Radiology, Pathology & Surgery* 4 (2017): 1-3.

13 D. Christie-David, C. Girgis, and C. Gunton, "Effects of Vitamins C and D in Type 2 Diabetes Mellitus," *Nutrition and Dietary Supplements* 7 (Feb. 2015): 21-28.

14 https://www.eurekalert.org/pub_releases/2015-02/tes-vdd021815.php. Accessed Nov. 26, 2018.

15 https://www.ncbi.nlm.nih.gov/pmc/articles/PMC3761874/#R150.

16 T. Martin, RD, CDE, LD, and R.K. Campbell, "Vitamin D and Diabetes," *Diabetes Spectrum* 24, no. 2 (May 2011): 113-118. https://doi.org/10.2337/diaspect.24.2.113.

17 https://www.webmd.com/diabetes/news/20100621/low-vitamin-d-linked-to-poor-diabetes-control#1. Accessed Nov. 26, 2018.

18 E.A. Sotaniemi et al., "Ginseng Therapy in Non-Insulin Dependent Diabetic Patients," *Diabetes Care* 18 (1995): 1373-1375.

19 M. Barbagallo and L.J. Dominguez, "Magnesium and Type 2 Diabetes," *World J Diabetes* 6, no. 10 (Aug. 2015): 1152-1157.

20 F. Guerrero-Romero et al., "Oral Magnesium Supplementation Improves Insulin Sensitivity in Non-Diabetic Subjects with Insulin Resistance: A Double-Blind Placebo-Controlled Randomized Trial," *Diabetes Metab* 30 (2004): 253-258.

21 F. Guerrero-Romero and M. Rodríguez-Morán, "Complementary Therapies for Diabetes: The Case for Chromium, Magnesium, and Antioxidants," *Arch Med Res* 36 (2005): 250-257.

22 M. Rodríguez-Morán and F. Guerrero-Romero, "Oral Magnesium Supplementation Improves Insulin Sensitivity and Metabolic Control in Type 2 Diabetic Subjects: A Randomized Double-Blind Controlled Trial," *Diabetes Care* 26 (2003): 1147-1152.

23 K. Yokota et al., "Clinical Efficacy of Magnesium Supplementation in Patients with Type 2 Diabetes," *J Am Coll Nutr* 23 (2004): 506S-509S.

24 H.W. de Valk et al., "Oral Magnesium Supplementation in Insulin-Requiring Type 2 Diabetic Patients," *Diabet Med* 15 (1998): 503-507.

25 https://www.ncbi.nlm.nih.gov/pmc/articles/PMC4549665/#B54. Accessed Feb. 29, 2019.

26 https://www.ncbi.nlm.nih.gov/pmc/articles/PMC4549665/. Accessed May 13, 2020.

27 G. Paolisso et al., "Pharmacologic Doses of Vitamin E Improved Insulin Action in Healthy Subjects and Non-Insulin Dependent Diabetic Patients," *Am J Clin Nutr* 57 (1993): 650-656.

28 *Free Radical Biology and Medicine* (Nov. 15, 2000).

29 http://internalmedicine.medscape.com/r11/4/2000. Accessed Nov. 17, 2018.

30 K.H. Thompson et al., "Vanadium Treatment of Type 2 Diabetes: A View to the Future," *Journal of Inorganic Biochemistry* 103, no. 4 (Apr. 2009): 554-558.

31 https://www.ncbi.nlm.nih.gov/pmc/articles/PMC3249697/. Accessed Nov. 5, 2021.

32 M. Urberg and M.B. Zemel, "Evidence for Synergism Between Chromium and Nicotinic Acid in the Control of Glucose Tolerance in Elderly Humans," *Metabolism* (1987): 896-899.

33 https://www.webmd.com/diet/supplement-guide-alpha-lipoic-acid#1. Accessed Nov. 26, 2018.

34 https://www.webmd.com/vitamins/ai/ingredientmono-932/chromium. Accessed Nov. 14, 2018.

35 https://www.webmd.com/vitamins/ai/ingredientmono-965/thiamine-vitamin-b1. Accessed Nov. 14, 2018.

36 M. Maebashi et al., "Therapeutic Evaluation of the Effect of Biotin on Hyperglycemia in Patients with Non-Insulin Dependent Diabetes Mellitus," *J Clin Biochem Nutr* 14 (1993): 211-218.

37 W.R. Dick, E.A. Fletcher, and S.A. Shah, "Reduction of Fasting Blood Glucoses and Hemoglobin A1C Using Oral Aloe Vera: A Meta-Analysis," *J Altern and Complem Med* 22, no. 6 (June 2016). https://doi.org/10.1089/acm.2015.0122.

38 S. Yongchaiyudha et al., "Anti-Diabetic Activity of Aloe Vera L. Juice. I. Clinical Trial in New Cases of Diabetes Mellitus," *Phytomedicine* 3 (1996): 241-243.

39 D. Brunk, "Carbohydrate Restriction a Viable Choice for Reversal of Type 2 Diabetes, Experts Say," *MDEdge Endocrinology* (Jan. 9, 2020). Accessed Jan. 9, 2020.

40 https://www.mdedge.com/dermatology/article/215102/acne/ketogenic-diet-and-dermatology-primer-current-literature/page/0/.

41 https://www.medicalnewstoday.com/articles/325798#benefits. Accessed May 6, 2020.

42 https://www.ncbi.nlm.nih.gov/pmc/articles/PMC2410097/. Accessed May 6, 2020.

43 https://pubmed.ncbi.nlm.nih.gov/14633804/. Accessed Apr. 2, 2021.

44 *The Washington Manual for Medical Therapeutics*, 34th ed., 1118.

Diabetic Neuropathy

1 V.J. McCann and R.E. Davis, "Serum Pyridoxal Concentrations in Patients with Diabetic Neuropathy," *Aust N Z J Med* 8, no. 3 (June 1978): 259-261.

2 E.R. Levin et al., "The Influence of Pyridoxine in Diabetic Peripheral Neuropathy," *Diabetes Care* 4, no. 6 (Nov.-Dec. 1981): 606-609.

3 H. Keen et al., "Treatment of Diabetic Neuropathy with Gamma-Linolenic Acid," *Diabetes Care* 16 (1993): 8-15.

4 https://onlinelibrary.wiley.com/doi/abs/10.1111/j.1464-5491.1990.tb01397.x. Accessed Jan. 22, 2019.

5 https://www.ncbi.nlm.nih.gov/pmc/articles/PMC4192992/. Accessed Jan. 22, 2019.

6 S.C. Sweetman, ed., *Martindale: The Complete Drug Reference* (London: Pharmaceutical Press, 2009), 1976-1977.

7 H. Kinoshita and I. Nonaka, "Recurrent Muscle Weakness and Ataxia in Thiamine-Responsive Pyruvate Dehydrogenase Complex Deficiency," *J Child Neurology* 12, no. 2 (Feb. 1997): 141-144.

8 D. De Grandis and C. Minardi, "Acetyl-L-Carnitine (Levacecarnine) in the Treatment of Diabetic Neuropathy," *Drugs R&D* (2002): 3: 223. https://doi.org/10.2165/00126839-200203040-00001.

9 A.A. Sima et al., "Acetyl-L-Carnitine Improves Pain, Nerve Regeneration, and Vibratory Perception in Patients with Chronic Diabetic Neuropathy: An Analysis of Two Randomized Placebo-Controlled Trials," *Diabetes Care* 28, no. 1 (2005): 89-94.

10 D. DeGrandis and C. Minardi, "Acetyl-L-Carnitine (Levacecarnine) in the Treatment of Diabetic Neuropathy: A Long-Term, Randomized, Double-Blind, Placebo-Controlled Study," *Drugs R D* 3, no. 4 (2002): 223-231.

11 D. Koutsikos, "Biotin for Diabetic Peripheral Neuropathy," *Biomed and Pharmacotherapy* 44 (1990): 511-514.

12 H.N. Santosh and Chaya M. David, "Role of Ascorbic Acid in Diabetes Mellitus: A Comprehensive Review," *Journal of Medicine, Radiology, Pathology & Surgery* 4 (2017): 1-3.

13 J.M. Keppel Hesselink and T.A.M. Hekker, "Therapeutic Utility of Palmitoylethanolamide in the Treatment of Neuropathic Pain Associated with Various Pathological Conditions: A Case Series," *J Pain Res* (2012): 5: 437-442. Published online Oct. 26, 2012. DOI: 10.2147/JPR.S32143.

14 https://www.ncbi.nlm.nih.gov/pmc/articles/PMC3221300/. Accessed Nov. 27, 2018.

15 https://www.webmd.com/diet/supplement-guide-alpha-lipoic-acid#1. Accessed Nov. 26, 2018.

16 K.J. Ruhnau et al., "Effects of 3-Week Oral Treatment with the Antioxidant Thioctic Acid (Alpha-Lipoic Acid) in Symptomatic Diabetic Polyneuropathy," *Diabet Med* 16, no. 12 (1999): 1040-1043. (PubMed)

17 D. Ziegler et al., "Oral Treatment with Alpha-Lipoic Acid Improves Symptomatic Diabetic Polyneuropathy: The SYDNEY 2 Trial," *Diabetes Care* 29, no. 11 (2006): 2365-2370.

18 https://www.webmd.com/vitamins/ai/ingredientmono-938/coenzyme-q10. Accessed Nov. 18, 2018.

19 G. Devathasan, W.L. Teo, and A. Mylvaganam. "Methylcobalamin in Chronic Diabetic Neuropathy: A Double-Blind Clinical and Electrophysiological Study," *Clinical Trials Journal* 23, no. 2 (1986): 130-140.

20 S. Kuwabara et al., "Intravenous Methylcobalamin Treatment for Uremic and Diabetic Neuropathy in Chronic Hemodialysis Patients," *Internal Medicine* 38, no. 6 (1999): 472-475.

21 H. Ishihara et al., "Efficacy of Intravenous Administration of Methylcobalamin for Diabetic Peripheral Neuropathy," *Med Consult N Remedies* 29, no. 1 (1992): 1720-1725.

22 *BMJ Open Diabetes Res Care* 4 (2016): e000148. https://drc.bmj.com/content/bmjdrc/4/1/e000148.full.pdf?with-ds=yes. Accessed June 15, 2021.

23 https://www.medscape.com/viewarticle/871621#vp_2. Accessed Jan. 8, 2019.

24 https://www.ncbi.nlm.nih.gov/pmc/articles/PMC4549665/. Accessed May 13, 2020.

Diaper Rash/Diaper Dermatitis/Contact Dermatitis

1 https://www.dermis.net/dermisroot/en/15645/diagnose.htm. Accessed Jan. 7, 2022.

2 https://www.mayoclinic.org/diseases-conditions/diaper-rash/doagnosis-treatment/drc-20371641. Accessed Dec. 16, 2018.

3 M. Gupta et al., "Zinc Therapy in Dermatology: A Review," *Dermatol Res Pract* 2014 (2014): 709152. Published online July 10, 2014. DOI: 10.1155/2014/709152.

4 P. Manzoni. "Effectiveness of Topical Acetate Tocopherol for the Prevention and Treatment of Skin Lesions in Newborns: A 5 Years Experience in a 3rd Level Italian Neonatal Intensive Care Unit," *Minerva Pediatr* 57, no. 5 (Oct. 2005): 305-311.

5 https://www.mayoclinic.org/diseases-conditions/diaper-rash/diagnosis-treatment/drc-20371641. Accessed Nov. 21, 2018.

6 https://www.webmd.com/vitamins/ai/ingredientmono-235/calendula. Accessed Nov. 21, 2018.

7 https://www.mayoclinic.org/diseases-conditions/diaper-rash/diagnosis-treatment/drc-20371641. Accessed Nov. 21, 2018.

8 https://newsnetwork.mayoclinic.org/discussion/home-remedies-dealing-with-that-darn-diaper-rash/. Accessed Dec. 16, 2018.

9 https://www.webmd.com/vitamins/ai/ingredientmono-982/zinc. Accessed Jan. 29, 2019.

10 https://www.medicalnewstoday.com/articles/322472#ten-treatments-and-home-remedies. Accessed Jan. 7, 2022.

Diarrhea (Acute)

1 D. Hui, *Approach to Internal Medicine: A Resource Book for Clinical Practice*, 3rd ed. (Springer, 2011), 119.

2 https://www.medicinenet.com/diarrhea/article.htm#what_is_the_treatment_for_diarrhea_in_older_children_and_adults. Accessed Nov. 15, 2018.

3 https://www.merckmanuals.com/professional/gastrointestinal-disorders/symptoms-of-gi-disorders/diarrhea. Accessed Mar. 24, 2019.

4 https://www.medscape.com/answers/2038394-35961/what-types-of-cardiac-arrhythmia-are-caused-by-hypomagnesemia. Accessed May 14, 2020.

5 M.A. Chisolm-Burns et al., *Pharmacotherapy Principles & Practice* (McGraw-Hill Medical, 2008), 313.

6 D. Hui, *Approach to Internal Medicine: A Resource Book for Clinical Practice*, 3rd ed. (Springer, 2011), 123.

7 B.G. Wells et al., *Pharmacotherapy Handbook*, 9th ed. (McGraw Hill Education), 200.

8 https://www.medicalnewstoday.com/articles/320124.php. Accessed Oct. 24, 2019.

9 http://www.nmihi.com/d/diarrhea.htm. Accessed Mar. 24, 2019.

10 https://www.medicinenet.com/diarrhea/article.htm#what_is_the_treatment_for_diarrhea_in_older_children_and_adults. Accessed Nov. 15, 2018.

11 S. Sazawal et al., "Zinc Supplementation in Young Children with Acute Diarrhea in India," *N Engl J Med* 333 (1995): 389-344.

12 https://www.webmd.com/lung/news/19991207/zinc-reduces-pneumonia-diarrhea-children#1. Accessed Nov. 1, 2019.

13 https://www.ncbi.nlm.nih.gov/pmc/articles/PMC3625079/. Accessed Nov. 15, 2018.

14 https://www.webmd.com/vitamins/ai/ingredientmono-790/lactobacillus. Accessed Jan. 12, 2019.

15 A. Sullivan and C.E. Nord, "Probiotics and Gastrointestinal Disease," *J Intern Med* 257 (2005): 78-92.

16 https://www.webmd.com/digestive-disorders/chronic-diarrhea-16/diarrhea-more-fiber. Accessed Nov. 11, 2019.

Diarrhea (Chronic)

1 D. Hui, *Approach to Internal Medicine: A Resource Book for Clinical Practice*. 3rd ed. (Springer, 2011), 124.

2 https://www.medicalnewstoday.com/articles/319995.php. Accessed Nov. 20, 2018.

3 http://www.nmihi.com/d/diarrhea.htm. Accessed Mar. 24, 2019.

4 https://www.drugs.com/imodium.html. Accessed Nov. 15, 2018. Accessed Nov. 15, 2018.

5 L.B. Carruthers, "Chronic Diarrhea Treated with Folic Acid," *Lancet* 1 (1946): 849-850.

Diarrhea (Traveler's)

1 A. Sullivan and C.E. Nord, "Probiotics and Gastrointestinal Disease," *J Intern Med* 257 (2005): 78-92.

2 https://www.medicinenet.com/9_tips_to_prevent_travelers_diarrhea/views.htm. Accessed Nov. 15, 2018.

3 G. Juckett, MD, "Prevention and Treatment of Traveler's Diarrhea," *Am Fam Physician* 60, no. 1 (July 1, 1999): 119-124.

4 https://www.medscape.com/viewarticle/887515. Accessed Nov. 15, 2018.

5 https://www.webmd.com/vitamins/ai/ingredientmono-1502/bismuth. Accessed Nov. 15, 2018.

Digitalis Toxicity

1 http://pennstatehershey.adam.com/content.aspx?productId=117&pid=1&gid=000165. Accessed Feb. 8, 2019.

Disc Desiccation/Disk Degeneration

1 D.J. Bell et al., "Disk Desiccation." https://radiopaedia.org/articles/disc-desiccation. Accessed Feb. 8, 2019.

2 https://my.clevelandclinic.org/health/diseases/16912-degenerative-disk-disease. Accessed May 23, 2021.

3 J. Greenwood Jr., "Optimum Vitamin C Intake as a Factor in the Preservation of Disc Integrity," *Med Ann D.C.* 33 (1964): 274-276.

Diuretics (Loop and Thiazide Diuretics)

1 A. Travalto, D.N. Nuhlicik, and J.E. Midtling, "Drug-Nutrient Interactions," *Am Fam Phys* 44, no. 5 (Nov. 1991): 1651-1658.

2 https://medlineplus.gov/ency/article/000165.htm. Accessed Feb. 8, 2019.

Diverticulitis

1 https://www.medscape.com/viewarticle/822917_3. Accessed Feb. 17, 2019.

2 https://www.medicinenet.com/diverticulosis/article.htm#what_medications_treat_diverticulitis_and_diverticulosis. Accessed Feb. 17, 2019.

3 *The Merck Manual of Diagnosis and Therapy,* 19th ed., 242.

4 https://universityhealthnews.com/daily/digestive-health/break-the-diverticulitis-cycle/. Accessed Feb. 17, 2019.

5 A. Tursi, A Papa, and S. Danese, review article: "The Pathophysiology and Medical Management of Diverticulosis and Diverticular Disease of the Colon," *Alimentary Pharmacology and Therapeutics* 42, no. 6 (2015): 664-684.

6 https://www.healthline.com/health/diverticulitis. Accessed Feb. 17, 2019.

7 https://www.webmd.com/digestive-disorders/understanding-diverticulitis-treatment. Accessed July 25, 2021.

8 https://www.uspharmacist.com/article/diverticulitis-overview-and-management. Accessed Feb. 17, 2019.

Dizziness/Vertigo/Benign Paroxysmal Positional Vertigo (BPPV)

1 https://www.ncbi.nlm.nih.gov/pmc/articles/PMC6383320/.

2 E.T. Bope and R.D. Kellerman, *Conn's Current Therapy*, 14th ed. (Philadelphia: Elsevier/Saunders), 36.

3 J.C.M. Brust, *Current Diagnosis and Treatment Neurology*, 2nd ed. (McGraw-Hill, 2012): 44.

4 https://www.medicalnewstoday.com/articles/320492.php. Accessed Dec. 28, 2018.

5 R. Swartz and P. Longwell, "Treatment of Vertigo," *Am Fam Physician* 71, no. 6 (Mar. 15, 2005): 1115-1122.

6 L. Sokolova, R. Hoerr, and T. Mishchenko, "Treatment of Vertigo: A Randomized, Double Blind Trial Comparing Efficacy and Safety of Ginkgo Biloba Extract EG761 and Betahistine," *Int J Otolaryngol* 2014 (2014): 682439. Published online June 25, 2014. DOI: 10.1155/2014/682439.

7 https://www.medicalnewstoday.com/articles/320492.php. Accessed Nov. 17, 2018.

8 J.D. Kirschmann, *Nutrition Almanac* (1979), 60.

9 https://www.aafp.org/afp/2005/0315/p1115.html.

Dry Eye Syndrome/Keratoconjunctivitis Sicca/Xerophthalmia

1 https://www.mayoclinicproceedings.org/article/S0025-6196(12)01090-7/fulltext. Accessed June 16, 2021.

2 https://www.ncbi.nlm.nih.gov/pmc/articles/PMC1772141/. Accessed Mar. 22, 2019.

3 www.ncbi.nlm.nih.gov/pubmed/9537797. Accessed Nov. 15, 2018.

4 https://www.mayoclinicproceedings.org/article/S0025-6196(12)01090-7/fulltext. Accessed June 16, 2021.

5 J.C. Wojtowicz et al., "Pilot, Prospective, Randomized, Double-Masked, Placebo-Controlled Clinical Trial of an Omega-3 Supplement for Dry Eye," *Cornea* 30 (2011): 308-314.

6 https://www.ncbi.nlm.nih.gov/books/NBK431094/. Accessed Apr. 14, 2020.

7 A. Sommer, *Int Ophthalmol* 14 (1990): 195. https://doi.org/10.1007/BF00158318.

8 A. Sommer et al., "Oral versus Intramuscular Vitamin A in the Treatment of Xerophthalmia," *Lancet* 1, no. 8168, pt. 1 (Mar. 15, 1980): 557-559.

Duchenne Muscular Dystrophy

1 https://rarediseases.info.nih.gov/diseases/6291/duchenne-muscular-dystrophy. Accessed Nov. 17, 2020.

2 J. Seiler and E.T. Bope, "The Muscular Dystrophies," *Am Fam Phys* 34, no. 6 (July 1986): 128-130.

3 F. Cornelio et al., "Functional Evaluation of Duchenne Muscular Dystrophy: Proposal for a Protocol," *Ital J Neurol Sci* 3, no. 4 (Dec. 1982): 323-330.

4 https://www.webmd.com/vitamins/ai/ingredientmono-1078/idebenone. Accessed Nov. 14, 2018.

Dumping Syndrome

1 https://www.oregonclinic.com/diets-anti-dumping-post-gastrectomy. Accessed Dec. 10, 2018.

2 http://www.nchmd.org/education/mayo-health-library/details/CON-20028034. Accessed Dec. 10, 2018.

Dupuytren's Contracture/Palmar Fibromatosis

1 https://dupuytrens-contracture.com/dupuytren-contracture-treatment-options/dupuytren-contacture-vitamin-e/. Accessed Nov. 15, 2018.

2 G. Russel Thompson, "Treatment of Dupuytren's Contracture with Vitamin E," *Br J Med* 2 (July 1949): 1382.

3 *Br Med J* 1, no. 4772 (June 1952): 1328.

4 L.C. Hurst and M.A. Badalamente, "Nonoperative Treatment of Dupuytren's Disease," *Hand Clinics* 15, no. 1 (1999): 97-107, vii.

5 A.R. Parsons, "Dupuytren's Contracture: Treatment by Massive Doses of Vitamin E," *Ir J Med Sci* 19, no. 270 (1948): 272-274.

6 R.A. King, "Vitamin E Therapy in Dupuytren's Contracture: Examination of the Claim That Vitamin Therapy Is Successful," *J Bone Joint Surg Br* 31B, no. 3 (1949): 443.

7 G.R. Thompson, "The Treatment of Dupuytren's Contracture with Vitamin E: Report of a Case," *Glasgow Med J* 30, no. 9 (1949): 329-332.

8 C.L. Steunberg, "Tocopherols in Treatment of Primary Fibrositis; Including Dupuytren's Contracture, Periarthritis of the Shoulders, and Peyronie's Disease," *AMA Arch Surg* 63, no. 6 (1951): 824-833.

9 J.E. Kirk and M. Chieffi, "Tocopherol Administration to Patients with Dupuytren's Contracture: Effect on Plasma Tocopherol Levels and Degree of Contracture," *Proc Soc Exp Biol Med* 80, no. 4 (1952): 565-568.

10 https://www.ncbi.nlm.nih.gov/pmc/articles/PMC3351506/. Accessed July 23, 2020.

Dysgeusia/Abnormal Taste

1 https://www.colgate.com/en-us/oral-health/life-stages/adult-oral-care/dysgeusia--symptoms--causes-and-treatment. Accessed Mar. 3, 2019.

2 https://www.ncbi.nlm.nih.gov/pmc/articles/PMC3201003/#R133. Accessed Dec. 31, 2018.

3 S.M. Heckmann et al., "Zinc Gluconate in the Treatment of Dysgeusia: A Randomized Clinical Trial," *Journal of Dental Research* 84, no. 1 (2005): 35-38.

4 R. Devere, MD, "Dysosmia and Dysgeusia: A Patient's Nightmare and an Opportunity for Learning," *Practical Neurology* (2011). http://practicalneurology.com/2011/02/dysosmia-and-dysgeusia-a-patients-nightmare-and-an-opportunity-for-learning. Accessed Nov. 17, 2018.

5 F. Femiano and C. Scully, "Burning Mouth Syndrome (BMS): Double Blind Controlled Study of Alpha-Lipoic Acid Thioctic Acid Therapy," *J Oral Pathol Med* 31 (2002): 267-269.

Dysmenorrhea

1 Z. Harel et al., "Supplementation with Omega-3 Polyunsaturated Fatty Acids in the Management of Dysmenorrhea in Adolescents," *Am J Obstet Gynecol* 174 (1996): 1335-1338.

2 https://www.medicaldaily.com/menstrual-cramps-6-home-remedies-247558. Accessed Nov. 16, 2018.

3 https://pubmed.ncbi.nlm.nih.gov/30611908/.

4 B. Deutch, E. Bonefeld Jørgensen, and J.C. Hansen, "Menstrual Discomfort in Danish Women Reduced by Dietary Supplements of Omega-3 PUFA and B12 (Fish Oil or Seal Oil Capsules)," *Nutrition Research* 20, no. 5 (May 2000): 621-631.

5 https://www.hopkinsmedicine.org/healthlibrary/conditions/gynecological_health/dysmenorrhea_85,P00557. Accessed Nov. 16, 2018.

6 https://emedicine.medscape.com/article/253812-treatment#d10. Accessed Nov. 16, 2018.

7 L. French, "Dysmenorrhea," *Am Fam Phys* 71, no. 2 (Jan. 2005): 285-291.

8 S. Ziaei, M. Zakeri, and A. Kazemnejad, "A Randomized Controlled Trial of Vitamin E in the Treatment of Primary Dysmenorrhea," *BJOG* 112, no. 4 (Apr. 2005): 466-469.

9 M.M. Keifer, *Pocket Primary Care,* 2nd ed. (Wolters Kluver).

10 V.P. Arcangelo and A.M. Peterson, *Pharmacotherapeutics for Advanced Practice: A Practical Approach,* 3rd ed. (Wolters Kluwer/Lippincott Williams & Wilkins, 2013): 121.

11 M. Blumenthal and German Federal Institute for Drugs and Medical Devices Commission E, *The Complete German Commission E Monographs: Therapeutic Guide to Herbal Medicines* (Austin, Tex.: American Botanical Council, 1998).

12 https://pubmed.ncbi.nlm.nih.gov/2897319/. Accessed Apr. 9, 2021.

13 *PDR for Nonprescription Drugs* (Oradell, NJ: Medical Economics Co., 1988), 542.

14 https://www.livestrong.com/article/264715-magnesium-for-menstrual-cramps/. Accessed Nov. 16, 2018.

15 https://www.medicalnewstoday.com/articles/157333.php. Accessed Nov. 17, 2018.

16 https://www.webmd.com/vitamins/ai/ingredientmono-954/vitamin-e. Accessed Nov. 15, 2018.

17 https://www.webmd.com/vitamins/ai/ingredientmono-965/thiamine-vitamin-b1. Accessed Nov. 14, 2018.

18 https://medlineplus.gov/druginfo/natural/965.html. Accessed Jan. 6, 2019.

19 https://www.webmd.com/vitamins/ai/ingredientmono-894/boron. Accessed Nov. 18, 2018.

20 https://emedicine.medscape.com/article/253812-overview. Accessed Mar. 13, 2019.

21 https://www.aafp.org/afp/2005/0115/p285.html. Accessed Apr. 18, 2020.

Dyspraxia

1 https://dyspraxiafoundation.org.uk/about-dyspraxia/. Accessed Feb. 9, 2019.

2 https://www.webmd.com/vitamins/ai/ingredientmono-954/vitamin-e. Accessed Nov. 15, 2018.

Eczema/Atopic Dermatitis

1 https://www.ncbi.nlm.nih.gov/pmc/articles/PMC5582672/, Accessed July 25, 2021.

2 https://www.mayoclinic.org/diseases-conditions/atopic-dermatitis-eczema/symptoms-causes/syc-20353273. Accessed Oct. 24, 2019.

3 G. Faghihi et al., "The Efficacy of '0.05% Clobetasol + 2.5% Zinc Sulphate' Cream versus '0.05% Clobetasol Alone' Cream in the Treatment of the Chronic Hand Eczema: A Double-Blind Study," *Journal of the European Academy of Dermatology and Venereology* 22, no. 5 (2008): 531-536.

4 https://lpi.oregonstate.edu/mic/health-disease/skin-health/essential-fatty-acids. Accessed Nov. 15, 2018.

5 M.S. Manku et al., "Essential Fatty Acids in the Plasma Phospholipids of Patients with Atopic Eczema," *Br J Dermatol* 110, no. 6 (June 1984): 643-648.

6 D.F. Horrobin, "Essential Fatty Acid Metabolism and Its Modification in Atopic Eczema," *The American Journal of Clinical Nutrition* 71, no. 1 (Jan. 2000): 367s-372s.

7 M.H. Javanbakht et al., "Randomized Controlled Trial Using Vitamins E and D Supplementation in Atopic Dermatitis," *J Dermatolog Treat* 22, no. 3 (2011): 144-150. (PubMed)

8 M. Amestejani et al., "Vitamin D Supplementation in the Treatment of Atopic Dermatitis: A Clinical Trial Study," *J Drugs Dermatol* 11, no. 3 (2012): 327-330.

9 https://lpi.oregonstate.edu/mic/vitamins/vitamin-D#reference290. Accessed Dec. 28, 2018.

10 https://www.medicalnewstoday.com/articles/14417. Accessed May 27, 2020.

11 M. Stücker et al., "Topical Vitamin B12—A New Therapeutic Approach in Atopic Dermatitis: Evaluation of Efficacy and Tolerability in a Randomized Placebo-Controlled Multicenter Clinical Trial," *Br. J Dermatol* 150, no. 5 (May 2004): 977-983.

Ehlers-Danlos Syndrome

1 https://www.rightdiagnosis.com/e/ehlers_danlos_syndrome/complic.htm#complication_list. Accessed Mar. 3, 2019.

2 https://www.arthritis.org/about-arthritis/types/ehlers-danlos-syndrome-eds/. Accessed Nov. 17, 2018.

3 D. Mantle, R.M. Wilkins, and V. Preedy, "A Novel Therapeutic Strategy for Ehlers-Danlos Syndrome Based on Nutritional Supplements," *Medical Hypotheses* 64 (2005): 279-283.

4 W. Emser, "A Case of Ehlers-Danlos Syndrome and Its Zinc Therapy," *Klin Padiatr* 190, no. 4 (July 1978): 397-402. (author's transl)

Ehlers-Danlos Syndrome (Type VI)

1 https://www.sciencedirect.com/science/article/pii/003042208290295X. Accessed Nov. 16, 2018.

2 W.M. Ringsdorf Jr., DMD, MS, and E. Cheraskin, MD, DMD, "Vitamin C and Human Wound Healing," *Oral Surgery, Oral Medicine, Oral Pathology* 53, no. 3 (Mar. 1982): 231-236.

Eosinophilic Pneumonia/Acute Eosinophilic Pneumonia or AEP

1 B.W. Jhun, MD, et al., "Vitamin D Status in South Korean Military Personnel with Acute Eosinophilic Pneumonia: A Pilot Study," *Tuberc Respir Dis (Seoul)* 78, no. 3 (July 2015): 232-238. Published online June 30, 2015. DOI: 10.4046/trd.2015.78.3.232.

Epidermolysis Bullosa

1 https://www.mayoclinic.org/diseases-conditions/epidermolysis-bullosa/symptoms-causes/syc-20361062. Accessed Mar. 13, 2019.

2 S. Ingen-Housz-Oro et al., "Vitamin and Trace Metal Levels in Recessive Dystrophic Epidermolysis Bullosa," *J Euro Acad Derm and Venereology* 18, no. 6 (Sept. 2004): 649-653.

3 E.T. Bope and R.D. Kellerman, *Conn's Current Therapy*, 14th ed. (Philadelphia: Elsevier/Saunders), 246.

4 H. Degreef, "Epidermolysis Bullosa: Treatment with Vitamin E, Preliminary Results," *Archives Belges de Dermatologie* 30, no. 2 (Apr. 1974): 83-87.

5 J.D. Michelson et al., "Vitamin E Treatment of Epidermolysis Bullosa: Changes in Tissue Collagenase Levels," *Arch Dermatol* 109 (1974): 67-69.

6 E.B. Smith and V.M. Michener, "Vitamin E Treatment of Epidermolysis Bullosa: A Controlled Study," *Arch Dermatol* 108 (1973): 254-256.

Epilepsy/Seizures

1 V.P. Arcangelo and A.M. Peterson, *Pharmacotherapeutics for Advanced Practice: A Practical Approach*, 3rd ed. (Wolters Kluwer/Lippincott Williams & Wilkins, 2013): 595.

2 https://epilepsyjourney.com/2020/10/paternal-antiseizure-meds-have-little-impact-on-offspring/. Accessed Oct. 15, 2020.

3 https://www.nejm.org/doi/full/10.1056/NEJM198210213071717. Accessed Jan. 7, 2021.

4 A.O. Ogunmedan et al., "A Randomized Double-Blind, Placebo-Controlled, Clinical Trial Alpha-Tocopheryl Acetate (Vitamin E), as Add-On Therapy, for Epilepsy in Children," *Epilepsia* 30 (1989): 84-89.

5 J. Mehvari et al., "Effects of Vitamin E on Seizure Frequency, Electroencephalogram Findings, and Oxidative Stress Status of Refractory Epileptic Patients," *Adv Biomed Res* 5, no. 36 (Mar. 2016). DOI: 10.4103/2277-9175.178780.

6 G.F. Carl et al., "Association of Low Blood Manganese Concentrations with Epilepsy," *Neurology* 36 (1986): 1584-1587.

7 P.S. Papavasiliou et al., "Seizure Disorders and Trace Metals: Manganese Tissue Levels in Treated Epileptics," *Neurology* 29 (1979): 1466-1473.

8 P. Sampson, "Low Manganese Level May Trigger Epilepsy," *JAMA* 238 (1977): 1805.

9 A. Sohler and C.C. Pfeiffer, "A Direct Method for the Determination of Manganese in Whole Blood. Patients with Seizure Activity Have Low Blood Levels," *J Orthomol Psych* 8 (1979): 275-280.

10 *See also* Ellen C.G. Grant, "Epilepsy and Manganese," *Lancet* 363 (2004): 572.

11 R.S. Goldman and S.M. Finkbeiner, "Therapeutic Use of Magnesium Sulfate in Selected Cases of Cerebral Ischemia," *N Engl J Med* 319 (1988): 1224-1225.

12 U. Bonuccelli et al., "Plasma Levels of Ca, Mg and Phenobarbital in Epileptic and Brain Trauma Patients on Chronic Therapy," *Res Commun Psychol Psychiatr Behav* 7 (1982): 369-375.

13 C. Otsuki, "Studies on Serum Ca, P and Mg Metabolism in Children with Special Emphasis on Their Relationship with Anticonvulsant Therapy," *Acta Paediatr Jpn* 8 (1973): 24-26.

14 C. Christiansen, N.S. Pors, and P. Rodro, "Anticonvulsant Hypomagnesemia," *Br Med J* ii (1974): 198-199.

15 R. Yassa and C. Schwartz, "Plasma Mg and Anticonvulsant Therapy," *NY State J Med* 84 (1984): 114-116.

16 A. Barbeau et al., "Zinc, Taurine, and Epilepsy," *Arch Neurol* 30 (1974).

17 E.S. Roach et al., "N,N-Dimethylglycine for Epilepsy," *N Engl J Med* 30 (1982): 1081-1082.

18 https://www.nejm.org/doi/full/10.1056/NEJM198210213071717. Accessed Jan. 7, 2021.

19 A.R. Gaby, "Natural Approaches to Epilepsy," *Altern Med Rev* 12, no. 1 (Mar. 2007): 9-24.

20 https://www.sciencedirect.com/science/article/pii/092012119390030B. Accessed Mar. 3, 2019.

21 https://onlinelibrary.wiley.com/doi/full/10.1046/j.1528-1157.2003.26102.x. Accessed Nov. 25, 2018.

22 B. Jansen, "Ketogenic Diets Are What's Cooking for Drug-Refractory Epilepsy," *MDEdge Internal Medicine* (Aug. 14, 2019). Accessed Aug. 14, 2019.

23 F. Lefevre and N. Aronson, "Ketogenic Diet for the Treatment of Refractory Epilepsy in Children: A Systematic Review of Efficacy," *Pediatrics* 105 (2000): 1-7.

24 E.H. Kossoff et al., "Optimal Clinical Management of Children Receiving Dietary Therapies for Epilepsy: Updated Recommendations of the International Ketogenic Diet Study Group," *Epilepsia Open* 3, no. 2 (2018): 175-192.

25 J. Remaly, "Celiac May Underlie Seizures," *MDEdge Family Medicine* (Oct. 28, 2019). Accessed Nov. 6, 2019.

26 J. Mehvari et al., "Effects of Vitamin E on Seizure Frequency, Electroencephalogram Findings, and Oxidative Stress Status of Refractory Epileptic Patients," *Adv Biomed Res* 5 (Mar. 2016): 36.

27 https://www.webmd.com/vitamins/ai/ingredientmono-436/choline. Accessed Nov. 23, 2018.

28 https://www.rxlist.com/gaba_gamma-aminobutyric_acid/supplements.htm. Accessed Nov. 27, 2018.

29 R. Gilroy and J.S. Meyer, *Medical Neurology*, 3rd ed. (Macmillan Publishing, 1979), 280.

30 R.W. Manville and G.W. Abbott, "Cilantro Leaf Harbors a Potent Potassium Channel-Activating Anticonvulsant," *The FASEB Journal*. Published online: Oct. 1, 2019. https://doi.org/10.1096/fj.201900485R.

31 https://www.ncbi.nlm.nih.gov/pmc/articles/PMC1123448/. Accessed May 15, 2020.

32 *The Washington Manual for Medical Therapeutics*, 34th ed., 1257.

Epilepsy—Status Epilepticus (Children)

1 C.E. Sanders and M.T. Ho, *Current Emergency Diagnosis and Treatment*, 4th ed., A Lange Medical Book (1993), 826.

Erectile Dysfunction

1 https://www.mayoclinic.org/diseases-conditions/erectile-dysfunction/in-depth/erectile-dysfunction-herbs/art-20044394. Accessed Nov. 29, 2018.

2 A.W. Zorgniotti and E.F. Lizza, "Effect of Large Doses of the Nitric Oxide Precursor, L-Arginine, on Erectile Dysfunction," *Int J Impot Res* 6, no. 1 (1994): 33-36.

3 T. Klotz et al., "Effectiveness of Oral L-Arginine in First-Line Treatment of Erectile Dysfunction in a Controlled Crossover Study," *Urol Int* 63 (1999): 220-223.

4 R. Stanislavov and V. Nikolov, "Sexual and Reproductive Parameters in Aging Males after Treatment with Pycnogenol® and L-Arginine," *Int J Impot Res* 14, suppl. 4 (2002): S65.

5 R. Stanislavov, V. Nikolova, and P. Rohdewald, "Improvement of Erectile Function with Prelox: A Randomized, Double-Blind, Placebo-Controlled, Crossover Trial," *Int J Impot Res* 20, no. 2 (Mar. 2008): 173.

6 J. Chen et al., "Effect of Oral Administration of High-Dose Nitric Oxide Donor L-Arginine in Men with Organic Erectile Dysfunction: Results of a Double-Blind, Randomized Study," *BJU Int* 83, no. 3 (1999): 269-273.

7 K.P. Kuhn et al., "Oral Citrulline Effectively Elevates Plasma Arginine Levels for 24 Hours in Normal Volunteers," *Circulation* 106, no. II (2002): 1-766.

8 L. Cormio et al., "Oral L-Citrulline Supplementation Improves Erection Hardness in Men with Mild Erectile Dysfunction," *Urology* 77, no. 1 (2011): 119-122.

9 V. Gentile et al., "Effect of Propionyl-L-Carnitine, L-Arginine and Nicotinic Acid on the Efficacy of Vardenafil in the Treatment of Erectile Dysfunction in Diabetes," *Curr Med Res Opin* 25, no. 9 (2009): 2223-2228. PMID: 19624286.

10 https://www.mayoclinic.org/diseases-conditions/erectile-dysfunction/in-depth/erectile-dysfunction-herbs/art-20044394. Accessed Nov. 29, 2018.

11 https://www.sciencedirect.com/science/article/pii/S0090429598005718. Accessed Nov. 29, 2018.

Erythema Nodosum (EN)

1 https://www.webmd.com/skin-problems-and-treatments/erythema-nodosum. Accessed Dec. 17, 2018.

2 https://www.medicalnewstoday.com/articles/320829.php. Accessed Dec. 17, 2018.

3 https://www.skinsight.com/skin-conditions/adult/erythema-nodosum. Accessed Dec. 17, 2018.

4 https://emedicine.medscape.com/article/1081633-medication. Accessed Dec. 17, 2018.

5 T. Horio, MD, et al., "Potassium Iodide in the Treatment of Erythema Nodosum and Nodular Vasculitis," *Arch Dermatol* 117, no. 1 (1981): 29-31. DOI: 10.1001/archderm.1981.01650010035020.

6 https://www.aocd.org/page/PotassiumIodide. Accessed Dec. 18, 2018.

Erythropoietic Protoporphyria (EPP)

1 https://www.dermnetnz.org/topics/erythropoietic-protoporphyria/. Accessed Apr. 18, 2020.

2 https://www.webmd.com/vitamins/ai/ingredientmono-999/beta-carotene. Accessed Dec. 18, 2018.

3 https://rarediseases.org/rare-diseases/x-linked-protoporphyria/. Accessed Nov. 2, 2018.

4 https://medlineplus.gov/ency/article/001208.htm. Accessed Nov. 1, 2018.

5 https://rarediseases.org/rare-diseases/erythropoietic-protoporphyria/. Accessed Apr. 20, 2020.

6 https://www.medicaljournals.se/acta/download/10.1080/00015550310016535/. Accessed Dec. 18, 2018.

7 M.M. Mathews-Roth, "Treatment of Erythropoietic Protoporphyria with Beta-Carotene," *Photodermatol* 1, no. 6 (Dec. 1984): 318-321.

8 M.M. Mathews-Roth, MD, et al., "Beta Carotene Therapy for Erythropoietic Protoporphyria and Other Photosensitivity Diseases," *Arch Dermatol* x113 (Sept. 1977): 1229-1232.

9 https://porphyriafoundation.org/for-patients/types-of-porphyria/EPP-XLP/. Accessed May 21, 2020.

Facial Neuralgia (Atypical)

1 https://www.practicalpainmanagement.com/pain/maxillofacial/atypical-facial-neuralgias. Accessed Oct. 24, 2019.

2 R.A. Abma, "Facial Neuralgia May Be Linked to Vitamin B12 Deficiency," *Neurology Reviews* 17, no. 11 (Nov. 2009).

Familial Mediterranean Fever (FMF)

1 L.M. Tierney Jr., S.J. McPhee, and M.A. Papadakis, *Current Medical Diagnosis and Treatment*, 34th ed., A Lange Medical Book (1995), 495.

2 https://www.ncbi.nlm.nih.gov/pmc/articles/PMC4848823/. Accessed Dec. 8, 2018.

3 https://www.tandfonline.com/doi/full/10.3109/0886022X.2015.1056064. Accessed Dec. 8, 2018.

4 http://www.clinexprheumatol.org/abstract.asp?a=6637. Accessed Dec. 8, 2018.

Fanconi Syndrome

1 https://rarediseases.info.nih.gov/diseases/9118/fanconi-syndrome. Accessed May 15, 2020.

2 https://www.merckmanuals.com/home/kidney-and-urinary-tract-disorders/disorders-of-kidney-tubules/fanconi-syndrome. Accessed Dec. 18, 2018.

3 https://www.webmd.com/drugs/2/drug-56979/shohls-modified-oral/details.

4 https://emedicine.medscape.com/article/981774-treatment. Accessed Dec. 18, 2018.

Fatigue/Chronic Fatigue Syndrome

1 I.M. Cox, M.J. Campbell, and D. Dowson, "Red Blood Cell Magnesium and Chronic Fatigue Syndrome," *The Lancet* 337 (Mar. 30, 1991): 757-760,

2 https://medicin.net.com/magnesium/supplements-vitamins.htm. Accessed Dec. 16, 2018.

3 F.J. Crescent, "Treatment of Fatigue in a Surgical Practice," *J Abdominal Surg* 4 (1962): 73-76.

4 C.A. Kruse, "Treatment of Fatigue with Aspartic Acid Salts," *Northwest Med* 60 (1961): 597-604.

5 J.T. Hicks, "Treatment of Fatigue in General Practice: A Double-Blind Study," *Clin Med* (Jan. 1964): 85-90.

6 D.L. Shaw Jr. et al., "Management of Fatigue: A Physiologic Approach," *Am J Med Sci* (1962): 243.

7 P.E. Formica, "The Housewife Syndrome: Treatment with the Potassium and Magnesium Salts of Aspartic Acid," *Curr Ther Res* 4 (1962): 98-106.

8 A.R. Gaby, "Potassium-Magnesium Aspartate: A Special Supplement for Tired People," *Nutrition and Healing* 2 (1995).

9 L.C. Heap, T.J. Peters, and S. Wessely, "Vitamin B Status in Patients with Chronic Fatigue Syndrome," *J R Soc Med* 92, no. 4 (Apr. 1999): 183-185.

10 M. Le Gal, P. Cayhebra, and K. Struby, "Pharmaton Capsules in the Treatment of Functional Fatigue: A Double Blind Study versus Placebo Evaluated by a New Methodology," *Phytother Res* 10 (1996): 49-53.

11 A. Costantini and M.I. Pala, "Thiamine and Fatigue in Inflammatory Bowel Diseases: An Open Label Pilot Study." *J Altern Complement Med.* Published online first Feb. 4, 2013. DOI: 10.1089/acm.2011.0840.

12 A. Costantini et al., "Thiamine and Spinocerebellar Ataxia Type 2," *BMJ Case Reports.* Published online Jan. 10, 2013.

13 https://www.emedicinehealth.com/l-carnitine/vitamins-supplements.htm. Accessed Nov. 26, 2018.

14 https://examine.com/supplements/glycine/#hem-fatigue. Accessed Jan. 7, 2019.

Fibrocystic Breasts/Cystic Mastitis/Mammary Dysplasia

1 J.K. Pye, R.E. Mansel, and L.E. Hughes, "Clinical Experience of Drug Treatments for Mastalgia," *Lancet* 2 (1985): 373-377.

2 https://www.mayoclinic.org/deseases-conditiond/fibrocystic-breasts/diagnosis-treatment/drc-20350442. Accessed Nov. 26, 2018.

3 K.L. Cheung, "Management of Cyclical Mastalgia in Oriental Woman Pioneer Experience of Using Gamolenic Acid (Efamast) in Asia," *Aust NZ J Surg* 69 (1999): 492-494.

4 K.D. Tripathi, *Essentials of Medical Pharmacology*, 7th ed. (2013), 912.

5 R.S. London et al., "Mammary Dysplasia: Endocrine Parameters and Tocopherol Therapy," *Nutrition Research* 2, no. 3 (June 1982): 243-247.

6 A.A. Abrahms, "Use of Vitamin E in Chronic Mastitis," *N Engl J Med* 272 (May 1965): 1080-1081.

7 W.R. Ghent et al., "Iodine Replacement in Fibrocystic Disease of the Breast," *Can J Surg* 36, no. 5 (Oct. 1993): 453-460.

8 J.H. Kessler, "The Effect of Supraphysiologic Levels of Iodine on Patients with Cyclic Mastalgia," *Breast J* 10, no. 4 (July-Aug. 2004): 328-336.

9 D.N. Ader et al., "Cyclical Mastalgia: Prevalence and Associated Health and Behavioral Factors," *J Psychosom Obstet Gynecol* 22 (2001): 71-76.

10 https://www.webmd.com/vitamins/ai/ingredientmono-333/ginkgo. Accessed Nov. 26, 2018.

11 B. Wasi, *Standard Treatment Guidelines: A Manual for Medical Therapeutics*, 1st ed. (2014), 379.

Fibromyalgia

1 https://www.cdc.gov/arthritis/basics/fibromyalgia.htm. Accessed Oct. 24, 2019.

2 J. Eisinger et al., "Selenium and Magnesium Status in Fibromyalgia," *Magnesium Research* 7, no. 3-4 (1994): 285-288.

3 G.E. Abraham and J.D. Flechas, "Management of Fibromyalgia: Rationale for the Use of Magnesium and Malic Acid," *J Nutr Med* 3 (1992): 49-59.

4 https://www.webmd.com/vitamins/ai/ingredientmono-998/magnesium. Accessed Nov. 18, 2018.

5 D. Amital et al., "Posttraumatic Stress Disorder, Tenderness, and Fibromyalgia Syndrome: Are They Different Entities?," *Journal of Psychosomatic Research* 61, no. 5 (2006): 663-669.

6 Institute of Medicine, "10 Creatine," *Nutrition and Traumatic Brain Injury: Improving Acute and Subacute Health Outcomes in Military Personnel* (Washington DC: The National Academies Press, 2011). DOI: 17226/13121.

7 C.R. Alves et al., "Creatine Supplementation in Fibromyalgia: A Randomized, Double-Blind, Placebo-Controlled Trial," *Arthritis Care Res (Hoboken)* 65 (2013): 1449-1459.

8 https://www.webmd.com/fibromyalgia/guide/fibromyalgia-herbs-and-supplements#1. Accessed Nov. 18, 2018.

9 A.L. Hassett and R.N. Gevirtz, "Nonpharmacologic Treatment for Fibromyalgia: Patient Education, Cognitive-Behavioral Therapy, Relaxation Techniques, and Complementary and Alternative Medicine," *Rheum Dis Clin North Am* 35, no. 2 (2009): 393-407.

10 R.G. Gamber et al., "Osteopathic Manipulative Treatment in Conjunction with Medication Relieves Pain Associated with Fibromyalgia Syndrome: Results of a Randomized Clinical Pilot Project," *J Am Osteopath Assoc* 102, no. 6 (2002): 321-325.

11 https://www.webmd.com/vitamins/ai/ingredientmono-938/coenzyme-q10. Accessed Nov. 18, 2018.

12 A. Costantini et al., "High-Dose Thiamine Improves the Symptoms of Fibromyalgia," *BMJ Case Reports* 2013 (2013): bcr2013009019. Published online May 20, 2013. DOI: 10.1136/bcr-2013-009019.

Fire Ant Bites

1 T. Devlin, MD, "Postgraduate Medicine Pearls," *Postgraduate Medicine* 99, no. 3 (1996): 6.

Fish Odor Syndrome/Trimethylaminuria

1 J. Messenger et al., "A Review of Trimethylaminuria (Fish Odor Syndrome)," *J Clin Aesthet Dermatol* 6, no. 11 (Nov. 2013): 45-48.

2 H. Yamazaki et al., "Effects of the Dietary Supplements, Activated Charcoal and Copper Chlorophyllin, on Urinary Excretion of Trimethylamine in Japanese Trimethylaminuria Patients," *Life Sci* 74, no. 22 (2004): 2739-2747.

3 https://www.epainassist.com/genetic-disorders/fish-odor-syndrome-or-trimethylaminuria. Accessed Nov. 22, 2018.

4 https://rarediseases.org/rare-diseases/trimethylaminuria/. Accessed Nov. 22, 2018.

5 https://www.genome.gov/Genetic-Disorders/Trimethylaminuria. Accessed Nov. 5, 2020.

Folic Acid Deficiency

1 https://www.ncbi.nlm.nih.gov/pmc/articles/PMC1123448/. Accessed Feb. 11, 2019.

2 https://www.drugs.com/dosage/folic-acid.html#Usual_Adult_Dose_for_Megaloblastic_Anemia. Accessed May 15, 2020.

3 https://www.medicalnewstoday.com/articles/219853.php. Accessed Feb. 11, 2019.

Foot Odor/Bromodosis

1 *Postgraduate Medicine* 96, no. 3 (Sept. 1994): 23.

2 K.E. Sharquie, A.A. Noaimi, and S.D. Hameed, "Topical 15% Zinc Sulfate Solution Is an Effective Therapy for Feet Odor," *Journal of Cosmetics, Dermatological Sciences and Applications* 3 (2013): 203-208.

3 M. Gupta et al., "Zinc Therapy in Dermatology: A Review," *Dermatol Res Pract* 2014 (2014): 709152. Published online July 10, 2014. DOI: 10.1155/2014/709152.

4 https://www.medicalnewstoday.com/articles/319002.php. Accessed Mar. 13, 2019.

Friedreich's Ataxia

1 https://www.ninds.nih.gov/Disorders/Patient-Caregiver-Education/Fact-Sheets/Friedreichs-Ataxia-Fact-Sheet. Accessed Feb. 9, 2019.

2 J.C.M. Brust, *Current Diagnosis and Treatment Neurology*, 2nd ed. (McGraw-Hill, 2012): 240.

3 J.M. Cooper et al., "Coenzyme Q10 and Vitamin E Deficiency in Friedreich's Ataxia: Predictor of Efficacy of Vitamin E and Coenzyme Q10 Therapy," *Eur J Neurol* 15, no. 12 (2008): 1371-1379. DOI: 10.1111/j.1468-1331.2008.02318.x.

4 https://www.medicalnewstoday.com/articles/162368.php. Accessed Nov. 22, 2018.

5 I.R. Livingstone and F.L. Mastiglia, "Choline Chloride in the Treatment of Ataxia," *British Medical Journal* 2 (1979): 939.

6 I.R. Livingstone et al., "Choline Chloride in the Treatment of Cerebellar and Spinocerebellar Ataxia," *J Neurol Sci* 50, no. 2 (May 1981): 161-174.

7 S.B. Melancon et al., "Oral Lecithin and Linoleic Acid in Friedreich's Ataxia: II. Clinical Results," *Canadian J of Neuro Sci* 9, no. 2 (May 1982): 155-164.

8 P.C. Kruger et al., "Abundance and Significance of Iron, Zinc, Copper, and Calcium in the Hearts of Patients with Friedreich Ataxia," *The American Journal of Cardiology* 118, no. 1 (July 2016): 127-131.

Gallbladder-Biliary Dyskinesia/Functional Gallbladder Disorder/ Cystic Duct Syndrome

1 https://en.medicine-worlds.com/diskineziya-zhelchevyvodyashih-putej.htm. Last accessed Nov. 14, 2018.

2 R.J. Sokol et al., "Multicenter Trial of D-Alpha-Tocopheryl Polyethylene Glycol 1000 Succinate for Treatment of Vitamin E Deficiency in Children with Chronic Cholestasis," *Gastroenterology* 104 (1993): 1727-1735.

3 https://www.ncbi.nlm.nih.gov/pubmed/12495265. Accessed May 14, 2020.

4 https://www.ncbi.nlm.nih.gov/pubmed/10499460. Accessed May 14, 2020.

Gallstone Disease/Cholelithiasis/Cholecystitis

1 *Andreoli and Carpenter's Cecil Essentials of Medicine*, 8th ed. (Saunders/Elsevier, 2010), 488.

2 J.C. Breneman, "Allergy Elimination Diet as the Most Effective Gall Bladder Diet," *Ann Allergy* 26 (1968): 83-87.

3 J.R. Thornton et al., "Diet and Gall Stones: Effects of Refined Carbohydrate Diets on Bile Cholesterol Saturation and Bile Acid Metabolism," *Gut* 24 (1983): 2.

4 W.M. Capper et al., "Gallstones, Gastric Secretion and Flatulent Dyspepsia. *Lancet* 1 (1967): 413-415.

5 S.A. Tuzhilin et al., "The Treatment of Patients with Gall Stones by Lecithin," *Am J Gastroenterol* 65 (1976): 104-114.

6 A.R. Gaby, "Commentary," *Nutrition and Healing* 5, no. 7 (Aug. 1995): 10-11.

7 N.P. Dorvil et al., "Taurine Prevents Cholestasis Induced by Lithocholic Acid Sulfate in Guinea Pigs," *Am J Clin Nutr* 37 (1983): 221-232.

8 Y. Yamanaka et al., "Stimulation of Chenoxycholic Acid Excretion in Hypercholesterolemic Mice by Dietary Taurine," *J Nutr Sci Vitaminol* 32 (1986): 296.

9 A.R. Gaby, "Taurine: The Cellular Buffer," *Nutrition & Healing* 4, no. 1 (Jan. 1997): 4.

10 R.J. Sokol et al., "Multicenter Trial of D-Alpha-Tocopheryl Polyethylene Glycol 1000 Succinate for Treatment of Vitamin E Deficiency in Children with Chronic Cholestasis," *Gastroenterology* 104 (1993): 1727-1735.

11 U. Gustafsson, "The Effect of Vitamin C in High Doses on Plasma and Biliary Lipid Composition in Patients with Cholesterol Stones," *Eur J Clin Invest* 27 (1997): 387-391.

12 https://www.webmd.com/digestive-disorders/news/20000411/vitamin-c-may-help-protect-women-from-gallbladder-disease#1. Accessed Dec. 11, 2018.

13 T. Walcher et al., "Vitamin C Supplement Use May Protect Against Gallstones: An Observational Study on a Randomly Selected Population," *BMC Gastroenterol* 9 (Oct. 2009): 74. Published online Oct. 8, 2009. DOI: 10.1186/1471-230X-9-74.

14 https://www.drugs.com/uk/rowachol-capsules-leaflet.html. Accessed Jan. 22, 2019.

Gastritis

1 https://www.mayoclinic.org/diseases-conditions/gastritis/diagnosis-treatment/drc-20355813. Accessed Nov. 16, 2018.

2 A. Aditi and D.Y. Graham, "Vitamin C, Gastritis, and Gastric Disease: A Historical Review and Update," *Dig Dis Sci* 57, no. 10 (Oct. 2012). DOI: 10.1007/s10620-012-2203-7.

Gastroenteritis (Viral)

1 https://www.ncbi.nlm.nih.gov/pmc/articles/PMC3625079/#b2-0590363. Accessed Jan. 2, 2019.

2 *The Merck Manual of Diagnosis and Therapy,* 19th ed., 209.

3 https://www.ncbi.nlm.nih.gov/pmc/articles/PMC3113371/. Accessed Feb. 29, 2019.

4 https://www.webmd.com/drugs/2/drug-4086/zinc-sulfate-oral/details.

5 K.H. Brown et al., "Preventive Zinc Supplementation among Infants, Preschoolers, and Older Prepubertal Children," *Food Nutr Bull* 30, (suppl. 1 (2009): S12-S40.

Genital Herpes/Herpes Genitalis

1 https://www.cdc.gov/std/herpes/stdfact-herpes.htm. Accessed Mar. 25, 2019.

2 M. Gupta et al., "Zinc Therapy in Dermatology: A Review," *Dermatol Res Pract* 2014 (2014): 709152. Published online July 10, 2014. DOI: 10.1155/2014/709152.

3 B.B. Mahajan, M. Dhawan, and R. Singh, "Herpes Genitalis. Topical Zinc Sulfate: An Alternative Therapeutic and Modality," *Indian J Sex Transm Dis AIDS* 34, no. 1 (Jan.-June 2013): 32-34. DOI: 10.4103/2589-0557.112867.

4 https://www.webmd.com/vitamins/ai/ingredientmono-607/aloe. Accessed Jan. 5, 2019.

Geographic Tongue

1 https://www.statpearls.com/articlelibrary/viewarticle/22216/. Accessed Mar. 20, 2021.

2 https://medlineplus.gov/ency/article/001049.htm. Accessed Nov. 17, 2018.

3 https://www.statpearls.com/articlelibrary/viewarticle/22216/.

4 https://www.webmd.com/oral-health/guide/geographic-tongue#2. Accessed Nov. 17, 2018.

5 https://www.medicalnewstoday.com/articles/319342.php. Accessed Nov. 17, 2018.

6 https://medicalpoint.org/geographic-tongue/. Accessed Nov. 17, 2018.

7 https://www.rightdiagnosis.com/g/geographic_tongue/treatments.htm. Accessed Nov. 17, 2018.

8 https://geographictongue.org/tag/folate/. Accessed Mar. 20, 2021.

Gingivitis

1 Pirkko J. Pussinen et al., "Periodontitis Is Associated with a Low Concentration of Vitamin C in Plasma," *Clin Diagn Lab Immunol* 10, no. 5 (Sept. 2003): 897-902.

2 https://www.ncbi.nlm.nih.gov/pubmed/6748685. Accessed Sept. 17, 2018.

3 T. Nakamoto, M. McCroskey, and H.M. Mallek, "The Role of Ascorbic Acid Deficiency in Human Gingivitis—A New Hypothesis," *J Theor Biol* 108, no. 2 (May 21, 1984): 163-171.

4 https://www.webmd.com/oral-health/bleeding-gums-other-conditions#2. Accessed Sept. 17, 2018.

5 H.G. Campbell and R.P. Cook, "Treatment of Gingivitis with Ascorbic Acid," *The British Medical Journal* 1 (Mar. 1941): 360-361.

6 A. Amaliya, A.S. Risdiana, and U. Van der Velden, "Effect of Guava and Vitamin C Supplementation on Experimental Gingivitis: A Randomized Clinical Trial," *J Clinical Periodontology* 45, no. 8 (May 2018): 959-967.

7 https://www.webmd.com/vitamins/ai/ingredientmono-235/calendula. Accessed Nov. 21, 2018.

8 https://www.webmd.com/vitamins/ai/ingredientmono-982/zinc. Accessed Jan. 29, 2019.

9 https://www.medicalnewstoday.com/articles/318591#dental-plaque. Accessed Nov. 30, 2020.

Glaucoma

1 https://nei.nih.gov/health/glaucoma/glaucoma_facts. Accessed Mar. 3, 2019.

2 https://www.mayoclinic.org/diseases-conditions/glaucoma/diagnosis-treatment/drc-20372846. Accessed May 1, 2021.

3 H.H. Boyd, "Eye Pressure Lowering Effect of Vitamin C," *J Orthomolec Med* 10 (1995): 165-168.

4 V. Parisi, "Electrophysiological Assessment of Glaucomatous Visual Dysfunction during Treatment with Cytidine-5'-Diphosphocholine (Citicoline): A Study of 8 Years of Follow-Up," *Doc Ophthalmol* 110, no. 1 (2005): 91-102.

5 L. Ottobelli et al., "Citicoline Oral Solution in Glaucoma: Is There a Role in Slowing Disease Progression?," *Ophthalmologica* 229, no. 4 (2013): 219-226.

6 V. Parisi et al., "Cytidine-5'-Diphosphocholine (Citicoline): A Pilot Study in Patients with Non-Arteritic Ischemic Optic Neuropathy," *Eur J Neurol* 15, no. 5 (2008): 465-474.

7 https://www.webmd.com/vitamins/ai/ingredientmono-202/bilberry. Accessed Feb. 3, 2020.

Glomerulosclerosis

1 https://pubmed.ncbi.nlm.nih.gov/16828231/. Accessed Dec. 28, 2021.

2 https://www.webmd.com/vitamins/ai/ingredientmono-954/vitamin-e. Accessed Nov. 17, 2018.

Glossalgia

1 *Am Fam Phys* 30, no. 1 (July 1984): 160.

2 http://medicalj-center.info/stomatology/glossalgia-causes-symptoms-treatment.html. Accessed Nov. 13, 2018.

Glucose-6-Phosphate Dehydrogenase (G6PD) Deficiency

1 https://ghr.nlm.nih.gov/condition/glucose-6-phosphate-dehydrogenase-deficiency. Accessed Mar. 3, 2019.

2 https://www.aafp.org/afp/2005/1001/p1277.pdf. Accessed Nov. 14, 2018.

3 https://www.webmd.com/vitamins/ai/ingredientmono-954/vitamin-e. Accessed Nov. 15, 2018.

4 https://www.webmd.com/vitamins/condition-1219/glucose-6-phosphate+dehydrogenase+g6pd+deficiency.aspx. Accessed Dec. 18, 2018.

5 DOI: 10.3329/jbsp.v6i1.8088. Accessed Dec. 18, 2018.

6 K.D. Tripathi, *Essentials of Medical Pharmacology*, 7th ed. (2013), 911.

Glutaric Acidemia/Glutathione Synthetase Deficiency

1 https://rarediseases.org/rare-diseases/glutaricaciduria-i/. Accessed Feb. 9, 2019.

2 https://rarediseases.info.nih.gov/diseases/6522/glutaric-acidemia-type-i. Accessed Nov. 26, 2021.

3 https://ghr.nlm.nih.gov/condition/glutaric-acidemia-type-i.

4 https://www.ncbi.nlm.nih.gov/pmc/articles/PMC3210240/. Accessed Nov. 6, 2021.

5 https://pubmed.ncbi.nlm.nih.gov/8300996.

6 https://pubmed.ncbi.nlm.nih.gov/3951704/. Accessed Nov. 21, 2021.

7 https://rarediseases.info.nih.gov/diseases/10047/glutathione-synthetase-deficiency.

8 A. Larsson, "Glutathione Synthetase Deficiency," *National Organization for Rare Disorders* (2015). https://rarediseases.org/rare-diseases/glutathione-synthetase-deficiency/.

9 G. Elmer, "Vitamins: Part 4," *Nurse Pract* 7, no. 2 (Feb. 1982): 26-29.

10 "Council on Scientific Affairs: Vitamin Preparations as Dietary Supplements and as Therapeutic Agents," *JAMA* 257, no. 14 (Apr. 10, 1987): 1929-1936.

11 L.A. Boxer et al., "Protection of Granulocytes by Vitamin E in Glutathione Synthetase Deficiency," *N Eng J Med* 301 (1979): 901-905.

Goiter (Endemic Goiter)

1 https://www.medicinenet.com/goiter_causes_symptoms_and_treatment/views.htm. Accessed Nov. 17, 2018.

2 https://www.mayoclinic.org/diseases-conditions/goiter/symptoms-causes/syc 20351829. Accessed Nov. 27, 2018.

3 https://emedicine.medscape.com/article/122714-treatment. Accessed Nov. 17, 2018.

4 G. Hintze, D. Emrich, and J. Kobberling, "Controlled Study on the Effect of Iodine and Thyroxine," *Horm Metabol Res* 17, no. 7 (1985): 362-365.

Gout

1 E.T. Bope and R.D. Kellerman, *Conn's Current Therapy*, 14th ed. (Philadelphia: Elsevier/Saunders), 747.

2 W.L. Nyhan, *Rosenberg's Molecular and Genetic Basis of Neurological and Psychiatric Disease*, 5th ed. (2015). https://www.sciencedirect.com/topics/medicine-and-dentistry/purine-metabolism. Accessed May 15, 2020.

3 https://www.arthritis.org/about-arthritis/types/gout/. Accessed Mar. 3, 2019.

4 Myers R. Allen, National Medical Series for Independent Study (NMS), "Gout," *Medicine*, 3rd ed., 532-727.

5 B.G. Wells et al., *Pharmacotherapy Handbook*, 9th ed. (McGraw Hill Education, 2012), 2, 5.

6 M.A. Chisolm-Burns et al., *Pharmacotherapy Principles & Practice* (McGraw-Hill Medical, 2008), 893.

7 K.A. Oster, "Evaluation of Serum Cholesterol Reduction in Xanthine Oxidase Inhibition in the Treatment of Atherosclerosis," *Recent Advances in Studies on Cardiac Structure* 3, ed. N.S. Dhalla (1973): 73-80.

8 K.A. Oster, "Zanthine Oxidase and Folic Acid," *Ann Intern Med* 87 (1977): 252-253.

9 H.B. Stein et al., "Ascorbic Acid-Induced Uricosuria: A Consequence of Megavitamin Therapy," *Ann Intern Med* 84 (1976): 385-388.

10 H.K. Choi, X. Gao, and G. Curhan, "Vitamin C Intake and the Risk of Gout in Men: A Prospective Study," *Arch Int Med* 169, no. 5 (2009): 502-507.

11 https://www.webmd.com/arthritis/news/20090309/vitamin-c-may-help-prevent-gout. Accessed Nov. 18, 2018.

12 L.W. Blau, "Cherry Diet Control for Gout and Arthritis," *Tex Rep Biol Med* 8 (1950): 309-311.

13 https://www.webmd.com/arthritis/news/20101110/cherries-may-cut-risk-of-gout-flare-ups#1. Accessed June 25.

14 B.L. Hainer, E. Matheson, and R.T. Wilkes, "Diagnosis, Treatment, and Prevention of Gout," *Am Fam Physician* 90 (2014): 831-836.

15 https://www.mayoclinic.org/healthy-lifestyle/nutrition-and-healthy-eating/in-depth/gout-diet/art-20048524. Accessed Jan. 22, 2019.

16 https://www.webmd.com/arthritis/gout-diet-curb-flares. Accessed Jan. 22, 2019.

17 https://www.ncbi.nlm.nih.gov/pmc/articles/PMC3413920/. Accessed Apr. 29, 2019.

Granuloma Annulare (Localized)

1 https://www.webmd.com/vitamins/condition-1220/granuloma-annulare. Accessed Nov. 19, 2018.

2 T. Bogenrieder, M. Landthaler, and R-M. Szeimies, "Successful Treatment of Granuloma Annulare with a Topically Applied Vitamin E Emulsion: A Retrospective Study," *Journal of Dermatological Treatment* 9, no. 3 (July 2009): 169-173.

3 https://www.researchgate.net/publication/288594821_Generalized_granuloma_annulare_Improvement_with_vitamin_E_therapy. Accessed Nov. 19, 2018.

4 A.S. Boyd, "Granuloma Annulare Responsive to Oral Calcitriol," *Int J Dermatol* 51, no. 1 (Jan. 2012): 120-122. DOI: 10.1111/j.1365-4632.2010.04510.x.

Gray Hair

1 https://www.medicalnewstoday.com/articles/320288#causes-of-white-hair. Accessed Apr. 18, 2020.

2 https://www.disabled-world.com/health/dermatology/hair/gray-hair-causes.php. Accessed Feb. 9, 2019.

3 https://www.emedicinehealth.com/para-aminobenzoic_acid_paba/vitamins-supplements.htm. Accessed Dec. 26, 2018.

4 C. Zarafonetis, "Darkening of Gray Hair During Para-Aminobenzoic Acid Therapy," *J Investig Dermatology* 15, no. 6 (Dec. 1950): 399-401.

5 B.F. Sieve, "Clinical Achromotrichia," *Sci* 94 (1941): 257.

6 http://www.winchesterhospital.org/health-library/article?id=21831. Accessed Dec. 26, 2018.

7 https://www.webmd.com/beauty/features/abcs-premature-graying#2. Accessed Apr. 18, 2020.

Gynecomastia

1 https://emedicine.medscape.com/article/120858-overview. Accessed Nov. 19, 2018.

2 https://www.medicalnewstoday.com/articles/266129.php. Accessed Nov. 19, 2018.

3 https://www.ncbi.nlm.nih.gov/pmc/articles/PMC3987263/.

4 *The Merck Manual of Diagnosis and Therapy,* 19th ed., 2494.

5 https://www.gynecoma.com/gynecomastia-diagnosis-treatment/#anti-estrogen-diet. Accessed May 16, 2020.

6 https://www.aafp.org/afp/2012/0401/afp20120401p716.pdf. Accessed Apr. 11, 2021.

7 R.E. Johnson, and M. Hassan Murad, "Gynecomastia: Pathophysiology, Evaluation, and Management," *Mayo Clin Proc* 84, no. 11 (Nov. 2009): 1010-1015.

8 S.C. Cunnane, *Zinc: Clinical and Biochemical Significance* (Boca Raton, FL: CRC Press, Inc., 1988).

9 R.S. London, G.S. Sundaram, and P.J. Goldstein, "Medical Management of Mammary Dysplasia," *Obstet Gynecol* 59, no. 4 (Apr. 1982): 519-523.

10 https://www.ncbi.nlm.nih.gov/pmc/articles/PMC3071351/. Accessed Apr. 13, 2020.

Gyrate Atrophy of the Choroid and Retina

1 https://medlineplus.gov/genetics/condition/gyrate-atrophy-of-the-choroid-and-retina/. Accessed Apr. 25, 2021.

2 htpps://www.dovemed.com/diseases-conditions/gyrate-atrophy-choroid-and-retina/. Accessed Nov. 20, 2018.

3 https://www.aao.org/bcscsnippetdetail.aspx?id=4e9c5446-a64a-4cd2-874b-cafb19b8d2c3. Accessed Oct. 2, 2018.

4 https://www.ncbi.nlm.nih.gov/pmc/articles/PMC1312141/. Accessed Oct. 2, 2018.

5 A. Javadzadeh and D. Gharabaghi, "Gyrate Atrophy of the Choroid and Retina with Hyper-Ornithinemia Responsive to Vitamin B6: A Case Report," *Journal of Medical Case Reports* 1, no. 27 (June 2007). https://doi.org/10.1186/1752-1947-1-27. Accessed Oct. 2, 2018.

H. Pylori Infection

1 *The Washington Manual of Medical Therapeutics*, 33rd ed., 847.

2 R. Urgesi, R. Cianci, and M.E. Riccion, "Update on Triple Therapy for Eradication of *H. pylori*: Current Status of the Art," *Clin Exp Gastroenterol* 5 (2012): 151-157. Published online Sept. 17, 2012. DOI: 10.2147/CEG.S25416.

3 https://www.webmd.com/vitamins/ai/ingredientmono-1001/vitamin-c-ascorbic-acid. Accessed Nov. 14, 2018.

4 https://www.ncbi.nlm.nih.gov/pmc/articles/PMC3229773/. Accessed Dec. 4, 2018.

5 M. Sezikli et al., "Oxidative Stress in *Helicobacter pylori* Infection: Does Supplementation with Vitamins C and E Increase the Eradication Rate?," *Helicobacter* 14 (2009): 280-285.

6 https://www.medicinenet.com/diarrhea/article.htm#which_medications_treat_diarrhea. Accessed Nov. 15, 2018.

7 https://www.medicinenet.com/taurine/supplements-vitamins.htm. Accessed Nov. 28, 2018.

8 H. Szajewska, A. Horvath, and A. Piwowarczyk, "Meta-Analysis: The Effects of *Saccharomyces boulardii* Supplementation on *Helicobacter pylori* Eradication Rates and Side Effects during Treatment," *Aliment Pharmacol Ther* 32, no. 9 (2010): 1069-1079.

9 G. Cammarota et al., "Biofilm Demolition and Antibiotic Treatment to Eradicate Resistant *Helicobacter pylori*: A Clinical Trial," *Clin Gastroenterol Hepatol* 8, no. 9 (2010): 817-820.

10 *World J Gastrointestinal Pharmacol Ther* 6, no. 4 (Nov. 6, 2015): 183-198. https://universityhealthnews.com/daily/digestive-health/4-step-h-pylori-natural-treatment-protocol/. Accessed Dec. 4, 2018.

11 https://www.webmd.com/heartburn-gerd/news/20021230/with-beer-wine-stomachs-fine. Accessed Dec. 4, 2018.

12 https://www.hpyloridiet.org/foods-to-avoid-with-h-pylori/. Accessed Feb. 9, 2019.

13 S. Park et al., "Rescue of *Helicobacter pylori*-Induced Cytotoxicity by Red Ginseng," *Dig Dis Sci* 50 (2005): 1218-1227. DOI: 10.1007/s10620-005-2763-x.

14 https://www.ncbi.nlm.nih.gov/pmc/articles/PMC6406303/#B84-jcm-08-00179. Accessed May 12, 2020.

15 O. Ustün et al., "Flavonoids with Anti-*Helicobacter pylori* activity from *Cistus laurifolius* Leaves," *J Ethnopharmacol* 108 (2006): 457-461. DOI: 10.1016/j.jep.2006.06.001.

16 https://www.medicalnewstoday.com/articles/322627#natural-treatments. Accessed July 25, 2021.

Hailey-Hailey Disease

1 https://rarediseases.info.nih.gov/diseases/6559/hailey-hailey-disease. Accessed Dec. 18, 2018.

2 https://rarediseases.org/rare-diseases/hailey-hailey-disease/. Accessed Mar. 13, 2019.

3 S. Ayres Jr., "Hailey-Hailey Disease: Response to Vitamin E Therapy," *Arch Dermatol* 119, no. 6 (1983): 450. DOI: 10.1001/archderm.1983.01650300004002.

Hartnup Disease

1 https://rarediseases.org/rare-diseases/hartnup-disease/. Accessed Nov. 17, 2020.

2 https://www.britannica.com/science/Hartnup-disease. Accessed Oct. 4, 2018.

3 https://ghr.nlm.nih.gov/condition/hartnup-disease. Accessed Oct. 4, 2018.

4 https://emedicine.medscape.com/article/1115549-medication. Accessed June 14, 2021.

5 K.J. Isselbacher et al., *Harrison's Principles of Internal Medicine*, 13th ed., 473.

6 https://emedicine.medscape.com/article/1115549-treatment. Accessed Oct. 4, 2018.

7 A.J. Jonas and I.J. Biutler, "Circumvention of Defective Neutral Amino Acid Transport in Hartnup Disease Using Tryptophan Ethyl Ester," *J Clin Invest* 84, no. 1 (July 1989): 200-204.

Hay Fever/Allergic Rhinitis

1 https://www.medicalnewstoday.com/articles/160665. Accessed May 15, 2020.

2 M.A. Chisolm-Burns et al., *Pharmacotherapy Principles & Practice* (McGraw-Hill Medical, 2008), 931.

3 http://pennstatehershey.adam.com/content.aspx?productId=107&pid=33&gid=000328. Accessed Nov. 16, 2018.

4 https://www.webmd.com/vitamins/ai/ingredientmono-662/turmeric. Accessed Nov. 14, 2018.

5 C. Bachert, MD, et al., "Influence of Oral Calcium Medication on Nasal Resistance in the Nasal Allergen Provocation Test," *Journal of Allergy and Clinical Immunology* 91, no. 2 (Feb. 1993): 599-604.

6 R.R. Widmann and J.D. Keye, "Epinephrine Precursors in Control of Allergy," *Northwest Med* 51 (1952): 588-590.

7 https://www.webmd.com/vitamins/ai/ingredientmono-790/lactobacillus. Accessed Oct. 4, 2018.

8 https://www.medicalnewstoday.com/articles/323276.php. Accessed Mar. 2, 2019.

9 https://www.webmd.com/allergies/news/20050822/butterbur-may-be-effective-hay-fever-remedy#1. Accessed Mar. 2, 2019.

10 https://www.medicalnewstoday.com/articles/264667.php. Accessed May 8, 2019.

11 M.A. Chisolm-Burns et al., *Pharmacotherapy Principles & Practice* (McGraw-Hill Medical, 2008), 932.

Hearing Loss/Presbycusis

1 https://medical-dictionary.thefreedictionary.com/presbycusis%20Last%20Accessed%2012-23-2018. https://medical-dictionary.thefreedictionary.com/presbycusis. Accessed Oct. 1, 2018.

2 *The Merck Manual of Diagnosis and Therapy*, 19th ed., 533.

3 https://www.nidcd.nih.gov/health/noise-induced-hearing-loss. Accessed May 23, 2021.

4 Z. Shemesh et al., "Vitamin B12 Deficiency in Patients with Chronic-Tinnitus and Noise-Induced Hearing Loss," *Am J Otolaryngol* 14, no. 2 (Mar.-Apr. 1993): 94-99.

5 D.K. Houston et al., "Age-Related Hearing Loss, Vitamin B-12, and Folate in Elderly Women," *The American Journal of Clinical Nutrition* 69, no. 3, (Mar. 1, 1999): 564-571.

6 A. Gordin et al., "Magnesium: A New Therapy for Idiopathic Sudden Sensorineural Hearing Loss," *Otology & Neurotology* 23, no. 4 (July 2002): 447-451.

7 https://www.webmd.com/vitamins/ai/ingredientmono-998/magnesium. Accessed Oct. 5, 2018.

8 G.B. Brookes. "Vitamin D Deficiency and Deafness: 1984 Update," *Am J Otol* 6, no. 1 (Jan. 1985): 102-107.

9 S.G. Curhan et al., "Fish and Fatty Acid Consumption and the Risk of Hearing Loss in Women," *The American Journal of Clinical Nutrition* 100, no. 5 (Nov. 1, 2014): 1371-1377.

10 https://www.sciencedaily.com/releases/2009/02/090212093704.htm. Accessed Oct. 4, 2018.

11 https://www.medicalnewstoday.com/articles/219853.php. Accessed Feb. 11, 2019.

12 *The Merck Manual of Diagnosis and Therapy,* 19th ed., 528.

Heart Disease

1 https://www.mayoclinic.org/diseases-conditions/heart-disease/diagnosis-treatment/drc-20353124. Accessed Mar. 6, 2020.

2 A.R. Gaby, "Magnesium: An Inexpensive, Safe and Effective Treatment for Cardiovascular Disease," *J Advancement Med* 1 (1988): 179-181.

3 N. Boyce, "Homocysteine Screening for Heart Disease on Horizon," *Clinical Laboratory News* 22, no. 5 (May 1996): 1, 3.

4 *JAMA* 270 (1993): 2693-2698.

5 K.L. Tucker et al., "Folic Acid Fortification of the Food Supply: Potential Benefits and Risks for the Elderly Population," *JAMA* 276 (1996): 1879-1885.

6 https://www.webmd.com/heart-disease/news/20021122/folic-acid-for-your-heart. Accessed Nov. 14, 2018.

7 https://www.webmd.com/vitamins/ai/ingredientmono-957/riboflavin. Accessed Nov. 14, 2018.

8 https://medlineplus.gov/druginfo/natural/957.html. Accessed Nov. 16, 2018.

9 J.J. DiNicolantonio et al., "L-Carnitine in the Secondary Prevention of Cardiovascular Disease: Systematic Review and Meta-Analysis," *Mayo Clin Proc* (2013). DOI: 10.1016/j.mayocp.2013.02.007. Available at: http://www.mayoclinicproceedings.org.

Heart Failure/Congestive Heart Failure

1 https://www.aafp.org/afp/2004/1201/p2145.html. Accessed Feb. 28, 2021.

2 https://my.clevelandclinic.org/health/diseases/17069-heart-failure-understanding-heart-failure. Accessed May 4, 2021.

3 https://pubmed.ncbi.nlm.nih.gov/21861070/. Accessed May 9, 2021.

4 A.B.M. Abdullah, *Practical Manual in Clinical Medicine* (Philadelphia: Jaypee—The Health Sciences Publisher, 2017): 63.

5 https://www.sciencedirect.com/science/article/pii/S0735109721005775?via%3Dihub. Accessed June 15, 2021.

6 M.M. Keifer, *Pocket Primary Care,* 2nd ed. (Wolters Kluver).

7 Kasper et al., *Harrison's Manual of Medicine,* 19th ed. (McGraw Hill Education), 688.

8 T. Eshenhagen, "Therapy of Heart Failure," in *Gilbert & Goodman's: The Pharmacological Basis of Therapeutics,* 13th ed. (2018), 531.

9 P.A. Heidenreich et al., "2020 ACC/AHA Clinical Performance and Quality Measures for Adults with Heart Failure: A Report of The American College of Cardiology/American Heart Association Task Force on Performance Measures," *J Am Coll Cardiol* 76 (2020): 2527-2564.

10 R.A. Bonakdar and E. Guarneri, "Coenzyme Q10," *Am Fam Physician* 72, no. 6 (Sept. 15, 2005): 1065-1070.

11 S.A. Mortensen et al., "The Effect of Coenzyme Q10 on Morbidity and Mortality in Chronic Heart Failure: Results From Q-SYMBIO: A Randomized Double-Blind Trial," *J Am College Cardiology: Heart Failure* 2, no. 6 (Dec. 2014). DOI: 10.1016/j.jchf.2014.06.008.

12 J.J. DiNicolantonio et al., "Coenzyme Q10 for the Treatment of Heart Failure: A Review of the Literature," *Open Heart* 2, no. 1 (2015): e000326. Published online Oct. 19, 2015. DOI: 10.1136/openhrt-2015-000326.

13 A.M. Soja and S.A. Mortensen, "Treatment of Congestive Heart Failure with Coenzyme Q10 Illuminated by Meta-Analyses of Clinical Trials," *Mol Aspects Med* 18 (1997): 159-168.

14 https://www.rxlist.com/consumer_coenzyme_q10_coq10_ubiquinone/drugs-condition.htm. Accessed Jan. 21, 2019.

15 H.L. Sacher et al., "The Clinical and Hemodynamic Effects of Coenzyme Q10 in Congestive Cardiomyopathy," *American Journal of Therapeutics* 4, no. 2 (Feb.-Mar. 1997): 61. Published online Oct. 19, 2015. DOI: 10.1136/openhrt-2015-000326.

16 V.P. Arcangelo and A.M. Peterson, *Pharmacotherapeutics for Advanced Practice: A Practical Approach.* 3rd ed. (Wolters Kluwer/Lippincott Williams & Wilkins, 2013): 121.

17 C. Morisco, B. Trimarco, and M. Condorelli, "Effect of Coenzyme Q10 Therapy in Patients with Congestive Heart Failure: A Long-Term Multicenter Randomized Study," *Clin Investig* 71, suppl. 8 (1993): S134-S136.

18 M. Jafari et al., "Coenzyme Q10 in the Treatment of Heart Failure: A Systematic Review of Systematic Reviews," *Indian Heart Journal* 70, suppl. 1 (July 2018): S111-S117.

19 https://onlinelibrary.wiley.com/doi/full/10.1111/chf.12037. Accessed Apr. 13, 2020.

20 https://lcm.amegroups.com/article/view/5448/html. Accessed Apr. 11, 2021.

21 https://onlinelibrary.wiley.com/doi/full/10.1111/chf.12037. Accessed Apr. 11, 2021.

22 I. Shimon et al., *Am J Med* 98, no. 5 (1995): 485-490.

23 K. Takihara, "Beneficial Effect of Taurine in Rabbits with Chronic Congestive Heart Failure," *Am Heart J* 112, no. 6 (Dec. 1986): 1278-1184.

24 J. Azuma et al., "Taurine for Treatment of Congestive Heart Failure. International," *Journal of Cardiology* 2, no. 2 (1982): 303-304.

25 J. Azuma et al., "Therapy of Congestive Heart Failure with Orally Administered Taurine," *Clin Ther* 5, no. 4 (1983): 398-408.

26 J. Azuma et al., "Usefulness of Taurine in Chronic Congestive Heart Failure and Its Prospective Application," *Japanese Circ J* 56 (Jan. 1992): 95-99.

27 M. Reza et al., "Effect of Taurine Supplementation on Exercise Capacity of Patients with Heart Failure," *Journal of Cardiology* 57, no. 3 (2011): 333-337.

28 J. Azuma et al., "Double-Blind Randomized Crossover Trial of Taurine in Congestive Heart Failure," *Curr Ther Res* 34 (1983): 534.

29 A.R. Gaby, "Taurine: The Cellular Buffer," *Nutrition and Healing* 4 (Jan. 1997): 3, 11.

30 https://www.emedicinehealth.com/taurine/vitamins-supplements.htm. Accessed Nov. 21, 2018.

31 Y. Wen-qiu and C. Shan-wan, *Acta Academiae Medicinae Wuhan* 5 (1985): 38. https://doi.org/10.1007/BF02856908.

32 W.H. Liu, H.J. Wang, and H.B. Jing, "Treatment of Congestive Heart Failure Complicating Chronic Keshan Disease with Magnesium Sulfate and Captopril," *Chinese Journal of Internal Medicine* 32, no. 1 (Jan. 1993): 49-51.

33 https://openheart.bmj.com/content/5/2/e000775. Accessed Mar. 20, 2021.

34 J.C. Fuentes, A.A. Salmon, and M.A. Silver, "Acute and Chronic Oral Magnesium Supplementation: Effects on Endothelial Function, Exercise Capacity, and Quality of Life in Patients with Symptomatic Heart Failure," *Heart Failure* 12, no. 1 (2006): 9-13.

35 O.B. Stepura and A.I. Martynow, "Magnesium Orotate in Severe Congestive Heart Failure," *International Journal of Cardiology* 131, no. 2 (Jan. 2009): 293-295.

36 M.C. Cave et al., "Obesity, Inflammation, and the Potential Application of Pharmaconutrition," *Nutr Clin Pract* 23, no. 1 (Feb. 2008). DOI: 10.1177/011542650802300116.

37 I. Rizos, "Three-Year Survival of Patients with Heart Failure Caused by Dilated Cardiomyopathy and L-Carnitine Administration," *Am Heart J* 139, no. 2, pt. 3 (2000): S120-S123.

38 https://www.medicinenet.com/l-carnitine/supplements-vitamins.htm#Dosing. Accessed Nov. 26, 2018.

39 B. Bednarz et al., "L-Arginine Supplementation Prolongs Exercise Capacity in Congestive Heart Failure," *Kardiol Pol* 60, no. 4 (2004): 348-353. PMID: 15226784. [in English, Polish]

40 E.A. Bocchi et al., "L-Arginine Reduces Heart Rate and Improves Hemodynamics in Severe Congestive Heart Failure," *Clin Cardiol* 23, no. 3 (2000): 205-210. PMID: 10761810.

41 T.C. Wascher et al., "Vascular Effects of L-Arginine: Anything Beyond a Substrate for the NO-Synthase?," *Biochem Biophys Res Commun* 234, no. 1 (1997): 35-38. PMID: 9168955.

42 B. Koifmany et al., "Improvement of Cardiac Performance by Intravenous Infusion of L-Arginine in Patients with Moderate Congestive Heart Failure," *J Amer Coll Cardiol* 26, no. 5 (Nov. 1995). DOI: 10.1016/0735-1097(95)00318-5.

43 E.A. Bocci et al., "L-Arginine Reduces Heart Rate and Improves Hemodynamics in Severe Congestive Heart Failure," *Clinical Cardiology* 23 (2000): 205-210.

44 T.S. Rector et al., "Randomized, Double-Blind, Placebo-Controlled Study of Supplemental Oral L-Arginine in Patients with Heart Failure," *Circulation* 93 (1996): 2135-2141.

45 J.L. Anderson et al., "Relation of Vitamin D Deficiency to Cardiovascular Risk Factors, Disease Status, and Incident Events in a General Healthcare Population," *Am J Cardiol* 106, no. 7 (2010): 963-968.

46 https://www.emedicinehealth.com/vitamin_d/vitamins-supplements.htm. Accessed Dec. 28, 2018.

Heartburn/Acid Reflux/Indigestion/Dyspepsia/Pyrosis/GERD

1 https://www.mdedge.com/podcasts/daily-medical-news/half-patients-report-resistant-gerd?utm_source=News_Power_eNL_052419_F&utm_medium=email&utm_content=Postcall%20Podcast:%20Movies%20for%20interns%20and%20residents. Accessed May 25, 2019.

2 J.T. DiPiro et al., *Pharmacotherapy: A Pathophysiologic Approach*, 6th ed. (McGraw-Hill, 2005), 623.

3 B.G. Wells et al., *Pharmacotherapy Handbook*, 9th ed. (McGraw Hill Education, 2012), 206.

4 https://www.medicinenet.com/heartburn_reflux/article.htm#lifestyle_changes. Accessed Nov. 21, 2018.

5 M.A. Chisolm-Burns et al., *Pharmacotherapy Principles & Practice* (McGraw-Hill Medical, 2008), 259.

6 B.G. Wells et al., *Pharmacotherapy Handbook*, 9th ed. (McGraw Hill Education, 2012), 210.

7 K.A. Sharkey and W.K. MacNaughton, "Pharmacotherapy for Gastric Acidity, Peptic Ulcers, and Gastroesophageal Reflux Disease," in *Gilbert & Goodman's: The Pharmacological Basis of Therapeutics*, 13th ed. (2018), 914.

8 https://www.webmd.com/drugs/2/drug-11325/sodium-bicarbonate-oral/details. Accessed Dec. 16, 2018.

9 J.T. DiPiro et al., *Pharmacotherapy: A Pathophysiologic Approach*, 6th ed. (McGraw-Hill, 2005), 621.

10 M.A. Chisolm-Burns et al., *Pharmacotherapy Principles & Practice* (McGraw-Hill Medical, 2008), 262.

11 J.T. DiPiro et al., *Pharmacotherapy: A Pathophysiologic Approach*, 6th ed. (McGraw-Hill, 2005), 613.

12 *Gastroenterology* 135 (2008): 1392.

13 https://www.aafp.org/afp/2009/0715/p157.html. Accessed June 15, 2021.

14 https://reference.medscape.com/drug/milk-of-magnesia-magnesium-hydroxide-342018. Accessed Mar. 25, 2021.

15 https://www.webmd.com/vitamins/ai/ingredientmono-998/magnesium. Accessed Dec. 16, 2018.

16 https://www.webmd.com/vitamins/ai/ingredientmono-881/licorice. Accessed Mar. 2, 2019.

Heat Intolerance/Heat Stroke

1 https://www.webmd.com/fitness-exercise/heat-exhaustion#1. Accessed Dec. 18, 2018.

2 W.L. Weaver, "The Prevention of Heat Prostration by Use of Vitamin C," *Southern Medical J* 51, no. 5 (1948): 479-481.

3 https://www.mayoclinic.org/diseases-conditions/heat-exhaustion/diagnosis-treatment/drc-20373253. Accessed Dec. 18, 2018.

4 "Everything You Need to Know About Heat Intolerance," *MNT Weekly Newsletter* (May 22, 2019). medicalnewstoday.com.

Heavy Metal Poisoning

1 https://www.ncbi.nlm.nih.gov/pmc/articles/PMC3783921/. Accessed Nov. 16, 2018.

2 R.A. Goyer and M.G. Cherian, "Ascorbic Acid and EDTA Treatment of Lead Toxicity in Rats," *Life Sci* 24 (1979): 433-438. DOI: 10.1016/0024-3205(79)90215-7.

3 https://www.ncbi.nlm.nih.gov/pmc/articles/PMC3783921/. Accessed Nov. 16, 2018.

4 http://pennstatehershey.adam.com/content.aspx?productId=107&pid=33&gid=000285. Accessed Nov. 16, 2018.

Hemorrhoids

1 https://www.ncbi.nlm.nih.gov/pubmed/24881480. Accessed May 16, 2020.

2 *The Merck Manual of Diagnosis and Therapy,* 19th ed., 250.

3 https://www.aafp.org/afp/2011/0715/p204.html. Accessed Oct. 12, 2019.

4 https://www.health.harvard.edu/diseases-and conditions/hemorrhoids_and_what_to_do_about_them. Accessed Nov. 19, 2018.

5 American Gastroenterological Association Medical Position Statement, "Diagnosis and Treatment of Hemorrhoids," *Gastroenterology* 126 (2004): 1461-1462.

6 https://www.aafp.org/afp/2018/0201/p172.html. Accessed June 7, 2021.

7 S.R. Gorfine, "Treatment of Benign Anal Disease with Topical Nitroglycerin," *Dis Colon Rectum* 38 (1995): 453-457.

8 S.R. Gorfine, "Topical Nitroglycerin Therapy for Anal Fissures and Ulcers [letter]," *N Engl J Med* 333 (1995): 1156-1157.

9 W.R. Schouten et al., "Intra-Anal Application of Isosorbide Dinitrate in Chronic Anal Fissure," *Ned Tijdschr Geneeskd* 139 (July 15, 1995): 1447-1449.

10 J.N. Lund, N.C. Armitage, and J.H. Scholefield, "Use of Glyceryl Trinitrate Ointment in the Treatment of Anal Fissure," *Br J Surg* 83 (1996): 776-777.

11 https://www.webmd.com/vitamins/ai/ingredientmono-522/msm-methylsulfonylmethane. Accessed Nov. 18, 2018.

Hepatic Encephalopathy

1 http://wwwclevelandclinicmeded.com/medicalpubs/diseasemanagement/hepatology/hepatic-encephalopathy/. Accessed Mar. 3, 2019.

2 D. Hui, *Approach to Internal Medicine: A Resource Book for Clinical Practice*, 3rd ed. (Springer, 2011), 129.

3 N.J. Shores and E.B. Keeffe, "Is Oral L-Acyl Carnitine an Effective Therapy for Hepatic Encephalopathy? Review of the Literature," *Dig Dis Sci* (2008).

4 https://www.ncbi.nlm.nih.gov/pmc/articles/PMC2861661/#B58. Accessed Oct. 29, 2018.

5 Thorne Research, Inc., "Monograph on L-Carnitine," *Alternative Medicine Review* 10, no. 1 (2005): 45. Available from, as of February 22, 2008: http://www.thorne.com/altmedrev/. fulltext/10/1/42.pdf. Accessed Nov. 29, 2018.

6 https://www.webmd.com/vitamins/ai/ingredientmono-200/ornithine. Accessed Nov. 29, 2018.

7 K. Mullin, "Nutrition in Hepatic Encephalopathy," *Nutr Clin Pract* 25 (2010): 257.

Hexane Inhalation

1 https://www.medicinenet.com/script/main/art.asp?articlekey=19085. Accessed Nov. 16, 2018.

2 *PDR for Nutritional Supplements*, 2nd ed. (Montvale, NJ: Thomson Reuters, 2008), 25.

3 https://pubchem.ncbi.nlm.nih.gov/compound/dl-Thioctic_acid#section=Therapeutic-Uses. Accessed Nov. 16, 2018.

Hiccups (Persistent)

1 https://www.cghjournal.org/article/S1542-3565(12)01047-6/fulltext. Accessed Jan. 5, 2019.

2 M.A. Papadakis and S.J. McPhee, *Current Medical Diagnosis & Treatment* (2019): ch. 15, 595.

3 https://www.medscape.com/viewarticle/815243_5. Accessed Jan. 4, 2019.

4 https://www.ncbi.nlm.nih.gov/pmc/articles/PMC3006663/. Accessed Aug. 20, 2021.

5 "Practice Tips," *Postgraduate Medicine* 1197, no. 101(a): 50.

6 A.J. Bredenoord, "Management of Belching, Hiccups and Aerophagia," *Clinical Gastroenterology and Hepatology* 11, no. 1 (Jan. 2013): 6-12. Reprinted with permission from Elsevier.

Homocystinuria

1 https://www.ncbi.nlm.nih.gov/pmc/articles/PMC5203861/. Accessed May 29, 2020.

2 https://www.ncbi.nlm.nih.gov/pmc/articles/PMC2020308/pdf/archdisch01552-0099.pdf. Accessed May 29, 2020.

3 https://www.researchgate.net/publication/18479899_Homocystinuria. Accessed May 29, 2020.

4 J.A. Thomas, "Homocystinuria: Diagnosis and Management," *Nutrition Management of Inherited Metabolic Diseases*, eds. L. Bernstein, F. Rohr, and J. Helm (Cham: Springer, 2015).

5 https://www.cigna.com/individuals-families/health-wellness/hw/medical topics/ homocystinuria-tu2113. Accessed Oct. 8, 2018.

6 M.A. Papadakis and S.J. McPhee, *Current Medical Diagnosis & Treatment* (2019): ch. 10, 1686.

7 https://www.aao.org/disease-review/homocystinuria-3. Accessed May 29, 2021.

Hot Flashes/Hot Flushes/Menopausal Symptoms

1 https://www.healthline.com/health/menopause/understanding-hot-flashes#triggers. Accessed Dec. 18, 2018.

2 M.A. Hollinger, *Introduction to Pharmacology*, 2nd ed. (Tayor & Francis, 2003), 845.

3 E.S. Ginsburg, "Hot Flashes—Physiology, Hormonal Therapy and Alternative Therapies. Menopause and Mood," *Postgraduate Medicine* 108, no. 3 (Sept. 1, 2000).

4 https://www.webmd.com/menopause/guide/menopause-hot-flashes#2-6.

5 ACOG Practice Bulletin, Clinical Management Guidelines for Obstetrician-Gynecologists, "Use of Botanicals for Management of Menopausal Symptoms," *Obstet Gynecol* 97, suppl. 1-11 (2001). https://www.aafp.org/afp/2003/0701/p114.html. Accessed Jan. 29, 2021.

6 https://www.webmd.com/menopause/news/20000209/natural-alternatives-hormone-therapy#2. Accessed Feb. 29, 2019.

7 https://www.aafp.org/afp/2006/0201/p457.html. Accessed July 28, 2021.

8 https://www.mayoclinic.org/diseases-conditions/hot-flashes/diagnosis-treatment/drc-20352795. Accessed Nov. 16, 2018.

9 S. Ziaei, A. Kazemnejad, and M. Zareai, "The Effect of Vitamin E on Hot Flashes in Menopausal Women," *Gynecol Obstet Invest* 64, no. 4 (2007): 204-207. Epub July 30, 2007.

10 https://mayoclinic.pure.elsevier.com/en/publications/prospective-evaluation-of-vitamin-e-for-hot-flashes-in-breast-can. Accessed Nov. 16, 2018.

11 B.G. Katzung, *Basic & Clinical Pharmacology*, 14th ed., A Lange Medical Book (2018), 1140.

12 https://www.aafp.org/afp/2006/0201/p457.html. Accessed July 28, 2021.

Huntington's Chorea

1 https://www.webmd.com/vitamins/ai/ingredientmono-954/vitamin-e. Accessed Oct. 9, 2018.

2 https://www.sciencedaily.com/releases/2014/02/140208080705.htm. Accessed Nov. 16, 2018.

3 J. Alpha, A. Caro, and S. Caro, "Vitamin E in Treatment of Huntington's Chorea," *British Medical Journal* 1 (1978): 153. DOI: 10.1136/bmj.1.6116.859-c.

4 https://web.stanford.edu/group/hopes/cgi-bin/hopes_test/coenzyme-q10/. Accessed Nov. 16, 2018.

5 http://hdsa.org/wp-content/uploads/2015/04/Nutrition-and-HD.pdf. Accessed Nov. 16, 2018.

Hypertension/High Blood Pressure

1 https://www.nia.nih.gov/health/high-blood-pressure.

2 https://www.ncbi.nlm.nih.gov/pubmed/20550499. Accessed Feb. 23, 2020.

3 https://journals.lww.com/co-cardiology/Citation/2016/07000/Impact_of_comorbidities_in_hypertension.6.aspx. Accessed Oct. 12, 2019.

4 Y.R. Wang et al., "Outpatient Hypertension Treatment, Treatment Intensification, and Control in Western Europe and the United States," *Arch Intern Med* 167 (2007): 141-147.

5 T. Eshenhagen, "Treatment of Hypertension," in *Gilbert & Goodman's: The Pharmacological Basis of Therapeutics*, 13th ed. (2018), 521.

6 *The Merck Manual of Diagnosis and Therapy*, 19th ed., 2226.

7 M. Poplawski, N.K. Nelson, and J.S. Earwood, "Rethinking Daily Aspirin for Primary Prevention," *J Fam Pract* 69, no. 9 (2020): 461-462. DOI: 10.12788/jfp.0092.

8 L.J. Appel et al., "A Clinical Trial of the Effects of Dietary Patterns on Blood Pressure: DASH Collaborative Research Group," *N Engl J Med* 336 (1997): 1117-1124.

9 E.B. Rimm et al., "Vegetable, Fruit and Cereal Fiber Intake and Risk of Coronary Heart Disease among Men," *JAMA* 275 (1996): 447-451.

10 M.W. Gillman et al., "Protective Effect of Fruits and Vegetable on Development of Stroke in Men," *JAMA* 273 (1995): 1113-1117.

11 https://emedicine.medscape.com/article/241381-treatment#d9. Accessed Feb. 3, 2020.

12 B. Wasi, *Standard Treatment Guidelines: A Manual for Medical Therapeutics*, 1st ed. (2014), 101.

13 N.L. Benowitz, "Cardiovascular-Renal Drugs" in B.G. Katzung, S.B. Masters, and A.J. Trevor, *Basic and Clinical Pharmacology*, 12th ed. (McGrawHill/Lange, 2010): 186.

14 P.K. Whelton et al., "Sodium Reduction and Weight Loss in the Treatment of Hypertension in Older Persons: A Randomized, Controlled Trial of Nonpharmacologic Interventions in the Elderly (TONE)," *JAMA* 279, TONE Collaborative Research Group (1998): 839-846.

15 M.A. Papadakis and S.J. McPhee, *Current Medical Diagnosis & Treatment* (2019): ch. 9, 453.

16 https://pubmed.ncbi.nlm.nih.gov/22051430/. Accessed Mar. 20, 2021.

17 M.T. Tran et al., "Role of Coenzyme Q10 in Chronic Heart Failure, Angina, and Hypertension," *Pharmacotherapy* 21 (2001): 797-806.

18 V. Digiesi et al., "Coenzyme QIO in Essential Hypertension," *Molec Aspects Med* 15, Suppl. (1994): S257-S263.

19 V.P. Arcangelo and A.M. Peterson, *Pharmacotherapeutics for Advanced Practice: A Practical Approach*, 3rd ed. (Wolters Kluwer/Lippincott Williams & Wilkins, 2013): 121.

20 S.P. Juraschek et al., "Effects of Vitamin C Supplementation on Blood Pressure: A Meta-Analysis of Randomized Controlled Trials," *Am J Clin Nutr* 95, no. 5 (2012): 1079-1088.

21 S.J. Duffy et al., "Treatment of Hypertension with Ascorbic Acid," *Lancet* 354 (1999): 2048-2049.

22 https://www.ncbi.nlm.nih.gov/pmc/articles/PMC4963920/. Accessed May 17, 2020.

23 G.D. Miller et al., "Benefits of Dairy Product Consumption on Blood Pressure in Humans: A Summary of the Biomedical Literature," *J Am Coll Nutr* 19, Suppl. 2 (2000): 147S-164S.

24 https://www.webmd.com/vitamins/ai/ingredientmono-1017/folic-acid. Accessed Nov. 19, 2018.

25 https://pubmed.ncbi.nlm.nih.gov/28912716/. Accessed Apr. 11, 2021.

26 https://www.webmd.com/vitamins/ai/ingredientmono-1024/taurine. Accessed Nov. 28, 2018.

27 S.K. Kunutsor, T.A. Apekey, and M. Steur, "Vitamin D and Risk of Future Hypertension: Meta-Analysis of 283,537 Participants," *Eur J Epidemiol* 28, no. 3 (2013): 205-221.

28 A. Burgaz et al., "Blood 25-Hydroxyvitamin D Concentration and Hypertension: A Meta-Analysis," *J Hypertens* 29, no. 4 (2011): 636-645.

29 https://restorativemedicine.org/journal/cardiovascular-effects-berberine/. Accessed May 6, 2020.

30 https://www.sciencedirect.com/science/article/abs/pii/S037887411400871X. Accessed May 6, 2020.

31 L.M. Gibbs, R.J. Nair, and J. Nashelsky, "Does Evidence Support the Use of Supplements to Aid in BP Control," *J Fam Pract* 69, no. 7 (Sept. 2020): E14-E16. DOI: 10.12788/jfp.0055.

Hyperthyroidism

1 https://www.winchesterhospital.org/health-library/article?id=19617. Accessed Apr. 13, 2020.

2 https://familydoctor.org/condition/hyperthyroidism/. Accessed Nov. 22, 2018.

3 https://pubmed.ncbi.nlm.nih.gov/25514898/. Accessed Mar. 20, 2021.

4 https://www.mayoclinic.org/diseases-conditions/hyperthyroidism/diagnosis-treatment/drc-20373665. Accessed Nov. 22, 2018.

5 *JAMA* 123, no. 16 (1943): 1049-1050. DOI: 10.1001/jama.1943.02840510043011.

6 https://www.merckmanuals.com/professional/nutritional-disorders/vitamin-deficiency,-dependency,-and-toxicity/thiamin. Accessed Nov. 22, 2018.

7 S. Benvenga et al., "Usefulness of L-Carnitine, a Naturally Occurring Peripheral Antagonist of Thyroid Hormone Action, in Iatrogenic Hyperthyroidism: A Randomized, Double-Blind, Placebo-Controlled Clinical Trial," *J Clin Endocrinol Metab* 86 (2001): 3579-3594.

8 J.R. Reid and S.F. Wheeler, "Hyperthyroidism: Diagnosis and Treatment," *Am Fam Physician* 72, no. 4 (Aug. 15, 2005): 623-630.

9 https://www.medicalnewstoday.com/articles/326275#foods-to-eat. Accessed May 17, 2020.

10 C. Marcocci et al., "Selenium and the Course of Mild Graves' Orbitopathy," *N Engl J Med* 364 (2011): 1920-1931.

11 https://www.sciencedirect.com/science/article/pii/S0929664612002719. Accessed May 17, 2020.

Hypoglycemia/Low Blood Sugar

1 D. Hui, *Approach to Internal Medicine: A Resource Book for Clinical Practice*, 3rd ed. (Springer, 2011), 342.

2 https://www.nhs.uk/conditions/low-blood-sugar-hypoglycaemia/. Accessed May 17, 2020.

3 https://www.ncbi.nlm.nih.gov/pubmed/3550373. Accessed May 17, 2020.

4 A. Shansky, "Vitamin B3 in the Alleviation of Hypoglycemia," *Drug and Cosmetic Industry* 129, no. 4 (1981): 68-69.

5 https://www.webmd.com/diabetes/guide/diabetes-hypoglycemia#2. Accessed Nov. 19, 2018.

6 https://www.mayoclinic.org/diseases-conditions/hypoglycemia/diagnosis-treatment/drc-20373689. Accessed Nov. 19, 2018.

Hypomagnesemia

1 https://www.merckmanuals.com/professional/endocrine-and-metabolic-disorders/electrolyte-disorders/hypomagnesemia. Accessed Nov. 16, 2018.

2 https://www.ncbi.nlm.nih.gov/pmc/articles/PMC1855626/. Accessed Jan. 22, 2019.

3 https://www.ncbi.nlm.nih.gov/pmc/articles/PMC2464251/. Accessed Nov. 25, 2018.

4 M.A. Krupp and M.J. Chatton, *Current Medical Diagnosis & Treatment* (1983): 30.

5 J. Soar et al., "European Resuscitation Council Guidelines for Resuscitation 2010 Section 8. Cardiac Arrest in Special Circumstances: Electrolyte Abnormalities, Poisoning, Drowning, Accidental Hypothermia, Hyperthermia, Asthma, Anaphylaxis, Cardiac Surgery, Trauma, Pregnancy, Electrocution," *Resuscitation* 81, no. 10 (Oct. 2010): 1400-1433.

Hypothyroidism

1 https://www.aafp.org/afp/2015/0315/p359.html. Accessed Nov. 17, 2020.

2 A. Costantini and M.I. Pala, "Thiamine and Hashimoto's Thyroiditis: A Report of Three Cases," *J Altern Complement Med* 20, no. 3 (Mar. 2014): 208-211. DOI: 10.1089/acm.2012.0612. Epub Sept. 25, 2013.

3 I.A.Al-Juboori, R.Al-Rawi, and H.K. A-Hakeim, "Estimation of Serum Copper, Manganese, Selenium and Zinc in Hypothyroidism Patients," *IUFS Journal of Biology* 68, no. 2 (2009): 121-126.

4 https://www.webmd.com/vitamins/ai/ingredientmono-1003/selenium. Accessed Nov. 25, 2018.

Ichthyosis Vulgaris

1 *The Merck Manual of Diagnosis and Therapy*, 16th ed. (1992), 2447.

2 https://www.mayoclinic.org/diseases-conditions/ichthyosis-vulgaris/symptoms-causes/syc-20373754. Accessed Dec. 18, 2018.

3 https://www.mayoclinic.org/diseases-conditions/ichthyosis-vulagaris/symptoms-causes-syc-20373754. Accessed Dec. 16, 2018.

4 https://www.dermnetnz.org/topics/ichthyosis/. Accessed May 17, 2020.

5 https://wwwwebmd.com-skin-problems-and-treatments/what-is-ichthyosis#3. Accessed Dec. 16, 2018.

6 G. Sethuramany et al., "Vitamin D: A New Promising Therapy for Congenital Ichthyosis," *Pediatrics* 137, no. 1 (Jan. 2016). http://pediatrics.aappublications.org/content/137/1/e20151313.

7 W. Levy, "Effect of Vitamin B12 on Ichthyosis," *Lancet* 2 (1952): 144.

8 A. Lodin et al., "Vitamin B12 in the Treatment of Congenital Ichthyosiform Eryththroderma," *Acta Derm Veneral* 38 (1958): 51-67.

9 A.R. Gaby, "Nutrient of the Month: Vitamin B12, Part 11," *Nutrition and Healing* 5, no. 7 (Aug. 1995): 4.

10 H.G. Rapaport, H. Herman, and E. Lehman, "Treatment of Ichthyosis with Vitamin A," *J Pediatrics* 21, no. 6 (1942): 733-746.

Immune System Dysfunction/Immunodeficiency

1 https://www.niaid.nih.gov/research/immune-system-overview. Accessed Feb. 8, 2021.

2 W.R. Beisel et al., "Single-Nutrient Effects on Immunologic Functions." Report of a workshop sponsored by the Department of Food and Nutrition and its nutrition advisory group of the American Medical Association, *JAMA* 245, no. 1 (Jan. 2, 1981): 53-58.

3 J. Duchateau et al., "Beneficial Effects of Oral Zinc Supplementation on the Immune Response of Old People," *Am J Med* 70, no. 5 (May 1981): 1001-1004.

Incontinence (Bowel)

1 https://www.ncbi.nlm.nih.gov/pmc/articles/PMC2780124/. Accessed Nov. 16, 2018.

2 https://www.ncbi.nlm.nih.gov/pmc/articles/PMC4020129/. Accessed Nov. 16, 2018.

3 https://www.niddk.nih.gov/health-information/digestive-diseases/bowel-control-problems-fecal-incontinence/treatment. Accessed Nov. 16, 2018.

4 L.H. Siegel, "The Control of Ileostomy and Colostomy Odors," *Gastroenterology* 38 (1960): 634-636.

5 M. Weingarten and B. Payson, "Deodorization of Colostomies with Chlorophyll," *Rev Gastroenterol* 18, no. 8 (1951): 602-604.

6 https://lpi.oregonstate.edu/mic/dietary-factors/phytochemicals/chlorophyll-chlorophyllin #reference24. Accessed Nov. 20, 2018.

7 S. Badvie and H.J.N. Andreyev, "Topical Phenylephrine in the Treatment of Radiation-Induced Fecal Incontinence," *Clinical Oncology* [Royal College of Radiologists (Great Britain)] 17, no. 2 (2005): 122-126. DOI: 10.1016/j.clon.2004.07.011.

Incontinence (Urinary)

1 B.G. Wells et al., *Pharmacotherapy Handbook*, 9th ed. (McGraw Hill Education, 2012), 866.

2 Ibid., 867.

3 https://www.nia.nih.gov/health/urinary-incontinence-older-adults. Accessed Apr. 19, 2020.

4 https://www.news-medical.net/news/20100720/Benefits-of-drug-L-methionine-for-neurogenic-bladder-disorders-unclear.aspx. Accessed Nov. 14, 2018.

5 G. Rosenberg, "Dl-Methionine in Urinary Incontinence," *Can Med Assoc J* 79, no. 2 (July 1958): 123, 148.

6 https://www.webmd.com/urinary-incontinence-oab/urinary-incontinence-diet-medications-chart#1. Accessed Nov. 14, 2018.

7 P.S. Vasavada and R.R. Rackley, "Electrical Stimulation in Storage and Emptying Failure," *Campbell-Walsh Urology*, 10th ed., eds. A.J. Wein et al. (Philadelphia: Elsevier Health Science, Inc., 2011), 377-381.

Infantile Colic

1 https://www.mayoclinic.org/diseases-conditions/colic/symptoms-causes/syc-20371074. Accessed Dec. 10, 2018.

2 American Academy of Pediatrics, Committee on Nutrition, "Soy Protein-Based Formulas: Recommendations for Use in Infant Feeding," *Pediatrics* 101, no. 1 (1998): 149-153.

3 A.E.M. Khier, "Infantile Colic, Facts and Fiction," *Ital J Pediatr* 38 (2012): 34.

4 F. Savino et al., "Lactobacillus Reuteri (American Type Culture Strain 55730) versus Simethicone in the Treatment of Infantile Colic: A Prospective Randomized Study," *Pediatrics* 119, no. 1 (2007): 2124-2130.

5 F. Savino et al., "*Lactobacillus reuteri* DSM 17938 in Infantile Colic: A Randomized, Double-Blind, Placebo-Controlled Trial," *Pediatrics* 126, no. 3 (2010): e526-e533.

6 D.M. Roberts, M. Ostapchuk, and J.G. O'Brien, "Infantile Colic," *Am Fam Physician* 70, no. 4 (2004): 735-740.

7 D. Dobson et al., "Manipulative Therapies for Infantile Colic," *Cochrane* (2012). https://www.cochrane.org/CD004796/BEHAV_manipulative-therapies-for-infantile-colic. Accessed Dec. 10, 2018.

8 J.M.M. Wiberg, J. Nordsteen, and N. Nilsson, "Short-Term Effect of Spinal Manipulation in the Treatment of Infantile Colic: A Randomized Controlled Clinical Trial with a Blinded Observer," *J Manipulative Physiol Ther* 22, no. 8 (Oct. 1999): 517-522.

9 C. Mercer and B. Nook, "The Efficacy of Chiropractic Spinal Adjustments as a Treatment Protocol in the Management of Infantile Colic," *5th Biennial Congress of the World Federation of Chiropractic*, eds. S. Haldeman and B. Murphy (Auckland, New Zealand: 1999), 170-171.

10 https://www.webmd.com/vitamins/ai/ingredientmono-311/fennel. Accessed Mar. 2, 2019.

11 https://wwwrxlist.com/fennel/supplements.htm. Accessed Mar. 2, 2019.

Infections

1 https://www.medicalnewstoday.com/articles/325798#benefits. Accessed May 6, 2020.

2 https://www.liebertpub.com/doi/abs/10.1089/fpd.2018.2594?rfr_dat=cr_pub%3Dpubmed&url_ver=Z39.88-2003&rfr_id=ori%3Arid%3Acrossref.org&journalCode=fpd&. Accessed June 5, 2020.

3 https://www.drugs.com/npp/oregano.html. Accessed June 5, 2020.

4 https://www.ncbi.nlm.nih.gov/pmc/articles/PMC4659158/. June 5, 2020.

5 A. Murkies, "Phytoestrogens—What Is the Current Knowledge?," *Aust Fam Physician*, Brighton Medical Clinic, Victoria 27, Suppl. 1 (Jan. 1998): S47-S51.

6 https://www.ncbi.nlm.nih.gov/pmc/articles/PMC3609166/. Accessed June 14, 2020.

7 https://www.medicalnewstoday.com/articles/321108#seven-best-natural-antibiotics. Accessed June 14, 2020.

8 https://pubmed.ncbi.nlm.nih.gov/32319538/. Accessed July 27, 2020.

9 https://www.researchgate.net/publication/7605866_Zinc_and_infection_A_review. Accessed July 27, 2020.

10 https://medicalxpress.com/news/2020-07-scientists-perspectives-zinc-intake-covid-.html. Accessed July 27, 2020.

Infertility

1 https://www.mayoclinic.org/diseases-conditions/infertility/symptoms-causes/syc-20354317. Accessed Dec. 20, 2018.

2 P.A. Regidor and A.E. Schindler, "Myoinositol as a Safe and Alternative Approach in the Treatment of Infertile PCOS Women: A German Observational Study," *Int J Endocrinol* (2016). Published online Aug. 23, 2016. DOI: 10.1155/2016/9537632.

3 H. Henmi et al., "Effects of Ascorbic Acid Supplementation on Serum Progesterone Levels in Patients with a Luteal Phase Defect," *Fertil Steril* 80 (2002): 459-461.

4 https://link.springer.com/article/10.1007/s10815-020-01906-3. Accessed Dec. 10, 2020.

5 G. Vitali, R. Parente, and C. Melotti, "Carnitine Supplementation in Human Idiopathic Asthenospermia: Clinical Results," *Drugs Exp Clin Res* 21, no. 4 (1995): 157-159. (PubMed)

6 M. Costa et al., "L-Carnitine in Idiopathic Asthenozoospermia: A Multicenter Study. Italian Study Group on Carnitine and Male Infertility," *Andrologia* 26, no. 3 (1994): 155-159.

7 A.R. Gaby, "Nutrient of the Month: The Study of L-Carnitine," *Nutrition and Healing* 2, no. 4 (1995): 4.

8 A. Fallah et al., "Zinc Is an Essential Element for Male Fertility: A Review of Zn Roles in Men's Health, Germination, Sperm Quality, and Fertilization," *J Reprod & Infert* 19, no. 2 (2018): 69-79.

9 https://www.ncbi.nlm.nih.gov/pmc/articles/PMC3783921/. Accessed Dec. 20, 2018.

10 E.T. Donnelly, N. McClure, and S.E. Lewis, "Glutathione and Hypotaurine in Vitro: Effects on Human Sperm Motility, DNA Integrity and Production of Reactive Oxygen Species," *Mutagenesis* 15 (2000): 61-68.

11 H. Kodama et al., "Increased Oxidative Deoxyribonucleic Acid Damage in Spermatozoa of Infertile Male Patients," *Fertil Steril* 68 (1997): 519-524.

12 E. Donnelly, N. McClure, and S.E.M. Lewis, "The Effect of Ascorbate and Alpha-Tocopherol Supplementation in Vitro on DNA Integrity and Hydrogen Peroxide Induced DNA Damage in Human Spermatozoa," *Mutagenesis* 14 (1999): 505-512.

13 https://ods.od.nih.gov/factsheets/Selenium-HealthProfessional/. Accessed Nov. 19, 2018.

14 T.K. Jensen et al., "Associations of Fish Oil Supplement Use with Testicular Function in Young Men," *JAMA Netw Open* 3, no. 1 (2020): e1919462. DOI: 10.1001/jamanetworkopen.2019.19462. Accessed Feb. 6, 2020.

Influenza

1 M. Mumcuoglu et al., "Inhibition of Several Strains of Influenza Virus and Beneficial Effect of Sambucol in the Treatment of Naturally Occurring Influenza B in a Double-Blind Preliminary Study," *International Congress for Infectious Diseases*, Abstract #1271 (Prague: Apr. 1994), 392.

2 https://www.webmd.com/vitamins/ai/ingredientmono-434/elderberry. Accessed May 23, 2021.

3 https://pubmed.ncbi.nlm.nih.gov/9230243/. Accessed May 23, 2021.

4 J. Beran, E. Salapova, and M. Spajdel, "Inosine Pranobex Is Safe and Effective for the Treatment of Subjects with Confirmed Respiratory Viral Infections: Analysis and Subgroup Analysis from a Phase 4, Randomized, Placebo-Controlled, Double-Blind Study," *BMC Infect Dis* 16 (Nov. 2016): 648. DOI: 10.1186/s12879-016-1965-5.

Insect Stings and Bites (Prevention)

1 http://www.bestonlinemd.com/insect-bites-and-stings-treament-symptoms-and-prevention/. Accessed Nov. 16, 2018.

2 https://www.cdc.gov/niosh/docs/2010-117/pdfs/2010-117.pdf. Accessed Nov. 16, 2018.

3 https://www.webmd.com/first-aid/understanding-insect-bites-spider-bites-prevention. Accessed Nov. 16, 2018.

4 M.D. Scribner, "Zinc Sulfate and Axillary Perspiration Odor," *Arch Dermatol* 113, no. 9 (1977): 1302.

5 https://pubchem.ncbi.nlm.nih.gov/compound/vitamin_B1#section=Therapeutic-Uses. Accessed Nov. 17, 2018.

Insomnia

1 https://www.medicalnewstoday.com/articles/9155.php. Accessed Feb. 19, 2019.

2 T. Carr, "Sick and Tired," *Consumer Reports* 84, no. 3 (Mar. 2019): 35-37.

3 https://www.aafp.org/afp/2017/0701/p29.html. Accessed Jan. 29, 2021.

4 E. Ferracioli-Oda, A. Qawasmi, and M.H. Bloch, "Meta-Analysis: Melatonin for the Treatment of Primary Sleep Disorders," *PLoS ONE* 8, no. 5 (2013): e63773. https://doi.org/10.1371/journal.pone.0063773.

5 A.G. Wade et al., "Efficacy of Prolonged Release Melatonin in Insomnia Patients Aged 55-80: Quality of Sleep and Next Alertness Outcomes," *Current Medical Research and Opinion* 27, no. 10 (Aug. 2007): 2597-2605.

6 B. Alvarez et al., "The Delayed Sleep Phase Syndrome: Clinical and Investigative Findings in 14 Subjects," *Neurol Neurosurg Psychiatry* 55 (1992): 665-670.

7 M. Dahlitz et al., "Delayed Sleep Phase Syndrome Response to Melatonin," *Lancet* 337 (1991): 1121-1124.

8 https://www.medicinenet.com/melatonin-oral/article.htm#which_drugs_or_supplements_interact_with_melatonin-oral. Accessed Nov. 17, 2018.

9 B.G. Katzung, *Basic & Clinical Pharmacology*, 14th ed., A Lange Medical Book (2018), 1144.

10 V.P. Arcangelo and A.M. Peterson, *Pharmacotherapeutics for Advanced Practice: A Practical Approach*, 3rd ed. (Wolters Kluwer/Lippincott Williams & Wilkins, 2013), 124.

11 https://www.mayoclinic.org/diseases-conditions/insomnia/diagnosis-treatment/drc20355173. Accessed Nov. 17, 2018.

12 https://www.medicalnewstoday.com/articles/318088.php. Accessed Nov. 17, 2018.

13 S. Bent et al., "Valerian for Sleep: A Systematic Review and Meta-Analysis," *Am J Med* 119, no. 12 (Dec. 2006): 1005-1012. DOI: 10.1016/j.amjmed.2006.02.026.

14 V.P. Arcangelo and A.M. Peterson, *Pharmacotherapeutics for Advanced Practice: A Practical Approach*, 3rd ed. (Wolters Kluwer/Lippincott Williams & Wilkins, 2013): 125.

15 K. Inagawa et al., "Subjective Effects of Glycine Ingestion before Bedtime on Sleep Quality," *Sleep Biol. Rhythms* 4 (2006): 75-77. DOI: 10.1111/j.1479-8425.2006.00193.x.

16 W. Yamadera et al., "Glycine Ingestion Improves Subjective Sleep Quality in Human Volunteers, Correlating with Polysomnographic Changes," *Sleep Biol Rhythms* 5 (2007): 126-131. DOI: 10.1111/j.1479-8425.2007.00262.x.

17 https://www.webmd.com/vitamins/ai/ingredientmono-1072/glycine. Accessed Nov. 28, 2018.

18 https://web.stanford.edu/~dement/delayed.html. Accessed Jan. 23, 2019.

19 https://pubmed.ncbi.nlm.nih.gov/3090582/. Accessed July 23, 2021.

Intermittent Claudication (IC)

1 https://www.ncbi.nlm.nih.gov/pmc/articles/PMC1635612/. Accessed May 17, 2020.

2 https://www.aafp.org/afp/2006/0601/p1971.html. Accessed Feb. 14, 2021.

3 P. Neglen, P. Qvarfordt, and B. Eklof, "Peroral Magnesium Hydroxide Therapy and Intermittent Claudication," *Vasa* 14, no. 3 (1985): 285-288.

4 G. Brevetti et al., "Propionyl-L-Carnitine in Intermittent Claudication: Double-Blind, Placebo-Controlled, Dose Titration, Multicenter Study," *J Am Coll Cardiol* 26, no. 6 (1995): 1411-1416.

5 G. Brevetti, C. Diehm, and D. Lambert, "European Multicenter Study on Propionyl-L-Carnitine in Intermittent Claudication," *J Am Col Cardiol* 34, no. 5 (1999): 1618-1624.

6 https://lpi.oregonstate.edu/mic/health-disease/intermittent-claudication. Accessed Nov. 19, 2018.

7 G. Brevetti et al., "Increases in Walking Distance in Patients with Peripheral Vascular Disease Treated with L-Carnitine: A Double-Blind, Cross-Over Study," *Circulation* 77 (1988): 767-773.

8 A.R. Gaby, "Nutrient of the Month: The Story of L-Carnitine," *Nutrition & Healing* 2, no. 4 (1995): 4.

9 K.D. Tripathi, *Essentials of Medical Pharmacology*, 7th ed. (2013), 912.

10 J. Kleijnen and D. Mackerras, "Vitamin E for Intermittent Claudication," *Cochrane Database of Systematic Reviews* (Feb. 2000). DOI: 10.1002/14651858.CD000987.

11 https://www.medscape.com/viewarticle/456944. Accessed Nov. 19, 2018.

12 H.S. Smulski et al., "Placebo-Controlled, Double-Blind Trial to Determine the Efficacy of the Tibetan Plant Preparation Padma 28 for Intermittent Claudication," *Alternative Ther* 1, no. 3 (1995): 44-49.

13 http://altmedrev.com/archive/publications/3/3/222.pdf. Accessed Nov. 27, 2018.

14 J. O'Hara, "A Double-Blind Placebo-Controlled Study of Hexopal in the Treatment of Intermittent Claudication," *J Int Med Res* 13, no. 6 (1985): 322-327.

15 J. O'Hara, P.N. Jolly, and C.G. Nicol, "The Therapeutic Efficacy of Inositol Nicotinate (Hexopal) in Intermittent Claudication: A Controlled Trial," *Br J Clin Practice* 42 (1988): 377-383.

16 V.C.H. Tyson, "Treatment of Intermittent Claudication," *Practitioner* 223 (1979): 121-126.

17 H. Seckfort, "Treating Circulatory Problems with Inositol Nicotinic Acid Ester," *Med Klin* 10 (1959): 416-418.

18 R. Murphy, "The Effect of Inositol Nicotinate (Hexopal) in Patients with Raynaud's Phenomenon," *Clinical Trials Journal* 22, no. 6 (1985): 521-529.

19 https://openheart.bmj.com/content/6/1/e001011. Accessed Feb. 14, 2021.

Irritable Bowel Syndrome (IBS)

1 https://www.mayoclinic.org/diseases-conditions/irritable-bowel-syndrome/symptoms-causes/syc-20360016. Accessed Nov. 20, 2018.

2 https://emedicine.medscape.com/article/180389-treatment#d10. Accessed Nov. 20, 2018.

3 https://www.medicalnewstoday.com/articles/319995.php. Accessed Nov. 20, 2018.

4 W.D.W. Rees, B.K. Evan, and J. Rhodes, "Treating Irritable Bowel Syndrome with Peppermint Oil," *Br Med J* 2 (1979): 835.

5 J.H. Liu et al., "Enteric-Coated Peppermint-Oil Capsules in the Treatment of Irritable Bowel Syndrome: A Prospective, Randomized Trial," *J Gastroenterol* 32, no. 6 (Dec. 1997): 765-768.

6 G. Cappello et al., "Peppermint Oil (Mintoil) in the Treatment of Irritable Bowel Syndrome: A Prospective Double Blind Placebo-Controlled Randomized Trial," *Dig Liver Dis* 39, no. 6 (June 2007): 530-536.

7 S. Merat et al., "The Effect of Enteric-Coated, Delayed-Release Peppermint Oil on Irritable Bowel Syndrome," *Dig Dis Sci* 55, no. 5 (May 2010): 1385-1390.

8 H.G. Grigoleit and P. Grigoleit, "Peppermint Oil in Irritable Bowel Syndrome," *Phytomedicine* 12, no. 8 (Aug. 2005): 601-606.

9 C. Cremon et al., "Randomized Clinical Trial: The Analgesic Properties of Dietary Supplementation with Palmitoylethanolamide and Polydatin in Irritable Bowel Syndrome," *Ailment Pharmoacol Ther* 45, no. 7 (Apr. 2017): 909-922.

10 Y. Khayyat and S. Attar, "Vitamin D Deficiency in Patients with Irritable Bowel Syndrome: Does it Exist?," *Oman Med J* 30, no. 2 (Mar. 2015): 115-118. DOI: 10.5001/omj.2015.25.

11 https://www.webmd.com/vitamins/ai/ingredientmono-881/licorice. Accessed Mar. 2, 2019.

Kidney Failure/Renal Insufficiency/Chronic Kidney Disease (CKD)

1 T.K. Chen, D.H. Knicely, and M.E. Grams, "Chronic Kidney Disease Diagnosis and Management: A Review," *JAMA* 322, no. 13 (2019): 1294-1304. DOI: 10.1001/jama.2019.14745. Accessed Oct. 11, 2019.

2 J.T. DiPiro et al., *Pharmacotherapy: A Pathophysiologic Approach*, 6th ed. (McGraw-Hill, 2005), 821.

3 https://www.ncbi.nlm.nih.gov/pmc/articles/PMC2474786/. Accessed Mar. 15, 2019.

4 https://www.niddk.nih.gov/health-information/kidney-disease/chronic-kidney-disease-ckd/managing. Accessed May 4, 2021.

5 *The Merck Manual of Diagnosis and Therapy*, 14th ed. (1982), 895.

6 I. de Brito-Ashurst et al., "Bicarbonate Supplementation Slows Progression of CKD and Improves Nutritional Status," *J Am Soc Nephrol* 20 (July 16, 2009): 2075-2084.

7 R.K. Singh et al., "Randomized, Double-Blind, Placebo-Controlled Trial of Coenzyme Q10 in Patients with End-Stage Renal Failure," *Journal of Nutritional & Environmental Medicine* 13, no. 1 (2003): 13-22.

8 S.B. Jing et al., "Effect of Chitosan on Renal Function in Patients with Chronic Renal Failure," *J Pharm Pharmacol* 49 (1997): 721-723.

9 https://www.medscape.org/viewarticle/551577. Accessed Nov. 14, 2018.

10 https://www.webmd.com/vitamins/ai/ingredientmono-1026/l-carnitine. Accessed Nov. 14, 2018.

11 https://lpi.oregonstate.edu/mic/dietary-factors/L-carnitine#reference57. Accessed Nov. 14, 2018.

12 https://www.ncbi.nlm.nih.gov/pmc/articles/PMC3155231/. Accessed Jan. 6, 2019.

13 https://www.webmd.com/vitamins/ai/ingredientmono-662/turmeric. Accessed Nov. 14, 2018.

14 https://www.webmd.com/vitamins/ai/ingredientmono-1018/n-acetyl-cysteine. Accessed Nov. 17, 2018.

15 M. Walser, W.E. Mitch, and E. Abras, "Supplements Containing Amino Acids and Keto Acids in the Treatment of Chronic Uremia," *Kidney Int Suppl* 16 (Dec. 1983): S285-S289.

16 https://pubmed.ncbi.nlm.nih.gov/3090582/. Accessed July 23, 2021.

17 S.K. Mahajan et al., "Zinc Deficiency: A Reversible Complication of Uremia," *The American Journal of Clinical Nutrition* 35, no. 6 (1982): 1177-1183. DOI: 10.1093/ajcn/36.6.1177.

18 https://www.webmd.com/vitamins/ai/ingredientmono-1017/folic-acid. Accessed Feb. 11, 2019.

19 https://www.ncbi.nlm.nih.gov/pmc/articles/PMC3413920/. Accessed Apr. 29, 2019.

20 S. Klahr et al., "The Effects of Dietary Protein Restriction and Blood-Pressure Control on the Progression of Chronic Renal Disease," Modification of Diet in Renal Disease Study Group, *N Engl J Med* 330, no. 13 (1994): 877-884.

21 N. Goraya et al., "Dietary Acid Reduction with Fruits and Vegetables or Bicarbonate Attenuates Kidney Injury in Patients with a Moderately Reduced Glomerular Filtration Rate Due to Hypertensive Nephropathy," *Kidney Int* 81, no. 1 (2012): 86-93.

22 T. Banerjee et al., "High Dietary Acid Load Predicts ESRD among Adults with CKD," Centers for Disease Control and Prevention Chronic Kidney Disease Surveillance Team, *J Am Soc Nephrol* 26, no. 7 (2015): 1693-1700.

23 "KDIGO 2012 Clinical Practice Guideline for the Evaluation and Management of Chronic Kidney Disease," Kidney Disease: Improving Global Outcomes (KDIGO) CKD Work Group, *Kidney Int Suppl* 3, no. 1 (2013): 1-150.

24 M.B. Vieira et al., "Caffeine Consumption and Mortality in Chronic Kidney Disease: A Nationally Representative Analysis," *Nephrology Dialysis Transplantation* 34, no. 6 (Sept. 12, 2018). https://academic.oup.com/ndt/advance-article/doi/10.1093/ndt/gfy234/5063554.

25 T.D. Nolan and P.A. Friedman, "Agents Affecting Mineral Ion Homeostasis and Bone Turnover," in *Gilbert & Goodman's: The Pharmacological Basis of Therapeutics*, 13th ed. (2018), 896.

Kidney Stones

1 M.A. Papadakis and S.J. McPhee, *Current Medical Diagnosis & Treatment* (2019): ch. 23, 976.

2 G. Johansson et al., "Effects of Magnesium Hydroxide in Renal Stone Disease," *J Am Coll Nutr* 1 (1982): 179-185.

3 J.K. Aikana, "CRC Series on Cations of Biological Significance," *Magnesium: Its Biologic Significance* (1981): 97.

4 B. Ettinger et al., "Potassium-Magnesium Is an Effective Prophylaxis against Recurrent Calcium Oxalate Nephrolithiasis," *J Urol* 158 (Dec. 1997): 2069-2073.

5 K.E. Miller, "Tips from Other Journals: Magnesium-Potassium Citrate to Prevent Nephrolithiasis," *Am Fam Physician* 57, no. 8 (1998).

6 E.L. Prien Sr. and S.N. Gershoff, "Magnesium Oxide-Pyridoxine Therapy for Recurrent Calcium Oxalate Calculi," *J Urol* 112 (1974): 509-512.

7 T. Ohkawa et al., "Rice Bran Treatment for Patients with Hypercalciuric Stones: Experimental and Clinical Studies," *J Urol* 132 (1984): 1140-1145.

8 A.R. Gaby, "Study Shows Rice Bran Prevents Kidney Stones," *Nutrition & Healing* (Aug. 1995): 8.

9 T. Hirvonen et al., "Nutrient Intake and Use of Beverages and the Risk of Kidney Stones among Male Smokers," *Am J Epidem* 150, no. 2 (July 1999): 187-194.

10 G.C. Curhan et al., "Intake of Vitamins B6 and C and the Risk of Kidney Stones in Women," *JASN* 10, no. 4 (Apr. 1999): 840-845.

11 https://www.ncbi.nlm.nih.gov/pubmed/10625946. Accessed May 11, 2020.

12 https://www.renalandurologynews.com/home/departments/commentary/kidney-stone-prevention-fact-versus-fiction/.

13 https://pubmed.ncbi.nlm.nih.gov/18845701/. Accessed June 30, 2021.

14 https://www.medicinenet.com/kidney_stones_and_calcium/views.htm. Accessed June 30, 2021.

15 T.D. Nolan and P.A. Friedman, "Agents Affecting Mineral Ion Homeostasis and Bone Turnover," in *Gilbert & Goodman's: The Pharmacological Basis of Therapeutics*, 13th ed. (2018), 896.

16 https://www.renalandurologynews.com/home/departments/commentary/kidney-stone-prevention-fact-versus-fiction/.

17 https://www.ncbi.nlm.nih.gov/pmc/articles/PMC3413920/. Accessed Apr. 29, 2019.

18 A.D. Rule, J.C. Lieske, and V.M. Pais, "Management of Kidney Stones in 2020," *JAMA* 323, no. 19 (2020): 1961-1962. DOI: 10.1001/jama.2020.0662. Accessed Nov. 26, 2018.

Lead Poisoning

1 https://www.michigan.gov/lead/0,5417,7-310-65222_65234---,00.html. Accessed Nov. 15, 2018.

2 J.A. Simon and E.S. Hudes, "Relationship of Ascorbic Acid to Blood Lead Levels," *JAMA* 281, no. 24 (June 1999): 2289-2293.

3 https://www.ncbi.nlm.nih.gov/pubmed/510231. Accessed Nov. 15, 2018.

4 M.B. Zimmermann et al., "Iron Fortification Reduces Blood Lead Levels in Children in Bangalore, India," *Pediatrics* 117, no. 6 (2006): 2014-2021.

5 A.W. Wolf, E. Jimenez, and B. Lozoff, "Effects of Iron Therapy on Infant Blood Lead Levels," *J Pediatr* 143, no. 6 (2003): 789-795.

6 https://www.sciencedaily.com/releases/2016/10/161026135432.htm. Accessed Nov. 15, 2018.

7 https://www.ncbi.nlm.nih.gov/pmc/articles/PMC4303853/#B58-nutrients-07-00552. Accessed Nov. 16, 2018.

8 https://pubmed.ncbi.nlm.nih.gov/1304229/, Accessed Jan. 19, 2022.

Leber's Hereditary Optic Neuropathy (LHON)/Leber's Optic Neuropathy (LOA)

1 https://ghr.nlm.nih.gov/condition/leber-hereditary-optic-neuropathy. Accessed Mar. 25, 2019.

2 https://www.ncbi.nlm.nih.gov/pubmed/2685705. Accessed Sept. 3, 2018.

3 J.C.M. Brust, *Current Diagnosis and Treatment Neurology*, 2nd ed. (McGraw-Hill, 2012): 389-390.

4 https://www.webmd.com/vitamins/ai/ingredientmono-1078/idebenone. Accessed Nov. 14, 2018.

5 Y. Mashima et al., "Do Idebenone and Vitamin Therapy Shorten the Time to Achieve Visual Recovery in Leber Hereditary Optic Neuropathy?," *J Neuroophthalmol* 20 (2000): 166-170.

6 J. Gilroy and John Stirling Meyer, *Medical Neurology*, 3rd ed. (New York: Macmillan, 1975), 174.

7 W.S. Foulds et al., "Hydroxocobalamin in the Treatment of Leber's Hereditary Optic Atrophy," *The Lancet* 291, no. 7548 (Apr. 27, 1968): 896-897.

8 A. Sadun et al., "Effect of EPI-743 on the Clinical Course of the Mitochondrial Disease Leber's Hereditary Optic Neuropathy," *Arch Neurol* 69 (2012): 331-338.

Leigh Syndrome (Encephalopathy)

1 https://ghr.nlm.nih.gov/condition/leigh-syndrome. Accessed Mar. 25, 2019.

2 "Vitamin Deficiency and Excess," *Harrison's Principles of Internal Medicine*, 13th ed., 475.

3 https://rarediseases.org/rare-diseases/leigh-syndrome/. Accessed Jan. 3, 2019.

4 https://www.news-medical.net/health/Leighs-Syndrome-Management.aspx. Accessed May 11, 2020.

5 https://jnnp.bmj.com/content/85/3/257. Accessed Apr. 13, 2020.

6 *BMJ Case Reports* (2013). Published online Oct. 7, 2013.

Leiner Disease

1 https://www.dermnetnz.org/topics/leiner-disease/. Accessed Dec. 19, 2018.

2 A. Nisenson, "Seborrheic Dermatitis of Infants and Leiner's Disease: A Biotin Deficiency," *The Journal of Pediatrics* 51, no. 5 (Nov. 1957): 537-548.

Leprosy

1 M. Gupta et al., "Zinc Therapy in Dermatology: A Review," *Dermatol Res Pract* (2014). Published online July 10, 2014. DOI: 10.1155/2014/709152.

Leukemia

1 https://www.medicinenet.com/leukemia/article.htm. Accessed Dec. 19, 2018.

2 https://www.medicalnewstoday.com/articles/319017.php. Accessed Sept. 3, 2018.

3 L. Cimmino et al., "Restoration of TET2 Function Blocks Self-Renewal in Leukemia Progression," *Cell* 170, no. 6 (Sept. 2017): 1079-1095. DOI: https://doi.org/10.1016/j.cell.2017.07.032.

4 K. Schonberger and N. Cabezas-Wallsheid, "Vitamin C: C-ing a New Way to Fight Leukemia," *Stem Cell* 5, no. 2 (2017): 561-563.

5 *Cleveland Clinic Journal of Medicine* 18, no. 1 (Jan. 1951): 35-41.

6 https://www.mdedge.com/ccjm/article/89984/cutaneous-sensitivity-monoglycerol-para-aminobenzoate. Accessed Dec. 26, 2018.

7 http://scienceinfoworld.blogspot.com/2012/11/para-aminobenzoic-acid-paba.html. Accessed Dec. 26, 2018.

8 http://www.winchesterhospital.org/health-library/article?id=21831. Accessed Sept. 13, 2018.

Leukoplakia

1 https://www.rxlist.com/consumer_lycopene/drugs-condition.htm. Accessed May 10, 2019.

Liver Disease—Alcoholic Hepatitis/Cirrhosis

1 *The Washington Manual of Medical Therapeutics*, 34th ed., 879.

2 J.T. DiPiro et al., *Pharmacotherapy: A Pathophysiologic Approach*, 6th ed. (McGraw-Hill, 2005), 693.

3 E.T. Bope and R.D. Kellerman, *Conn's Current Therapy*, 14th ed. (Philadelphia: Elsevier/Saunders), 546.

4 https://www.healthguideinfo.com/liver-disease/p17200/. Accessed Feb. 10, 2019.

5 A.B.M. Abdullah, *Practical Manual in Clinical Medicine* (Philadelphia: Jaypee—The Health Sciences Publisher, 2017), 350.

6 A.B.M. Abdullah, *Practical Manual in Clinical Medicine* (Philadelphia: Jaypee—The Health Sciences Publisher, 2017): 314.

7 https://pubmed.ncbi.nlm.nih.gov/27979049/. Accessed Jan. 7, 2021.

8 S. Khan et al., "Current Therapies in Alleviating Liver Disorders and Cancers with a Special Focus on the Potential of Vitamin D," *Nutr & Metab* (Lond) 15, no. 13 (Dec. 15, 2018). https://doi.org/10.1186/s12986-018-0251-5.

9 https://www.academia.edu/33028477/Clinical_Nutrition_Fourth_Edition?email_work_card=view-paper. p.127. Accessed May 15, 2020.

10 https://www.webmd.com/vitamins/ai/ingredientmono-1026/l-carnitine. Accessed Nov. 14, 2018.

11 https://www.webmd.com/vitamins/ai/ingredientmono-1018/n-acetyl-cysteine. Accessed Nov. 17, 2018.

12 P.J. Thuluvath and D.R. Triger, "Selenium in Chronic Liver Disease," *J Hepatol* 14, no. 2-3 (Mar. 1992): 176-182.

13 https://www.researchgate.net/publication/19443808_Selenium_alcohol_and_liver_diseases. Accessed Nov. 26, 2018.

14 G. Wenzel et al., "Alkoholtoxische Hepatitis—Eine 'Frei Radikale' Assoziierte Erkrankung. Letalitatssenkung Durch Adjuvante Antioxidantientherapie," *Inn Med* 48 (1993): 490-496.

15 https://www.ncbi.nlm.nih.gov/pmc/articles/PMC3959115/. Accessed July 15, 2020.

16 "Milk Thistle: Effects on Liver Disease and Cirrhosis and Clinical Adverse Effects," *Summary, Evidence Report/Technology Assessment* 21 (Rockville, MD: Agency for Healthcare Research and Quality, Sept. 2000). AHRQ Publication Number 01-E024. http://text.nlm.nih.gov/ftrs/directBrowse.pl?collect=epc&dbName=milktsum. Accessed Sept. 2, 2019.

17 P. Ferenci et al., "Randomized Controlled Trial of Silymarin Treatment in Patients with Cirrhosis of the Liver," *J Hepatol* 9 (1989): 105-113.

Liver Disease—Viral Hepatitis

1 Hepatitis C Technical Advisory Group, National Hepatitis C Program Office, "Complementary and Integrative Medicine for Hepatitis C," 2005. https://www.hepatitis.va.gov/provider/reviews/alternative-medicine.asp. Accessed Nov. 28, 2018.

2 https://zeenews.india.com/exclusive/hepatitis-b-is-100-times-more-infectious-than-hiv_3278.html. Accessed Sept. 2, 2020.

3 https://pubmed.ncbi.nlm.nih.gov/27979049/. Accessed Jan. 7, 2021.

4 G. Rasi et al., "Combination Thymosin-Alpha 1: A Lymphoblastoid Interferon Treatment in Chronic Hepatitis C," *Gut* 39 (1996): 679-683.

5 A.R. Gaby, "Nutrient of the Month: Vitamin B12, Part 11," *Nutrition and Healing* 5, no. 7 (Aug. 1995): 3-4.

6 https://www.webmd.com/vitamins/ai/ingredientmono-1024/taurine. Accessed Nov. 28, 2018.

Low Birth Weight Infants

1 https://www.child-encyclopedia.com/prematurity/according-experts/effective-early-intervention-programs-low-birth-weight-premature. Accessed Apr. 29, 2021.

2 https://pediatrics.aappublications.org/content/102/Supplement_E1/1293. Accessed Apr. 29, 2021.

3 https://www.pregnancycorner.com/giving-birth/complications/low-birth-weight.html. Accessed May 28, 2019.

4 J. Tyson et al., "Vitamin A Supplementation for Extremely Low Birth Weight Infants," *New Engl J of Med* 340, no. 25 (June 24, 1999): 1962-1968.

5 "Anemia Due to Other Nutritional Deficiencies," *Williams Hematology* (2011): ch. 39.

6 A. Slomski, "More Folic Acid for Pregnant Smokers," *JAMA* 321, no. 2 (2019): 1965. DOI: 10.1001/jama.2019.6681. Accessed May 28, 2019.

Lupus (Discoid)

1 https://www.medicalnewstoday.com/articles/319472. Accessed May 11, 2020.

2 https://www.ncbi.nlm.nih.gov/pubmed/759121. Accessed May 11, 2020.

3 C. Yildirim-Toruner and B. Diamond, "Current and Novel Therapeutics in the Treatment of Systemic Lupus Erythematosus," *The Journal of Allergy and Clinical Immunology* 127, no. 2 (2011): 303-412, quiz 313-314.

Lupus (Systemic Lupus Erythematosus)

1 *The Washington Manual of Medical Therapeutics*, 33rd ed., 1226.

2 https://www.ncbi.nlm.nih.gov/books/NBK535405/. Accessed Apr. 29, 2021.

3 https://www.lupus.org/resources/common-symptoms-of-lupus. Accessed Mar. 16, 2019.

4 *The Washington Manual of Medical Therapeutics*, 34th ed., 1228.

5 http://www.winchesterhospital.org/health-library/article?id=21831. Accessed Dec. 26, 2018.

6 https://www.rheumatologyadvisor.com/2017/03/06/lupus-using-diet-and-nutrition-to-improve-symptoms-and-outcomes/. Accessed Oct. 21, 2019.

7 https://www.medicalnewstoday.com/articles/323665.php. Accessed Dec. 26, 2018.

8 R.F. Van Vollenhoven et al., "Dehydroepiandrosterone in Systemic Lupus Erythematosus," *Arthritis Rheum* 38 (1995): 1826-1831.

9 https://www.hopkinslupus.org/lupus-treatment/lupus-medications/. Accessed Jan. 12, 2019.

10 https://www.mayoclinic.org/diseases-conditions/lupus/diagnosis-treatment/drc-20365790. Accessed Sept. 3, 2018.

11 https://www.ncbi.nlm.nih.gov/pubmed/17143589. Accessed May 11, 2020.

12 C. Lourdudoss et al., "The Association Between Diet and Glucocorticoid Treatment in Patients with SLE," *Lupus Science & Medicine* 3 (2016): e000135. DOI: 10.1136/lupus2015-000135.

13 https://www.emedicinehealth.com/para-aminobenzoic_acid_paba/vitamins-supplements.htm. Accessed Dec. 26, 2018.

14 https://www.mdedge.com/ccjm/article/89984/cutaneous-sensitivity-monoglycerol-para-aminobenzoate. Accessed Dec. 26, 2018.

15 *Cleveland Clinic Journal of Medicine* 18, no. 1 (Jan. 1951): 35-41.

16 D.F. Bradley, "Subacute Disseminated Lupus Erythematosus; Report of a Case Treated with Para-Aminobenzoic Acid," *New Orleans Med Surg J* 102, no. 2 (Aug. 1949): 83-85.

17 H. Black, "The Treatment of Lupus Erythematosus with Mepacrine and Para-Amino-Benzoic Acid," *Brit J Dermatol* 65, no. 6 (June 1952): 195-203.

18 https://www.sciencedirect.com/science/article/abs/pii/S1568997219301995?via%3Dihub. Accessed Dec. 1, 2019.

19 https://www.ncbi.nlm.nih.gov/pmc/articles/PMC4185297/. Accessed Jan. 23, 2019.

Macular Degeneration/Age-Related Macular Degeneration (AMD)

1 A.A. Khan et al., "Resveratrol Regulates Pathologic Angiogenesis by a Eukaryotic Elongation Factor-2 Kinase-Regulated Pathway," *American Journal of Pathology* (2010). DOI: 10.2353/ajpath.2010.090836.

2 "Clinical Briefs," *Am Fam Phys* (1989): 275.

3 A.F. Shaughnessy, "Lutein Improves Vision in Men with Macular Degeneration," *Am Fam Physician* 70, no. 8 (Oct. 15, 2004): 1556-1557.

4 https://www.emedicinehealth.com/vitamin_c_ascorbic_acid/vitamins-supplements.htm. Accessed Sept. 11, 2018.

5 https://www.webmd.com/eye-health/macular-degeneration/age-related-macular-degeneration-treatment#1. Accessed Nov. 18, 2018.

6 https://nccih.nih.gov/health/vitamins. Accessed Nov. 18, 2018.

7 https://www.webmd.com/vitamins/ai/ingredientmono-938/coenzyme-q10. Accessed Nov. 18, 2018.

8 https://www.macular.org/latest-research. Accessed May 31, 2020.

9 https://pubmed.ncbi.nlm.nih.gov/25091551/. Accessed Mar. 22, 2021.

10 Robert Abel Jr., MD, *Age Related Macular Degeneration in Integrative Medicine*, 4th ed. (2018) 838-846. https://www.mountsinai.org/health-library/supplement/vitamin-b9-folic-acid. Accessed Jan. 22, 2021.

Maple Syrup Urine Disease (MSUD)

1 https://rarediseases.org/rare-diseases/maple-syrup-urine-disease/. Accessed Feb. 10, 2019.

2 https://rarediseases.org/rare-diseases/maple-syrup-urine-disease/. Accessed Sept. 11, 2018.

3 *The Merck Manual of Diagnosis and Therapy*, 14th ed. (1982), 964.

4 https://www.msud-support.org/newsletters/113-volume-31-2/592-thiamin-responsive-maple-syrup-urine-disease. Accessed Apr. 13, 2020.

Measles/Rubeola

1 https://www.cdc.gov/measles/about/complications.html. Accessed Mar. 18, 2019.

2 https://www.ncbi.nlm.nih.gov/books/NBK448068/. Accessed Jan. 6, 2022.

3 D.A. Ross, "Recommendations for Vitamin A Supplementation," *The Journal of Nutrition* 132, no. 9 (Sept. 2002): 2902S-2906S. https://doi.org/10.1093/jn/132.9.2902S. Accessed Sept. 12, 2018.

4 https://www.webmd.com/vitamins/ai/ingredientmono-964/vitamin-a.

5 https://www.cochrane.org/CD001479/ARI_vitamin-a-for-measles-in-children. Accessed Jan. 5, 2022.

6 https://www.cdc.gov/measles/hcp/index.html. Accessed Jan. 5, 2022.

Melanoma

1 https://www.ncbi.nlm.nih.gov/pubmed/17505263. Accessed Mar. 24, 2019.

2 C.A. Gamba et al., "Aspirin Is Associated with Lower Melanoma Risk among Postmenopausal Caucasian Women: The Women's Health Initiative," *Cancer* 119 (2013): 1562-1569.

3 https://www.ncbi.nlm.nih.gov/pmc/articles/PMC4314970/. Accessed May 23, 2019.

4 "Vitamins and Cancer," *Postgraduate Medicine* 82, no. 3 (Sept. 1987): 149.

5 *Journal of Investigative Dermatology.* https://www.webmd.com/melanoma-skin-cancer/news/20120301/vitamin-a-may-help-reduce-melanoma-risk. Accessed Nov. 20, 2018.

6 https://www.mdedge.com/dermatology/article/215102/acne/ketogenic-diet-and-dermatology-primer-current-literature/page/0/1. Accessed Jan. 30, 2020.

7 L.C. Clark et al., "Effects of Selenium Supplementation for Cancer Prevention Inpatients with Carcinoma of the Skin," *JAMA* 276 (1996): 1957-1963.

Melasma/Chloasma

1 S.W. Yenny and W. Lestari, "A Study Comparing the Use of 10% L-Ascorbic Acid and 10% Zinc Sulfate Solution in the Treatment of Melasma," *Malaysian Journal of Dermatology (Dermatology Therapeutics)* 29 (Dec. 2012): 38-50.

2 J. Navarrete-Solís et al., "A Double-Blind, Randomized Clinical Trial of Niacinamide 4% versus Hydroquinone 4% in the Treatment of Melasma," *Dermatology Research and Practice*, Article ID 379173 (2011). DOI: 10.1155/2011/379173.

3 https://www.drugs.com/npp/emblica.html. Accessed Feb. 5, 2021.

4 https://www.webmd.com/vitamins/ai/ingredientmono-881/licorice. Accessed Mar. 2, 2019.

Memory Loss/Forgetfulness

1 J.J. Secades, "Citicoline: Pharmacological and Clinical Review, 2010 Update," *Rev Neurol* 52, Suppl. 2 (2011): S1-S62.

2 https://www.medscape.com/viewarticle/780283. Accessed Mar. 16, 2021.

3 M. Fioravanti and M. Yanagi, "Cytidinediphosphocholine (CDP-Choline) for Cognitive and Behavioral Disturbances Associated with Chronic Cerebral Disorders in the Elderly," *Cochrane Database Syst Rev* (Apr. 20, 2005). CD000269.

4 A.M. Cotroneo et al., "Effectiveness and Safety of Citicoline in Mild Vascular Cognitive Impairment: The IDEALE Study," *Clin Interv Aging* 8 (2013): 131-137.

5 J. Alvarez-Sabin et al., "Long-Term Treatment with Citicoline May Improve Poststroke Vascular Cognitive Impairment," *Cerebrovasc Dis* 35, no. 2 (2013): 146-154.

6 X.A. Alvarez et al., "Double-Blind Placebo-Controlled Study with Citicoline in APOE Genotyped Alzheimer's Disease Patients. Effects on Cognitive Performance, Brain Bioelectrical Activity and Cerebral Perfusion," *Methods Find Exp Clin Pharmacol* 21, no. 9 (1999): 633-644.

7 Oregon State University, "Choline." https://lpi.oregonstate.edu/mic/other-nutrients/choline. Accessed Nov. 2, 2018.

8 C. Poly et al., "The Relation of Dietary Choline to Cognitive Performance and White-Matter Hyperintensity in the Framingham Offspring Cohort," *Am J Clin Nutr* 94, no. 6 (2011): 1584-1591. (PubMed)

9 E. Nurk et al., "Plasma Free Choline, Betaine and Cognitive Performance: The Hordaland Health Study," *Br J Nutr* 109, no. 3 (2013): 511-519.

10 G.P. Vecchi et al., "Acetylcarnitine Treatment of Mental Impairment in the Elderly: Evidence from a Multi-Center Study," *Arch Gerontol Geriatr* Suppl 2 (1991): 159-168.

11 G. Vorberg, "Ginkgo Biloba Extract (GBE): A Long-Term Study of Chronic Cerebral Insufficiency in Geriatric Patients," *Clin Trials J* 22 (1985): 149-157.

12 J. Taillandier et al., "Ginkgo Biloba Extract in the Treatment of Cerebral Disorders Due to Aging," *Presse Med* 15 (1986): 1583-1587.

13 https://www.webmd.com/brain/memory-loss#1. Accessed Nov. 4, 2018.

14 https://www.webmd.com/vitamins/ai/ingredientmono-1072/glycine. Accessed Nov. 28, 2018.

15 https://www.mdedge.com/neurology/article/244147/alzheimers-cognition/flavonoids-dietary-powerhouses-cognitive-decline? Accessed Aug. 14, 2021.

16 R. Voelker, "How Certain Foods Affect Cognition, Seizures, and Cardiometabolic Disease: Food for Thought," *JAMA* 322, no. 18 (2019): 1753-1754. DOI: 10.1001/jama.2019.16477.

17 M.G. Miller, D.A. Hamilton, and J.A. Joseph, "Dietary Blueberry Improves Cognition among Older Adults in a Randomized, Double-Blind, Placebo-Controlled Trial," *Eur J Nutr* 57, no. 3 (Apr. 2018): 1169-1180. DOI: 10.1007/s00394-017-1400-8. Epub Mar. 10, 2017.

18 https://www.mdedge.com/neurology/article/216430/alzheimers-cognition/dietary-flavonol-intake-linked-reduced-risk-alzheimers. Accessed Mar. 15, 2021.

19 https://pubmed.ncbi.nlm.nih.gov/26635191/.

Meningitis

1 https://www.cdc.gov/meningitis/bacterial.html. Accessed Mar. 18, 2019.

2 https://www.researchgate.net/publication/16996741_Low_CSF_GABA_concentration_in_children_with_febrile_convulsions_untreated_epilepsy_and_meningitis. Accessed Jan. 3, 2019.

3 https://www.webmd.com/vitamins/ai/ingredientmono-464/gaba-gamma-aminobutyric-acid. Accessed Jan. 3, 2019.

4 https://www.rxlist.com/gaba_gamma-aminobutyric_acid/supplements.htm. Accessed Jan. 3, 2019.

Menkes Kinky Hair Syndrome

1 https://rarediseases.info.nih.gov/diseases/1521/menkes-disease. Accessed May 24, 2021.

2 https://emedicine.medscape.com/article/1180460-treatment#d9. Accessed Oct. 11, 2018.

3 https://www.ninds.nih.gov/Disorders/All-Disorders/Menkes-Disease-Information-Page. Accessed Oct. 11, 2018.

Menorrhagia

1 https://www.cdc.gov/ncbddd/blooddisorders/women/menorrhagia.html. Accessed Apr. 2, 2021.

2 https://www.medicalnewstoday.com/articles/295202.php. Accessed Dec. 20, 2018.

3 M.A. Chisolm-Burns et al., *Pharmacotherapy Principles & Practice* (McGraw-Hill Medical, 2008), 760.

4 https://pubmed.ncbi.nlm.nih.gov/7005780/. Accessed Sept. 27, 2020.

5 S.N. Lewin, MD, in Arielle Tschinkel, "Can Ibuprofen Really Reduce Your Period Flow." https://www.shape.com/lifestyle/mind-and-body/ibuprofen-heavy-period-flow. Accessed Sept. 27, 2020.

6 A. Lethaby, K. Duckitt, and C. Farquhar, "Non-Steroidal Anti-Inflammatory Drugs for Heavy Menstrual Bleeding," *Cochrane Database Syst Rev* 1 (2013). CD000400.

7 N.I.L. Taymor et al., "The Etiological Role of Chronic Iron Deficiency in Production of Menorrhagia," *JAMA* 187 (1964): 323-327.

8 A.J. Samuels, "Studies in Patients with Functional Menorrhagia: The Antihemorrhagic Effect of the Adequate Repletion of Iron Stores," *Isr J Med Sci* 1 (1965): 851-853.

9 https://www.medicalnewstoday.com/articles/295202.php. Accessed Nov. 14, 2018.

10 https://www.webmd.com/vitamins/ai/ingredientmono-1001/vitamin-c-ascorbic-acid. Accessed Nov. 14, 2018.

11 D.M. Lithgow et al., "Vitamin A in the Treatment of Menorrhagia," *S Afr Med J* 51 (1977): 191-193.

12 J. Keough, "Common Herbal Therapies" in *Shaum's Outlines in Pharmacology* (The McGraw-Hill Companies, Inc., 2010), 72.

13 https://www.webmd.com/vitamins/ai/ingredientmono-954/vitamin-e. Accessed Nov. 15, 2018.

Methylmalonic Acidemia

1 https://ghr.nlm.nih.gov/condition/methylmalonic-acidemia. Accessed Dec. 20, 2018.

2 https://medlineplus.gov/ency/article/001162.htm. Accessed May 24, 2021.

3 https://rarediseases.org/rare-diseases/acidemia-methylmalonic/. Accessed Dec. 9, 2018.

Migraine

1 https://www.medscape.org/viewarticle/946235?src=mkmcmr_driv_cust_mscpedu_210804-US-ANES-946235-cta. Accessed Aug. 4, 2021.

2 D.C. Buse et al., "Comorbid and Co-Occurring Conditions in Migraine and Associated Risk of Increasing Headache Pain Intensity and Headache Frequency: Results of the Migraine in America Symptoms and Treatment (MAST) Study," *J Headache Pain* 21, no. 1 (2020): 23.

3 C. Locher et al., "Efficacy, Safety, and Acceptability of Pharmacologic Treatments for Pediatric Migraine Prophylaxis: A Systematic Review and Network Meta-Analysis," *JAMA Pediatr.* Published online February 10, 2020. DOI: 10.1001/jamapediatrics.2019.5856.

4 B.G. Wells et al., *Pharmcotherapy Handbook*, 9th ed. (McGraw Hill Education), 545-546.

5 A. Mauskop et al., "Intravenous Magnesium Sulphate Relieves Migraine Attacks in Patients with Low Serum Ionized Magnesium Levels: A Pilot Study," *Clin Sci* 89 (1995): 633-636.

6 http://www.nyheadache.com/blog/emergency-treatment-of-headaches-with-intravenous-magnesium/. Accessed Feb. 3, 2020.

7 K. Weaver, "Magnesium and Migraine," *Headache* 30 (1990): 169.

8 T.L. Kopjas, "The Use of Folic Acid in Vascular Headache of the Migraine Type," *Headache* 8 (1969): 167-170.

9 C. Andrad, "Ginger for Migraine," *J Clin Psychiatry* 82, no. 6 (2021): 21f14325. https://doi.org/10.4088/JCP.21f14325.

10 K. Weaver, "Magnesium and Migraine," *Headache* 30 (1990): 168.

11 F. Faccinetti et al., "Magnesium Prophylaxis of Menstrual Migraine: Effects on Intracellular Magnesium," *Headache* 3, no. 1 (1991): 298-304.

12 M.M. Keifer, *Pocket Primary Care,* 2nd ed. (Wolters Kluver).

13 A. Peikert, C. Wilimzig, and R. Kohne-Volland, "Prophylaxis of Migraine with Oral Magnesium, Results from a Prospective, Multi-Center, Placebo-Controlled and Double-Blind Randomized Study," *Cephalgia* 16: (1996): 247-263.

14 B. Baker, "New Research Approach Helps Clarify Magnesium Migraine Link," *Family Pract News* (Aug. 15, 1993): 16.

15 W. Stoll, "Teen Headaches Disappear," *Med Tribune* (Mar. 31, 1982): 23.

16 J. Robblee, and A.J. Starling, "SEEDS for Success: Lifestyle Management in Migraine," *Cleve Clin J Med* 86, no. 11 (2019): 741-749. Accessed Feb. 24, 2020.

17 T.D. Rozen et al., "Open Label Trial of Coenzyme Q10 as a Migraine Preventive," *Cephalalgia* 22, no. 2 (Mar. 2002): 137-141. DOI: 10.1046/j.1468-2982.2002.00335.x.

18 V.P. Arcangelo and A.M. Peterson, *Pharmacotherapeutics for Advanced Practice: A Practical Approach*, 3rd ed. (Wolters Kluwer/Lippincott Williams & Wilkins, 2013): 121.

19 J. Schoenen, J. Jacquy, and M. Lenaerts, "Effectiveness of High-Dose Riboflavin in Migraine Prophylaxis. A Randomized Controlled Trial," *Neurology* 50 (1998): 466-470.

20 M. Condo et al., "Riboflavin Prophylaxis in Pediatric and Adolescent Migraine," *J Headache Pain* 10 (2009): 361-365.

21 A. Talebian et al., "Prophylactic Effect of Riboflavin on Pediatric Migraine: A Randomized, Double Blind, Placebo-Controlled Trial," *Electronic Physician* 10, no. 2 (Feb. 25, 2018): 6279-6285.

22 A. Rahimdel et al., "Effectiveness of Vitamin B2 versus Valproate in Migraine Prophylaxis: A Randomized Clinical Trial," *Electronic Physician* 7, no. 6 (Oct. 19, 2015): 1344-1348.

23 D. Magis et al., "A Randomized Double-Blind Placebo-Controlled Trial of Thioctic Acid in Migraine Prophylaxis," *Headache* 47 (2007): 47: 52-57.

24 https://medlineplus.gov/drufinfo/natural/957.html. Accessed Nov. 16, 2018.

25 F. Cerritelli et al., "Clinical Effectiveness of Osteopathic Treatment in Chronic Migraine: 3-Armed Randomized Controlled Trial," *Complementary Therapies in Medicine* 23, no. 2 (Apr. 2015): 149-156.

26 G.B. Parker, H. Tupling, and D.S. Prior, "A Controlled Trial of Cervical Manipulation for Migraine," *Aust NZ J Med* 8 (1978): 589-593.

27 J. Lance, *Migraine and Other Headaches* (New York: Scribner, 1986).

28 https://americanmigrainefoundation.org/resource-library/occipital-nerve-blocks/. Accessed Apr. 11, 2020.

29 https://www.sciencedirect.com/science/article/abs/pii/S1521689620300641?via%3Dihub.

30 W. Grossman and H. Schmidramsl, "An Extract of Petasites Hybridus Is Effective in the Prophylaxis of Migraine," *Alternative Medicine Review* 6, no. 3 (2001): 303-310.

31 J.C. Cash and C.A. Glass, *Family Practice Guidelines*, 4th ed. (Springer, 2017), 585.

32 https://pubmed.ncbi.nlm.nih.gov/32903062/.

33 G. Bono et al., "L5HT Treatment in Primary Headaches: An Attempt at Clinical Identification of Responsive Patients," *Cephalgia* 4 (1984): 163.

34 https://medlineplus.gov/druginfo/natural/794.html.

35 C. Theisler, *Migraine Headache Disease: Diagnostic and Management Strategies* (Aspen Publishers, 1990), 119.

36 P. Kangasniemi et al., "Levotryptophan Treatment in Migraine," *Headache: The Journal of Head and Face Pain* 18, no. 3 (1978): 161-166.

37 N.H. Raskin, *Headache*, 2nd ed. (Churchill Livingstone, 1980), 187.

38 https://pubmed.ncbi.nlm.nih.gov/16961791/. Accessed July 23, 2021.

Miscarriages (Habitual and Unexplained Losses)

1 www.ncbi.nlm.nih.gov/pmc/articles/PMC4229790. Accessed Nov. 17, 2018.

2 H. Shi et al., "NAD Deficiency, Congenital Malformations, and Niacin Supplementation," *N Engl J Med* 377 (2017): 544-552. DOI: 10.1056/NEJMoa1616361.

3 H. Baker et al., "Vitamin Profile of 563 Gravidas during Trimesters of Pregnancy," *J Am Coll Nutr* 21, no. 1 (Feb. 2002): 33-37.

4 M. D'Uva et al., "Hyperhomocysteinemia in Women with Unexplained Sterility or Recurrent Early Pregnancy Loss from Southern Italy: A Preliminary Report," *Thrombosis Journal* 5 (2007). DOI: 10.1186/1477-9560-5-10. Accessed Nov. 17, 2018.

Mitral Valve Prolapse

1 https://emedicine.medscape.com/article/759004-clinical. Accessed Feb. 5, 2021.

2 https://www.webmd.com/vitamins/ai/ingredientmono-998/magnesium. Accessed Nov. 18, 2018.

3 https://www.webmd.com/heart/mitral-valve-prolapse-symptoms-causes-and-treatment#1. Accessed Nov. 18, 2018.

4 M. Trivellato et al., "Carnitine Deficiency as the Possible Etiology of Idiopathic Mitral Valve Prolapse: Case Study with Speculative Annotation," *Texas Heart Inst J* 11 (1984): 370-376.

5 A.R. Gaby, "Nutrient of the Month: The Story of L-Carnitine," *Nutrition and Healing* 2, no. 4 (1995): 4.

Morning Sickness/Nausea of Pregnancy/Hyperemesis Gravidarum

1 https://www.acog.org/Patients/FAQs/Morning-Sickness-Nausea-and-Vomiting-of-Pregnancy. Accessed Nov. 19, 2018.

2 https://www.aafp.org/afp/2003/0701/p121.html. Accessed Nov. 19, 2018.

3 *Clinician Reviews* 9, no. 6 (1999): 1-16. Williams & Wilkins.

4 J.R. Niebyl and T. Murphy Goodwin, "Understanding and Treating Nausea and Vomiting of Pregnancy: Overview of Nausea and Vomiting of Pregnancy with an Emphasis on Vitamins and Ginger," *American Journal of Obstetrics and Gynecology* 186, no. 5, suppl. 2 (2002): S253-S255.

5 J.D. Quinlan and D. Ashley Hill, "Nausea and Vomiting of Pregnancy," *Am Fam Physician* 68, no. 1 (July 1, 2003): 121-128.

6 W. Fischer-Rasmussen et al., "Ginger Treatment of Hyperemesis Gravidarum," *Eur J Obstet Gynecol Reprod Biol* 38 (1991): 19-24.

7 T. Vutyavanich, S. Wongtra-ngan, and R. Ruangsri, "Pyridoxine for Nausea and Vomiting of Pregnancy: A Randomized, Double-Blind, Placebo-Controlled Trial," *American Journal of Obstetrics and Gynecology* 173, no. 3, pt. 1 (Sept. 1995): 881-884.

8 ACOG (American College of Obstetrics and Gynecology), "Practice Bulletin: Nausea and Vomiting of Pregnancy," *Obstet Gynecol* 103 (2004): 803-814.

9 American College of Obstetricians and Gynecologists. https://www.acog.org/Patients/FAQs/Morning-Sickness-Nausea-and-Vomiting-of-Pregnancy#feel. Accessed Nov. 19, 2018.

10 https://www.babycenter.com/morning-sickness#articlesection8. Accessed Nov. 19, 2018.

11 https://www.ncbi.nlm.nih.gov/pubmed/24829772/. Accessed Jan. 23, 2020.

Morphea

1 https://rarediseases.info.nih.gov/diseases/10485/morphea. Accessed Nov. 17, 2020.

2 www.medicalnewstoday.com/articles/320708.php. Accessed Nov. 19, 2018.

3 http://jddonline.com/articles/dermatology/S1545961613P0014X/1. Accessed Nov. 19, 2018.

4 S. Ayres Jr. and R. Mihan, "Vitamin E and Dermatology," *Cutis* 16 (1975): 1017-1021.

Motion Sickness/Travel Sickness/Car Sickness

1 R.R. Campitelli, "Motion Sickness Remedy from Postgraduate Medicine Pearls," *Postgraduate Medicine* 95, no. 6 (1994): 37.

2 *The Merck Manual of Diagnosis and Therapy*, 36th ed. (1992), 2522.

3 https://www.rxlist.com/gaba_gamma-aminobutyric_acid/supplements.htm. Accessed Jan. 3, 2019.

4 https://www.webmd.com/first-aid/how-to-beat-motion-sickness#2. Accessed Dec. 20, 2018.

5 https://www.webmd.com/drugs/2/drug-5680/benadryl-oral/details. Accessed Dec. 20, 2018.

Multiple Sclerosis

1 M.C. Levin, "Multiple Sclerosis (MS); Neurologic Disorders," *Merck Manuals Professional Edition* (Merck & Co., Inc., rev. Dec. 2019). https://www.merckmanuals.com/professional/neurologic-disorders/demyelinating-disorders/multiple-sclerosis-ms?query=multiple sclerosis.

2 https://www.mdedge.com/neurology/article/236681/multiple-sclerosis/vitamin-d-deficiency-linked-early-cognitive-impairment?ecd=wnl_evn_210303_mdedge_8pm&uac=.

3 E. Kočovská et al., "Vitamin-D Deficiency as a Potential Environmental Risk Factor in Multiple Sclerosis, Schizophrenia, and Autism," *Front Psychiatry* 8 (2017): 47. Accessed July 21, 2017.

4 S.M. Kimball, "Safety of Vitamin D_3 in Adults with Multiple Sclerosis," *The American Journal of Clinical Nutrition* 86, no. 3 (Sept. 2007): 645-651. https://doi.org/10.1093/ajcn/86.3.645.

5 J. Swanson, MD, "Vitamin D and MS: Is There Any Connection?." https://www.mayoclinic.org/diseases-conditions/multiple-sclerosis/expert-answers/vitamin-d-and-ms/faq-20058258. Accessed Nov. 20, 2018.

6 https://www.sciencedaily.com/releases/2016/01/160104080559.htm. Accessed Nov. 20, 2018.

7 A. Minkovsky et al., "High-Dose Biotin Treatment for Secondary Progressive Multiple Sclerosis May Interfere with Thyroid Assays," *AACE Clinical Case Reports* 2, no. 4 (Autumn 2016): e370-e373.

8 F. Sedel et al., "High Doses of Biotin in Chronic Progressive Multiple Sclerosis: A Pilot Study," *Mult Scler Relat Disord* 4, no. 2 (Mar. 2015): 159-169.

9 https://www.webmd.com/vitamins/ai/ingredientmono-313/biotin. Accessed Jan. 5, 2019.

10 http://n.neurology.org/content/86/16_Supplement/S49.005. Last accessed Jan. 5, 2019.

11 http://n.neurology.org/content/84/14_Supplement/PL2.002. Accessed Jan. 5, 2019.

12 T. Korwin-Piotrowska et al., "Experience of Padma 28 in Multiple Sclerosis," *Phytother Res* 6 (1992): 133-136.

13 A.R. Gaby, "Research Review," *Nutrition and Healing* 3, no. 3 (1996): 8.

14 https://www.webmd.com/vitamins/ai/ingredientmono-807/glucosamine-sulfate. Accessed Nov. 18, 2018.

15 https://n.neurology.org/content/90/15_Supplement/P2.349.abstract. Accessed Jan. 4, 2021.

Muscle Cramps/Leg Cramps

1 https://www.ncbi.nlm.nih.gov/books/NBK499895/. Accessed Mar. 7, 2021.

2 G.L. Young and D. Jewell, "Interventions for Leg Cramps in Pregnancy," *Cochrane Database Syst Rev* 1 (2002). CD000121.

3 C. Roffe et al., "Randomized, Cross-Over, Placebo Controlled Trial of Magnesium Citrate in the Treatment of Chronic Persistent Leg Cramps," *Med Sci Monit* 8, no. 5 (May 2002). CR326-30.

4 D.L. Bilbey and V.M. Prabhakaran, "Muscle Cramps and Magnesium Deficiency: Case Reports," *Canadian Family Physician* 42 (July 1996): 1348-1351.

5 L.O. Dahle et al., "The Effect of Oral Magnesium Substitution on Pregnancy Induced Leg Cramps," *Am J Obstet Gynecol* 173 (1995): 175-180.

6 *Physician's Desk Reference*, 36th ed. (1982), 1338.

7 G.L. Young and D. Jewell, "Interventions for Leg Cramps in Pregnancy," Cochrane Satabase of Systematic Reviews (Online). (2000). CD000121.

8 *Physician's Desk Reference*, 36th ed. (1982), 761.

9 https://www.webmd.com/diet/supplement-guide-potassium#1. Accessed Nov. 18, 2018.

10 https://www.webmd.com/sleep-disorders/leg-cramps.

11 R.E. Allen and K.A. Kirby, "Nocturnal Leg Cramps," *Am Fam Physician* 86, no. 4 (Aug. 15 2012): 350-355.

12 L. Butcher, "FDA Warns against Quinine for Muscle Cramps—Some Neurologists Ask Why," *Neurology Today* 10, no. 18 (Sept. 2010): 1-8.

13 K.C. Miller et al., "Reflex Inhibition of Electrically Induced Muscle Cramps in Hypohydrated Humans," *Med Sci Sports Exerc* 42, no. 5 (May 2010): 953-961. DOI: 10.1249/MSS.0b013e3181c0647e.

14 P. Chan et al., "Randomized, Double-Blind, Placebo-Controlled Study of the Safety and Efficacy of Vitamin B Complex in the Treatment of Nocturnal Leg Cramps in Elderly Patients with Hypertension," *J Clin Pharmacol* 38 (1998): 1151-1154.

15 https://www.cdc.gov/niosh/topics/heatstress/heatrelillness.html.

Muscle Cramps/Night (Nocturnal) Cramps

1 R.E. Allen and K.A. Kirby, "Nocturnal Leg Cramps," *Am Fam Physician* 86, no. 4 (Aug. 15, 2012): 350-355.

2 https://www.medicinenet.com/muscle_cramps/article.htm. Accessed Nov. 13, 2018.

3 https://www.emedicinehealth.com/muscle_cramps/article_em.htm#what_causes_muscle_cramps. Accessed Nov. 13, 2018.

4 https://www.medicalnewstoday.com/articles/180160.php. Accessed Nov. 13, 2018.

5 J.M. Hallegraeff et al., "Stretching Before Sleep Reduces the Frequency and Severity of Nocturnal Leg Cramps in Older Adults: A Randomised Trial," *J Physiother* 58, no. 1 (2012): 17-22.

6 https://www.medicinenet.com/muscle_cramps/article.htm#body_fluid_shifts_low_blood_calcium_and_low_potassium_muscle_cramps. Accessed Nov. 14, 2018.

7 https://www.medicalnewstoday.com/articles/321865.php. Accessed Nov. 13, 2018.

8 M. Hammar, L. Larsson, and L. Tegler, "Calcium Treatment of Leg Cramps in Pregnancy. Effect on Clinical Symptoms and Total Serum and Ionized Serum Calcium Concentrations," *Acta Obstet Gynecol Scand* 60, no. 4 (1981): 345-347.

9 K. Zhou et al., "Interventions for Leg Cramps during Pregnancy," *Cochrane Database of Systematic Reviews* 8 (Aug. 2015). CD010655. DOI: 10.1002/14651858.CD010655.pub2.

10 https://www.webmd.com/diet/supplement-guide-calcium#1. Accessed Nov. 13, 2018.

11 R.E. Allen and K.A. Kirby, "Nocturnal Leg Cramps," *Am Fam Physician* 86, no. 4 (Aug. 15, 2012): 350-355.

12 K.D. Tripathi, *Essentials of Medical Pharmacology*, 7th ed. (2013), 912.

13 S. Ayers and R. Mikan, "Nocturnal Leg Cramps (Systremma): A Progress Report on Response to Vitamin E," *S Calif Med* 111 (1969): 87-91.

14 M. Serrao et al., "Gabapentin Treatment for Muscle Cramps: An Open-Label Trial," *Clin Neuropharmacol* 23 (2000): 45-49.

15 http://n.neurology.org/content/74/8/691. Accessed Nov. 14, 2018.

16 L. Butcher, "FDA Warns against Quinine for Muscle Cramps—Some Neurologists Ask Why," *Neurology Today* 10, no. 18 (Sept. 2010): 1-8.

Muscle Pain (Myalgia)

1 https://pubmed.ncbi.nlm.nih.gov/12766976/. Accessed June 16, 2021.

2 J. Durlach, *Magnesium in Clinical Practice* (London: John Libbey, 1988), 360.

3 C. Zeana and G. Radu, "Magnesium in Preventing Muscular Cramps in Swimmers (Abstr)," *Magnes Res* 6 (1993): 73.

4 G.E. Abraham and J.D. Flechas, "Management of Fibromyalgia: Rationale for the Use of Magnesium and Malic Acid," *J Nutr Med* 3 (1992): 49-59.

5 https://www.webmd.com/vitamins/ai/ingredientmono-1024/taurine. Accessed Nov. 28, 2018.

6 https://www.medscape.com/viewarticle/876941. Accessed Dec. 20, 2018.

Muscle Performance and Damage (Related to Exercise)

1 D.M. Ahrendt, "Ergogenic Aids: Counseling the Athlete," *Am Fam Physician* 63 (2001): 913-923.

2 S.W. Muir and M. Montero-Odasso, "Effect of Vitamin D Supplementation on Muscle Strength, Gait and Balance in Older Adults: A Systematic Review and Meta-Analysis," *J Am Geriatr Soc* 59, no. 12 (2011): 2291-2300.

3 *The Merck Manual of Diagnosis and Therapy*, 19th ed., 1774.

4 https://www.ncbi.nlm.nih.gov/pmc/articles/PMC3761874/#R70. Accessed Dec. 14, 2020.

5 https://www.webmd.com/vitamins/ai/ingredientmono-522/msm-methylsulfonylmethane. Accessed Nov. 14, 2018.

6 https://www.ncbi.nlm.nih.gov/pmc/articles/PMC2579450/. Accessed Dec. 20, 2018.

7 M. Kaminski and R. Boal, "An Effect of Ascorbic Acid on Delayed-Onset-Muscle-Soreness," *Pain* 50, no. 3 (1992): 317-321.

8 P. Barlas et al., "Effects of Ascorbic and Acetylsalicylic Acids upon Objective Signs and Symptoms of Delayed Onset Muscle Soreness (DOMS) in Man." https://www.ncbi.nlm.nih.gov/pmc/articles/PMC1157831/pdf/jphysiol00328-0075.pdf. Accessed Dec. 20, 2018.

9 W.M. Staton, "The Influence of Ascorbic Acid Supplementation in Minimizing Post-Exercise Muscle Soreness in Young Men. *Res Q* 23 (1952): 356-360.

10 https://www.ncbi.nlm.nih.gov/pmc/articles/PMC3665020/. Accessed Dec. 20, 2018.

Myasthenia Gravis

1 https://www.ninds.nih.gov/Disorders/Patient-Caregiver-Education/Fact-Sheets/Myasthenia-Gravis-Fact-Sheet. Accessed Feb. 10, 2019.

2 https://www.ncbi.nlm.nih.gov/pmc/articles/PMC4734680/. Accessed Nov. 26, 2018.

3 https://www.webmd.com/vitamins/ai/ingredientmono-764/huperzine-a. Accessed Nov. 26, 2018.

Myocardial Infarction/Heart Attack

1 https://www.nhlbi.nih.gov/health-topics/heart-attack. Accessed Aug. 31, 2020.

2 N.G. Stephens et al., "Randomized Controlled Trial of Vitamin E in Patients with Coronary Disease: Cambridge Heart Antioxidant Study (CHAOS)," *The Lancet* 347 (Mar. 23, 1996): 781-786.

3 M.J. Stampfer et al., "Vitamin E Consumption and the Risk of Coronary Disease in Women," *N Engl J Med* 328 (1993): 1444-1449.

4 E.B. Rimm et al., "Vitamin E Consumption and the Risk of Coronary Heart Disease in Men," *N Engl J Med* 328 (1993): 1450-1456.

5 https://lpi.oregonstate.edu/mic/vitamins/vitamin-E. Accessed Nov. 20, 2018.

6 P. Knekt et al., "Antioxidant Vitamin Intake and Coronary Mortality in a Longitudinal Population Study," *Am J Epidemiol* 139 (1994): 1180-1189.

7 J.J. DiNicolantonio et al., "L-Carnitine in the Secondary Prevention of Cardiovascular Disease: Systematic Review and Meta-Analysis," *Mayo Clin Proc* 88, no. 6 (2013): 544-551.

8 P. Colonna and S. Iliceto, "Myocardial Infarction and Left Ventricular Remodeling: Results of the CEDIM Trial. Carnitine Ecocardiografia Digitalizzata Infarto Miocardico," *Am Heart J* 139 (2000): S124-S130. DOI: 10.1067/mhj.2000.103918.

9 P. Davini et al., "Controlled Study on L-Carnitine Therapeutic Efficacy in Post-Infarction," *Drugs Exp Clin Res* 18, no. 8 (1992): 355-365.

10 R.B. Singh et al., "A Randomized, Double-Blind, Placebo-Controlled Trial of L-Carnitine in Suspected Acute Myocardial Infarction," *Postgrad Med J* 72 (1996): 45-50. DOI: 10.1136/pgmj.72.843.45.

11 Y.X. Xue et al., "L-Carnitine as an Adjunct Therapy to Percutaneous Coronary Intervention for Non-ST Elevation Myocardial Infarction," *Cardiovasc Drugs Ther* 21 (2007): 445-448. DOI: 10.1007/s10557-007-6056-9.

12 J.L. Anderson et al., "Relation of Vitamin D Deficiency to Cardiovascular Risk Factors, Disease Status, and Incident Events in a General Healthcare Population," *Am J Cardiol* 106, no. 7 (2010): 963-968.

13 Ohio University, "Vitamin D3 Could Help Heal or Prevent Cardiovascular Damage," *ScienceDaily* (Jan. 30, 2018). www.sciencedaily.com/releases/2018/01/180130140242.htm.

14 Y.L. Le Thi et al., "Vitamin D Improves Cardiac Function after Myocardial Infarction through Modulation of Resident Cardiac Progenitor Cells," *Heart, Lung and Circulation* (2018). DOI: 10.1016/j.hlc.2018.01.006.

15 Y. Arnson et al., "Vitamin D inflammatory Cytokines and Coronary Events: A Comprehensive Review," *Clin Rev Allergy Immunol* (Jan. 12, 2013).

16 Daniel Weitz, MD, et al., "Fish Oil for the Treatment of Cardiovascular Disease," *Cardiol Rev* 18, no. 5 (Sept.-Oct. 2010): 258-263.

17 B.G. Brown et al., "Simvastatin and Niacin, Antioxidant Vitamins, or the Combination for the Prevention of Coronary Disease," *N Engl J Med* 345 (2001): 1583-1592.

18 https://www.researchgate.net/publication/8191782_Niacin_therapy_in_atherosclerosis. Accessed Nov. 19, 2018.

19 P.L. Canner et al., "Fifteen Year Mortality in Coronary Drug Project Patients: Long-Term Benefit with Niacin," *J Am Coll Cardiol* 8 (1986): 1245-1255.

20 G. Brown et al., "Regression of Coronary Artery Disease as a Result of Intensive Lipid-Lowering Therapy in Men with High Levels of Apolipoprotein B," *N Engl J Med* 323 (1990): 1289-1298.

21 H.A. Nieper, "Decrease in Incidence of Coronary Infarct by Mg- and K-Orotate and Bromelain," *Acta Med Empirica* 12 (1977): 614-618.

22 N.J. Talley, B. Frankum, and D. Currow, *Essentials of Internal Medicine*, 3rd ed. (Churchill Livingstone/Elsevier, 2015), 181.

23 https://www.medicinenet.com/heart_attack/article.htm#what_causes_a_heart_attack. Accessed Feb. 10, 2019.

24 Naval Branch Clinic Diego Garcia (Dr. Smith), Penn State University Family and Community Medicine Residency Program (Dr. Demetriou), Naval Hospital Okinawa (Dr. Weber), "Aspirin for Primary Prevention: USPSTF Recommendations for CVD and Colorectal Cancer," *J Fam Pract* 68, no. 3 (Apr. 2019): 146-151.

25 J.M. Guirguis-Blake et al., "Aspirin for the Primary Prevention of Cardiovascular Events: A Systematic Evidence Review for the U.S. Preventive Services Task Force," *Ann Intern Med* 164 (2016): 804-813.

26 Y. Ikeda et al., "Low-Dose Aspirin for Primary Prevention of Cardiovascular Events in Japanese Patients 60 years or Older with Atherosclerotic Risk Factors: A Randomized Clinical Trial," *JAMA* 312 (2014): 2510-2520.

27 M. Poplawski, N.K. Nelson, and J.S., "Rethinking Daily Aspirin for Primary Prevention," *J Fam Pract* 69, no. 9 (2020): 461-462. DOI: 10.12788/jfp.0092.

Myocarditis

1 *The Merck Manual of Diagnosis and Therapy*, 16th ed. (1992), 538.

2 http://jpma.org.pk/full_article_text.php?article_id=4257. Accessed Dec. 22, 2018.

3 https://www.webmd.com/vitamins/ai/ingredientmono-1026/l-carnitine. Accessed Nov. 14, 2018.

4 https://www.medicinenet.com/l-carnitine/supplements-vitamins.htm#Dosing. Accessed Nov. 26, 2018.

Nails—Beau's Lines/Onychorrhexis

1 "Toenail Ridges," *J Fam Pract* 71, no. 1 (Jan. 2022). DOI: 10.12788/jfp.0368.

2 https://www.webmd.com/skin-problems-and-treatments/what-to-know-about-onychorrhexis.

3 N. Scheinfeld, M.J. Dahdah, and R. Scher, "Vitamins and Minerals: Their Role in Nail Health and Disease," *J Drugs Dermatol* 6 (2007): 782-787.

4 G. Singh, "Nail Changes and Disorders in Elderly," *Nail and Its Disorders*, eds. S. Sacchidanand and A.S. Savitha (London: Jaypee Brothers Medical, 2013), ch. 6, 221-237.

5 D. Seshadri and D. De, "Nails in Nutritional Deficiencies," *Indian J Dermatol Venereol Leprol* 78, no. 3 (2012): 237-241.

6 R. Sarkany et al., "Metabolic and Nutritional Disorders," *Rook's Textbook of Dermatology*, eds. T. Burns et al. (John Wiley and Sons, 2010), 58-59, 76.

7 M.W Cashman and S.B Sloan, "Nutrition and Nail Disease," *Clin Dermatol* 28 (2010): 420-425.

8 *JAMA* (June 1990): 1753.

9 K. Weismann and H. Hoyer, "Zinc Deficiency Dermatoses. Etiology, Clinical Aspects and Treatment," *Hautarzt* 33, no. 8 (Aug. 1982): 405-410. [article in German]

Nails—Brittle Nail Syndrome/Onychoschizia

1 https://link.springer.com/article/10.1007/s13555-019-00338-x. Accessed May 28, 2021.

2 https://share.upmc.com/2018/03/brittle-nails-causes-treatments/.

3 https://www.aocd.org/page/BrittleSplittingNail. Accessed May 29, 2021.

4 https://www.mayoclinic.org/healthy-lifestyle/adult-health/expert-answers/split-fingernails/faq-20058182. Accessed Dec. 20, 2018.

5 https://www.webmd.com/vitamins/ai/ingredientmono-313/biotin. Accessed Jan. 5, 2019.

6 V.E. Colombo et al., "Treatment of Brittle Fingernails and Onychoschizia with Biotin: Scanning Electron Microscopy," *J Am Acad Dermatol* 23, no. 6, pt. 1 (Dec. 1990): 1127-1132.

7 L.G. Hochman et al., "Brittle Nails: Response to Daily Biotin Supplementation," *Cutis* 51 (1993): 303-305.

8 https://www.aocd.org/page/BrittleSplittingNail. Accessed Mar. 6, 2019.

9 M.W. Cashman and S.B. Sloan, "Nutrition and Nail Disease," *Clin Dermatol* 28 (2010): 420-425.

10 https://www.medicalnewstoday.com/articles/zinc-deficiency-and-nails#symptoms. Accessed May 30, 2021.

11 https://ods.od.nih.gov/factsheets/Zinc-HealthProfessional/. Accessed May 30, 2021.

Nails—Brown-Gray Discoloration

1 M.E. Williams, "Examining the Fingernails when Evaluating Presenting Symptoms in Elderly Patients: Observing the Nail Shape and Surface," *Medscape Family Medicine*. http://www.medscape.com/viewarticle/712251_2. Published Nov. 3, 2009. Accessed Dec. 4, 2014.

2 https://www.podiatrytoday.com/when-vitamin-and-nutritional-deficiencies-cause-skin-and-nail-changes. Accessed Nov. 20, 2018.

Nails—Fungal Infection/Onychomycosis

1 https://www.ncbi.nlm.nih.gov/books/NBK441853/. Accessed Feb. 28, 2021.

2 D.A. Stolmeier et al., "Utility of Laboratory Test Result Monitoring in Patients Taking Oral Terbinafine or Griseofulvin for Dermatophyte Infections," *JAMA Dermatol* 154 (2018): 1409-1416. DOI: 10.1001/jamadermatol.2018.3578.

3 D.S. Buck et al., "Comparison of Two Topical Preparations for the Treatment of Onychomycosis: Melaleuca Alternifolia (Tea Tree) Oil and Cloirimazole," *J Family Pract* 38 (1994): 601-605.

4 J.V. Wright, MD, *Nutrition and Healing* 5, no. 9 (Sept. 1998): 4.

Nails—Koilonychia

1 https://www.ncbi.nlm.nih.gov/pmc/articles/PMC3038811/. Accessed Nov. 21, 2018.

2 https://www.podiatrytoday.com/when-vitamin-and-nutritional-deficiencies-cause-skin-and-nail-changes. Accessed Nov. 21, 2019.

Nails—Paronychia/Infection

1 D. Rigopoulo et al., "Acute and Chronic Paronychia," *Am Fam Physician* 77 (2008): 339-346.

2 J. Karnes, MD, "Separation and Discoloration of Thumb Nail" *MDEdge Family Medicine* (July 22, 2021). Accessed July 23, 2021.

3 *Rosen & Barkin's 5 Minute Emergency Medicine Consult*, 5th ed. (Wolters Kluwer), 2828.

4 https://www.aafp.org/afp/2017/0701/afp20170701p44.pdf. Accessed July 22, 2021.

5 C.E. Heidelberger, MD, "Practice Tips," *Postgraduate Medicine* 101, no. 3 (1997): 55.

Nails—Transverse Leukonychia/Mees' Lines

1 B. Ahmed, MD, "Mees' Lines," *Medicalopedia* (Oct. 13, 2011. https://www.medicalopedia.org/1801/mees-lines/.

2 https://www.thelancet.com/article/S0140-6736(08)61587-1/fulltext. Accessed Jan. 6, 2021.

3 C. Foti et al., "Transverse Leukonychia in Severe Hypocalcemia," *Eur J Dermatol* 14 (2004): 67-68.

4 J.A. Simpson, "Dermatological Changes in Hypocalcemia," *Br J Dermatol* 66 (1954): 1-15.

5 M.W. Cashman and S.B. Sloan, "Nutrition and Nail Disease," *Clin Dermatol* 28 (2010): 420-425.

Nails—Yellow Nail Syndrome

1 https://www.aafp.org/afp/2004/0315/p1417.html. Accessed Feb. 11, 2019.

2 M.A. Keen and I. Hassan, "Vitamin E in Dermatology," *Indian Dermatol Online J* 7, no. 4 (July-Aug. 2016): 311-315. DOI: 10.4103/2229-5178.185494.

3 https://www.ncbi.nlm.nih.gov/pmc/articles/PMC5327582/. Accessed Apr. 12, 2021.

Necrolytic Migratory Erythema

1 M. Gupta et al., "Zinc Therapy in Dermatology: A Review," *Dermatol Res Pract* (2014). Published online July 10, 2014. DOI: 10.1155/2014/709152.

2 https://www.ncbi.nlm.nih.gov/pmc/articles/PMC2664208/. Accessed Dec. 22, 2018.

3 S.A. Sinclair and N.J. Reynolds, "Necrolytic Migratory Erythema and Zinc Deficiency," *The British Journal of Dermatology* 136, no. 5 (1997): 783-785.

4 U. Patel et al., "Necrolytic Acral Erythema," *Dermatology* 16, no. 11 (2010): 15.

5 E.A. Mullans and P.R. Cohen, "Iatrogenic Necrolytic Migratory Erythema: A Case Report and Review of Nonglucagonoma-Associated Necrolytic Migratory Erythema," *Journal of the American Academy of Dermatology* 38 (1998): 866-873.

6 E. Delaporte, B. Catteau, and F. Piette, "Necrolytic Migratory Erythema-Like Eruption in Zinc Deficiency Associated with Alcoholic Liver Disease," *British Journal of Dermatology* 137 (1997): 1027-1028.

Neural Tube Defects (NTDs)

1 https://www.nichd.nih.gov/health/topics/ntds/conditioninfo. Accessed Nov. 21, 2018.

2 R.W. Smithells, S. Sheppard, and C.J. Schorah, "Vitamin Deficiencies and Neural Tube Defects," *Arch Dis Child* 51 (1976): 944-950.

3 A.E. Czeizel and I. Dudas, "Prevention of the First Occurrence of Neural-Tube Defects by Periconceptional Vitamin Supplementation," *N Engl J Med* 327 (1992): 1832-1835.

4 MRC Vitamin Study Research Group, "Prevention of Neural Tube Defects: Results of the Medical Research Council Vitamin Study," *Lancet* 338 (1991): 131-137.

5 https://www.webmd.com/baby/guide/prenatal-vitamins#1. Accessed Nov. 21, 2018.

6 Federal Register, *Food Standards: Amendment of Standards of Identity for Enriched Grain Products to Require Addition of Folic Acid; Final Rule* (Washington, DC: Food and Drug Administration, Mar. 5, 1996).

7 "Three of the B Vitamins: Folate, Vitamin B6 and Vitamin B12," Harvard T.H. Chan School of Public Health. https://www.hsph.harvard.edu/nutritionsource/what-should-you-eat/vitamins/vitamin-b/. Accessed Nov. 21, 2018.

8 https://www.nhs.uk/conditions/pregnancy-and-baby/vitamins-minerals-supplements-pregnant/. Accessed Nov. 21, 2018.

9 https://www.webmd.com/vitamins/ai/ingredientmono-436/choline. Accessed Nov. 23, 2018.

Nitroglycerine

1 https://www.webmd.com/vitamins/ai/ingredientmono-1001/vitamin-c-ascorbic-acid. Accessed Nov. 14, 2018.

2 https://www.ncbi.nlm.nih.gov/pmc/articles/PMC509066/. Accessed Mar. 18, 2019.

Nonalcoholic Fatty Liver Disease (NAFLD)

1 https://www.ncbi.nlm.nih.gov/pmc/articles/PMC3612568/. Accessed July 15, 2020.

2 G.A. Michelotti, M.V. Machado, and A.M. Diehl, "NAFLD, NASH and Liver Cancer," *Nat Rev Gastroenterol Hepatol* 10, no. 11 (2013): 656-665.

3 S.H. Zeisel, "Choline," *Modern Nutrition in Health and Disease*, 11th ed., eds. A. Ross et al. (Lippincott Williams & Wilkins, 2014), 416-426.

4 V. Parisi et al., "Cytidine-5'-Diphosphocholine (Citicoline): A Pilot Study in Patients with Non-Arteritic Ischemic Optic Neuropathy," *Eur J Neurol* 15, no. 5 (2008): 465-474.

5 L. Ottobelli et al., "Citicoline Oral Solution in Glaucoma: Is There a Role in Slowing Disease Progression?," *Ophthalmologica* 229, no. 4 (2013): 219-226.

6 https://www.webmd.com/hepatitis/fatty-liver-disease#4. Accessed Nov. 22, 2018.

7 http://patients.gi.org/topics/fatty-liver-disease-nafld/. Accessed Nov. 22, 2018.

8 N.P. Chalasani et al., "Pioglitazone versus Vitamin E versus Placebo for the Treatment of Non-Diabetic Patients with Non-Alcoholic Steatohepatitis: PIVENS Trial Design," *Contemp Clin Trials* 30, no. 1 (2009): 88-96.

9 H.F. Ji, "Vitamin E Therapy on Aminotransferase Levels in NAFLD/NASH Patients," *Nutrition* 31, no. 6 (2015): 899.

10 https://lpi.oregonstate.edu/mic/vitamins/vitamin-E. Accessed Nov. 22, 2018.

11 L.M. Fischer et al., "Sex and Menopausal Status Influence Human Dietary Requirements for the Nutrient Choline," *Am J Clin Nutr* 85, no. 5 (2007): 1275-1285.

12 https://lpi.oregonstate.edu/mic/other-nutrients/choline#reference16. Accessed Nov. 23, 2018.

13 S. Khan et al., "Current Therapies in Alleviating Liver Disorders and Cancers with a Special Focus on the Potential of Vitamin D," *Nutr & Metab* (Lond) 15 (Dec. 15, 2018): 13. https://doi.org/10.1186/s12986-018-0251-5.

14 https://www.aafp.org/afp/2017/1201/ol1.html. Accessed Jan. 6, 2019.

15 https://www.webmd.com/vitamins/ai/ingredientmono-881/licorice. Accessed Mar. 2, 2019.

16 https://www.ncbi.nlm.nih.gov/pubmed/27270872. Accessed Feb. 27, 2019.

17 https://www.medicaldaily.com/turmeric-can-treat-liver-disease-233928. Accessed Feb. 27, 2019.

18 "Alcohol Use Linked to NAFLD," *MDEdge Internal Medicine* (Feb. 20, 2020). Accessed Feb. 23, 2020.

19 S. Chen et al., "Resveratrol Improves Insulin Resistance, Glucose and Lipid Metabolism in Patients with Non-Alcoholic Fatty Liver Disease: A Randomized Controlled Trial," *Digestive Liver Dis* 47, no. 3 (2015): 226-232. PMID: 25577300.

Obsessive-Compulsive Disorder

1 https://www.nimh.nih.gov/health/topics/obsessive-compulsive-disorder-ocd/index.shtml. Accessed Feb. 11, 2019.

2 C.B. Brink et al., "Effects of Myo-Inositol versus Fluoxetine and Imipramine Pretreatments on Serotonin 5HT2A and Muscarinic Acetylcholine Receptors in Human Neuroblastoma Cells," Conference Paper, Stellenbosch University Library (2004). http://handle.net/10019.1/11468. Accessed Nov. 23, 2018.

3 J.A. Yaryura-Tobias and H.N. Bhagavan, "L-Tryptophan in Obsessive-Compulsive Disorders," *Am J Psychiatry* 134, no. 11 (1977): 1298-1299.

4 A. Szegedi et al., "Acute Treatment of Moderate to Severe Depression with Hypericum Extract WS 5570 (St. John's Wort): Randomized Controlled Double Blind Non-Inferiority Trial Versus Paroxetine," *British Medical Journal* 330, no. 7494 (2005): 759.

5 M. Fava et al., "A Double-Blind, Randomized Trial of St. John's Wort, Fluoxetine, and Placebo in Major Depressive Disorder," *J Clin Psychopharmacol* 25, no. 5 (2005): 441-447.

6 W. Louis Cleveland et al., "High Dose Glycine Treatment of Refractory Obsessive-Compulsive Disorder and Body Dysmorphic Disorder in a 5-Year Period," *Neural Plast* (2009). DOI: 10.1155/2009/768398.

Olivopontocerebellar Atrophy (OA)/Multiple System Atrophy

1 https://rarediseases.org/rare-diseases/olivopontocerebellar-atrophy/. Accessed Jan. 3, 2019.

2 H. Sarva and V.L. Shanker, "Treatment Options in Degenerative Cerebellar Ataxia: A Systematic Review," *Movement Disorders Clinical Practice* 1, no. 4 (2014). DOI: 10.1002/mdc3.12057.

3 https://www.mayoclinic.org/diseases-conditions/multiple-system-atrophy/diagnosis-treatment/drc-20356157. Accessed Jan. 3, 2018.

4 *Medical World News* (Nov. 8, 1982): 26.

5 https://jnnp.bmj.com/content/jnnp/45/3/257.full.pdf. Accessed Jan. 3, 2019.

Operative Nutritional Status (Preoperative and Postoperative)

1 https://www.ncbi.nlm.nih.gov/pmc/articles/PMC4143525/. Accessed Mar. 18, 2019.

2 https://www.ncbi.nlm.nih.gov/pmc/articles/PMC5144568/. Accessed Mar. 18, 2019.

3 D. Hui, *Approach to Internal Medicine: A Resource Book for Clinical Practice*, 3rd ed. (Springer, 2011), 406.

4 J.H. Crandon et al., "Ascorbic Acid Economy in Surgical Patients as Indicated by Blood Ascorbic Acid Levels," *N Engl J Med* 258 (1958): 105-113.

5 R. Fukushima and E. Yamazaki, "Vitamin C Requirement in Surgical Patients," *Curr Opin Clin Nutr Metab Care* 13, no. 6 (Nov. 2010): 669-676.

6 https://dailymed.nlm.nih.gov/dailymed/fda/fdaDrugXsl.cfm?setid=d05200cb-cf29-4bc7-bf0c-b42ab2d20958. Accessed Nov. 24, 2018.

7 https://www.sciencedirect.com/science/article/pii/003042208290295X. Accessed Nov. 24, 2018.

8 K.D. Tripathi, *Essentials of Medical Pharmacology*, 7th ed. (2013), 918.

9 https://www.naturalnews.com/2017-02-10-vitamin-c-is-a-powerful-heart-healer-especially-after-surgery.html.

10 https://www.webmd.com/vitamins/ai/ingredientmono-1001/vitamin-c-ascorbic-acid. Accessed Nov. 14, 2018.

11 Y. Jeon et al., "Effect of Intravenous High Dose Vitamin C on Postoperative Pain and Morphine Use after Laparoscopic Colectomy: A Randomized Controlled Trial," *Pain Research and Management* (2016). http://dx.doi.org/10.1155/2016/9147279. Accessed Nov. 24, 2018.

12 *The Washington Manual of Medical Therapeutics*, 34th ed., 70.

13 https://www.sciencedaily.com/releases/2011/11/111103081429.htm. Accessed Nov. 24, 2018.

14 G.C. Tassman, J.N. Zafran, and G.M. Zayon, "Evaluation of a Plate Proteolytic Enzyme for the Control of Inflammation and Pain," *Journal of Dental Medicine* 19 (1964): 73-77. [Google Scholar]

15 G.C. Tassman, J.N. Zafran, and G.M. Zayon, "A Double-Blind Crossover Study of a Plant Proteolytic Enzyme in Oral Surgery," *The Journal of Dental Medicine* 20 (1965): 51-54.

16 R.C.L. Howat and G.D. Lewis, "The Effect of Bromelain Therapy on Episiotomy Wounds—A Double Blind Controlled Clinical Trial," *Journal of Obstetrics and Gynaecology of the British Commonwealth* 79, no. 10 (1972): 951-953.

17 https://www.mdedge.com/dermatology/article/7813/wounds/bromelain-pineapple-extract/page/0/1. Accessed Oct. 14, 2019.

18 https://www.emedicinehealth.com/glutamine/vitamins-supplements.htm. Accessed Nov. 28, 2018.

19 https://www.webmd.com/vitamins/ai/ingredientmono-878/glutamine. Accessed Nov. 28, 2018.

Optic Neuritis/Retrobulbar Neuropathy

1 https://www.mdedge.com/ccjm/article/89860/retrobulbar-neuritis. Accessed Dec. 23, 2018.

2 https://www.ncbi.nlm.nih.gov/pmc/articles/PMC3414716/. Accessed Mar. 6, 2019.

3 https://www.ncbi.nlm.nih.gov/pmc/articles/PMC2701125/. Accessed Mar. 6, 2019.

4 https://journal.opted.org/article/vitamin-b12-deficiency-optic-neuropathy-a-teaching-case-report/. Accessed Mar. 6, 2019.

5 https://www.ncbi.nlm.nih.gov/pmc/articles/PMC4581115/. Accessed Mar. 6, 2019.

6 https://www.medicinenet.com/optic_neuritis/article.htm#what_is_the_prognosis_for_optic_neuritis.

7 R.G. Petersdorf et al., *Harrison's Principles of Internal Medicine*, 10th ed., 2151.

8 http://www.aetna.com/cpb/medical/data/500_599/0536.html. Accessed Dec. 9, 2018.

Osteitis Fibrosa Cystica

1 https://www.symptoma.com/en/info/osteitis-fibrosa-cystica. Accessed Mar. 19, 2019.

2 E.D. Tamiegra, "Hyperparathyroidism," *Am Fam Physician* 69, no. 2 (Jan. 15, 2004): 333-339.

3 S.J. Silverberg and S. Kramer, "Vitamin Deficiency and Primary Hyperparathyroidism," *J Bone Miner Res* 22, suppl. 2 (Dec. 2007): V100-V104. DOI: 10.1359/jbmr.07s202. https://emedicine.medscape.com/article/874690-overview. Accessed Dec. 18, 2018.

4 https://www.emedicinehealth.com/vitamin_d/vitamins-supplements.htm. Accessed Dec. 18, 2018.

Osteoarthritis (OA)

1 Medscape_CME_Recap@mail.medscape.org. Accessed May 12, 2021.

2 B.G. Gilmer et al., "Which Oral Nonopioid Agents Are Most Effective for OA Pain?," *J Fam Pract* 68, no. 7 (Sept. 2019): 417-418.

3 https://www.ncbi.nlm.nih.gov/pubmed/6373158. Accessed Jan. 23, 2020.

4 https://pubmed.ncbi.nlm.nih.gov/28850416/. Accessed Feb. 25, 2021.

5 https://www.mdedge.com/familymedicine/quiz/8523/rheumatology/osteoarthritis-test-your-skills-these-5-questions. Accessed Oct. 20, 2019.

6 J.T. DiPiro et al., *Pharmacotherapy: A Pathophysiologic Approach*, 6th ed. (McGraw-Hill, 2005), 1693.

7 https://www.emedicinehealth.com/vitamin_c_ascorbic_acid/vitamins-supplements.htm. Accessed Dec. 19, 2018.

8 https://www.webmd.com/vitamins/ai/ingredientmono-1001/vitamin-c-ascorbic-acid. Accessed Nov. 14, 2018.

9 https://www.medicinenet.com/osteoarthritis/views.htm. Accessed Dec. 19, 2018.

10 B.G. Wells et al., *Pharmacotherapy Handbook*, 9th ed. (McGraw Hill Education), 17.

11 M.A. Flynn et al., "The Effect of Folate and Cobalamin on Osteoarthritic Hands," *J Am Coll Nutr* 13 (1994): 351-356.

12 W. McCarty, "Osteoarthritis," *Med Hypothesis* 92 (1994): 323-327.

13 https://www.webmd.com/vitamins/ai/ingredientmono-807/glucosamine-sulfate. Accessed Nov. 18, 2018.

14 M.C. Magaña-Villa et al., "B-Vitamin Mixture Improves the Analgesic Effect of Diclofenac in Patients with Osteoarthritis: A Double Blind Study," *Drug Res (Stuttg)* 63 (2013): 289-292.

15 G. Blankenhorn, "Clinical Effectiveness of Spondyvit (Vitamin E) in Activated Arthroses. A Multicenter Placebo-Controlled Double-Blind Study," *Z Orthop* 124 (1986): 340-343.

16 Z. Mahmud and S.M. Ali, "Role of Vitamin A and E in Spondylosis," *Bangladesh Med Res Counc Bull* 18 (1992): 47-59.

17 N.M. Akhtar et al., "Oral Enzyme Combination versus Diclofenac in the Treatment of Osteoarthritis of the Knee—A Double-Blind Prospective Randomized Study," *Clinical Rheumatology* 23, no. 5 (2004): 410-415.

18 S. Brien et al., "Bromelain as a Treatment for Osteoarthritis: A Review of Clinical Studies," *Evidence-Based Complementary and Alternative Medicine* 1, no. 3 (2004): 251-257.

19 B. Wasi, *Standard Treatment Guidelines: A Manual for Medical Therapeutics*, 1st ed. (2014), 346.

20 S. Baxter, "Healing with Chiropractic Medicine," The Arthritis Foundation. http://www.arthritis.org/living-with-arthritis/treatments/natural/othertherapies/chiropractic-medicine.php.

21 A. Qaseem et al., "Noninvasive Treatments for Acute, Subacute and Chronic Low Back Pain: A Clinical Practice Guideline from the American College of Physicians," *Annals of Internal Medicine* 166, no. 4 (Feb. 14, 2017). DOI 10.7326/M16-2367.

22 A.I. Binder, "Cervical Spondylosis and Neck Pain," *BMJ* 334 (2007): 527.

Osteoarthritis (Knee and Hip)

1 https://www.nih.gov/news-events/nih-research-matters/intensive-weight-loss-helps-knee-arthritis. Accessed Aug. 15, 2020.

2 B.G. Wells et al., *Pharmacotherapy Handbook*, 9th ed. (McGraw Hill Education), 10.

3 https://www.medicinenet.com/osteoarthritis/views.htm. Accessed Dec. 19, 2018.

4 R.K. Chaganti et al., "Association of 25-Hydroxyvitamin D with Prevalent Osteoarthritis of the Hip in Elderly Men: The Osteoporotic Fractures in Men Study," *Arthritis Rheum* 62, no. 2 (Feb. 2010): 511-514. DOI: 10.1002/art.27241.

5 R. Marcholongo et al., "Double-Blind, Multicenter Study of Activity of S-Adenosyl-Methionine in Hip and Knee Osteoarthritis," *Curr Ther Res* 37 (1985): 82-94.

6 https://pubmed.ncbi.nlm.nih.gov/3318442/.

7 https://www.ncbi.nlm.nih.gov/pmc/articles/PMC387830/.

8 https://www.webmd.com/vitamins/ai/ingredientmono-807/glucosamine-sulfate. Accessed Nov. 18, 2018.

9 J.M. Ritter et al., "Alternative Medicines: Herbals and Nutraceuticals," in *A Textbook of Pharmacology and Clinical Therapeutics*, 5th ed. (UK: Hodder Arnold, 2008): 101.

10 http://pennstatehershey.adam.com/content.aspx?productId=107&pid=33&gid=000328. Accessed Jan. 7, 2019.

11 W. McCarty, "Osteoarthritis," *Med Hypothesis* 92 (1994): 323-327.

12 Philip Gregory, Morgan Sperry, and Amy Friedman Wilson, "Dietary Supplements for Osteoarthritis," *Am Fam Physician* 77, no. 2 (Jan. 15, 2008): 177-184.

13 L. Raith, The Arthritis Foundation. http://blog.arthritis.org/osteoarthritis/pharmaceutical-chondroitin-helps-knee-oa-pain/. Accessed June 16, 2021.

Osteogenesis Imperfecta (OI)

1 https://medlineplus.gov/osteogenesisimperfecta.html#summary. Accessed Mar. 25, 2019.

2 https://www.nichd.nih.gov/health/topics/osteogenesisimp/conditioninfo/symptoms. Accessed Mar. 25, 2019.

3 http://www.oif.org/site/PageServer?pagename=Nutrition. Accessed Oct. 22, 2018.

4 https://www.bones.nih.gov/health-info/bone/osteoporosis/conditions-behaviors/osteoporosis-oi. Accessed Oct. 22, 2018.

5 https://www.nap.edu/read/13050/chapter/7#349. Accessed Feb. 27, 2019.

6 E.A. Winterfeldt, E.J. Eyring, and V.M. Vivian, "Ascorbic Acid Treatment for Osteogenesis Imperfecta," *The Lancet* 295, no. 7660 (June 1970): 1347-1348. Letters to the editor.

7 E.A. Winterfeldt, *The Effects of Ascorbic Acid Treatment for Osteogenesis Imperfecta*. Ohio State University. 1970. https://www.researchgate.net/publication/34981378_The_effects_of_ascorbic_acid_treatment_for_Osteogenesis_imperfecta. Accessed Dec. 22, 2018.

Osteomalacia

1 https://www.ncbi.nlm.nih.gov/pmc/articles/PMC3215492/. Accessed Mar. 19, 2019.

2 https://www.cedars-sinai.edu/Patients/Health-Conditions/Osteomalacia.aspx. Accessed Mar. 25, 2019.

3 M.A. Papadakis and S.J. McPhee, *Current Medical Diagnosis & Treatment* (2019): ch. 26, 1176.

4 https://www.webmd.com/osteoporosis/what-is-osteomalacia#2. Accessed Dec. 23, 2018.

5 https://www.mayoclinic.org/diseases-conditions/osteomalacia/symptoms-causes/syc-20355514. Accessed Dec. 23, 2018.

6 https://rarediseases.info.nih.gov/diseases/7285/osteomalacia. Accessed Dec. 22, 2018.

7 https://my.clevelandclinic.org/health/diseases/13017-osteomalacia. Accessed Dec. 23, 2018.

8 *The Washington Manual for Medical Therapeutics*, 34th ed., 1192.

9 R.S. Weinstein and P. Madhavaram, *Osteomalacia Endocrinology Advisor.* https://www.endocrinologyadvisor.com/endocrinology-metabolism/osteomalacia/article/595381/. Accessed Dec. 23, 2018.

Osteoporosis

1 B.G. Wells et al., *Pharmacotherapy Handbook*, 9th ed. (McGraw Hill Education), 16-17.

2 https://www.medicinenet.com/osteoporosis/article.htm#what_is_osteoporosis. Accessed Mar. 19, 2019.

3 https://www.medicalnewstoday.com/articles/155646.php. Accessed Dec. 22, 2018.

4 M.M. Keifer, *Pocket Primary Care,* 2nd ed. (Wolters Kluver).

5 Cleveland Clinic, "Osteoporosis: Prevention with Calcium Treatment." https://my.clevelandclinic.org/health/articles/15049-osteoporosis-prevention-with-calcium-treatment. Accessed Aug. 22, 2018.

6 M.A. Chisolm-Burns et al., *Pharmacotherapy Principles & Practice* (McGraw-Hill Medical, 2008), 858.

7 https://www.mayoclinic.org/diseases-conditions/osteoporosis/symptoms-causes/syc-20351968. Accessed Aug. 22, 2018.

8 https://my.clevelandclinic.org/health/articles/15049-osteoporosis-prevention-with-calcium-treatment. Accessed Aug. 22, 2018.

9 International Osteoporosis Foundation, "Osteoporosis and Musculoskeletal Disorders." https://www.iofbonehealth.org/osteoporosis-musculoskeletal-disorders/osteoporosis/prevention/vitamin-d. Accessed Aug. 23, 2018.

10 D.D. Bikle, "Agents That Affect Bone Mineral Homeostasis" in B.G. Katzung, S.B. Masters, and A.J. Trevor, *Basic and Clinical Pharmacology,* 12th ed. (McGrawHill/Lange, 2010): 781.

11 H. Aydin et al., "Short-Term Oral Magnesium Supplementation Suppresses Bone Turnover in Postmenopausal Osteoporotic Women," *Biol Trace Elem Res* 133 (2010): 136-143.

12 https://ods.od.nih.gov/factsheets/Magnesium-HealthProfessional/. Accessed Sept. 23, 2018.

13 L. Cohen and R. Kitzes, "Infrared Spectroscopy and Magnesium Content of Bone Mineral in Osteoporotic Women," *Isr J Med Sci* 17 (1981): 1123-1125.

14 L.E. Vikhanski, "Magnesium May Slow Bone Loss," *Med Tribune* (July 23, 1993.

15 https://www.webmd.com/vitamins/ai/ingredientmono-998/magnesium. Accessed Nov. 18, 2018.

16 https://www.mayoclinic.org/diseases-conditions/osteoporosis/diagnosis-treatment/drc-20351974. Accessed Nov. 18, 2018.

17 J.M. Ritter et al., *A Textbook of Clinical Pharmacology and Therapeutics*, 5th ed. (2008), 269.

18 J. Eaton-Evans et al., "Copper Supplementation and Bone Mineral Density in Middle-Aged Women," *Proc Nutr Soc* 54 (1995): 191A.

19 F.H. Nielsen et al., "Effect of Dietary Boron on Mineral, Estrogen and Testosterone Metabolism in Postmenopausal Women," *FASEB J* 5 (Nov. 1, 1987): 394-397.

20 https://www.medscape.com/viewarticle/440898. Accessed Nov. 19, 2018.

21 https://www.webmd.com/vitamins/ai/ingredientmono-310/ipriflavone. Accessed Nov. 18, 2018.

22 https://www.webmd.com/vitamins/ai/ingredientmono-182/manganese. Accessed Nov. 19, 2018.

Otitis Externa/Swimmer's Ear

1 A. Kothari, "Treatment of 'Resistant' Otorrhea with Acetic Acid," *Laryngoscope* 79, no. 3 (1969): 494-498. Available from PM 5776741.

2 *The Merck Manual of Diagnosis and Therapy,* 19th ed., 513.

3 https://www.aafp.org/afp/2001/0301/p927.html. Accessed Apr. 29, 2019.

4 T. Bjarnsholt et al., "Antibiofilm Properties of Acetic Acid," *Adv Wound Care (New Rochelle)* 4, no. 7 (July 1, 2015): 363-372. DOI: 10.1089/wound.2014.0554.

5 https://www.drugs.com/pro/acetic-acid.html. Accessed Apr. 29, 2019.

Otitis Media

1 https://emedicine.medscape.com/article/994656-overview. Accessed June 16, 2021.

2 https://pediatrics.aappublications.org/content/131/3/e964#xref-ref-66-1. Accessed Apr. 19, 2021.

3 https://www.healthline.com/health/ear-infection-acute#treatments. Accessed Feb. 11, 2019.

4 https://pubmed.ncbi.nlm.nih.gov/16856108/. Accessed Apr. 19, 2021.

5 https://www.rxlist.com/calendula/supplements.htm. Accessed Dec. 16, 2018.

6 R.M. Froehle, "Ear Infection: A Retrospective Study Examining Improvement from Chiropractic Care and Analyzing for Influencing Factors," *J Manip Physiol Ther* 19, no. 3 (Mar.-Apr. 1996): 169-177.

7 https://www.medicalnewstoday.com/articles/312634.php. Accessed Mar. 5, 2019.

Otosclerosis

1 http://www.emedmd.com/content/otosclerosis. Accessed Oct. 14, 2018.

2 A.S. Cruise, A. Singh, and R.E. Quiney, "Sodium Fluoride in Otosclerosis Treatment: Review," *J Laryngology and Otology* 124, no. 6 (Feb. 2010): 583-586.

3 B.D. Forquer, F.H. Linthicum, and C. Bennett, "Sodium Fluoride: Effectiveness of Treatment for Cochlear Otosclerosis," *Am J Otol* 7, no. 2 (Mar. 1986): 121-125.

4 G.B. Brookes, "Vitamin Deficiency in Otosclerosis," *Otolaryngol Head Neck Surg* 93, no. 3 (June 1985): 313-321.

5 https://medlineplus.gov/ency/article/001036.htm. Accessed Oct. 14, 2018.

6 https://emedicine.medscape.com/article/994891-medication#2. Accessed Oct. 14, 2018.

Overweight/Obesity

1 https://edhub.ama-assn.org/jn-learning/video-player/18655763?utm_source=silverchair&utm_medium=email&utm_campaign=article_alert-jama&utm_content=olf&utm_term=111721. Accessed Nov. 17, 2021.

2 V.P. Arcangelo and A.M. Peterson, *Pharmacotherapeutics for Advanced Practice: A Practical Approach*, 3rd ed. (Wolters Kluwer/Lippincott Williams & Wilkins, 2013): 861.

3 W.O. Pickrell, "Idiopathic Intracranial Hypertension Is on the Rise," *MDEdge Neurology* (Jan. 28, 2021).

4 M. Frellick, "Time to Embrace Growing Array of Options," *MDEdge Family Medicine* (Feb. 27, 2020). Accessed Mar. 11, 2020.

5 D. Hui, *Approach to Internal Medicine: A Resource Book for Clinical Practice*, 3rd ed. (Springer, 2011), 403-404.

6 M.M. Keifer, *Pocket Primary Care,* 2nd ed. (Wolters Kluver).

7 https://link.springer.com/article/10.1007/s13668-021-00353-5. Accessed May 16, 2021.

8 L.H. Leung, "Pantothenic Acid as a Weight-Reducing Agent: Fasting without Hunger, Weakness and Ketosis," *Med Hypotheses* 44 (1995): 403-405.

9 A.A. Conte, "A Non-Prescription Alternative in Weight Reduction Therapy," *The Bariatrician* (Summer 1993): 17-19.

10 A.A. Conte, "The Allendale Study," in *Citrin: A Revolutionary, Herbal Approach to Weight Management*, eds. R. Rosen et al. (Burlingame, CA: New Editions Publ., 1994).

11 A.A. Conte, "The Hilton Head Study II: Citrin 75," in *Citrin: A Revolutionary, Herbal Approach to Weight Management*, eds. R. Rosen et al. (Burlingame, CA: New Editions Publ., 1994).

12 A.A. Conte, "The Effects of (-) Hydroxycitrate and Chromium (GTF) on Obesity," Abstract 60, 35th Annual Meeting Amer. Coll. Nutr., Atlanta (Oct. 1994).

13 http://www.healthy.net/Health/Interview/Americas_No_1_Health_Problem_Overweight_but_Undernourished/161/2. Accessed Nov. 27, 2018.

14 https://www.webmd.com/vitamins/ai/ingredientmono-767/alpha-lipoic-acid. Accessed Nov. 19, 2018.

15 https://www.ncbi.nlm.nih.gov/pmc/articles/PMC3744050/. Accessed Nov. 27, 2018.

16 https://www.webmd.com/vitamins/ai/ingredientmono-607/aloe. Accessed Jan. 5, 2019.

17 J. Abbasi, "Interest in the Ketogenic Diet Grows for Weight Loss and Type 2 Diabetes," *JAMA* 319, no. 3 (2018): 215-217. DOI: 10.1001/jama.2017.20639. Accessed Mar. 27, 2019.

18 J. Herness et al., "Vitamin Supplementation in Healthy Patients: What Does the Evidence Support?," *J Fam Pract* 70, no. 8 (Oct. 2021): 386-398d. DOI: 10.12788/jfp.0288.

19 https://www.medicalnewstoday.com/articles/325798#benefits. Accessed May 6, 2020.

20 https://www.webmd.com/diet/health-benefits-gaba#1. Accessed Jan. 20, 2021.

21 V.P. Arcangelo and A.M. Peterson, *Pharmacotherapeutics for Advanced Practice: A Practical Approach*, 3rd ed. (Wolters Kluwer/Lippincott Williams & Wilkins, 2013): 865.

22 https://pubmed.ncbi.nlm.nih.gov/28689741/. Accessed Mar. 12, 2021.

23 https://pubmed.ncbi.nlm.nih.gov/25636220/. Accessed Mar. 12, 2021.

24 https://med.virginia.edu/ginutrition/wp-content/uploads/sites/199/2014/06/Parrish-February-17.pdf. Accessed Nov. 18, 2018.

25 W. Eichorn and S. Jevert-Eichorn, "Helping Your Obese Patient Achieve a Healthier Weight," *J Fam Pract* 70, no. 3 (Apr. 2021): 131-136. DOI: 10.12788/jfp.0169.

Paget's Disease/Osteitis Deformans

1 E.T. Bope and R.D. Kellerman, *Conn's Current Therapy*, 14th ed. (Philadelphia: Elsevier/Saunders, 2014), 633.

2 https://www.mayoclinic.org/diseases-conditions/pagets-disease-of-bone/symptoms-causes/syc-20350811. Accessed Aug. 30, 2020.

3 https://www.aafp.org/afp/2002/0515/p2069.html. Accessed Nov. 5, 2020.

4 https://www.nhs.uk/conditions/pagets-disease-bone/complications/. Accessed Mar. 25, 2019.

5 E.S. Siris et al., "Medical Management of Paget's Disease of Bone: Indications for Treatment and Review of Current Therapies," *J Bone and Mineral Research* 21, suppl. 2 (Dec. 2009): 94-98.

6 https://www.belmarrahealth.com/pagets-disease-bone-causes-symptoms-treatment/. Accessed Oct. 17, 2018.

7 https://www.bones.nih.gov/health-info/bone/pagets/patient-info. Accessed Oct. 17, 2018.

8 https://emedicine.medscape.com/article/334607-treatment. Accessed Oct. 17, 2018.

9 https://www.webmd.com/vitamins/ai/ingredientmono-310/ipriflavone. Accessed Oct. 17, 2018.

10 https://www.medicinenet.com/ipriflavone/supplements-vitamins.htm. Accessed Oct. 18, 2018.

11 D. Agnusdei et al., "Short-Term Treatment of Paget's Disease of Bone with Ipriflavone," *Bone and Mineral* 19, no. 1 (Oct. 1992): S35-S42.

12 T.K. Basu et al., "Ascorbic Acid Therapy for the Relief of Bone Pain in Paget's Disease," *Acta Vitaminol Enzymol* 32, no. 1-4 (1978): 45-49.

Pain—Acute

1 J.M. Stevans et al., "Risk Factors Associated with Transition from Acute to Chronic Low Back Pain in US Patients Seeking Primary Care," *JAMA Netw Open* 4, no. 2 (2021): e2037371. DOI: 10.1001/jamanetworkopen.2020.37371.

2 https://www.jwatch.org/fw116946/2020/08/17/guideline-calls-topical-nsaids-first-line-therapy-acute. Accessed Jan. 7, 2021.

3 M. Moss, "Effects of Molybdenum on Pain and General Health: A Pilot Study," *J Nutr Environ Med* 5 (1995): 5.

4 *Ann Intern Med* 166 (2017): 166. *Lancet* 384 (2014): 1586.

5 M.A. Mibielli et al., "Diclofenac Plus B Vitamins Versus Diclofenac Monotherapy in Lumbago: The DOLOR Study," *Curr Med Res Opin* 25, no. 11 (Nov. 2009): 2589-2599.

6 https://www.ncbi.nlm.nih.gov/pmc/articles/PMC3888748/#B12. Accessed Nov. 27, 2018.

7 I.Y. Hanai et al., "Clinical Study of Methylcobalamin on Cervicales," *Drug Therapy* 13, no. 4 (1980): 29.

8 C.K Chiu et al., "The Efficacy and Safety of Intramuscular Injections of Methylcobalamin in Patients with Chronic Nonspecific Low Back Pain: A Randomized Controlled Trial," *Singapore Medical Journal* 52, no. 12 (2011): 868-873.

9 https://www.ncbi.nlm.nih.gov/pmc/articles/PMC3726845/. Accessed Mar. 4, 2019.

10 https://www.medicine.net.com/magnesium/supplements-vitamins.htm. Accessed Dec. 16, 2018.

11 T.O. Seyhan et al., "Effects of Three Different Dose Regimens of Magnesium on Propofol Requirements, Haemodynamic Variables and Postoperative Pain Relief in Gynaecological Surgery," *Br J Anaesth* 96 (2006): 247-252.

12 Reported to the annual conference of the German Society of Cardiologists by Dr. Eberhard Bassenge of the University of Freiburg.

13 M.A. Hollinger, *Introduction to Pharmacology*, 2nd ed. (Tayor & Francis, 2003), 845.

14 R.L. Sahu, "Non-Drug Non-Invasive Treatment in the Management of Low Back Pain," *Ann Med Health Sci Res* 4, no. 5 (Sept.-Oct. 2014): 780-785.

15 https://nccih.nih.gov/health/pain/spinemanipulation.htm. Accessed Dec. 13, 2018.

16 B.W. Koes et al., "Spinal Manipulation and Mobilization for Back and Neck Pain: A Blinded Review," *Br Med J* 303 (1991): 1298-1303.

17 J.L. Hoving et al., "Manual Therapy, Physical Therapy, or Continued Care by a General Practitioner for Patients with Neck Pain a Randomized, Controlled Trial," *Ann Intern Med* 136, no. 10 (May 21, 2002): 713-722.

18 S. Bigos et al., *Clinical Practice Guidelines: Acute Low Back Problems in Adults*, pub. no. 95-0642 (U.S. Dept. of Health and Human Services, Agency for Health Care Policy and Research, Dec. 1994).

19 https://www.practicalpainmanagement.com/treatments/manipulation/efficacy-chiropractic-care-back-pain-clinical-summary. Accessed May 27, 2021.

20 J. Jordan, K. Konstantinou, and J. O'Dowd, "Herniated Lumbar Disk," *BMJ Clin Evid* 2009 (2009): 1118. Published online Mar. 26, 2009.

21 https://www.spineuniverse.com/conditions/back-pain/low-back-pain/lumbar-radiculopathy-low-back-leg-pain. Accessed on Dec. 13, 2018.

22 G. McMorland et al., "Manipulation or Microdiskectomy for Sciatica? A Prospective Randomized Clinical Study," *Journal of Manip and Physiol Ther* 33, no. 8 (Oct. 2010): 576-584.

23 C.C. Apfel et al., "Restoration of Disk Height through Non-Surgical Spinal Decompression Is Associated with Decreased Discogenic Low Back Pain: A Retrospective Cohort Study," *BMC Musculoskelet Disord* 11 (2010): 155.

24 E. Gose and L. Naguszewski, "Vertebral Axial Decompression Therapy: An Outcome Study," *J Neuro Res* 20, no. 3 (1998).

25 https://www.emedicinehealth.com/bromelain/vitamins-supplements.htm. Accessed Dec. 21, 2018.

26 K. Weber et al., "Perioperative Bromelain Therapy after Wisdom Teeth Extraction—A Randomized, Placebo-Controlled, Double-Blinded, Three-Armed, Cross-Over Dose-Finding Study: Bromelain Therapy after Wisdom Teeth Extraction," *Phytotherapy Research* 30, no. 12 (Sept. 2016). DOI: 10.1002/ptr.5707. Accessed Dec. 30, 2018.

27 https://www.ncbi.nlm.nih.gov/pmc/articles/PMC5778900/. Accessed May 18, 2020.

28 https://www.webmd.com/oral-health/qa/can-clove-oil-help-a-toothache. Accessed Sept. 14, 2020.

Pain—Chronic

1 A.M. Dydyk and S. Grandhe, "Pain Assessment," in *StatPearls* [Internet], (Treasure Island, FL: StatPearls Publishing, Jan. 2021). Available from: https://www.ncbi.nlm.nih.gov/books/NBK556098/.

2 J.M. Stevans et al., "Risk Factors Associated with Transition from Acute to Chronic Low Back Pain in US Patients Seeking Primary Care," *JAMA Netw Open* 4, no. 2 (2021): e2037371. DOI: 10.1001/jamanetworkopen.2020.37371.

3 D. Cherkin et al., "Effect of Mindfulness-Based Stress Reduction vs Cognitive Behavioral Therapy or Usual Care on Back Pain and Functional Limitations in Adults with Chronic Low Back Pain," *JAMA* 315, no. 12 (2016): 1240-1249.

4 A. Qaseem et al., for the Clinical Guidelines Committee of the American College of Physicians, "Noninvasive Treatments for Acute, Subacute, and Chronic Low Back Pain: A Clinical Practice Guideline from the American College of Physicians," *Ann Intern Med.* Published online ahead of print Feb. 14, 2017. Accessed Feb. 17, 2017.

5 M. Kasovic et al., "Analgesic Properties of Vitamin K," *Proc Soc Exp Biol Med* 90 (1955): 660-662.

6 https://www.researchgate.net/publication/327904950_Chronic_Pain_and_the_Use_of_Palmitoylethanolamide. Accessed Oct. 10, 2018.

7 A.A. Yousef and A.E. Al-deeb, "A Double-Blinded Randomized Controlled Study of the Value of Sequential Intravenous and Oral Magnesium Therapy in Patients with Chronic Low Back Pain with a Neuropathic Component," *Anaesthesia* 68, no. 3 (Mar. 2013): 260-266. DOI: 10.1111/anae.12107.

Pancreatic Exocrine Insufficiency (PEI)

1 https://www.medscape.org/viewarticle/709097. Accessed Dec. 18, 2018.

2 http://archive.foundationalmedicinereview.com/publications/13/4/307.pdf. Accessed Dec. 30, 2020.

3 http://archive.foundationalmedicinereview.com/publications/13/4/307.pdf.

4 R. Pezzilli, "Chronic Pancreatitis: Maldigestion, Intestinal Ecology and Intestinal Inflammation," *World J Gastroenterol* 15, no. 14 (2009): 1673-1676.

5 https://www.ncbi.nlm.nih.gov/pmc/articles/PMC3831207/. Accessed May 15, 2020.

6 https://www.webmd.com/digestive-disorders/epi-treatment.

Pancreatitis—Acute

1 M.A. Mederos, H.A. Reber, and M.D. Girgis, "Acute Pancreatitis: A Review," *JAMA* 325, no. 4 (2021): 382-390. DOI: 10.1001/jama.2020.20317.

2 https://www.medscape.com/answers/2038394-35984/how-does-acute-pancreatitis-cause-magnesium-levels. Accessed Nov. 6, 2018.

3 M. Brenner and M. Safani, "Acute Pancreatitis," in *Clinical Care and Cardiac Medicine: Current Clinical Strategies* (CCS Publishing, 2005).

4 https://www.pancreapedia.org/reviews/pain-management-in-acute-pancreatitis. Accessed Mar. 4, 2019.

5 https://www.ncbi.nlm.nih.gov/pmc/articles/PMC4810896/. Accessed Mar. 4, 2019.

6 V. Schick et al., "Effect of Magnesium Supplementation and Depletion on the Onset and Course of Acute Experimental Pancreatitis," *Gut* 63 (Oct. 2014): 1469-1480.

7 "Low Intracellular Magnesium in Patients with Acute Pancreatitis and Hypocalcemia." https://www.researchgate.net/publication/20749138_Low_intracellular_magnesium_in_patients_with_acute_pancreatitis_and_hypocalcemia. Accessed Sept. 15, 2018.

8 G. Fluhr et al., "Pre-Study Protocol MagPEP: A Multicentre Randomized Controlled Trial of Magnesium Sulphate in the Prevention of Post-ERCP Pancreatitis," *BMC Gastroenterol* 13 (2013): 11. PMID: 23320650.

9 https://www.ncbi.nlm.nih.gov/pmc/articles/PMC3726845/. Accessed Mar. 4, 2019.

10 https://www.sciencedirect.com/science/article/pii/S1567576920309772?via%3Dihub. Accessed Dec. 10, 2020.

Pancreatitis—Chronic

1 https://www.emedicinehealth.com/pancreatitis/article_em.htm. Accessed Mar. 6, 2019.

2 E.T. Bope and R.D. Kellerman, *Conn's Current Therapy*, 14th ed. (Philadelphia: Elsevier/Saunders, 2014), 519.

3 https://health.clevelandclinic.org/best-and-worst-foods-for-pancreatitis-pain/. Accessed May 24, 2021.

4 https://www.medicalnewstoday.com/articles/160459.php. Accessed Dec. 28, 2018.

5 R.J. Nair, L. Lawler, and M.R. Miller, "Chronic Pancreatitis," *Am Fam Physician* 76, no. 11 (Dec. 1, 2007): 1679-1688.

6 I.M. Papazachariou et al., "Magnesium Deficiency in Patients with Chronic Pancreatitis Identified by an Intravenous Loading Test," *Clin Chim Acta* 302, no. 1-2 (Dec. 2000): 145-154.

7 https://www.ncbi.nlm.nih.gov/pmc/articles/PMC3132852/. Accessed Dec. 28, 2018.

Parkinson's Disease

1 https://pubmed.ncbi.nlm.nih.gov/17588236/. Accessed Nov. 10, 2021.

2 https://www.medicalnewstoday.com/articles/314486#causes-and-risk-factors.

3 T.H. Mertsalmi et al., *Mov Disord* (Nov. 18, 2019). DOI: 10.1002/mds.27924.

4 B. Nogrady, "Antibiotic Use May Increase the Risk of Parkinson's Disease," *MDEdge Family Medicine* (Dec, 3, 2019). Accessed Dec. 3, 2019.

5 S. Zafar, "Parkinson Disease" in *Stat Pearls* (2021). https://www.ncbi.nlm.nih.gov/books/NBK470193/. Accessed Jan. 14, 2022.

6 J.C. Cash and C.A. Glass, *Family Practice Guidelines*, 4th ed. (Springer, 2017), 598.

7 D. Belvisi et al., "Modifiable Risk and Protective Factors in Disease Development, Progression and Clinical Subtypes of Parkinson's Disease: What Do Prospective Studies Suggest?," *Neurobiol Dis* 134 (2020): 104671. Accessed Mar. 24, 2020.

8 S. Fahn, "A Pilot Trial of High-Dose Alpha-Tocopherol and Ascorbate in Early Parkinson's Disease," *Ann Neurol* 32 (1992): S128-S132.

9 https://n.neurology.org/content/96/6/e895. Accessed Feb. 18, 2021.

10 https://www.webmd.com/parkinsons-disease/news/20020117/folic-acid-linked-to-parkinsons-disease#1. Accessed Nov. 11, 2018.

11 https://www.webmd.com/vitamins/ai/ingredientmono-42/methionine. Accessed Nov. 14, 2018.

12 https://www.researchgate.net/publication/16063801_L-methionine_treatment_of_Parkinson's_disease_Preliminary_results. Accessed Jan. 7, 2019.

13 J.R. Smythies and J.H. Halsey, "Treatment of Parkinson's Disease with L-Methionine," *South Med J* 77 (1984): 1577.

14 https://www.news-medical.net/news/20160617/Natural-molecule-NAC-could-benefit-patients-with-Parkinsons-disease.aspx.

15 L.D. Coles et al., "Oral NAC in Parkinson's Disease: Brain Glutathione and Oxidative Stress," *Journal of Clinical Pharmacology* (Sept. 2017). https://accp1.onlinelibrary.wiley.com/doi/abs/10.1002/jcph.1008. Accessed Feb. 24, 2019.

16 C. Pellicano et al., "Prodromal Non-Motor Symptoms of Parkinson's Disease," *Neuropsychiat Dis Treat* 3 (2007): 145-152. DOI: 10.2147/nedt.2007.3.1.145.

17 L. Stefanis, "α-Synuclein in Parkinson's Disease," *Cold Spring Harb Perspec Med* 2, no. 2 (2012): a009399. DOI: 10.1101/cshperspect.a009399.

18 https://www.ncbi.nlm.nih.gov/pmc/articles/PMC4899466/#B35. Accessed Jan. 3, 2019.

19 https://www.ncbi.nlm.nih.gov/pmc/articles/PMC3068871/. Accessed Jan. 7, 2019.

20 https://medlineplus.gov/magazine/issues/winter14/articles/winter14pg8-10.html. Accessed Feb. 11, 2019.

21 https://pubmed.ncbi.nlm.nih.gov/26343714/. Accessed June 14, 2021.

22 https://www.webmd.com/vitamins/condition-1460/parkinson%27s+disease.aspx. Accessed Dec. 22, 2018.

23 "New Strategies in the Management of Parkinson's Disease: A Biological Approach Using a Phospholipid Precursor (CDP-Choline)." https://www.ncbi.nlm.nih.gov/pubmed/7162583. Accessed Mar. 7, 2021.

24 https://pubmed.ncbi.nlm.nih.gov/12821288/. Accessed June 14, 2021.

Pellagra

1 https://www.webmd.com/diet/niacin-deficiency-symptoms-and-treatments#1. Accessed Nov. 4, 2018.

2 https://emedicine.medscape.com/article/985427-treatment. Accessed Nov. 4, 2018.

3 https://www.dermatologyadvisor.com/dermatology/pellagra/article/691369/. Accessed Nov. 4, 2018.

4 R. Gilroy and J.S. Meyer, *Medical Neurology*, 3rd ed. (New York: Macmillan Publishing, 1979), 279.

5 https://emedicine.medscape.com/article/1095845-treatment. Accessed Nov. 5, 2018.

Pemphigus Vulgaris

1 https://rarediseases.info.nih.gov/diseases/7355/pemphigus-vulgaris. Accessed May 11, 2020.

2 https://www.nhs.uk/conditions/pemphigus-vulgaris/treatment/. Accessed Jan. 7, 2021.

3 *Clin Exp Rheumatol* 13, no. 3 (May-June 1995): 34.

4 S. Ayres and R. Mihan, "Vitamin E and Dermatology," *Cutis* 16 (1975): 1017-1021.

Periodic Paralysis—Hyperkalemic/Hypokalemic

1 https://www.webmd.com/brain/primary-periodic-paralysis#1. Accessed Dec. 22, 2018.

2 https://medlineplus.gov/ency/article/000316.htm. Accessed Dec. 22, 2018.

3 https://www.sciencedirect.com/topics/neuroscience/periodic-paralysis. Accessed Dec. 18, 2018.

4 D. DeJong, "Calcium Alleviates Symptoms in Hyperkalemic Periodic Paralysis by Reducing the Abnormal Sodium Influx," https://ruor.uottawa.ca/bitstream/10393/23487/3/DeJong_Danica_2012_thesis.pdf. Accessed Dec. 18, 2018.

5 https://emedicine.medscape.com/article/240903-medication. Accessed Dec. 18, 2018.

6 https://emedicine.medscape.com/article/240903-medication#2. Accessed Dec. 19, 2018.

7 http://hkpp.org/patients/hyperkpp-FAQ. Accessed Dec. 19, 2018.

8 https://www.ncbi.nlm.nih.gov/pubmed/20301669/. Accessed Dec. 19, 2018.

9 https://www.webmd.com/brain/primary-periodic-paralysis#4. Accessed Dec. 20, 2018.

10 https://medlineplus.gov/ency/article/000312.htm. Accessed Dec. 18, 2018.

11 J. Levitt, MD, "Managing Periodic Paralysis 101." http://www.periodicparalysis.org/CMFiles/Managing%20PP%20101.pdf.

Periodontal Disease

1 P.J. Pussinen et al., "Periodontitis Is Associated with a Low Concentration of Vitamin C in Plasma," *Clin Diagn Lab Immunol* 10, no. 5 (Sept. 2003): 897-902. DOI: 10.1128/CDLI.10.5.897-902.2003.

2 *JAMA* 246, no. 7 (1981): 730.

3 https://onlinelibrary.wiley.com/doi/abs/10.1111/j.1600-051X.2007.01053.x. Accessed Dec. 1, 2018.

Peripheral Neuropathy

1 J.C.M. Brust, *Current Diagnosis and Treatment Neurology,* 2nd ed. (McGraw-Hill, 2012): 492.

2 https://www.diabetesselfmanagement.com/blog/prediabetes-nerve-damage/. Accessed Mar. 24, 2019.

3 https://www.mayoclinic.org/diseases-conditions/diabetic-neuropathy/diagnosis-treatment/drc-20371587.

4 https://www.empr.com/features/peripheral-neuropathy-neurologic-condition-diagnosing-symptoms/article/750880/2/. Accessed Sept. 6, 2018.

5 *The Merck Manual of Diagnosis and Therapy,* 19th ed., 1798.

6 N. Vallianou, A. Evangelopoulos, and P. Koutalas, "Alpha-Lipoic Acid and Diabetic Neuropathy," *Rev Diabet Stud* 6, no. 4 (Winter 2009): 230-236. Published online Feb. 10, 2010. DOI: 10.1900/RDS.2009.6.230.

7 https://pubchem.ncbi.nlm.nih.gov/compound/dl-Thioctic_acid#section=Therapeutic-Uses. Accessed Nov. 27, 2018.

8 https://www.medicinenet.com/peripheral_neuropathy/article.htm#what_causes_peripheral_neuropathy. Accessed Sept. 6, 2018.

9 https://www.medicalnewstoday.com/articles/147963.php. Accessed Sept. 6, 2018.

10 K. Scherer, MD, "Neurologic Manifestations of Vitamin B_{12} Deficiency," *N Engl J Med* 348 (2003): 2208. DOI: 10.1056/NEJMicm020588.

11 *The Merck Manual of Diagnosis and Therapy,* 16th ed. (1992), 1434.

12 https://www.webmd.com/vitamins/condition-1148/diabetic-neuropathy. Accessed Sept. 6, 2018.

13 D. De Grandis and C. Minardi, "Acetyl-L-Carnitine (Levacecarnine) in the Treatment of Diabetic Neuropathy," *Drugs R&D* 3 (2002): 223. https://doi.org/10.2165/00126839-200203040-00001. Accessed Sept. 7, 2018.

14 M.G. Traber et al., "Lack of Tocopherol in Peripheral Nerves of Vitamin E-Deficient Patients with Peripheral Neuropathy," *N Engl J Med* 317 (1987): 262-265.

15 W.Y. Zhang and A.L. Wan Po, "The Effectiveness of Topically Applied Capsaicin: A Meta-Analysis," *Eur J Clin Pharmacol* 45 (1994): 517-522.

16 J.M. Keppel Hesselink and T.A.M. Hekker, "Therapeutic Utility of Palmitoylethanolamide in the Treatment of Neuropathic Pain Associated with Various Pathological Conditions: A Case Series," *J Pain Res* 5 (2012): 437-442. Published online Oct. 26, 2012. DOI: 10.2147/JPR.S32143.

17 https://www.webmd.com/vitamins/ai/ingredientmono-934/pyridoxine-vitamin-b6. Accessed Dec. 12, 2018.

18 *The Merck Manual of Diagnosis and Therapy*, 16th ed. (1992), 969.

19 *The Merck Manual of Diagnosis and Therapy*, 16th ed. (1992), 1435.

20 J.M. Ritter et al., *A Textbook of Clinical Pharmacology and Therapeutics*, 5th ed. (2008), 267.

Peyronie's Disease

1 https://www.urologyhealth.org/urologic-conditions/peyronies-disease/treatment. Accessed Oct. 2, 2018.

2 https://www.niddk.nih.gov/health-information/urologic-diseases/penile-curvature-peyronies-disease. Accessed Oct. 2, 2018.

3 G. Biagiotti and G. Cavallini, "Acetyl-L-Carnitine vs Tamoxifen in the Oral Therapy of Peyronie's Disease: A Preliminary Report," *BJU Int* 88 (2001): 63-67.

4 G. Cavallini et al., "Oral Propionyl-L-Carnitine and Intraplaque Verapamil in the Therapy of Advanced and Resistant Peyronie's Disease," *BJU Int* 89 (2002): 895-900.

5 https://www.webmd.com/vitamins/ai/ingredientmono-1004/para-aminobenzoic-acid-paba. Accessed Oct. 2, 2018.

6 C.J. Zarafonetis and T.N. Horrax, "Treatment of Peyronie's Disease with Potassium Paraaminobenzoate (Potaba)," *J Urol* 81, no. 6 (June 1959): 770-772.

7 C.C. Carson, "Potassium Para-Aminobenzoate for the Treatment of Peyronie's Disease: Is It Effective?," *Tech Urol* 3, no. 3 (1997): 145-149.

8 R. Hasche-Klunder, "Treatment of Peyronie's Disease with Para-Aminobenzoacidic Potassium," *Urologe A* 17 (1978): 224-247 [in German; English abstract].

9 G. Ludwig, "Evaluation of Conservative Therapeutic Approaches to Peyronie's Disease (Fibrotic Induration of the Penis)," *Urol Int* 47 (1991): 236-239.

Pick's Disease/Frontotemporal Dementia/Lobar Atrophy

1 https://rarediseases.info.nih.gov/diseases/8436/frontotemporal-dementia. Accessed Apr. 20, 2020.

2 J. Gilroy and J.S. Meyer, *Medical Neurology*, 3rd ed. (New York: Macmillan, 1975), 170.

Pityriasis Lichenoides Chronica

1 https://rarediseases.info.nih.gov/diseases/7400/pityriasis-lichenoides-chronica.

2 R. Massimiliano et al., "Role of Bromelain in the Treatment of Patients with Pityriasis Lichenoides Chronica," *J Dermatolog Treat* 18 (2007): 219-222.

Pityriasis Versicolor/Tinea Versicolor

1 M. Gupta et al., "Zinc Therapy in Dermatology: A Review," *Dermatol Res Pract* 2014 (2014): 709152. Published online July 10, 2014. DOI: 10.1155/2014/709152.

2 "Chronic Truncal Rash" *MDEdge Family Medicine* (Feb. 10, 2022). https://www.mdedge.com/familymedicine/article/251630/dermatology/chronic-truncal-rash?

Pneumonia

1 https://www.cdc.gov/pneumonia/index.html. Accessed Oct. 14, 2019.

2 https://www.medicalnewstoday.com/articles/151632#treatment. Accessed Apr. 20, 2020.

3 https://www.ncbi.nlm.nih.gov/pmc/articles/PMC4998156/. Accessed Oct. 14, 2019.

4 R.A. Neubauer, "A Plant Protease for Potentiation of and Possible Replacement of Antibiotics," *Exp Med Surg* 19 (1961): 143-160.

5 http://www.altmedrev.com/archive/publications/15/4/361.pdf. Accessed Oct. 14, 2019.

6 https://www.ncbi.nlm.nih.gov/pmc/articles/PMC2854541/. Accessed Nov. 1, 2019.

7 https://medicalxpress.com/news/2019-08-dietary-zinc-streptococcus-pneumoniae-infection.html. Accessed Nov. 1, 2019.

8 https://www.ncbi.nlm.nih.gov/pmc/articles/PMC2323679/. Accessed Nov. 1, 2019.

9 https://www.drugs.com/npp/zinc.html. Accessed Nov. 1, 2019.

10 https://www.who.int/elena/titles/zinc_pneumonia_children/en/. Accessed Nov. 1, 2019.

11 Johns Hopkins University Bloomberg School of Public Health, "Zinc Therapy Accelerates Recovery From Pneumonia," *Science Daily*, May 21, 2004. www.sciencedaily.com/releases/2004/05/040521072802.htm. Accessed Nov. 1, 2019.

12 https://www.webmd.com/lung/news/19991207/zinc-reduces-pneumonia-diarrhea-children#1. Accessed Nov. 1, 2019.

13 https://www.cochrane.org/CD005532/ARI_vitamin-c-for-preventing-and-treating-pneumonia. Accessed Nov. 1, 2019.

14 https://www.ncbi.nlm.nih.gov/pmc/articles/PMC4110863/. Accessed Nov. 1, 2019.

15 L. Leow et al., "Vitamin D, Innate Immunity and Outcomes in Community Acquired Pneumonia," *Respirology* 16, no. 4 (2011): 611. DOI: 10.1111/j.1440-1843.2011.01924.x.

Poison Ivy/Oak/Sumac

1 https://www.medicalnewstoday.com/articles/318059#Ten-poison-ivy-home-remedies. Accessed Feb. 11, 2021.

2 G. Litchman et al., "Contact Dermatitis," *NCBI Bookshelf, StatPearls* [Internet] (Treasure Island, FL: StatPearls Publishing, 2021).

3 https://zanfel.com/help/info.html. Accessed Oct. 6, 2018.

4 https://www.medicalnewstoday.com/articles/318059.php. Accessed Oct. 6, 2018.

5 https://ic.steadyhealth.com/poison-ivy-and-home-treatment. Accessed Oct. 6, 2018.

6 https://www.medicinenet.com/poison_ivy_oak_and_sumac/article.htm#what_is_the_treatment_for_a_poison_ivy_oak_or_sumac_rash. Accessed Oct. 6, 2018.

7 https://www.mayoclinic.org/diseases-conditions/poison-ivy/diagnosis-treatment/drc-20376490. Accessed Oct. 6, 2018.

8 http://www.foxnews.com/health/2012/07/24/natural-remedies-for-treating-poison-ivy-oak-and-sumac.html. Accessed Oct. 5, 2018.

9 https://www.sciencedirect.com/science/article/abs/pii/0190962295902376.

10 https://www.medicalnewstoday.com/articles/apple-cider-vinegar-for-poison-ivy-rash#other-remedies. Accessed Feb. 11, 2021.

11 D.H. Klasson, "Ascorbic Acid in the Treatment and Prevention of Poison Oak Dermatitis," *Arch Derm and Syph* 56 (Dec. 1947): 864-867.

Polycystic Ovarian Syndrome (PCOS)

1 https://ghr.nlm.nih.gov/condition/polycystic-ovary-syndrome. Accessed Mar. 19, 2019.

2 https://www.pcosaa.org/pcos-health-complications. Accessed Apr. 20, 2020.

3 https://www.aafp.org/afp/2000/0901/p1079.html. Accessed Feb. 8, 2021.

4 https://www.mayoclinic.org/diseases-conditions/pcos/symptoms-causes/syc-20353439. Accessed Feb. 8, 2021.

5 E. Benelli et al., "A Combined Therapy with Myo-Inositol and D-Chiro-Inositol Improves Endocrine Parameters and Insulin Resistance in PCOS Young Overweight Women," *Int J Endocrinol* 2016 (2016): 3204083. Published online July 14, 2016. DOI: 10.1155/2016/3204083.

6 https://www.medicalnewstoday.com/articles/325798#benefits. Accessed May 6, 2020.

Polyneuritis/Guillain-Barre Syndrome

1 M.A. Krupp and M.J. Chatton, *Current Medical Diagnosis & Treatment* (Lange Medical Publications, 1983), 600.

2 http://medicalency.com/polyneuritis.htm. Accessed Oct. 8, 2018.

3 www.cabdirect.org/cabdirect/abstract/19402700618. Accessed Oct. 8, 2018.

4 www.cabdirect.org/cabdirect/abstract/19361403992. Accessed Oct. 8, 2018.

Postherpetic Neuralgia (Pain Following Shingles)

1 https://www.mayoclinic.org/diseases-conditions/postherpetic-neuralgia/diagnosis-treatment/drc-20376593. Accessed Oct. 11, 2018.

2 J.Y. Chen et al., "Plasma Vitamin C Is in Postherpetic Neuralgia Patients and Administration of Vitamin C Reduces Spontaneous Pain but Not Brush-Evoked Pain," *Clin J Pain* 25, no. 7 (Sept. 2009): 562-569.

3 S.H. Byun and Y. Jeon, "Administration of Vitamin C in a Patient with Herpes Zoster—A Case Report," *Korean J Pain* 24, no. 2 (2011): 108-111.

4 J. Kauffman, "New Vaccine for Shingles: Is Prevention Really Better Than Treatment?," *J Am Phys Sur* 10 (2005): 117.

5 J.M. Orient, "Treating Herpes Zoster with Vitamin C: Two Case Reports," *Am J Phys & Surg* 11, no. 1 (2006): 26-27.

6 S. Ayers Jr. and R. Mihan, "Post-Herpes Zoster Neuralgia: Response to Vitamin E Therapy," *Arch Dermatol* 108 (1973): 855-866.

7 S. Ayres Jr. and R. Mihan, "Post-Herpes Zoster Neuralgia: Response to Vitamin E Therapy," *Arch Dermatol* 111 (1975): 396.

8 Z-W Lv and W-Z Tang, "Thiamine, Cobalamin, Locally Injected Alone or Combination for Herpetic Itching: A Single-Center Randomized Controlled Trial," *The Clinical Journal of Pain* 30, no. 3 (July 2013):. DOI: 10.1097/AJP.0b013e3182a0e085.

9 https://www.webmd.com/vitamins/condition-1498/postherpetic-neuralgia. Accessed Oct. 12, 2018.

10 https://www.mdmag.com/journals/pain-management/2012/february-2012/clinicians-have-several-options-for-treating-postherpetic-neuralgia. Accessed Oct. 12, 2018.

11 J.E. Bernstein et al., "Topical Capsaicin Treatment of Chronic Postherpetic Neuralgia," *J Amer Acad Dermatol* 21, no. 2, pt. 1 (1989): 265-270.

12 J. Bernstein et al., "Treatment of Chronic Postherpetic Neuralgia with Topical Capsaicin," *J Amer Acad Dermatol* 17 (1987): 93-96.

13 https://wa.kaiserpermanente.org/kbase/topic.jhtml?docId=hn-1272002. Accessed Oct. 12, 2018.

14 https://www.jpsmjournal.com/article/S0885-3924(04)00297-0/fulltext. Accessed Oct. 12, 2018.

Preeclampsia

1 https://www.ncbi.nlm.nih.gov/pmc/articles/PMC3231891/. Accessed Feb. 11, 2019.

2 A.S. Minhas et al., "Mediterranean-Style Diet and Risk of Preeclampsia by Race in the Boston Birth Cohort," *Journal of the American Heart Association*. Originally published Apr. 20, 2022. https://doi.org/10.1161/JAHA.121.022589. 2022;0:e022589.

3 G. Carroli et al., "Calcium Supplementation Reduces Blood Pressure during Pregnancy: A Systematic Review of Randomly Controlled Trials," *Br J Obstet Gynecol* 101 (1994): 753-758.

4 H.C. Bucher et al., "Effect of Calcium Supplementation on Pregnancy-Induced Hypertension and Preeclampsia," *JAMA* 275, no. 14 (1996): 1113-1117.

5 A.N. Atallah, G.J. Hofmeyr, and L. Duley, "Calcium Supplementation during Pregnancy for Preventing Hypertensive Disorders and Related Problems," *Cochrane Database of Systemic Reviews* 1. (Chichester, UK: Cochrane Review, Wiley Interscience, 2006).

6 M.J. Lucas, Kenneth J. Leveno, and F. Gary Cunningham, "A Comparison of Magnesium Sulfate with Phenytoin for the Prevention of Eclampsia," *N Engl J Med* 333 (1995): 201-205.

7 D. Altman et al., "Do Women with Pre-Eclampsia, and Their Babies, Benefit from Magnesium Sulphate? The MAGPIE Trial: A Randomized Placebo-Controlled Trial," *Lancet* 359, no. 9321 (2002): 1877-1890.

8 J. Simon et al., "Cost-Effectiveness of Prophylactic Magnesium Sulphate for 9996 Women with Pre-Eclampsia from 33 Countries: Economic Evaluation of the MAGPIE Trial," *BJOG* 113, no. 2 (2006): 144-151.

9 ACOG Committee on Obstetric Practice, "Vitamin D: Screening and Supplementation during Pregnancy," ACOG Committee Opinion No. 495, *Obstet Gynecol* 118, no. 1 (2011): 197-198.

10 https://www.bmj.com/content/342/bmj.d2901. Accessed Dec. 28, 2018.

11 https://www.webmd.com/vitamins/ai/ingredientmono-957/riboflavin. Accessed Nov. 14, 2018.

12 https://pubmed.ncbi.nlm.nih.gov/17512048/. Accessed Mar. 23, 2021.

13 L. Duley et al., "Antiplatelet Agents for Preventing Pre-Eclampsia and Its Complications," *Cochrane Database Syst Rev* 2 (Apr. 18, 2007). DOI: CD004659. Includes 37,560 women and demonstrates the benefits of low-dose aspirin in preventing pre-eclampsia with the greatest absolute risk reduction in high-risk women.

14 National Collaborating Centre for Women's and Children's Health, *Hypertension in Pregnancy: The Management of Hypertensive Disorders During Pregnancy* (London: Royal College of Obstetricians and Gynaecologists, 2010).

15 L.C. Chappell et al., "Effect of Antioxidants on the Occurrence of Preeclampsia in Women at Increased Risk: A Randomised Trial," *Lancet* 354 (1999): 810-816.

16 https://www.nichd.nih.gov/health/topics/preeclampsia/conditioninfo/treatments. Accessed Dec. 27, 2018.

17 K.B. Nelson and J.K. Grether, "Can Magnesium Sulfate Reduce the Risk of Cerebral Palsy in Very Low Birth Weight Infants?," *Pediatrics* (1995): 95.

18 A.R. Gaby, "Research Review," *Nutrition and Healing* 2, no. 10 (1995): 8.

Premature Labor/Preterm Birth

1 https://www.nih.gov/news-events/nih-research-matters/exploring-induced-labor-full-term-pregnancy. Accessed Mar. 4, 2019.

2 https://www.cdc.gov/reprodivehealth/maternalinfanthealth/pretermbirth.htm. Accessed Mar. 4, 2019.

3 T.D. Nolin and P.A. Friedman, "Agents Affecting Mineral Ion Homeostasis and Bone Turnover" in *Gilbert & Goodman's The Pharmacological Basis of Therapeutics*, 13th ed. (2018), 896.

4 J.M. Ritter et al., *A Textbook of Clinical Pharmacology and Therapeutics*, 5th ed. (2008), 269.

5 G. Arikan et al., "Oral Magnesium Supplementation and the Prevention of Preterm Labor," SPO Abstracts, *Am J Obstet Gynecol* 176, no. 1, pt. 2 (Mar. 1997): S45.

6 https://www.webmd.com/baby/guide/premature-labor#1. Accessed Nov. 26, 2018.

7 https://www.webmd.com/vitamins/ai/ingredientmono-999/beta-carotene. Accessed Nov. 27, 2018.

8 https://pubmed.ncbi.nlm.nih.gov/12730475/. Accesses Jan. 8, 2021.

9 https://www.acog.org/Patients/FAQs/Preterm-Premature-Labor-and-Birth#magnesium.

10 https://americanpregnancy.org/labor-and-birth/premature-labor/. Accessed Mar. 4, 2019.

11 K.B. Nelson and J.K. Grether, "Can Magnesium Sulfate Reduce the Risk of Cerebral Palsy in Very Low Birth Weight Infants?," *Pediatrics* 95 (1995): 263-269.

Premenstrual Syndrome/Premenstrual Dysphoric Disorder

1 https://www.womenshealth.gov/menstrual-cycle/premenstrual-syndrome#13. Accessed Dec. 23, 2018.

2 https://www.webmd.com/vitamins/ai/ingredientmono-998/magnesium. Accessed Oct. 23, 2018.

3 F. Facchinetti et al., "Magnesium Prevention of Premenstrual Migraine: A Placebo-Controlled Study," *New Advances in Headache Research* 2, ed. Clifford Rose (London: Smith Gordon, 1991), 329-332.

4 *Cephalgia* 17, suppl. 20 (Dec. 1997).

5 J.K. Pye, R.E. Mansel, and L.E. Hughes, "Clinical Experience of Drug Treatments for Mastalgia," *Lancet* 2 (1985): 373-377.

6 R.S. London et al., "Efficacy of Alpha-Tocopherol in the Treatment of the Premenstrual Syndrome," *J Reprod Med* 32 (1987): 400-404.

7 https://www.webmd.com/vitamins/ai/ingredientmono-326/l-tryptophan. Accessed Oct. 23, 2018.

8 https://www.mayoclinic.org/diseases-conditions/premenstrual-syndrome/diagnosis-treatment/drc-20376787. Accessed Oct. 24, 2018.

9 https://www.webmd.com/vitamins/ai/ingredientmono-182/manganese. Accessed Nov. 19, 2018.

10 https://www.webmd.com/vitamins/ai/ingredientmono-333/ginkgo. Accessed Nov. 26, 2018.

11 S. Canning, M. Waterman, and L. Dye, "Dietary Supplements and Herbal Remedies for Premenstrual Syndrome (PMS): A Systematic Research Review of the Evidence for Their Efficacy," *Journal of Reproductive and Infant Psychology* 24, no. 4 (2006): 363-378.

12 Z. Ghanbari et al., "Effects of Calcium Supplement Therapy in Women with Premenstrual Syndrome," *Taiwanese Journal of Obstetrics and Gynecology* 48, no. 2 (2009): 124-129.

13 https://www.ncbi.nlm.nih.gov/pubmed/26608718. Accessed Jan. 28, 2019.

Prostatic Hypertrophy/Benign Prostatic Hypertrophy (BPH)

1 G. Champault, J.C. Patel, and A.M. Bonnard, "A Double-Blind Trial of an Extract of the Plant *Serenoa repens* in Benign Prostatic Hyperplasia," *Br J Clin Pharmacol* 18 (1984): 461-462.

2 M.M. Keifer, "BPH and Lower Urinary Tract Symptoms," in *Pocket Primary Care*, 2nd ed. (Wolters Kluver).

3 National Center for Complementary and Integrative Health https://nccih.nih.gov/health/providers/digest/BPH-science. Accessed Jan. 28, 2020.

4 J.P. Hart and W.L. Cooper, *Vitamin F in the Treatment of Prostatic Hypertrophy*, Report 1 (Milwaukee, WI: Lee Foundation for Nutritional Research, Nov. 1941).

5 M. Bush et al., *Zinc and the Prostate*, presented at the annual meeting of the American Medical Association, Chicago, 1974.

6 M.S. Fahim et al., "Zinc Treatment for Reduction of Hyperplasia of Prostate," *Fed Proc* 35 (1976): 361.

7 A.R. Gaby, "Commentary," *Nutrition and Healing* 1, no. 1 (1994).

8 https://www.medicalnewstoday.com/articles/321231.php#natural-remedies. Accessed Nov. 2, 2019.

9 https://www.ncbi.nlm.nih.gov/pmc/articles/PMC2809240/. Accessed Jan. 28, 2020.

10 https://www.webmd.com/vitamins/ai/ingredientmono-939/beta-sitosterol. Accessed Aug. 8, 2019.

11 T.J. Wilt, R. MacDonald, and A. Ishani, "Beta-Sitosterol for the Treatment of Benign Prostatic Hyperplasia: A Systematic Review," *BJU Int* 83, no. 9 (June 1999): 976-983.

12 https://www.ncbi.nlm.nih.gov/pmc/articles/PMC2907637/.

13 National Center for Complementary and Integrative Health. https://nccih.nih.gov/health/providers/digest/BPH-science. Accessed Jan. 28, 2020.

14 https://www.medicalnewstoday.com/articles/325244#bph. Accessed Oct. 24, 2020.

15 https://www.ncbi.nlm.nih.gov/pmc/articles/PMC3589769/. Accessed Feb. 29, 2020.

16 https://onlinelibrary.wiley.com/doi/abs/10.1111/ijun.12038. Accessed Jan. 29, 2020.

17 https://medlineplus.gov/ency/article/000381.htm. Accessed Dec. 23, 2018.

18 https://www.emedicinehealth.com/pygeum/vitamins-supplements.htm. Accessed Jan. 28, 2020.

19 https://clinicaltrials.gov/ct2/show/NCT00524680. Accessed Nov. 1, 2018.

Proton Pump Inhibitors (PPIs)

1 https://www.health.harvard.edu/diseases-and-conditions/proton-pump-inhibitors. Accessed May 12, 2020.

2 https://www.ncbi.nlm.nih.gov/pmc/articles/PMC4110863/. Accessed Nov. 1, 2019.

3 https://www.ncbi.nlm.nih.gov/pmc/articles/PMC3090427/. Accessed Apr. 13, 2020.

4 J.S. Lindberg et al., "Magnesium Bioavailability from Magnesium Citrate and Magnesium Oxide," *J Am Coll Nutr* 9, no. 1 (Feb. 1990): 48-55. DOI: 10.1080/07315724.1990.10720349.

Pseudotumor Cerebri/Idiopathic Intracranial Hypertension (IIH)

1 https://www.mdedge.com/neurology/article/235188/headache-migraine/idiopathic-intracranial-hypertension-rise.

2 W.O. Pickrell, "Idiopathic Intracranial Hypertension Is on the Rise," *MDEdge Neurology* (Jan. 28, 2021).

3 https://www.researchgate.net/publication/259354059_Vitamin_D_deficiency_rickets_presenting_as_pseudotumor_cerebri. Accessed Nov. 8, 2018.

4 S. Yetgin, O. Derman, and M. Dogan, "A Pediatric Patient with Recurrent Pseudotumor Cerebri and Vitamin B12 Deficiency," *Pediatric Hematology and Oncology* 23, no. 1 (2006): 39-43. DOI: 10.1080/08880010500313322.

5 G. Dotan et al., "Pediatric Pseudotumor Associated with Low Serum Levels of Vitamin A," *J Child Neur* 28, no. 11 (2013). https://doi.org/10.01177/0883073812474344.

6 https://n.neurology.org/content/early/2021/01/20/WNL.0000000000011463.

7 http://webeye.ophth.uiowa.edu/eyeforum/cases/99-Pseudotumor-Cerebri.htm. Accessed Nov. 8, 2018.

8 McC. Roach, MD, *Am Fam Phys* 114 (Jan. 1982).

9 https://www.ncbi.nlm.nih.gov/pmc/articles/PMC3858774/. Accessed Mar. 20, 2019.

10 https://journals.sagepub.com/doi/abs/10.1177/0883073812474344?journalCode=jcna. Accessed Mar. 20, 2019.

Pseudoxanthoma Elasticum

1 https://emedicine.medscape.com/article/1074713-treatment. Accessed Nov. 16, 2018.

2 https://www.dovemed.com/diseases-conditions/pseudoxanthoma-elasticum/. Accessed Nov. 16, 2018.

3 B. Marconi et al., "Pseudoxanthoma Elasticum and Skin: Clinical Manifestations, Histopathology, Pathomechanism, Perspectives of Treatment," *Intractable Rare Dis Res* 4, no. 3 (Aug. 2015): 113-122.

4 https://www.clinicaltrials.gov/ct2/show/NCT01525875. Accessed Nov. 15, 2018.

5 N. Chassaing et al., "Pseudoxanthoma Elasticum: A Clinical, Pathophysiological and Genetic Update Including 11 Novel ABCC6 Mutations," *J Med Genetics* 42, no. 12 (2004). DOI: http://dx.doi.org/10.1136/jmg.2004.030171.

6 https://www.emjreviews.com/dermatology/abstract/pseudoxanthoma-elasticum/. Accessed Nov. 16, 2018.

7 D.W. Sherer et al., "Oral Phosphate Binders in the Treatment of Pseudoxanthoma Elasticum," *J Am Acad Dermatol* 53 (2005): 610-615.

8 S. Ayres Jr. and R. Mihan, "Vitamin E and Dermatology," *Cutis* 16 (1975): 1017-1021.

9 https://www.ncbi.nlm.nih.gov/pmc/articles/PMC5424392/. Accessed May 12, 2020.

Psoriasis

1 https://www.webmd.com/skin-problems-and-treatments/psoriasis/understanding-psoriasis-basics#1. Accessed Dec. 23, 2018.

2 M. Krajewska-Wlodarczyk, A. Owczarczyk-Saczonek, and W. Placek, "Prevalence and Severity of Fatigue in Psoriasis and Psoriatic Arthritis," *Postepy Dermatol Alergol* 37, no. 1 (Feb. 2020): 46-51.

3 R. Parisi et al., "Alcohol-Related Mortality in Patients with Psoriasis: A Population-Based Cohort Study," *JAMA Dermatol* 153, no. 12 (2017): 1256-1262.

4 https://www.dermnetnz.org/topics/treatment-of-psoriasis/. Accessed Nov. 20, 2018.

5 https://emedicine.medscape.com/article/2196539-treatment#d10. Accessed Feb. 3, 2020.

6 E. Klingberg et al., "Weight Loss Is Associated with Sustained Improvement of Disease Activity and Cardiovascular Risk Factors in Patients with Psoriatic Arthritis and Obesity: A Prospective Intervention Study with Two Years of Follow-Up," *Arthritis Res Ther* 22 (2020): 254. https://doi.org/10.1186/s13075-020-02350-5.

7 https://emedicine.medscape.com/article/1943419-oerview. Accessed Nov. 19, 2018.

8 *The Merck Manual of Diagnosis and Therapy,* 19th ed., 792.

9 https://www.mayoclinic.org/diseases-conditions/psoriasis/diagnosis-treatment/drc-20355845. Accessed Nov. 20, 2018.

10 https://medlineplus.gov/ency/article/000434.htm. Accessed Nov. 20, 2018.

11 https://search.aol.com/aol/search?s_it=loki-windoid&ncid=aolsea00010000000041&q=niacinamide+for+psoriasis. Accessed Nov. 21, 2018.

12 *The Merck Manual of Diagnosis and Therapy,* 19th ed., 793.

13 A.H. Siadat et al., "Topical Nicotinamide in Combination with Calcipotriol for the Treatment of Mild to Moderate Psoriasis: A Double-Blind, Randomized, Comparative Study," *Adv Biomed Res* 2 (2013): 90. DOI: 10.4103/2277-9175.122520.

14 C.S. Ted Tse, "Niacin Is Not Niacinamide," *Am J Hosp Pharm* 38 (1981): 1662-1663.

15 M.C. Schanzer and J.K. Wilkin, "Diaper Dermatitis," *Am Fam Physician* (Apr. 1982): 123.

16 D.G. Ferderman, C.W. Froelich, and R.S. Kirsner, "Topical Psoriasis Therapy," *Am Fam Physician* 59, no. 4 (Feb. 15, 1999): 957-962.

17 G. Sadeghian, H. Ziaei, and M.A. Nilforoushzadeh, "Treatment of Localized Psoriasis with a Topical Formulation of Zinc Pyrithione," *Acta Dermatovenerologica Alpina, Pannonica et Adriatica* 20, no. 4 (2011): 187-190.

18 https://www.webmd.com/skin-problems-and-treatments/psoriasis/qa/what-overthecounter-products-are-approved-by-the-fda-to-treat-psoriasis. Accessed Dec. 17, 2018.

19 https://www.webmd.com/vitamins/ai/ingredientmono-607/aloe. Accessed Jan. 5, 2019.

20 https://pubmed.ncbi.nlm.nih.gov/30611908/. Accessed Dec. 13, 2020.

21 S. Morimoto et al., "An Open Study of Vitamin D3 Treatment in Psoriasis Vulgaris," *Br J Derm* 115 (1986): 421-429.

22 T. Kato et al., "Successful Treatment of Psoriasis with Topical Application of Active Vitamin D3 Analogue, 1 Alpha 24-Dihydroxycholecalciferol," *Br J Dermatol* 115 (1986): 432-433.

23 S. Takamoto et al., "Effect of 1 Alpha Hydroxycholecalciferol on Psoriasis Vulgaris: A Pilot Study," *Calcif Tis* 39 (1986): 360-364.

24 https://pubmed.ncbi.nlm.nih.gov/30611908/.

25 https://www.ncbi.nlm.nih.gov/pmc/articles/PMC4976416/. Accessed Nov. 21, 2018.

Psoriatic Arthritis (PsA)

1 https://allmedx.com/allmedicine/rheumatology/psoriatic+arthritis/Psoriatic+Arthritis/quiz_24?utm_source=Email2355&utm_medium=email&utm_campaign=Email2355&em_tag=686206%E2%80%8B%E2%80%8B%E2%80%8B#explanation-1. Accessed Apr. 6, 2020.

2 J.C. Cash and C.A. Glass, *Family Practice Guidelines*, 4th ed. (Springer, 2017), 663.

3 https://allmedx.com/allmedicine/rheumatology/psoriatic+arthritis/Psoriatic+Arthritis/quiz_4. Accessed Sept. 29, 2019.

4 O.J. Clemmensen et al., "Psoriatic Arthritis Treated with Oral Zinc Sulphate," *Br J Dermatol* 103, no. 4 (Oct. 1980): 411-415.

5 S.C. Cunnane, *Zinc: Clinical and Biochemical Significance* (Boca Raton, FL: CRC Press, Inc., 1988).

6 Spondylitis Association of America, "Treatment of Ankylosing Spondylitis & Related Diseases." Available at https://www.spondylitis.org/Treatment-Information. Last accessed Dec. 27, 2019.

Pulmonary Embolism

1 https://emedicine.medscape.com/article/300901-overview. Accessed Dec. 9, 2018.

2 https://www.medicalnewstoday.com/articles/153796. Accessed Apr. 20, 2020.

3 https://www.emedicinehealth.com/pulmonary_embolism/article_em.htm. Accessed Dec. 9, 2018.

4 M.A. Papadakis and S.J. McPhee, *Current Medical Diagnosis & Treatment* (2019): ch. 9, 308.

Raynaud's Phenomenon

1 https://www.medicalnewstoday.com/articles/176713. Accessed Apr. 20, 2020.

2 http://pennstatehershey.adam.com/content.aspx?productId=107&pid=33&gid=000140. Accessed Nov. 27, 2018.

3 https://www.nhsinform.scot/illnesses-and-conditions/heart-and-blood-vessels/conditions/raynauds-phenomenon. Accessed Dec. 23, 2018.

Respiratory Tract Infections

1 https://www.ncbi.nlm.nih.gov/books/NBK8142/. Accessed Dec. 14, 2018.

2 E.T. Bope and R.D. Kellerman, *Conn's Current Therapy*, 14th ed. (Philadelphia: Elsevier/Saunders), 437.

3 B.W. Jhun, MD, et al., "Vitamin D Status in South Korean Military Personnel with Acute Eosinophilic Pneumonia: A Pilot Study," *Tuberc Respir Dis (Seoul)* 78, no. 3 (July 2015): 232-238. Published online June 30, 2015. DOI: 10.4046/trd.2015.78.3.232.

4 D.A. Jolliffe, C.J. Griffiths, and A.R. Martineau, "Vitamin D in the Prevention of Acute Respiratory Infection: Systematic Review of Clinical Studies," *J Steroid Biochem Mol Biol* 136 (2013): 321-329.

5 P. Bergman et al., "Vitamin D and Respiratory Tract Infections: A Systematic Review and Meta-Analysis of Randomized Controlled Trials," *PLoS One* 8 (2013): e65835.

6 A. Aregbesola et al., "Serum 25-Hydroxyvitamin D3 and the Risk of Pneumonia in an Ageing General Population," *J Epidemiol Community Health* 67 (2013): 533-536.

7 H.H. Remmelts et al., "Addition of Vitamin D Status to Prognostic Scores Improves the Prediction of Outcome in Community-Acquired Pneumonia," *Clin Infect Dis* 55 (2012): 1488-1494.

8 https://www.emedicinehealth.com/vitamin_d/vitamins-supplements.htm. Accessed Dec. 28, 2018.

9 https://www.mdedge.com/hematology-oncology/article/233376/coronavirus-updates/vitamin-d-deficiency-covid-19-quadrupled?ecd=wnl_evn_201211_mdedge_.

10 https://pmj.bmj.com/content/early/2020/11/12/postgradmedj-2020-139065. Accessed Dec. 26, 2021.

11 https://pubmed.ncbi.nlm.nih.gov/30611908/. Accessed Dec. 13, 2020.

12 https://pubmed.ncbi.nlm.nih.gov/19341987/. Accessed July 27, 2020.

13 K.H. Brown et al., "Preventive Zinc Supplementation among Infants, Preschoolers, and Older Prepubertal Children," *Food Nutr Bull* 30, suppl. 1 (2009): S12-S40.

14 https://medicalxpress.com/news/2020-07-scientists-perspectives-zinc-intake-covid-.html. Accessed July 27, 2020.

15 J. Steckelberg, MD, "Is It True That Honey Calms Coughs Better Than Cough Medicine Does?." https://www.mayoclinic.org/diseases-conditions/common-cold/expert-answers/honey/faq-20058031. Last accessed May 8, 2019.

16 A. Schattner, "Colchinine—New Horizons for an Ancient Drug," *European Journal of Internal Medicine* (Dec. 2021). https://doi.org/10.1016/j.ejim.2021.10.002.

17 https://www.ncbi.nlm.nih.gov/pmc/articles/PMC3486425/.

18 https://www.ncbi.nlm.nih.gov/pmc/articles/PMC8573830/. Accessed Dec. 26, 2021.

Restless Legs

1 https://www.ninds.nih.gov/Disorders/Patient-Caregiver-Education/Fact-Sheets/Restless-Legs-Syndrome-Fact-Sheet. Accessed Mar. 20, 2019.

2 *BMJ* 344 (2012): 3056.

3 J.C.M. Brust, *Current Diagnosis and Treatment Neurology,* 2nd ed. (McGraw-Hill, 2012): 228.

4 https://www.mayoclinic.org/diseases-conditions/restless-legs-syndrome/diagnosis-treatment/drc-20377174. Accessed Nov. 26, 2018.

5 www.ninds.nih.gov/Disorders/Patient-Caregiver-Education/Fact-Sheets/Restless-Legs-Syndrome-Fact-Sheet#5.

6 M.I. Botez, "Folate Deficiency and Neurological Disorders in Adults," *Med Hypotheses* 2, no. 1 (1976).

7 W. Pryse-Phillips and T.J. Murray, *Essential Neurology (A Concise Textbook)* (1982): 558.

8 M.I. Botez et al., "Folate Responsive Neurological and Mental Disorders: Report of 16 Cases. Neuropsychological Correlates of Computerized Transaxial Tomography and Radionuclide Cisternography in Folic Acid Deficiencies," *Eur Neurol* 16 (1977): 230-246.

9 R. Sandyk, "L-Tryptophan in the Treatment of Restless Legs Syndrome," *Am J Psych* 143 (Apr. 1986): 544-555.

10 http://altmedrev.com/archive/publications/3/3/222.pdf. Accessed Nov. 27, 2018.

11 A.L. Welsh and M. Eade, "Inositol Hexanicotinate for Improved Nicotinic Acid Therapy," *Int Record Med* 174 (1961): 9-15.

12 https://www.ncbi.nlm.nih.gov/pmc/articles/PMC3372025/. Accessed Nov. 27, 2018.

13 D. Koutsikos, "Biotin for Diabetic Peripheral Neuropathy," *Biomed and Pharmacotherapy* 44 (1990): 511-514.

Retinopathy (Diabetic)

1 A.B.M. Abdullah, *Practical Manual in Clinical Medicine* (Philadelphia: Jaypee—The Health Sciences Publisher, 2017): 386.

2 A.A. Khan et al., "Resveratrol Regulates Pathologic Angiogenesis by a Eukaryotic Elongation Factor-2 Kinase-Regulated Pathway," *American Journal of Pathology* (2010). DOI: 10.2353/ajpath.2010.090836.

3 https://nei.nih.gov/health/diabetic/. Accessed Feb. 12, 2019.

4 https://www.ncbi.nlm.nih.gov/pmc/articles/PMC3980167/. Accessed Nov. 30, 2018.

5 P. McNair et al., "Hypomagnesemia, a Risk Factor in Diabetic Retinopathy," *Diabetes* 27 (1978): 1075-1077.

6 T. Kornerup and L. Strom, "Vitamin B12 and Retinopathy in Juvenile Diabetics," *Acta Paediatr* 47 (1958): 646-651.

7 A.J. Cameron and G.J. Ahern, "Diabetic Retinopathy and Cyanocobalamin (Vitamin B12). A Preliminary Report," *Br J Ophthalmol* 42 (1958): 666-693.

8 A.R. Gaby, "Nutrient of the Month: Vitamin B12, Part 11," *Nutrition & Healing* 5, no. 7 (Aug. 1995): 4.

9 H.N. Santosh and C.M. David, "Role of Ascorbic Acid in Diabetes Mellitus: A Comprehensive Review," *Journal of Medicine, Radiology, Pathology & Surgery* 4 (2017): 1-3.

10 R.A. Kowluru, J. Tang, and T.S. Kern, "Abnormalities of Retinal Metabolism in Diabetes and Experimental Galactosemia. VII. Effect of Long-Term Administration of Antioxidants on the Development of Retinopathy," *Diabetes* 50 (2001): 1938-1942.

11 G.T. Mustata et al., "Paradoxical Effects of Green Tea (*Camellia sinensis*) and Antioxidant Vitamins in Diabetic Rats: Improved Retinopathy and Renal Mitochondrial Defects but Deterioration of Collagen Matrix Glycoxidation and Cross-Linking," *Diabetes* 4 (2005): 517-526.

12 J.S. Penn et al., "Vascular Endothelial Growth Factor in Eye Disease," *Prog Retin Eye Res* 27 (2008): 331-371.

13 https://link.springer.com/article/10.1007/s10792-019-01165-x. Accessed Mar. 28, 2021.

14 I. Ahmad and M. Hoda, "Attenuation of Diabetic Retinopathy and Neuropathy by Resveratrol: Review on Its Molecular Mechanisms of Action," *Life Sciences* (2020): 245. https://doi.org/10.1016/j.lfs.2020.117350.

15 https://www.researchgate.net/publication/235619917_Resveratrol_improves_diabetic_retinopathy_possibly_through_oxidative_stress_-_Nuclear_factor_kB_-_Apoptosis_pathway. Accessed May 16, 2020.

16 https://wa.kaiserpermanente.org/kbase/topic.jhtml?docId=hn-2042004. Accessed Feb. 3, 2020.

Retinopathy (Hypertensive)

1 https://www.merckmanuals.com/professional/eye-disorders/retinal-disorders/hypertensive-retinopathy. Accessed June 9, 2020.

2 https://wa.kaiserpermanente.org/kbase/topic.jhtml?docId=hn-2042004. Accessed Feb. 3, 2020.

3 https://emedicine.medscape.com/article/241381-treatment#d9. Accessed Feb. 3, 2020.

Rheumatoid Arthritis

1 Arthritis Foundation, "How Rheumatoid Arthritis Affects More Than Joints." https://www.arthritis.org/diseases/more-about/how-rheumatoid-arthritis-affects-more-than-joints. Accessed May 13, 2020.

2 D. Aletaha and J.S. Smolen, "Diagnosis and Management of Rheumatoid Arthritis," *JAMA* 320, no. 13 (2018): 1360. DOI: 10.1001/jama.2018.13103. Accessed Sept. 27, 2019.

3 https://www.ncbi.nlm.nih.gov/pmc/articles/PMC2745780/. Accessed Sept. 6, 2020.

4 https://www.ncbi.nlm.nih.gov/pmc/articles/PMC3891482/. Accessed Apr. 6, 2020.

5 J. Freeman, "RA Diet: What Foods to Eat if You Have Rheumatoid Arthritis?," *Rheumatoid Arthritis Support Network*. https://www.rheumatoidarthritis.org/living-with-ra/diet/. Oct. 27, 2018. Accessed Mar. 19, 2020.

6 https://www.hopkinsarthritis.org/patient-corner/disease-management/rheumatoid-arthritis-nutrition/. Accessed Jan. 12, 2019.

7 *Annals of the Rheumatic Diseases*, British Medical Association (May 1997).

8 M. James, S. Proudman, and L. Cleland, "Fish Oil and Rheumatoid Arthritis: Past, Present and Future," *Proceedings of the Nutrition Society* 69, no. 3 (Aug. 2010): 316-323.

9 S.M. Proudman et al., "Fish Oil in Recent Onset Rheumatoid Arthritis: A Randomized, Double-Blind Controlled Trial within Algorithm-Based Drug Use," *Ann Rheum Dis* 74, no. 1 (Jan. 2015): 89-95. DOI: 10.1136/annrheumdis-2013-204145. Epub Sept. 30, 2013.

10 https://www.webmd.com/rheumatoid-arthritis/vitamins-ra#1. Accessed Jan. 11, 2019.

11 https://pubmed.ncbi.nlm.nih.gov/30611908/. Accessed Dec. 13, 2020.

12 Q. Hong et al., "Associations Between Serum 25-Hydroxyvitamin D and Disease Activity, Inflammatory Cytokines and Bone Loss in Patients with Rheumatoid Arthritis," *Rheumatology* (2014).

13 M. Rossini et al., "Vitamin D Deficiency in Rheumatoid Arthritis: Prevalence, Determinants and Associations with Disease Activity and Disability," *Arthritis Res Ther* 12 (2010): R216.

14 P. Welsh et al., "Vitamin D Deficiency Is Common in Patients with RA and Linked to Disease Activity, but Circulating Levels Are Unaffected by TNFα Blockade: Results from a Prospective Cohort Study," *Ann Rheum Dis* 70 (2011): 1165-1167.

15 https://www.ncbi.nlm.nih.gov/pmc/articles/PMC3539179/. Accessed Jan. 11, 2019.

16 https://www.vitamindcouncil.org/severity-of-rheumatoid-arthritis-may-be-mediated-by-vitamin-d-status-according-to-recent-study/. Accessed Jan. 12, 2019.

17 P. Leventis and S. Patel, "Clinical Aspects of Vitamin D in the Management of Rheumatoid Arthritis," *Rheumatology* 47, no. 11 (Nov. 2008): 1617-1621. https://doi.org/10.1093/rheumatology/ken296.

18 J.L. Funk et al., "Efficacy and Mechanism of Action of Turmeric Supplements in the Treatment of Experimental Arthritis," *Arthritis and Rheumatology* 54, no. 11 (Oct. 2006): 3452-3464.

19 https://www.medicalnewstoday.com/articles/315492.php. Accessed Jan. 6, 2019.

20 A. Wittenborg et al., "Effectiveness of Vitamin E in Comparison with Diclofenac Sodium in Treatment of Patients with Chronic Polyarthritis," *Z Rheumatol* 57 (1998): 215-221.

21 T. Brabant and A. Wittenborg, "Anti-Phlogistical and Analgetical Effectivity of Vitamin E (D-Alpha-Tocopherol Acetate, Spondyvite) in Comparison to Diclofenac-Sodium in the Treatment of Patients with Chronic Arthritis," *Zeitschrift fur Rheumatologie* 52 (1993): 356.

22 https://www.webmd.com/vitamins/ai/ingredientmono-596/borage. Accessed Jan. 12, 2019.

23 https://www.webmd.com/vitamins/ai/ingredientmono-790/lactobacillus. Accessed Jan. 12, 2019.

24 https://onlinelibrary.wiley.com/doi/abs/10.1111/1756-185X.12333. Accessed Jan. 12, 2019.

Ringworm/Dermatophytosis/Tinea Infections

1 https://www.medicinenet.com/ringworm/article.htm. Accessed Dec. 17, 2018.

2 https://www.aafp.org/afp/2014/1115/p702.html. Accessed Jan. 19, 2021.

3 M. Gupta et al., "Zinc Therapy in Dermatology: A Review," *Dermatol Res Pract* 2014 (2014): 709152. Published online July 10, 2014. DOI: 10.1155/2014/709152.

Rosacea/Acne Rosacea

1 https://jamanetwork.com/journals/jamadermatology/article-abstract/531303. Accessed Jan. 24, 2019.

2 https://www.aafp.org/afp/2015/0801/p187.pdf. Accessed May 12, 2020.

3 https://www.rosacea.org/patients/skin-care/sunscreen-for-rosacea.

4 https://www.medicinenet.com/rosacea/article.htm#is_it_possible_to_prevent_rosacea. Accessed Jan. 4, 2019.

5 K.E. Sharquie, R.A. Najim, and H.N. Al-Salman, "Oral Zinc Sulfate in the Treatment of Rosacea: A Double-Blind, Placebo-Controlled Study," *International Journal of Dermatology* 45, no. 7 (2006): 857-861.

6 A. Brocard et al., "Hidradenitis Suppurativa and Zinc: A New Therapeutic Approach. A Pilot Study," *Dermatology* 214, no. 4 (2007): 325-327.

7 H. Kobayashi, S. Aiba, and H. Tagami, "Successful Treatment of Dissecting Cellulitis and Acne Conglobata with Oral Zinc," *British Journal of Dermatology* 141, no. 6 (1999): 1137-1138.

8 M. Gupta et al., "Zinc Therapy in Dermatology: A Review," *Dermatol Res Pract* 2014 (2014): 709152. Published online July 10, 2014. DOI: 10.1155/2014/709152.

9 M.A. Krupp and M.J. Chatton, *Current Medical Diagnosis and Treatment* (1982): 53.

10 M. McCarty, "High-Chromium Yeast for Acne?," *Med Hypotheses* 14, no. 3 (July 1984): 307-310.

Sarcoidosis

1 https://rarediseases.info.nih.gov/diseases/7607/sarcoidosis.

2 https://www.aafp.org/afp/1998/1201/p2041.html. Accessed May 24, 2021.

3 https://www.webmd.com/lung/arthritis-sarcoidosis#3. Accessed Mar. 20, 2019.

4 https://www.nejm.org/doi/full/10.1056/NEJMra071714. Accessed Dec. 22, 2018.

5 E.T. Bope and R.T. Kellerman, *Conn's Current Therapy*, 14th ed. (Elsevier/Saunders), 423.

6 M.L. Cagnoni et al., "Melatonin for Treatment of Chronic Refractory Sarcoidosis," *Lancet* 346 (Nov. 1995): 1230-1231.

7 https://my.clevelandclinic.org/health/articles/11867-sarcoidosis-treatment-options. Accessed Dec. 22, 2018.

8 L.M. Sandler et al., "Studies of the Hypercalcemia of Sarcoidosis: Effect of Steroids and Exogenous Vitamin D3 on the Circulating Concentrations of 1,25-Dihydroxy Vitamin D3," *Q J Med* 53, no. 210 (Spring 1984): 165-180.

9 N. Saidenberg-Kermanac'h et al., "Bone Fragility in Sarcoidosis and Relationships with Calcium Metabolism Disorders: A Cross Sectional Study on 142 Patients," *Arthritis Research & Therapy* 16, no. 2 (2014): R78. DOI: 10.1186/ar4519.

10 https://iytmed.com/sarcoidosis/. Accessed Dec. 23, 2018.

Schizophrenia

1 https://www.mayoclinic.org/diseases-conditions/schizophrenia/diagnosis-treatment/drc-20354449. Accessed Dec. 9, 2018.

2 J. Firth et al., "The Effects of Vitamin and Mineral Supplementation on Symptoms of Schizophrenia: A Systematic Review and Meta-Analysis," *Psychological Medicine* 47, no. 9 (2017): 1515-1527. DOI: 10.1017/S0033291717000022.

3 H.E. Brown, MD, and Joshua L. Roffman, MD, "Vitamin Supplementation in the Treatment of Schizophrenia," *CNS Drugs* 28, no. 7 (July 2014): 611-622. DOI: 10.1007/s40263-014-0172-4.

4 https://www.ncbi.nlm.nih.gov/pmc/articles/PMC3783921/. Accessed Dec. 9, 2018.

5 D.C. Javitt et al., "Adjunctive High-Dose Glycine in the Treatment of Schizophrenia," *International Journal of Neuropsychopharmacology* 4, no. 4 (2001): 385-391.

6 https://www.webmd.com/vitamins/ai/ingredientmono-1072/glycine. Accessed Nov. 28, 2018.

7 https://nutritionj.biomedcentral.com/articles/10.1186/1475-2891-7-2. Accessed Jan. 7, 2019.

Sciatica

1 https://www.medicinenet.com/sciatica/article.htm#what_is_sciatica. Accessed Dec. 26, 2018.

2 *BMJ* 367 (2019): l6273. https://www.bmj.com/content/367/bmj.l6273. Accessed Sept. 1, 2020.

3 https://www.ehealthme.com/ds/thiamine-hcl/sciatica/. Accessed Dec. 24, 2018.

4 https://www.merckmanuals.com/en-ca/professional/nutritional-disorders/vitamin-deficiency,-dependency,-and-toxicity/thiamin. Accessed Dec. 24, 2018.

5 P. Seror, "Sciatica Cured by Vitamin B12," *Rev Rhum Mal Osteoartic* 56, no. 4 (Mar. 15, 1989): 344.

6 https://www.laserspineinstitute.com/back_problems/nerve_pain/supplements. Accessed Dec. 24, 2018.

7 https://www.medicalnewstoday.com/articles/318216.php. Accessed Dec. 23, 2018.

8 https://www.researchgate.net/publication/283270427_Palmitoylethanolamide_a_neutraceutical_in_nerve_compression_syndromes_Efficacy_and_safety_in_sciatic_pain_and_carpal_tunnel_syndrome. Accessed Apr. 13, 2021.

9 L. Canteri, "Reduction of Analgesics in Patients Suffering from Lumbosciatic Pain, Treated with Palmitoylethanolamide," *Dolor* 25 (2010): 227-234.

10 https://www.ncbi.nlm.nih.gov/pmc/articles/PMC3500919/#b30-jpr-5-437. Accessed Dec. 24, 2018.

11 A. Qaseem et al., "Noninvasive Treatments for Acute, Subacute, and Chronic Low Back Pain: A Clinical Practice Guideline from the American College of Physicians," *Ann Intern Med* 166, no. 4 (Feb. 2017): 1-17. DOI: 10.7326/M16-2367.

Scleroderma

1 https://my.clevelandclinic.org/health/diseases/8979-scleroderma-an-overview.

2 https://www.merckmanuals.com/professional/pulmonary-disorders/interstitial-lung-diseases/overview-of-interstitial-lung-disease.

3 https://www.hopkinsscleroderma.org/patients/scleroderma-treatment-options/. Accessed Dec. 19, 2018.

4 K. Sawalha, "Treatment of Scleroderma with Para-Aminobenzoic Acid: Effect on Disease Morbidity," *Arch Gen Intern Med* 2, no. 3 (2018): 19-22. DOI: 10.4066/2591-7951.1000052.

5 C.J. Zarafonetis, "Para-Aminobenzoic Acid Therapy in Scleroderma and Lymphoblastoma Cutis," *The Journal of Laboratory and Clinical Medicine* 33 (1948): 1462.

6 C.J. Zarafonetis, "Clinical Use of Paraaminobenzoic Acid," *Texas State Journal of Medicine* 49 (1953): 666-672.

7 C.J. Zarafonetis et al., "Retrospective Studies in Scleroderma: Effect of Potassium Paraaminobenzoate on Survival," *J Clinical Epidemiology* 41 (1988): 193-205.

8 C.J. Zarafonetis et al., "Retrospective Studies in Scleroderma: Pulmonary Findings and Effect of Potassium P-Aminobenzoate on Vital Capacity," *Respiration; International Review of Thoracic Diseases* 56: 22-33.

9 https://www.webmd.com/vitamins/ai/ingredientmono-1004/para-aminobenzoic-acid-paba. Accessed Dec. 24, 2018.

10 http://www.winchesterhospital.org/health-library/article?id=21831. Accessed Dec. 26, 2018.

11 A.L. Welsh and M. Eade, "Inositol Hexanicotinate for Improved Nicotinic Acid Therapy," *Int Record Med* 174 (1961): 9-15.

Scorpion Stings

1 www.mayoclinic.org/diseases-conditions/scorpion-stings/. Accessed Dec. 26, 2018.

2 W.J. McCormick, "Ascorbic Acid as a Chemotherapeutic Agent," *Arch of Pediatrics* 69, no. 4 (Apr. 1952): 151-155.

Scurvy

1 https://www.medicalnewstoday.com/articles/155758.php. Accessed Dec. 26, 2018.

2 https://www.medicalnewstoday.com/articles/195878.php.

3 https://medical-dictionary.thefreedictionary.com/scurvy. Accessed Dec. 26, 2018.

Seborrhea/Seborrheic Dermatitis/Dandruff

1 https://www.aocd.org/page/SeborrheicDermatiti. Accessed Oct. 13, 2019.

2 https://www.aafp.org/afp/2000/0501/p2703.html. Accessed May 12, 2020.

3 https://www.medicinenet.com/script/main/art.asp?articlekey=5428. Accessed Dec. 27, 2018.

4 B.A. Johnson and J.R. Nunley, "Treatment of Seborrheic Dermatitis," *Am Fam Physician* 61, no. 9 (May 1, 2000): 2703-2710.

5 *The Merck Manual of Diagnosis and Therapy*, 19th ed., 784.

6 G.C. Andrews, C.F. Post, and A.N. Domonkos, "Seborrheic Dermatitis: Supplemental Treatment with Vitamin B12," *NY State Med J* 50 (1950): 1921-1925.

7 A.R. Gaby, "Nutrient of the Month: Vitamin B12, Part 11," *Nutrition and Healing* 5, no. 7 (Aug. 1995): 4.

8 https://www.merckmanuals.com/professional/nutritional-disorders/vitamin-deficiency,-dependency,-and-toxicity/riboflavin. Accessed Nov. 25, 2018.

9 https://www.podiatrytoday.com/when-vitamin-and-nutritional-deficiencies-cause-skin-and-nail-changes. Accessed Jan. 5, 2019.

10 https://www.webmd.com/vitamins-and-supplements/ss/slideshow-vitamins-vitamin-b6-deficiency. Accessed Jan. 21, 2021.

11 https://pubmed.ncbi.nlm.nih.gov/31638351/. Accessed Jan. 6, 2021.

12 https://www.mdedge.com/familymedicine/quiz/9968/obesity/obesity-test-your-skills-these-5-questions?ecd=wnl_fam_210121_mdedge_4am. Accessed Jan. 21, 2021.

13 A.W. Schreiner et al., "Seborrheic Dermatitis: A Local Metabolic Defect Involving Pyridoxine," *J Lab Clin Med* 40 (1952): 121.

14 R.A. Schwartz, C.A. Janusz, and C.K. Janniger, "Seborrheic Dermatitis: An Overview," *Am Fam Physician* 74 (2006): 125-130.

15 https://www.mayoclinic.org/diseases-conditions/seobrrheic-dernatitis/diagnosis-treatment/drc-20352714. Accessed Jan. 2, 2019.

16 https://www.medicalnewstoday.com/articles/319113.php. Accessed Jan. 2, 2019.

17 https://examine.com/supplements/aloe-vera/. Accessed Mar. 5, 2019.

18 N.S. Al-Waili, "Therapeutic and Prophylactic Effects of Crude Honey on Chronic Seborrheic Dermatitis and Dandruff," *Eur J Med Res* 6, no. 7 (July 2001): 306-308. https://skindrone.com/articles/seborrheic-dermatits-eyebrows/#raw-honey. Accessed Jan. 24, 2019.

19 *The Merck Manual of Diagnosis and Therapy,* 19th ed., 784.

20 https://www.ncbi.nlm.nih.gov/pubmed/14678527. Accessed Jan. 5, 2019.

21 A. Nisenson and L.A. Barness, "Treatment of Seborrheic Dermatitis with Biotin and Vitamin B Complex," *J Pediatrics* (Sept. 1972): 81, no. 3): 630-631.

22 A. Nisenson, "Seborrheic Dermatitis of Infants and Leiner's Disease: A Biotin Deficiency," *J Pediatrics* 51, no. 5 (Nov. 1957): 537-548.

23 https://www.medicalnewstoday.com/articles/318724.php. Accessed Jan. 5, 2019.

Sepsis/Septic Shock

1 https://www.nigms.nih.gov/education/fact-sheets/Pages/sepsis.aspx Accessed Sept. 21, 2020.

2 https://emedicine.medscape.com/article/168402-overview. Accessed Dec. 26, 2018.

3 https://link.springer.com/referenceworkentry/10.1007/3-540-29662-X_958. Accessed Feb. 5, 2019.

4 M.H. Zabet et al., "Effect of High-Dose Ascorbic Acid on Vasopressor's Requirement in Septic Shock," *J Res Pharm Pract* 5, no. 2 (Apr.-June 3, 2016): 94-100. DOI: 10.4103/2279-042X.179569.

5 A.A. Fowler 3rd et al., "Phase I Safety Trial of Intravenous Ascorbic Acid in Patients with Severe Sepsis," *J Transl Med* 12 (2014): 32.

6 W. Alhazzani et al., "The Effect of Selenium Therapy on Mortality in Patients with Sepsis Syndrome: A Systematic Review and Meta-Analysis of Randomized Controlled Trials," *Crit Care Med* 41, no. 6 (2013): 1555-1564.

7 T.S. Huang et al., "Effect of Parenteral Selenium Supplementation in Critically Ill Patients: A Systematic Review and Meta-Analysis," *PLoS One* 8, no. 1 (2013): e54431.

8 S.K Shahid et al., "Efficacy and Safety of Phlogenzym—A Protease Formulation, in Sepsis in Children," *J Assoc Physicians India* 50: 527-531.

9 https://emedicine.medscape.com/article/2038394-overview#a2. Accessed Mar. 19, 2021.

10 X. Peng et al., "Clinical and Protein Metabolic Efficacy of Glutamine Granules-Supplemented Enteral Nutrition in Severely Burned Patients," *Burns* 31, no. 3 (2005): 342-346.

11 https://academic.oup.com/jn/article/138/10/2040S/4670117.

12 https://pubchem.ncbi.nlm.nih.gov/compound/choline_chloride#section=Therapeutic-Uses. Accessed Feb. 5, 2019.

13 http://www.freepatentsonline.com/6013273.html. Accessed Feb. 5, 2019.

Sickle Cell Anemia/Hemoglobin SS Disease

1 https://www.nhlbi.nih.gov/health-topics/sickle-cell-disease. Accessed Dec. 26, 2018.

2 J.C.M. Brust, *Current Diagnosis and Treatment Neurology*, 2nd ed. (McGraw-Hill, 2012): 502.

3 www.cdc.gov/ncbddd/sicklecell/treatments.html. Accessed Dec. 26, 2018.

4 K. Kaushansky et al., "Anemia Due to Other Nutritional Deficiencies," *Williams Hematology* (2011): ch. 39.

5 M.T. Lee, M. Licursi, and D.J. McMahon, "Vitamin D Deficiency and Acute Vaso-Occlusive Complications in Children with Sickle Cell Disease," *Pediatr Blood Cancer* 62 (2015): 643-647.

6 https://www.webmd.com/vitamins/ai/ingredientmono-982/zinc. Accessed Jan. 29, 2019.

Sinusitis (Acute)

1 https://www.medicalnewstoday.com/articles/149941.php. Accessed Jan. 3, 2019.

2 E.T. Bope and R.D. Kellerman, *Conn's Current Therapy*, 14th ed. (Philadelphia: Elsevier/Saunders), 355.

3 F.L. Van Buchem et al., "Primary-Care-Based Randomized Placebo-Controlled Trial Antibiotic Treatment in Acute Maxillary Sinusitis," *Lancet* 349 (1997): 683-687.

4 "Quantum Sufficit," *Am Fam Phys* 56 (1997): 1941.

5 R.E. Ryan, "A Double-Blind Clinical Evaluation of Bromelains in the Treatment of Acute Sinusitis," *Headache* 7 (1967): 13-17.

7 https://www.webmd.com/vitamins/ai/ingredientmono-716/gentian.

Smell Perception/Anosmia/Parosmia

1 https://www.bmj.com/content/371/bmj.m4739.

2 T. Aiba et al., "Effect of Zinc Sulfate on Sensorineural Olfactory Disorder," *Acta Otolaryngol Stockh* Suppl. 538 (1998): 202-204.

3 K.J. Isselbacher et al., *Harrison's Principles of Internal Medicine*, 13th ed., 110.

4 https://www.ncbi.nlm.nih.gov/pmc/articles/PMC3201003/#R133. Accessed Dec. 31, 2018.

5 http://www.familydiagnosis.com/diseases/parosmia.html. Accessed Nov. 19, 2018.

Smoking (Cessation)

1 https://www.cdc.gov/tobacco/data_statistics/fact_sheets/health_effects/effects_cig_smoking/index.htm. Accessed Aug. 12, 2020.

2 https://www.webmd.com/vitamins/ai/ingredientmono-326/l-tryptophan. Accessed Dec. 13, 2018.

3 Y. Ohmura et al., "5-Hydroxytryptophan Attenuates Somatic Signs of Nicotine Withdrawal," *J Pharmacol Sci* 117, no. 2 (2011): 121-124.

4 D.J. Bowen, B. Spring, and E. Fox., "Tryptophan and High-Carbohydrate Diets as Adjuncts to Smoking Cessation Therapy," *J Behav Med* 14 (1991): 97-110.

5 M. Perugini et al., "Effects of Tryptophan Depletion on Acute Smoking Abstinence Symptoms and the Acute Smoking Response," *Pharmacology, Biochemistry & Behavior* 74, no. 3 (2003): 513-522.

6 https://link.springer.com/article/10.1007/BF00846173. Accessed Dec. 13, 2018.

7 American Thoracic Society, "Pregnant Smokers May Reduce Harm Done to Baby's Lungs by Taking Vitamin C," *ScienceDaily* (May 21, 2018). www.sciencedaily.com/releases/2018/05/180521184704.htm.

8 Oregon State University, "Study with Smokers Shows Vitamins Combine for Benefits." *ScienceDaily* (Feb. 25, 2006). www.sciencedaily.com/releases/2006/02/060224104219.htm.

9 https://news.osu.edu/quit-smoking-vitamin-e-may-give-extra-boost-to-heart-health/. Accessed Dec. 13, 2018.

10 U.S. Food and Drug Administration, "Deeming Tobacco Products to Be Subject to the Federal Food, Drug, and Cosmetic Act, as Amended by the Family Smoking Prevention and Tobacco Control Act; Restrictions on the Sale and Distribution of Tobacco Products and Required Warning Statements for Tobacco Products," *Fed Regist* 81 (2016): 28973-29106.

11 J. Hartmann-Boyce et al., "Electronic Cigarettes for Smoking Cessation," *Cochrane Database Syst Rev* 9 (2016): CD010216.

12 W.K. Al-Delaimy et al., "E-Cigarette Use in the Past and Quitting Behavior in the Future: A Population-Based Study," *Am J Public Health* 105 (2015): 1213-1219.

Solar Urticaria/Sun Allergy

1 https://www.dermnetnz.org/topics/solar-urticaria/. Accessed Mar. 21, 2019.

2 https://www.ncbi.nlm.nih.gov/pmc/articles/PMC4203568/. Accessed Dec. 29, 2018.

3 https://www.healthline.com/health/skin-disorders/solar-urticaria. Accessed Dec. 29, 2018.

4 https://www.ncbi.nlm.nih.gov/pubmed/4078439. Accessed May 18, 2020.

5 https://www.medicalnewstoday.com/articles/318969#management-and-treatment. Accessed May 18, 2020.

6 https://www.ncbi.nlm.nih.gov/pmc/articles/PMC3063367/. Accessed May 18, 2020.

Steatorrhea

1 https://www.medicalnewstoday.com/articles/320361. Accessed May 12, 2020.

2 https://www.medicalnewstoday.com/articles/320361.php. Accessed Dec. 20, 2018.

3 https://mddk.com/steatorrhea.html. Accessed May 12, 2020.

4 https://www.dhinfo.org/2016/01/what-is-steatorrhea-symptoms-causes-and-treatment/. Accessed Dec. 20, 2018.

5 J.S. Fordtran, F. Bunch, and G.R. Davis, "Ox Bile Treatment of Severe Steatorrhea in an Ileectomy-Ileostomy Patient," *Gastroenterology* 82, no. 3 (Mar. 1982): 564-568.

6 K.H. Little et al., "Treatment of Severe Steatorrhea with Ox Bile in an Ileectomy Patient with Residual Colon," *Digest Dis Sci* 37 (1992): 929. https://doi.org/10.1007/BF01300393.

Stroke

1 https://www.cdc.gov/stroke/index.htm. Accessed Apr. 20, 2020.

2 https://www.webmd.com/stroke/news/20070531/folic-acid-may-lower-stroke-risk#1. Accessed Nov. 16, 2018.

3 J.A. David et al., "Supplemental Vitamins and Minerals for CVD Prevention and Treatment," *J Am Coll Cardiol* 71, no. 22 (June 2018): 2570-2584. Accessed Dec. 22, 2018.

4 International Stroke Conference (2009). https://www.webmd.com/stroke/news/20090220/b-vitamins-may-cut-stroke-risk#1. Accessed Dec. 22, 2018.

5 *Journal of the American College of Cardiology (JACC)* (May 28, 2018).

6 https://www.ncbi.nlm.nih.gov/pubmed/8133587. Accessed May 12, 2020.

7 B.T. Altura, and B.M. Altura, "The Role of Magnesium in Etiology of Strokes and Cerebrovasospasm," *Magnes Trace Elem* 10 (1991-1992): 182-192.

8 N. Boyce, "Homocysteine Screening for Heart Disease on Horizon," *Clinical Laboratory News* (1996): 22.

9 https://www.webmd.com/vitamins/ai/ingredientmono-957/riboflavin. Accessed Nov. 14, 2018.

10 https://www.medscape.com/viewarticle/820660.

11 Naval Branch Clinic Diego Garcia (Dr. Smith); Penn State University Family and Community Medicine Residency Program (Dr. Demetriou); Naval Hospital Okinawa (Dr. Weber), "Aspirin for Primary Prevention: USPSTF Recommendations for CVD and Colorectal Cancer," *J Fam Pract* 68, no. 3 (Apr. 2019): 146-151.

12 J.M. Guirguis-Blake et al., "Aspirin for the Primary Prevention of Cardiovascular Events: A Systematic Evidence Review for the U.S. Preventive Services Task Force," *Ann Intern Med* 164 (2016): 804-813.

13 Y. Ikeda et al., "Low-Dose Aspirin for Primary Prevention of Cardiovascular Events in Japanese Patients 60 Years or Older with Atherosclerotic Risk Factors: A Randomized Clinical Trial," *JAMA* 312 (2014): 2510-2520.

14 https://www.mdedge.com/internalmedicine/article/217954/stroke/more-evidence-backs-ldl-below-70-reduce-recurrent-stroke. Accessed Mar. 1, 2020.

Post-Stroke Management (Brain Hypoxia/Ischemic Damage)

1 P.F. Smith, K. Maclennan, and C.L. Darlington, "The Neuroprotective Properties of the Ginkgo Biloba Leaf: A Review of the Possible Relationship to Platelet-Activating Factor (PAF)," *J Ethanopharmacol* 50, no. 3 (Mar. 1996): 131-139.

2 A.A. Selin et al., "Mechanism Underlying the Protective Effect of Glycine in Energetic Disturbances in Brain Tissues under Hypoxic Conditions," *Bull Exp Biol Med* 153, no. 1 (2012): 44-47.

3 E.I. Gusev et al., "Neuroprotective Effects of Glycine for Therapy of Acute Ischemic Stroke," *Cerebrovasc Dis* 10 (2000): 49-60.

4 E.E.A. Salamal et al., "The Role of Vitamin E in Cerebral Hypoxia: An Ultrastructural Study," *Surgical Science* 4 (2013): 100-106. http://dx.doi.org/10.4236/ss.2013.41018.

5 C. Inan et al., "The Effect of High Dose Antenatal Vitamin E on Hypoxia-Induced Changes in Newborn Rats," *Pediatr Res* 38, no. 5 (Nov. 1995): 685-689.

6 E. Salama et al., "The Role of Vitamin E in Cerebral Hypoxia: An Ultrastructural Study," *Surgical Science* 4 (2013): 100-106. DOI: 10.4236/ss.2013.41018.

7 R. Balden, A. Selvamani, and F. Sohrabji, "Vitamin D Deficiency Exacerbates Experimental Stroke Injury and Dysregulates Ischemia-Induced Inflammation in Adult Rats," *Endocrinology* 153 (2012): 2420-2435. PMID: 22408173.

8 S. Won et al., "Vitamin D Prevents Hypoxia/Reoxygenation-Induced Blood-Brain Barrier Disruption via Vitamin D Receptor-Mediated NF-*k*B Signaling Pathways," *Plos One* (2015). https://journals.plos.org/plosone/article?id=10.1371/journal.pone.0122821.

9 L. Belayev et al., "Docosahexaenoic Acid Therapy of Experimental Ischemic Stroke," *Translational Stroke Research* (2010). DOI: 10.1007/s12975-010-0046-0.

10 https://pubmed.ncbi.nlm.nih.gov/17171187/. Accessed Mar. 7, 2021.

11 https://www.medicinenet.com/citicoline/supplements-vitamins.htm. Accessed Mar. 16, 2021.

12 J.T. DiPiro et al., *Pharmacotherapy: A Pathophysiologic Approach*, 6th ed. (McGraw-Hill, 2005), 420.

13 https://www.ahajournals.org/doi/10.1161/STR.0000000000000375. Accessed Aug. 10, 2021.

14 https://www.mdedge.com/neurology/article/244293/stroke/exercise-tied-50-reduction-mortality-after-stroke? Accessed Aug. 13, 2021.

Subacute Combined Degeneration of the Spinal Cord

1 D.O. Agamanolis, "Nutritional CNS Disorders." July 2014. Retrieved Sept. 13, 2014. http://neuropathology-web.org/.html. Accessed Dec. 26, 2018.

2 N. Kumar, J.B. Gross Jr., and J.E. Ahlskog, "Copper Deficiency Myelopathy Produces a Clinical Picture Like Subacute Combined Degeneration," *Neurology* 63, no. 1 (July 13, 2004): 33-39.

3 https://www.merckmanuals.com/home/brain,-spinal-cord,-and-nerve-disorders/spinal-cord-disorders/subacute-combined-degeneration. Accessed Apr. 20, 2020.

4 https://www.merckmanuals.com/home/brain,-spinal-cord,-and-nerve-disorders/spinal-cord-disorders/subacute-combined-degeneration. Accessed June 10, 2020.

5 R. Gilroy and J.S. Meyer, *Medical Neurology*, 3rd ed. (Macmillan Publishing, 1979), 280-281.

6 https://www.mayoclinic.org/diseases-conditions/diabetic-neuropathy/in-depth/diabetic-neuropathy-and-dietary-supplements/art-20095406. Accessed Jan. 8, 2019.

7 L.M. Tierney Jr., S.J. McPhee, and M.A. Papadakis, *Current Medical Diagnosis and Treatment*, 34th ed., A Lange Medical Book (1995), 862.

8 https://pubmed.ncbi.nlm.nih.gov/17894634/. Accessed Jan. 9, 2021.

9 L.J. Kinsella and D.E. Riley, "Nutritional Deficiencies and Syndromes Associated with Alcoholism," *Textbook of Clinical Neurology*, 3rd ed., ed. Christopher Goetz (2007).

Subcorneal Pustular Dermatosis (SPD)

1 https://www.dermnetnz.org/topics/subcorneal-pustular-dermatosis/. Accessed Nov. 30, 2020.

2 https://emedicine.medscape.com/article/1124252-overview. Accessed Dec. 26, 2018.

3 S. Ayres Jr., and R. Mihan, "Vitamin E and Dermatology," *Cutis* 16 (1975): 1017-1021.

4 S. Ayres Jr. and R. Mihan, Letter: "Subcorneal Pustular Dermatosis Controlled by Vitamin E," *Arch Dermatol* 109, no. 6 (June 1974): 914.

Sunburn

1 https://www.emedicinehealth.com/sunburn/article_em.htm. Accessed Mar. 6, 2019.

2 https://www.webmd.com/beauty/features/whats-best-sunscreen#1. Accessed Dec. 13, 2018.

3 https://www.emedicinehealth.com/vitamin_c_ascorbic_acid/vitamins-supplements.htm. Accessed Sept. 12, 2018.

4 G. La Ruche and J.P. Cesarini, "Protective Effect of Oral Selenium Plus Copper Associated with a Vitamin Complex on Sunburn Cell Formation in Human Skin," *Photodermatol Photoimmunol Photomed* 8, no. 6 (Paris, France: Laboratoires Gresval, Foundation A. de Rothschild, Dec. 1991), 232-235.

5 A.C. Turner et al., "The Effect of Preparation of Vitamin A and Calcium Carbonate on Sunburn," *Practitioner* 206 (1971): 662-665.

6 https://www.webmd.com/vitamins/ai/ingredientmono-954/vitamin-e. Accessed Sept. 12, 2018.

7 https://www.medicalnewstoday.com/articles/323628#side-effects. Accessed Apr. 2, 2021.

Tardive Dyskinesia (TD)

1 https://www.webmd.com/schizophrenia/tardive-dyskinesia#1. Accessed Mar. 21, 2019.

2 V. Lerner et al., "Vitamin B(6) in the Treatment of Tardive Dyskinesia: A Double-Blind, Placebo-Controlled, Crossover Study," *Am J Psychiatry* 158, no. 9 (2001): 1511-1514.

3 J. DeVeaugh-Geiss and L. Manion, "High-Dose Pyridoxine in Tardive Dyskinesia," *J Clin Psychiatry* 39 (1978): 575.

4 https://www.webmd.com/vitamins/ai/ingredientmono-954/vitamin-e. Accessed Dec. 28, 2018.

5 https://www.drugs.com/dosage/vitamin-e.html. Accessed Dec. 29, 2018.

6 J.B. Lohr and M.P. Caligiuri, "A Double-Blind Placebo-Controlled Study of Vitamin E Treatment of Tardive Dyskinesia," *J Clin Psychiatry* 57, no. 167 (1996): 73.

7 G.T. Vatassery, Timothy Bauer, and Maurice Dysken, "High Doses of Vitamin E in the Treatment of Disorders of the Central Nervous System in the Aged," *The American Journal of Clinical Nutrition* 70, no. 5 (Nov. 1999): 793-801. https://doi.org/10.1093/ajcn/70.5.793.

8 R.A. Kunin, "Manganese and Niacin in the Treatment of Drug-Induced Dyskinesias," *Orthomolecular Psychiatry* 5, no. 1 (1976): 4-27.

9 https://www.webmd.com/vitamins/condition-1607/tardive+dyskinesia. Accessed Dec. 28, 2018.

10 https://www.webmd.com/vitamins/ai/ingredientmono-333/ginkgo. Accessed Nov. 26, 2018.

11 J.H. Growdon, *Adv Neurol* 1979):24:387. https://pubchem.ncbi.nlm.nih.gov/compound/choline_chloride#section=Therapeutic-Uses. Accessed Feb. 5, 2019.

Taste Disorders

1 G.M. Gonzales and M.J. Cook, "Chapter 13: Disorders of Smell and Taste," *Neurology and Clinical Neuroscience* (Mosby, 2007): 171-177.

2 https://www.medicinenet.com/taste_disorders/article.htm#how_common_are_taste_disorders. Accessed Mar. 14, 2019.

3 http://www.alabamaentassociates.com/smell-and-taste-disorders.html. Accessed Nov. 23, 2018.

4 S.M. Bromley, "Smell and Taste Disorders: A Primary Care Approach," *Am Fam Physician* 61, no. 2 (Jan. 2000): 427-436.

5 K. Mullin, "Nutrition in Hepatic Encephalopathy," *Nutr Clin Pract* 25 (2010): 257.

6 https://emedicine.medscape.com/article/861242-overview#a3. Accessed Nov. 23, 2018.

7 https://www.ncbi.nlm.nih.gov/pubmedhealth/PMH0070634/. Accessed Nov. 23, 2018.

8 https://www.webmd.com/vitamins/condition-1285/hypogeusia. Accessed Nov. 23, 2018.

Testosterone

1 https://www.oxforddictionaries.com/. Accessed Nov. 15, 2018.

2 https://www.health.harvard.edu/mens-health/treating-low-testosterone-levels. Accessed Apr. 20, 2020.

3 T.C. Liu et al., "Effect of Acute DHEA Administration on Free Testosterone in Middle-Aged and Young Men Following High-Intensity Interval Training," *Eur J Appl Physiol* 113, no. 7 (July 2013): 1783-1792. DOI: 10.1007/s00421-013-2607-x. Epub Feb. 17, 2013.

4 T.K. Jensen et al., "Associations of Fish Oil Supplement Use with Testicular Function in Young Men," *JAMA Netw Open* 3, no. 1 (2020): e1919462. DOI: 10.1001/jamanetworkopen.2019.19462. Accessed Feb. 6, 2020.

5 https://www.webmd.com/vitamins/ai/ingredientmono-664/stinging-nettle. Accessed Oct. 24, 2020.

6 J.M. Ritter et al., "Alternative Medicines: Herbals and Nutraceuticals," in *A Textbook of Pharmacology and Clinical Therapeutics*, 5th ed. (UK: Hodder Arnold, 2008): 100.

Thrombophlebitis/Superficial Vein Thrombosis

1 https://www.mountsinai.org/health-library/diseases-conditions/superficial-thrombophlebitis.

2 https://my.clevelandclinic.org/health/diseases/17523-superficial-thrombophlebitis/management-and-treatment.

3 https://www.mayoclinic.org/diseases-conditions/thrombophlebitis/diagnosis-treatment/drc-20354613. Accessed Oct. 14, 2019.

4 R.A. Neubauer, "A Plant Protease for Potentiation of and Possible Replacement of Antibiotics," *Exp Med Surg* 19 (1961): 143-160.

5 https://www.ncbi.nlm.nih.gov/pmc/articles/PMC4998156/. Accessed Oct. 14, 2019.

6 A.E. Gutfreund, S.J. Taussig, and A.K. Morris, "Effect of Oral Bromelain on Blood Pressure and Heart Rate of Hypertensive Patients," *Hawaii Med J* 37 (1978): 143-146.

7 http://www.altmedrev.com/archive/publications/15/4/361.pdf. Accessed Oct. 14, 2019.

Tick Bites

1 https://www.cdc.gov/vitalsigns/vector-borne/. Accessed May 31, 2019.

2 J.C.M. Brust, *Current Diagnosis and Treatment Neurology,* 2nd ed. (McGraw-Hill, 2012): 512.

3 http://theconversation.com/tackling-the-tricky-task-of-tick-removal-26306. Accessed May 31, 2019.

Tinnitus

1 https://www.mayoclinic.org/diseases-conditions/tinnitus/symptoms-causes/syc-20350156. Accessed Mar. 21, 2019.

2 https://www.webmd.com/a-to-z-guides/understanding-tinnitus-treatment#3. Accessed Dec. 15, 2018.

3 H.N. Arda, "The Role of Zinc in the Treatment of Tinnitus," *Otol Neurotol* 24, no. 1 (Jan. 2003): 86-89.

4 K. Ehrenberger and R. Brix, "Glutamic Acid and Glutamic Acid Diethylester in Tinnitus Treatment," *ACTA Otolaryngol* 95, no. 5-6 (1983): 599-605.

5 https://www.medscape.com/answers/856916-103336/what-is-the-role-of-niacin-in-the-treatment-of-tinnitus. Accessed Dec. 15, 2018.

6 *Physician's Desk Reference*, 36th ed. (1982), 761.

7 *Tinnitus: Facts, Theories, and Treatments* (Washington, DC: National Academies Press, 1982). https://www.ncbi.nlm.nih.gov/books/NBK217858/.

8 R.J. Goodey, "Drugs in the Treatment of Tinnitus," in *CIBA Foundation Symposium* 85, Tinnitus (London: Pitman, 1981), 263-273.

9 https://www.mayoclinic.org/diseases-conditions/tinnitus/diagnosis-treatment/drc-20350162. Accessed Dec. 15, 2018.

Tooth Loss

1 https://www.emedicinehealth.com/vitamin_d/vitamins-supplements.htm. Accessed Dec. 28, 2018.

2 https://www.webmd.com/oral-health/news/20000927/keep-that-smile-calcium-vitamin-d-prevent-tooth-loss#1. Accessed Dec. 28, 2018.

Traumatic Brain Injury

1 http://www.traumaticbraininjury.com/. Accessed Dec. 28, 2018.

2 G. Sakellaris et al., "Prevention of Complications Related to Traumatic Brain Injury in Children and Adolescents with Creatine Administration: An Open Label Randomized Pilot Study," *Journal of Trauma-Injury Infection & Critical Care* 61, no. 2 (2006): 322-329.

3 G. Sakellaris, "Prevention of Traumatic Headache, Dizziness and Fatigue with Creatine Administration. A Pilot Study," *Acta Paediatrica* 87, no. 1 (2008): 31-34.

4 S.R. Dager et al., "Brain Metabolic Alterations in Medication-Free Patients with Bipolar Disorder," *Archives of General Psychiatry* 61, no. 5 (2004): 450-458.

5 M. Segal et al., "Serum Creatine Kinase Level in Unmediated Nonpsychotic, Psychotic, Bipolar and Schizoaffective Depressed Patients," *European Neuropsychopharmacology* 17, no. 3 (2007): 194-198.

6 D. Amital et al., "Open Study of Creatine Monohydrate in Treatment-Resistant Posttraumatic Stress Disorder," *Journal of Clinical Psychiatry* 67, no. 5 (2006): 836-837.

7 S. Roitman et al., "Creatine Monohydrate in Resistant Depression: A Preliminary Study," *Bipolar Disorders* 9 (2007): 754-758.

8 Institute of Medicine, "10 Creatine," *Nutrition and Traumatic Brain Injury: Improving Acute and Subacute Health Outcomes in Military Personnel* (Washington DC: The National Academies Press, 2011). DOI: 17226/13121.

9 J.J. Secades, "Citicoline: Pharmacological and Clinical Review, 2010 Update," *Rev Neurol* 52, suppl. 2 (2011): S1-S62.

10 https://lpi.oregonstate.edu/mic/other-nutrients/choline#reference5. Accessed Nov. 23, 2018.

11 https://lpi.oregonstate.edu/mic/other-nutrients/choline#reference74. Accessed Nov. 23, 2018.

12 L. Xi et al., "Treatment with Ginseng Total Saponins Reduces the Secondary Brain Injury in Rat after Cortical Impact," *J Neurosci Res* 90 (2012): 1424-1436.

Transient Ischemic Attack (TIA)

1 https://medlineplus.gov/transientischemicattack.html. Accessed Nov. 30, 2018.

2 https://www.ncbi.nlm.nih.gov/pmc/articles/PMC3134717/. Accessed Nov. 30, 2018.

3 N.J. Solenski, MD, "Transient Ischemic Attacks: Part II. Treatment," *Am Fam Physician* 69 (2004): 1681-1688.

4 https://www.webmd.com/heart-disease/news/20030214/baby-aspirin-may-not-prevent-stroke.

5 J.A. González-Correa et al., "Influence of Vitamin E on the Antiplatelet Effect of Acetylsalicylic Acid in Human Blood," *Platelets* 16 (2005): 3-4, 171-179. DOI: 10.1080/09537100400016797.

6 www.medscape.com/viewarticle/790747. Accessed Nov. 30, 2018.

7 https://www.researchgate.net/publication/11424923_Vitamin_E_potentiates_the_antiplatelet_activity_of_aspirin_in_collagen-stimulated_platelets. Accessed Nov. 30, 2018.

8 "Could Omega-3 Fatty Acids Help in Tackling Clopidogrel Resistance?," *Medscape* (Apr. 12, 2010). https://www.medscape.com/viewarticle/720119. Accessed Dec. 1, 2018.

Tremors

1 J.C.M. Brust, *Current Diagnosis and Treatment Neurology,* 2nd ed. (McGraw-Hill, 2012): 211.

2 https://www.medicinenet.com/tremor/article.htm#what_are_the_characteristics_of_tremor. Accessed Dec. 26, 2018.

3 *PDR for Nonprescription Drugs* (Oradell, NJ: Medical Economics Co., Inc., 1988).

4 https://www.ncbi.nlm.nih.gov/pmc/articles/PMC4586582/. Accessed Mar. 25, 2021.

5 https://www.webmd.com/vitamins/condition-1460/parkinson%27s+disease.aspx. Accessed Dec. 22, 2018.

6 J. Jannicelli, "Riboflavin: A New Treatment Option for Essential Tremor?," *Neurology Reviews* 15, no. 7 (July 2007): 34.

7 http:/connection.ebscohost.com/c/articles/25818050/riboflavin-new-treatment-option-essential-tremor. Accessed Dec. 26, 2018.

8 https://www.hopkinsmedicine.org/neurology_neurosurgery/centers_clinics/movement_disorders/conditions/essential_tremor.html. Accessed Dec. 26, 2018.

9 S. Gupte, ed., "Infantile Tremor Syndrome," *The Short Textbook of Paediatrics*, 10th ed. (New Delhi: Jaypee Brothers, 2004), 716-719.

10 https://www.ncbi.nlm.nih.gov/pmc/articles/PMC4920912/. Accessed Dec. 26, 2018.

11 A. de Souza and M.W. Moloi, "Involuntary Movements Due to Vitamin B12 Deficiency," *Neurol Res* 36, no. 12 (Dec. 2014): 1121-1128.

Trigeminal Neuralgia

1 https://www.ninds.nih.gov/Disorders/Patient-Caregiver-Education/Fact-Sheets/Trigeminal-Neuralgia-Fact-Sheet. Accessed Dec. 28, 2018.

2 http://fpa-support.org/neuropathic-facial-pain-vitamin-b-12-myelin/. Accessed Dec. 28, 2018.

3 S.J. Surtees, M.B. Lpool, and R.R. Hughes, "The Treatment of Trigeminal Neuralgia with Vitamin B12," *The Lancet* 263, no. 6809 (Feb. 1954): 425-472.

4 Anonymous, "Trigeminal Neuralgia Treated with Nicotinic Acid," *Lancet* 2 (1943): 295-296.

5 W.E. Adams and W. Robinson, "Trigeminal Neuralgia," *Lancet* 2: (1941): 5.

6 https://www.mayoclinic.org/diseases-conditions/trigeminal-neuralgia/diagnosis-treatment/drc-20353347. Accessed Dec. 28, 2018.

7 S. Glore and A. Ricker, "Trigeminal Neuralgia: Case Study of Pain Cessation with a Low Caffeine Diet," *J Am Diet Assoc* 91 (1991): 1120-1121.

Triglycerides/Hypertriglyceridemia

1 R.C. Oh and J.B. Lanier, "Management of Hypertriglyceridemia," *Am Fam Physician* 75, no. 9 (May 1, 2007): 1365-1371.

2 https://www.mayoclinic.org/diseases-conditions/high-blood-cholesterol/in-depth/triglycerides/art-20048186. Accessed Dec. 26, 2018.

3 https://emedicine.medscape.com/article/126568-treatment. Accessed Mar. 21, 2019.

4 Z. Raza et al., "Hypertriglyceridemia: A Strategic Approach," *J Fam Pract* 69, no. 4 (May 202): 180-187. Accessed May 14, 2020.

5 https://www.medicinenet.com/script/main/art.asp?articlekey=9487. Accessed Nov. 23, 2018.

6 B.G, Brown et al., "Simvastatin and Niacin, Antioxidant Vitamins, or the Combination for the Prevention of Coronary Disease," *N Engl J Med* 345 (2001): 1583-1592.

7 https://www.webmd.com/cholesterol-management/supplements#1. Accessed Nov. 23, 2018.

8 https://www.mayoclinic.org/diseases-conditions/high-blood-cholesterol/in-depth/cholesterol-lowering-supplements/art-20050980. Accessed Nov. 28, 2018.

9 J. Herbert, "Replacement of Dehydroepiandrosierone Enhances T-Lymphocyte Insulin Binding in Postmenopausal Women," *Fertil Steril* 63, no. 5 (May 1995): 1027-1031.

10 C. Revilla-Monsalve et al., "Biotin Supplementation Reduces Plasma Triacylglycerol and VLDL in Type 2 Diabetic Patients and in Nondiabetic Subjects with Hypertriglyceridemia," *Biomed Pharmacother* 60, no. 4 (2006): 182-185.

Tropical Sprue

1 https://www.merckmanuals.com/professional/gastrointestinal-disorders/malabsorption-syndromes/tropical-sprue. Accessed Dec. 26, 2018.

2 G.G. Lopez et al., "Folic Acid in the Rehabilitation of Persons with Sprue," *JAMA* 132 (1946): 906-911.

3 M.A. Krupp and M.J. Chatton, *Current Medical Diagnosis and Treatment* (1983): 371.

4 https://rarediseases.org/rare-diseases/tropical-sprue/. Accessed May 18, 2020.

5 https://www.merckmanuals.com/professional/gastrointestinal-disorders/malabsorption-syndromes/tropical-sprue. Accessed Mar. 21, 2019.

Tuberculosis (TB)

1 https://pubmed.ncbi.nlm.nih.gov/29171444/. Accessed Nov. 22, 2021.

2 https://journals.lww.com/jaapa/pages/articleviewer.aspx?year=2016&issue=02000&article=00003&type=Fulltext. Accessed Oct. 13, 2019.

3 S.R. Venkata, D. Vemuri, and R. Natham, "Ascorbic Acid Improves Stability and Pharmacokinetics of Rifampicin in the Presence of Isoniazid," *Journal of Pharmaceutical and Biomedical Analysis* 100 (Nov. 2014): 103-108.

4 C. Vilchèze et al., "Mycobacterium Tuberculosis Is Extraordinarily Sensitive to Killing by a Vitamin C-induced Fenton Reaction," *Nat Commun* 4 (2013): 1881. DOI: 10.1038/ncomms2898.

5 https://www.ncbi.nlm.nih.gov/pmc/articles/PMC3698613/. Accessed Dec. 27, 2018.

6 A. Travalto, D.N. Nuhlicik, and J.E. Midtling, "Drug-Nutrient Interactions," *Am Fam Phys* 44, no. 5 (Nov. 1991): 1651-1658.

7 https://academic.oup.com/cid/article/65/6/900/3837010. Accessed Mar. 25, 2021.

8 https://www.webmd.com/vitamins/ai/ingredientmono-964/vitamin-a. Accessed Nov. 19, 2018.

9 https://pubmed.ncbi.nlm.nih.gov/29171444/. Accessed Nov. 22, 2021.

10 N. Salahuddin et al., "Vitamin D Accelerates Clinical Recovery from Tuberculosis: Results of the SUCCINCT Study [Supplementary Cholecalciferol in Recovery from Tuberculosis]. A Randomized, Placebo-Controlled, Clinical Trial of Vitamin D Supplementation in Patients with Pulmonary Tuberculosis," *BMC Infect Dis* 13 (2013): 22.

11 https://pubmed.ncbi.nlm.nih.gov/30611908/. Accessed Dec. 13, 2020.

Tyrosinemia

1 https://ghr.nlm.nih.gov/condition/tyrosinemia. Accessed June 10, 2020.

2 https://www.webmd.com/vitamins/ai/ingredientmono-1001/vitamin-c-ascorbic-acid. Accessed Nov. 14, 2018.

Ulcerative Colitis

1 https://www.cancer.org/cancer/colon-rectal-cancer/detection-diagnosis-staging/acs-recommendations.html. Accessed Feb. 8, 2021.

2 J.C. Cash and C.A. Glass, *Family Practice Guidelines*, 4th ed. (Springer, 2017), 332.

3 J.T. DiPiro et al., *Pharmacotherapy: A Pathophysiologic Approach*, 6th ed. (McGraw-Hill, 2005), 654.

4 M.A. Chisolm-Burns et al., *Pharmacotherapy Principles & Practice* (McGraw-Hill Medical, 2008), 285.

5 https://www.medicalnewstoday.com/articles/322751#Strawberries-and-inflammation. Accessed Nov. 14, 2018.

6 https://www.ncbi.nlm.nih.gov/pmc/articles/PMC2984332/. Accessed Nov. 14, 2018.

7 A. Aslan, and G. Triadafilopoulos, "Fish Oil Fatty Acid Supplementation in Active Ulcerative Colitis: A Double-Blind, Placebo-Controlled, Crossover Study," *American Journal of Gastroenterology* 87, no. 4 (Apr. 1992): 432-437.

8 W.F. Strnson et al., "Dietary Supplementation with Fish Oil in Ulcerative Colitis," *Annals of Int Med* 116, no. 8 (Apr. 1992): 609-614.

9 A.H. Steinhart et al., "Treatment of Refractory Ulcerative Proctosigmoiditis with Butyrate Enemas," *Am J Gastroenterol* 89 (1994): 179-183.

10 https://www.webmd.com/vitamins/ai/ingredientmono-895/bromelain. Accessed Nov. 19, 2018.

11 https://www.researchgate.net/publication/12549284_Use_of_bromelain_for_mild_ulcerative_colitis. Accessed Jan. 7, 2019.

12 S. Kane and M.J. Goldberg, "Use of Bromelain for Mild Ulcerative Colitis," *Ann Int Med* 132 (2000): 680.

13 A. Costantini et al., "Thiamine and Spinocerebellar Ataxia Type 2," *BMJ Case Reports.* Published online Jan. 10, 2013.

14 https://www.webmd.com/vitamins/ai/ingredientmono-790/lactobacillus. Accessed Jan. 12, 2019.

15 https://www.ncbi.nlm.nih.gov/pmc/articles/PMC4001731/. Accessed Feb. 27, 2019.

16 https://www.webmd.com/vitamins/ai/ingredientmono-662/turmeric. Accessed Feb. 27, 2019.

17 H. Hanai et al., "Curcumin Maintenance Therapy for Ulcerative Colitis: Randomized, Multicenter, Double-Blind, Placebo-Controlled Trial," *Clinical Gastroenterology and Hepatology* 4, no. 12 (2006): 1502-1506.

18 R. Ahamed et al., *J Clin Gastroenterol* (July 24, 2019). DOI: 10.1097/MCG.0000000000001233.

19 https://www.ulcerativecolitis.org.uk/aloevera.htm.

20 J.T. DiPiro et al., *Pharmacotherapy: A Pathophysiologic Approach*, 6th ed. (McGraw-Hill, 2005), 651.

21 T.D. Nolan and P.A. Friedman, "Agents Affecting Mineral Ion Homeostasis and Bone Turnover," in *Gilbert & Goodman's: The Pharmacological Basis of Therapeutics*, 13th ed. (2018), 896.

Ulcers—Leg/Foot

1 https://www.canadaveinclinics.ca/venous-ulcers-complications-of-varicose-veins/. Accessed Dec. 12, 2020.

2 https://my.clevelandclinic.org/health/diseases/17169-leg-and-foot-ulcers. Accessed May 12, 2020.

3 E.T. Bope and R.D. Kellerman, *Conn's Current Therapy*, 14th ed. (Philadelphia: Elsevier/Saunders), 324.

4 https://www.aafp.org/afp/2010/0415/p989.html. Accessed Dec. 12, 2020.

5 https://www.podiatrytoday.com/blogged/why-you-should-consider-use-supplements-management-diabetic-neuropathy. Accessed Jan. 8, 2019.

6 https://www.woundsresearch.com/article/nutrition-wound-care-management-comprehensive-overview. Accessed Apr. 17, 2021.

7 H.E. Strömberg and M.S. Ågren, "Topical Zinc Oxide Treatment Improves Arterial and Venous Leg Ulcers," *British Journal of Dermatology* 111 (1984): 461-468.

8 S.L. Husain, "Oral Zinc Sulphate in Leg Ulcers," *Lancet* 1: (1967): 1069-1071.

9 S.C. Cunnan, *Zinc: Clinical and Biochemical Significance* (Boca Raton, FL: CRC Press, Inc., 1988).

10 T.L. Kopjas, "Folic Acid for the Treatment of Chronic Leg Ulcers in Elderly Patients," *Am Soc* 16 (1968): 338-342.

11 K.A. Oster, "The Treatment of Bovine Xanthine Oxidase Initiated Atherosclerosis by Folic Acid," *Clin Res* 24 (1976): 512A.

12 https://www.webmd.com/vitamins/ai/ingredientmono-235/calendula. Accessed Nov. 21, 2018.

13 M. Buzzi, F. de Freitas, and M. de Barros Winter, "Therapeutic Effectiveness of a *Calendula officinalis* Extract in Venous Leg Ulcer Healing," *Journal of Wound Care* 25, no. 12 (Dec. 2016): 732. Published online Dec. 15, 2016. https://doi.org/10.12968/jowc.2016.25.12.732.

Ulcers—Peptic/Gastroduodenal

1 https://www.ncbi.nlm.nih.gov/pmc/articles/PMC6406303/.

2 https://www.niddk.nih.gov/health-information/digestive-diseases/peptic-ulcers-stomach-ulcers/treatment. Accessed Feb. 24, 2019.

3 *The Washington Manual of Medical Therapeutics*, 34th ed. (Lippincott Williams and Wilkins, 2010), 849.

4 https://www.mayoclinic.org/diseases-conditions/peptic-ulcer/diagnosis-treatment/drc-20354229. Accessed Jan. 24, 2019.

5 J.T. DiPiro et al., *Pharmacotherapy: A Pathophysiologic Approach*, 6th ed. (McGraw-Hill, 2005), 640.

6 https://www.webmd.com/vitamins/ai/ingredientmono-326/l-tryptophan.

7 J.T. DiPiro et al., *Pharmacotherapy: A Pathophysiologic Approach*, 6th ed. (McGraw-Hill, 2005), 636-637.

8 V. Schulz, R. Hansel, and V.E. Tyler, *Rational Phytotherapy: A Physicians' Guide to Herbal Medicine*, 3rd ed. (Berlin, Germany: Springer-Verlag, 1998), 185.

9 A.G. Morgan et al., "Comparison Between Cimetidine and Caved-S in the Treatment of Gastric Ulceration, and Subsequent Maintenance Therapy," *Gut* 23 (1982): 545-551.

10 W.D. Rees et al., "Effect of Deglycyrrhizinated Liquorice on Gastric Mucosal Damage by Aspirin," *Scand J Gastroenterol* 14 (1979): 605-607.

11 A.G. Turpie et al., "Clinical Trial of Deglycyrrhinized Liquorice in Gastric Ulcer," *Gut* 10 (1969): 299-302.

12 R.D. Montgomery and J.B. Cookson, "The Treatment of Gastric Ulcer. Comparative Trial of Carbenoxolone and a Deglycyrrhizinated Liquorice Preparation (Caved-S)," *Clin Trials J* 1 (1972): 33-35.

13 S.N. Tewari and A.K. Wilson, "Deglycyrrhizinated Liquorice in Duodenal Ulcer," *Practitioner* 210 (1972): 820-825.

14 Z.A. Kassir, "Endoscopic Controlled Trial of Four Drug Regimens in the Treatment of Chronic Duodenal Ulceration," *Irish Med J* 78 (1985): 153-156.

15 D.J. Frommer, "The Healing of Gastric Ulcers by Zinc Sulphate," *Med J Aust* 2 (1975): 793-796.

16 M. Miwa et al., "The Therapeutics of Peptic Ulcers: Clinical Evaluation of C-Fe Therapy," *Tokai J Ex Clin Med* 5, no. 1 (1980): 41-44.

17 S. Weiss, J. Weiss, and B. Weiss, "Gastrointestinal Hemorrhage: Therapeutic Evaluation of Bioflavonoids. Report on 55 Cases," *Am J Gastroenterol* 24 (1955): 523-532.

18 M.E. McAlindon et al., "Effect of Allopurinol, Sulphasalazine, and Vitamin C on Aspirin Induced Gastroduodenal Injury in Human Volunteers," *Gut* 38 (1996): 518-524.

19 A. Aditi and D.Y. Graham, "Vitamin C, Gastritis, and Gastric Disease: A Historical Review and Update," *Dig Dis Sci* 57, no. 10 (Oct. 2012). DOI: 10.1007/s10620-012-2203-7.

20 S.L. Gorbach, "Bismuth Therapy in Gastrointestinal Diseases," *Gastroenterology* 99, no. 3 (Sept. 1990): 863-875.

21 https://www.medicinenet.com/taurine/supplements-vitamins.htm. Accessed Nov. 28, 2018.

22 S.W. Ryan, "Management of Dyspepsia and Peptic Ulcer Disease," *Altern Ther Health Med* 11, no. 5 (2005): 26-29.

23 https://www.researchgate.net/publication/290693918_Management_of_peptic_ulcer_disease_using_osteopathic_manipulation. Accessed Jan. 19, 2022.

24 G. Cheney, "Vitamin U Therapy of Peptic Ulcer," *California Medicine* 77, no. 4 (Oct. 1952): 248-252.

25 G. Cheney, S.H. Waxler, and I.J. Miller, "Vitamin U Therapy of Peptic Ulcer; Experience at San Quentin Prison," *Calif Med* 84, no. 1 (Jan. 1956): 39-42.

26 A.D. Patel and N.K. Prajapati, "Review on Biochemical Importance of Vitamin-U," *Journal of Chemical and Pharmaceutical Research* 4, no. 1 (2012): 209-215.

27 A.S. Salim, *J Pharm Sci* 81, no. 7 (July 1992): 698-700.

28 *The Washington Manual of Medical Therapeutics*, 34th ed., 850.

Ulcers—Pressure Ulcers/Decubitus Ulcers/Bedsores

1 https://www.webmd.com/skin-problems-and-treatments/pressure-sores-4-stages#1. Accessed Dec. 26, 2018.

2 https://pubmed.ncbi.nlm.nih.gov/30664906/. Accessed Mar. 12, 2021.

3 https://www.ncbi.nlm.nih.gov/pmc/articles/PMC3217823/. Accessed Dec. 26, 2018.

4 D.R. Thomas, "Prevention and Treatment of Pressure Ulcers: What Works? What Doesn't?," *Cleveland Clinic Journal of Medicine* 68, no. 8 (2001): 704-722.

5 https://www.aafp.org/afp/2008/1115/p1186.html. Accessed Mar. 12, 2021.

6 *Am Fam Phys* 55 (Sept. 1983): 137.

7 https://emedicine.medscape.com/article/190115-treatment#d6. Accessed Nov. 21, 2018.

8 https://pubmed.ncbi.nlm.nih.gov/28272014/. Accessed Mar. 12, 2021.

9 C. Cohen, "Zinc Sulphate and Bedsores," *Br Med J* 2 (1968): 561.

10 T.V. Taylor et al., "Ascorbic Acid Supplementation in the Treatment of Pressure Sores," *Lancet* 2 (1974): 544-546.

11 J.C.L. Neyens et al., "Arginine-Enriched Oral Nutritional Supplementation in the Treatment of Pressure Ulcers: A Literature Review," *Wound Medicine* 16 (Mar. 2017): 46-51.

12 J.M. Schols, H. Heyman, and E.P. Meijer, "Nutritional Support in the Treatment and Prevention of Pressure Ulcers: An Overview of Studies with Arginine Enriched Oral Nutritional Supplement," *J Tissue Viability* 18, no. 3 (Aug. 2009): 72-79.

13 E. Cereda et al., "Disease-Specific, versus Standard, Nutritional Support for the Treatment of Pressure Ulcers in Institutionalized Older Patients: A Randomized Controlled Trial," *J Am Ger Soc* 57, no. 8 (Aug. 2009): 1395-1402.

14 https://www.woundsresearch.com/article/9064. Accessed Nov. 21, 2018.

15 https://www.woundsresearch.com/article/nutrition-wound-care-management-comprehensive-overview. Accessed Apr. 17, 2021.

16 M. Reddy et al., "Treatment of Pressure Ulcers: A Systematic Review," *JAMA* 300 (2009): 2647-2662. DOI: 10.1001/jama.2008.778.

Uremia/Uremic Syndrome

1 S.C. Cunnane, *Zinc: Clinical and Biochemical Significance* (Boca Raton, FL: CRC Press, Inc., 1988).

2 D. McGregor, B. Shand, and K. Lynn, "A Controlled Trial of the Effect of Folate Supplements on Homocysteine, Lipid, and Hemorheology in End Stage Renal Disease," *Nephron* 85 (2000): 215-220.

Urethritis

1 S.N. Rous, "Symptomatic Treatment in Selected Cases of Urethritis," *NY State J Med* 71, no. 24 (Dec. 1971): 2865-2866.

Urinary Tract Infection (UTI)

1 S. Mori et al., "The Clinical Effect of Proteolytic Enzyme Containing Bromelain and Trypsin on Urinary Tract Infection Evaluated by Double-Blind Method," *Acts Obstet Gynecol Jap* (1972): 19.

2 A.R. Gaby, "The Story of Bromelain: Powerful Healing from the Pineapple," *Nutrition and Healing* 2, no. 5 (1995): 4.

3 https://www.medicalnewstoday.com/articles/189953.php. Accessed Dec. 14, 2018.

4 J. Avorn et al., "Reduction of Bacteriuria and Pyuria after Ingestion of Cranberry Juice," *JAMA* 271, no. 10 (1994): 751-754.

5 https://www.ncbi.nlm.nih.gov/pmc/articles/PMC3878051/. Accessed Oct. 14, 2019.

6 I. Singh, L.K. Gautam, and I.R. Kaur, "Effect of Oral Cranberry Extract (Standardized Proanthocyanidin-A) in Patients with Recurrent UTI by Pathogenic *E. coli*: A Randomized Placebo-Controlled Clinical Research Study," *Int Urol Nephrol* 48, no. 9 (Sept. 2016): 1379-1386.

7 https://www.webmd.com/drugs/2/drug-92227/lactobacillus-acidophilus-bifidobacterium-longum-oral/details. Accessed Oct. 14, 2019.

8 G. Reid et al., "Influence of Three-Day Antimicrobial Therapy and Lactobacillus Vaginal Suppositories on Recurrence of Urinary Tract Infections," *Clin Ther* 14 (1992): 11-16.

9 M. Günther et al., "Harnwegsinfektprophylaxe—Urinansäuerung Mittels L-Methionin bei Neurogener Blasenfunktionsstörung," *Der Urologe (B)* (2002): 218-220.

10 http://www.winchesterhospital.org/health-library/article?id=21792. Accessed Jan. 7, 2019.

11 B. Kranjčec et al., *World J Urol* 32, no. 1 (Feb. 2014): 79-84.

Urticaria/Hives

1 https://www.webmd.com/allergies/hives-urticaria-angioedema#1. Accessed Dec. 27, 2018.

2 https://www.clinicaladvisor.com/features/what-to-look-for-with-drug-induced-urticaria/article/164958/. Accessed Dec. 28, 2018.

3 S.W. Simon and P. Edmonds, "Cyanocobalamin B12: Comparison of Aqueous and Respiratory Preparations in Urticaria; Possible Mode of Action," *J Am Geriatr Soc* 12 (1964): 79-85.

4 A.R. Gaby, "Nutrient of the Month: Vitamin B12, Part 11," *Nutrition & Healing* 5, no. 7 (Aug. 1995): 10.

5 A. Knapp, G. Wolfram, and W. Posch, "Chronic Urticaria and Vitamin B6 Dependent Disorders in Tryptophan Metabolism," *Dermatol Monatsschr* 156, no. 3 (1970): 175-183. [article in German]

6 *The Merck Manual of Diagnosis and Therapy*, 12th ed. (1973), 1055.

Uveitis

1 https://www.webmd.com/eye-health/uveitis-inflammation-eye#1. Accessed Dec. 28, 2018.

2 https://www.ncbi.nlm.nih.gov/pmc/articles/PMC3084581/. Accessed Nov. 28, 2018.

3 https://www.webmd.com/vitamins/ai/ingredientmono-954/vitamin-e. Accessed Dec. 28, 2018.

4 J. van Rooi et al., "Oral Vitamins C and E as Additional Treatment in Patients with Acute Anterior Uveitis: A Randomized Double Masked Study in 145 Patients," *Br J Ophthalmol* 83, no. 11 (Nov. 1999): 1277-1282.

5 L.A. Grotting, MD, et al., "Association of Low Vitamin D Levels with Noninfectious Anterior Uveitis," *JAMA Ophthalmol* 135, no. 2 (2017): 150-153. DOI: 10.1001/jamaophthalmol.2016.4888.

6 https://pennstatehershey.adam.com/content.aspx?productId=107&pid=000171. Accessed Dec. 27, 2018.

7 B. Kandi, D. Cicek, and N. Ilhan, "Vitamin Levels in Behcet's disease," *J Dermatolog Treat* 18, no. 2 (2007): 69-75.

8 U.C. Yadav, S. Subramanyam, and K.V. Ramana, "Prevention of Endotoxin-Induced Uveitis in Rats by Benfotiamine, I lipophilic Analogue of Vitamin B1," *Invest Ophthalmol Vis Sci* 50 (2009): 2276-2282.

Vaginal or Vulvovaginal Atrophy/Atrophic Vaginitis/Genitourinary Syndrome of Menopause (GSM)

1 N. Mili et al., "Genitourinary Syndrome of Menopause: A Systematic Review on Prevalence and Treatment," *Menopause* 28, no. 6 (2021): 706-716. DOI: 10.1097/GME.0000000000001752.

2 https://www.mayoclinic.org/diseases-conditions/vaginal-atrophy/symptoms-causes/syc-20352288. Accessed Nov. 19, 2018.

3 https://wwwhealthline.com/health/atrophic-vaginitis#risk-factors. Accessed Dec. 28, 2018.

4 F. Labrie et al., "Intravaginal Dehydroepiandrosterone (Prasterone): A Physiological and Highly Efficient Treatment of Vaginal Atrophy," *Menopause* 16, no. 5 (Sept.-Oct. 2009): 907-922. DOI: 10.1097/gme.0b013e31819e8e2d.

5 "DHEA for Urogenital Atrophy and Sexual Function," *Medscape*, Dec. 1, 2014.

6 A.D. Genazzani et al., "Long-Term Low-Dose Dehydroepiandrosterone Oral Supplementation in Early and Late Postmenopausal Women Modulates Endocrine Parameters and Synthesis of Neuroactive Steroids," *Fertil Steril* 80, no. 6 (Dec. 2003): 1495-1501.

7 https://blogs.webmd.com/womens-health/2012/01/is-dhea-the-next-wonder-drug-for-menopause.html. Accessed Dec. 28, 2018.

8 P. Rad et al., "The Effect of Vitamin D on Vaginal Atrophy in Postmenopausal Women," *Iran J Nurs Midwifery Res* 20, no. 2 (Mar.-Apr. 2015): 211-215.

9 https://pubmed.ncbi.nlm.nih.gov/32967068/. Accessed Feb. 3, 2021.

10 B. Yildirim et al., "The Effects of Postmenopausal Vitamin D Treatment on Vaginal Atrophy," *Maturitas* 49, no. 4 (2004): 334-337.

11 https://www.webmd.com/vitamins/ai/ingredientmono-235/calendula. Accessed Nov. 21, 2018.

12 https://www.sciencedirect.com/science/article/pii/S0378512214002394. Accessed Dec. 28, 2018.

Vaginitis (Candida/Yeast Infection)

1 https://www.cdc.gov/std/tg2015/candidiasis.htm. Accessed Nov. 23, 2018.

2 R.C.R. Martinez et al., "Improved Treatment of Vulvovaginal Candidiasis with Fluconazole Plus Probiotic *Lactobacillus rhamnosus* GR-1 and *Lactobacillus reuteri* RC-14," Feb. 9, 2009. https://doi.org/10.1111/j.1472-765X.2008.02477.x. Accessed Nov. 23, 2018.

3 D.J. Drutz, "Lactobacillus Prophylaxis for Candida Vaginitis," *Annals of Int Med* 116, no. 5 (1992): 419-420.

4 https://www.ncbi.nlm.nih.gov/pmc/articles/PMC4514959/. Accessed Nov. 23, 2018.

Varicose Veins/Venous Insufficiency

1 https://www.nhlbi.nih.gov/health-topics/varicose-veins.

2 https://my.clevelandclinic.org/health/diseases/16872-chronic-venous-insufficiency-cvi. Accessed June 19, 2020.

3 https://pubmed.ncbi.nlm.nih.gov/10474049/.

4 https://www.sciencedirect.com/science/article/abs/pii/S153718912030330X.

5 C. Diehm et al., "Comparison of Leg Compression Stocking and Oral Horse-Chestnut-Seed Extract Therapy in Patients with Chronic Venous Insufficiency," *Lancet* 347 (1996): 292-294.

6 M.H. Pittler and E. Ernst, *Cochrane Database Syst Rev* 11 (Nov. 14, 2012): CD003230.

7 https://www.mayoclinic.org/diseases-conditions/varicose-veins/diagnosis-treatment/drc-20350649. Accessed Nov. 18, 2018.

8 https://www.webmd.com/vitamins/ai/ingredientmono-522/msm-methylsulfonylmethane. Accessed Nov. 18, 2018.

9 https://www.webmd.com/skin-problems-and-treatments/features/new-treatments-for-varicose-veins#3.

10 https://www.webmd.com/vitamins/ai/ingredientmono-202/bilberry. Accessed Mar. 28, 2021.

11 https://pubmed.ncbi.nlm.nih.gov/10844161/.

12 https://pubmed.ncbi.nlm.nih.gov/28804235/. Accessed Mar. 28, 2021.

Vertigo—Cervical Vertigo/Cervicogenic Dizziness

1 M.A. Papadakis and S.J. McPhee, *Current Medical Diagnosis & Treatment* (2019): ch. 8, 223.

2 R. Galm, M. Rittmeister, and E. Schmitt, "Vertigo in Patients with Cervical Spine Dysfunction," *Eur Spine J* 7 (1998): 55-58.

3 M. Karlberg et al., "Postural and Symptomatic Improvement after Physiotherapy in Patients with Dizziness of Suspected Cervical Origin," *Arch Phys Med Rehabil* 77 (1996): 874-882.

4 L.W. Wing and W. Hargrave-Wilson, "Cervical Vertigo," *Aust N Z J Surg* 44 (1974): 275-277.

5 http://www.tchain.com/otoneurology/disorders/central/cervical.html. Accessed Dec. 12, 2018.

Vitamin E Deficiency

1 A.B.M. Abdullah, *Practical Manual in Clinical Medicine* (London: The Health Sciences Publisher), 742.

2 https://www.medicalnewstoday.com/articles/321800#causes. Accessed Apr. 21, 2020.

3 M. Tanyel and L. Mancano, "Neurologic Findings in Vitamin E Deficiency," *Am Fam Phys* (Jan. 1997): 197.

4 https://www.drugs.com/dosage/vitamin-e.html#Usual_Adult_Dose_for_Vitamin_E_Deficiency. Accessed Dec. 29, 2018.

Vitiligo

1 https://rarediseases.info.nih.gov/diseases/10751/vitiligo. Accessed Dec. 29, 2018.

2 B. Wasi, *Standard Treatment Guidelines: A Manual for Medical Therapeutics*, 1st ed. (2014), 240.

3 M. Gupta et al., "Zinc Therapy in Dermatology: A Review," *Dermatol Res Pract* 2014 (2014): 709152. Published online July 10, 2014. DOI: 10.1155/2014/709152.

4 https://www.emedicinehealth.com/alpha-lipoic_acid/vitamins-supplements.htm. Accessed Nov. 19, 2018.

5 https://www.webmd.com/vitamins/ai/ingredientmono-1017/folic-acid. Accessed Nov. 19, 2018.

6 https://www.webmd.com/vitamins/ai/ingredientmono-653/phenylalanine. Accessed Nov. 27, 2018.

7 https://www.emedicinehealth.com/picrorhiza/vitamins-supplements.htm. Accessed Dec. 29, 2018.

8 A. Jalel, G.S. Soumaya, and M.H. Hamdaoui, "Vitiligo Treatment with Vitamin, Minerals and Polyphenol Supplementation," *Indian J Dermatol* 54, no. 4 (Oct.-Dec. 2009): 357-360.

9 https://www.mayoclinic.org/diseases-conditions/vitiligo/diagnosis-treatment/drc-20355916. Accessed Dec. 29, 2018.

Warts

1 E.T. Bope and R.D. Kellerman, *Conn's Current Therapy*, 14th ed. (Philadelphia: Elsevier/Saunders), 332.

2 M. Gupta et al., "Zinc Therapy in Dermatology: A Review," *Dermatol Res Pract* 2014 (2014): 709152. Published online July 10, 2014. DOI: 10.1155/2014/709152.

3 K.E. Sharquie, A.A. Khorsheed, and A.A. Al-Nuaimy, "Topical Zinc Sulphate Solution for Treatment of Viral Warts," *Saudi Med J* 28 (2007): 1418-1421.

Wernicke-Korsakoff Syndrome

1 https://www.emedicinehealth.com/alcoholism/article_em.htm#what_is_the_treatment_for_alcoholism. Accessed Dec. 21, 2018.

2 https://www.medicalnewstoday.com/articles/220007#symptoms. Accessed May 12, 2020.

3 A.B.M. Abdullah, *Practical Manual in Clinical Medicine* (Philadelphia: Jaypee—The Health Sciences Publisher, 2017): 822.

4 J.C.M. Brust, *Current Diagnosis and Treatment Neurology*, 2nd ed. (McGraw-Hill, 2012): 518.

5 https://www.webmd.com/brain/wernicke-korsakoff-syndrome-facts#1. Accessed Dec. 21, 2018.

6 https://www.ncbi.nlm.nih.gov/pmc/articles/PMC4085800/. Accessed Dec. 21, 2018.

7 https://www.ncbi.nlm.nih.gov/pmc/articles/PMC4578911/. Accessed Dec. 21, 2018.

Whooping Cough/Pertussis

1 https://www.consumerreports.org/health/why-you-need-a-whooping-cough-vaccine/. Accessed Mar. 6, 2019.

2 https://www.cdc.gov/pertussis/surv-reporting/cases-by-year.html. Accessed May 12, 2020.

3 M.J. Ormerod and B.M. Unkauf, "Ascorbic Acid (Vitamin C) Treatment of Whooping Cough," *The Canadian Medical Association Journal* 37, no. 2 (Aug. 1937): 134-136.

4 *JAMA* (June 1950).

5 https://www.seanet.com/~alexs/ascorbate/193x/otani-t-klin_wchnschr-1936-v15-n51-p1884-eng.htm. Accessed Dec. 22, 2018.

Wilson's Disease

1 https://www.niddk.nih.gov/health-information/liver-disease/wilson-disease. Accessed Nov. 16, 2020.

2 https://rarediseases.org/rare-diseases/wilson-disease/. Accessed Mar. 25, 2019.

3 https://emedicine.medscape.com/article/183456-treatment. Accessed Dec. 19, 2018.

4 *PDR for Nutritional Supplements*, 2nd ed. (Montvale, NJ: Thomson Reuters, 2008), 25.

5 https://pubchem.ncbi.nlm.nih.gov/compound/dl-Thioctic_acid#section=Therapeutic-Uses. Accessed Dec. 19, 2018.

6 https://wilsonsdisease.org/about-wilson-disease/treatments. Accessed Apr. 21, 2020.

7 G.J. Brewer et al., "Oral Zinc Therapy for Wilson's Disease," *Ann Intern Med* 99 (1983): 314-319.

8 *The Washington Manual for Medical Therapeutics,* 34th ed., 923.

9 A. von Herbay et al., "Low Vitamin E Content in Plasma of Patients with Alcoholic Liver Disease, Hemochromatosis and Wilson's Disease," *J Hepatol* 20 (1994): 41-46.

10 R.J. Sokol et al., "Oxidant Injury to Hepatic Mitochondria in Patients with Wilson's Disease and Bedlington Terriers with Copper Toxicosis," *Gastroenterology* 107 (1994): 1788-1798.

11 H. Ogihara et al., "Plasma Copper and Antioxidant Status in Wilson's Disease," *Pediatr Res* 37 (1995): 219-226.

12 S. Sinha et al., "Is Low Serum Tocopherol in Wilson's Disease a Significant Symptom?," *J Neurol Sci* 228 (2005): 121-123.

13 H. Nagasaka et al., "Relationship Between Oxidative Stress and Antioxidant Systems in the Liver of Patients with Wilson Disease: Hepatic Manifestation in Wilson Disease as a Consequence of Augmented Oxidative Stress," *Pediatr Res* 60 (2006): 472-477.

14 *AASLD Practice Guidelines.* https://www.aasld.org/sites/default/files/guideline_documents/Wilson%20Disease2009.pdf. Accessed Dec. 19, 2018.

15 https://www.ncbi.nlm.nih.gov/pmc/articles/PMC4678372/. Accessed Dec. 20, 2018.

16 https://www.ncbi.nlm.nih.gov/pmc/articles/PMC3096115/. Accessed Dec. 20, 2018.

17 https://www.cincinnatichildrens.org/health/w/wilsons. Accessed Nov. 9, 2018.

18 https://www.nm.org/conditions-and-care-areas/neurosciences/movement-disorders/wilson-disease/treatments. Accessed Dec. 20, 2018.

19 https://onlinelibrary.wiley.com/doi/full/10.1002/mdc3.12003. Accessed Nov. 9, 2018.

Wound Care (Chronic)/Delayed Healing

1 https://www.aafp.org/afp/2020/0201/p159.html. Accessed May 25, 2021.

2 https://pubmed.ncbi.nlm.nih.gov/12822727/. Accessed Apr. 17, 2021.

3 https://www.woundsresearch.com/article/nutrition-wound-care-management-comprehensive-overview. Accessed Apr. 17, 2021.

4 https://pubmed.ncbi.nlm.nih.gov/20130158/. Accessed Apr. 17, 2021.

5 https://www.ncbi.nlm.nih.gov/pmc/articles/PMC2903966/. Accessed Dec. 29, 2018.

6 T. Bjarnsholt et al., "Antibiofilm Properties of Acetic Acid," *Adv Wound Care (New Rochelle)* 4, no. 7 (July 1, 2015): 363-372. DOI: 10.1089/wound.2014.0554.

7 A. Bikker et al., "Ascorbic Acid Deficiency Impairs Wound Healing in Surgical Patients: Four Case Reports," *International J Surgery Open* 2: (2016): 15-18. DOI: https://doi.org/10.1016/j.ijso.2016.02.009.

8 M.A. Costa et al., "Oral Glutamine and the Healing of Colonic Anastomoses in Rats," *JPEN J Parenter Enteral Nutr* 27 (2003): 182-185.

9 A.C. Campos, A.K. Groth, and A.B. Branco, "Assessment and Nutritional Aspects of Wound Healing," *Curr Opin Clin Nutr Metab Care* 11 (2008): 281-288.

10 J. Irish, S. Blair, and D.A. Carter, "The Antimicrobial Activity of Honey Derived from Australian Flora," *PLos One* 6 (2011): e18229.

11 T. Bjarnsholt et al., "Antibiofilm Properties of Acetic Acid," *Adv Wound Care (New Rochelle)* 4, no. 7 (July 1, 2015): 363-372. DOI: 10.1089/wound.2014.0554.

12 https://www.woundsresearch.com/article/nutrition-wound-care-management-comprehensive-overview. Accessed Apr. 17, 2021.

Wrinkles

1 https://www.medicinenet.com/wrinkles/article.htm#wrinkles_facts. Accessed Mar. 22, 2019.

2 https://www.mayoclinic.org/diseases-conditions/dry-skin/in-depth/moisturizers/art-20044232. Accessed Mar. 22, 2019.

3 https://www.webmd.com/beauty/features/23-ways-to-reduce-wrinkles#3. Accessed Mar. 22, 2019.

4 https://www.mdedge.com/dermatology/article/108137/aesthetic-dermatology/vitamin-c. Accessed Feb. 24, 2019.

5 https://www.emedicinehealth.com/vitamin_c_ascorbic_acid/vitamins-supplements.htm. Accessed Dec. 27, 2018.

6 Anonymous, "Topical Vitamin C Diminishes Wrinkles, Signs of Photoaging," *Geriatrics* 50, no. 11 (1995): 23.

7 *Clin Cosmet Investig Dermatol* 8 (Sept. 2, 2015): 463-470.

8 H. Beitner, *Br J Dermatol* 149, no. 4 (2003): 841-849.

9 https://pubchem.ncbi.nlm.nih.gov/compound/dl-Thioctic_acid#section=Therapeutic-Uses. Accessed Dec. 17, 2018.

10 D.L. Bissett et al., "Niacinamide: A B Vitamin That Improves Aging Facial Skin Appearance," *Dermatol Surg* 31 (2005): 860-865, discussion 865.

11 M.G. Mahoney et al., "Extracellular Matrix in Cutaneous Ageing: The Effects of 0.1% Copper-Zinc Malonate-Containing Cream on Elastin Biosynthesis," *Experimental Dermatology* 18, no. 3 (2009): 205-211.

12 https://lpi.oregonstate.edu/mic/health-disease/skin-health/essential-fatty-acids. Accessed Nov. 15, 2018.

13 https://www.emedicinehealth.com/para-aminobenzoic_acid_paba/vitamins-supplements.htm. Accessed Dec. 26, 2018.

14 https://www.webmd.com/vitamins/ai/ingredientmono-1004/para-aminobenzoic-acid-paba. Accessed Mar. 22, 2019.

15 https://rosemed.com/hl/?/21831/PABA--Para-Aminobenzoic-Acid-. Accessed Mar. 22, 2019.

16 D.H. McDaniel et al., "Clinical Efficacy Assessment in Photodamaged Skin of 0.5% and 1.0% Idebenone," *J Cosmetic Dermatology* 4 (2005): 167-173.

Xanthelasma

1 R.C.V. Robinson, "Treatment of Xanthelasma with Vitamin B12," *Invest Dermatol* 24 (1955): 111-113.

2 A.R. Gaby, "Nutrient of the Month: Vitamin B12, Part 11," *Nutrition and Healing* 5, no. 7 (Aug. 1995): 4.

3 https://www.dermetnz.org/topics/xanthoma. Accessed June 11, 2020.

Xeroderma Pigmentosum

1 https://ghr.nlm.nih.gov/condition/xeroderma-pigmentosum. Accessed Mar. 22, 2019.

2 K.E. Sharquie, A.A. Noaimi, and N.O. Kadir, "Topical Therapy of Xeroderma Pigmentosa with 20% Zinc Sulfate Solution," *Iraqi Journal of Postgraduate Medicine* 7 (2008): 231-237.

3 M. Gupta et al., "Zinc Therapy in Dermatology: A Review," *Dermatol Res Pract* 2014 (2014): 709152. Published online July 10, 2014. DOI: 10.1155/2014/709152.

Printed in the United States
by Baker & Taylor Publisher Services